SECOND EDITION

TOXICANTS OCCURRING NATURALLY IN FOODS

Committee on Food Protection
Food and Nutrition Board
National Research Council

NATIONAL ACADEMY OF SCIENCES
Washington, D.C. 1973

NOTICE: The project that is the subject of this report was approved by the Governing Board of the National Research Council, acting in behalf of the National Academy of Sciences. Such approval reflects the Board's judgment that the project is of national importance and appropriate with respect to both the purposes and resources of the National Research Council.

The members of the committee selected to undertake this project and prepare this report were chosen for recognized scholarly competence and with due consideration for the balance of disciplines appropriate to the project. Responsibility for the detailed aspects of this report rests with that committee.

Each report issuing from a study committee of the National Research Council is reviewed by an independent group of qualified individuals according to procedures established and monitored by the Report Review Committee of the National Academy of Sciences. Distribution of the report is approved, by the President of the Academy, upon satisfactory completion of the review process.

Library of Congress Cataloging in Publication Data
Main entry under title:

Toxicants occurring naturally in foods.

Includes bibliographical references.
1. Food contamination. 2. Food poisoning.
I. National Research Council. Food Protection
Committee. [DNLM: 1. Food Analysis. 2. Food
Poisoning. QU50 N277t 1973]
TX531.T6 1973   615.9   73-8968
ISBN 0-309-02117-0

Available from

Printing and Publishing Office
National Academy of Sciences
2101 Constitution Avenue, N.W.
Washington, D.C. 20418

Printed in the United States of America

PREFACE

Much new information on food safety has become available in the 7 years since the first edition of this report* was published, and significant changes in public attitude have occurred. A number of food components, both naturally occurring and introduced by man, that were "generally recognized as safe" at that time have now come under suspicion. Public apprehension concerning the food supply has reached a high point. At the same time, there is all too little recognition of some of the hazards associated with food.

To the extent feasible, the subject matter of this report has been organized on the basis of the chemical nature of the materials considered. Authors of individual chapters were selected as specialists on the particular topic covered and as recognized authorities in the field. The final compilation was then thoroughly reviewed by the subcommittee. We wish to acknowledge our deep indebtedness to the authors and to thank them for their contributions.

*Committee on Food Protection, NRC. 1966. Toxicants occurring naturally in foods. National Academy of Sciences, Washington, D.C. 301 p.

CONTENTS

Frank M. Strong

INTRODUCTION

Nutritious food is essential to life. It is also a mixture of thousands of chemicals, any one of which, in sufficient amounts, would be harmful, perhaps fatal, to the consumer. This holds even for essential nutrients such as zinc, copper, methionine, and vitamin A. Human beings cannot live without them, but in excess they are very toxic.

The great concern of the public in demanding an absolutely safe food supply, free of harmful "chemicals," is mistaken and misdirected. It is mistaken because the belief that foods can be free of "chemicals" is false; all foods consist exclusively of chemicals. It is equally mistaken to demand a food supply containing no harmful substances; all substances are toxic in some degree and therefore potentially harmful. As in all other aspects of human life, no absolute safety or security is possible. However, it is important to distinguish between toxicity and actual hazard. A particular food chemical may or may not be hazardous depending on many factors, chiefly the amount ingested. (See Chapter 26.)

The public concern is misdirected because the more important dangers associated with food consumption are of a different nature. In the United States today the chief food hazards probably result from overeating, particularly of foods rich in fats and sugars. The causes of some of the most serious public health problems in the country, e.g., obesity, cardiovascular disease, hypertension, and dental caries,[1] al-

1

most certainly have a significant nutritional component that is not in the nature of a deficiency of any essential nutrient or the presence in the food of "toxic chemicals" in the popular sense.

Assuming, however, that we escape overindulgence, ordinary foods taken in moderate amounts may still be hazardous to a degree because of certain other chemical substances they may contain. These may be added deliberately, introduced unintentionally as a consequence of human activities, or an intrinsic part of the plant or animal food material as it was formed in nature. The present volume, as its title indicates, is concerned mainly with substances in the last category.

Definitions seldom are absolute. Difficulties arise when one tries to decide whether a given substance should be regarded as a "toxicant," whether it is "natural," and what constitutes a "food." In general, this report has included only materials that are actually eaten by substantial numbers of people on a fairly regular basis at least in some part of the world. Toxicants present only in animal feeds have not been covered, unless there is a real likelihood that they may be carried over into the resulting meat, milk, or other product eaten by people, as for example, in the case of toxic honeys (Chapter 22). Also omitted are problems arising from toxic substances formed during cooking or processing of foods and specialized individual problems caused by allergy. However, favism and disaccharide intolerance, which have genetic bases, are included because large populations are affected.

Substances so obviously and severely toxic that they would not normally be eaten except by mistake are generally excluded. The more dangerous toxicants from the public health standpoint are those that act in a slower, more subtle fashion and may therefore not be recognized as being dangerous. Some compounds of this sort have been shown to occur naturally in foods; others probably remain to be discovered.

Finally, the difficult question of whether a substance is "natural" has in most cases been left to the discretion of the individual authors. Borderline cases are unavoidable; for example, mercury contamination of fish probably is primarily of natural origin, although industrial wastes obviously contribute. In doubtful cases, the decision has usually been to include the substance concerned. Microbial toxins, particularly mycotoxins, have been included but are not covered exhaustively, as this would have required many times the space available in a volume of this size.

Several considerations have prompted the writing of this report. Perhaps the main one is the hope that it may contribute to a more informed, realistic, and sensible attitude on the part of the public toward the food supply. People need to understand that there is no reason to fear a particular food chemical simply because an overwhelming excess of it may be harmful. Ingestion of chemicals that would be toxic if consumed in excessive amounts is a perfectly normal situation that mankind has always faced and inevitably always will. It is impossible for living organisms to avoid taking toxic substances into their body because all substances are toxic in the sense that excessive amounts are harmful. Gaseous oxygen provides an impressive example: Three to five times the normal atmospheric concentration is toxic.[2] The really relevant considerations are: How much of the substance is consumed, and what is the effect of this amount (the dose–response relationship)? Is the benefit derived from the material eaten sufficient to justify any speculative associated risk (the benefit–risk ratio)? These matters are discussed more fully in Chapter 26.

More specifically, knowledge of toxic substances naturally present in plants and animals that are or may be used as foods should be useful in several other ways. The plant breeder attempting to develop higher yielding or disease-resistant crop varieties must, at the same time, be alert to the possible production of undesirable components. The possibility that newly developed or exotic foods may contain natural toxicants must be taken into account in evaluating their usefulness. Dieticians must avoid recommending foods that their patients cannot tolerate, possibly because of inability to metabolize or detoxify certain substances therein. Amounts of certain substances that are relatively safe when consumed individually can sometimes, when taken together, have serious and even fatal effects. Examples of such interactions are pressor amines plus monoamine oxidase inhibitors (p. 174), tannins in a protein-marginal diet (p. 331), ethanol plus barbiturates, and potentiation of bacterial endotoxins by trace amounts of lead.[3] The converse may also occur; for example, selenium tends to counteract the toxicity of mercury.[4]

In a broader sense, public health authorities need to be informed about possible dangers related to widespread, longstanding practices previously regarded as safe. Some of the natural compounds reviewed in this book are carcinogenic; some may be related to high blood pressure or to the worldwide high incidence of goiter. Continued surveillance, based insofar as possible on exact knowledge, is essential to public health and is constantly in progress.

At the same time, a great deal of useful information may be derived from human experience with foods now known to carry certain toxicants. In effect, "megaman experiments" have been going on for centuries. A vast array of specific chemical compounds of presently known structures has been eaten by large numbers of human beings over long periods of time. A recently discovered example is the relatively high intake of aflatoxins by people in certain rural areas in Thailand.[5] Surely a great deal can be learned from this experience with respect to the effect of certain chemical structures on man. Clinical and biochemical observations on people consuming foods containing specific toxicants should provide much information about how individual substances affect the human species—exactly the type of information so badly needed and so difficult to obtain exclusively from animal experimentation.

The book is addressed primarily to public health workers, nurses, nutritionists, medical and paramedical personnel, members of governmental regulatory agencies, international bodies concerned with the food supply, food technologists, and members of the food industry. It may be of interest also to various research specialists; however, an effort has been made to keep the writing as simple and intelligible to nonspecialists as is feasible in a technical book.

Increased interest in naturally occurring food toxicants has resulted in several recent publications of a rather limited nature in this area. The book edited by Liener[6] includes very good coverage of certain toxicants occurring in plants, with particular reference to inhibitors of proteolytic enzymes, hemagglutinins, goitrogens, saponins, and several others. It does not cover toxicants in foods of animal or marine origin. Gontzea and Sutzescu[7] give quite complete coverage of a few groups of natural food toxicants selected from those regarded to be of the greatest practical importance. The book by Sapeika[8] covers a great many different chemicals in somewhat lesser detail: about half are not of natural origin. Another important publication is the report of a symposium on natural food toxicants,[9] available from the American Chemical Society, Washington, D.C.

Other source materials, of somewhat different but nevertheless relevant character, include books on poisonous plants in Great Britain[10] and in the United States and Canada.[11] The latter has a particularly well-documented account of the extensive loss of human life occasioned by ingestion of milk containing "tremetol" from white snake root (*Eupatorium rugosum* Houtt) eaten by dairy cattle. Fortunately this toxicosis, which was widespread in the eastern United States during the nineteenth century, is now of only historical interest. Finally, a highly informative symposium entitled "Mechanisms of Toxicity"[12] deals with a variety of toxins, several of natural occurrence, from the standpoint of their metabolic actions.

REFERENCES

1. H. W. Scherp, Dental caries: Prospects for prevention. Science *173*:1199–1205 (1971).
2. Anonymous, Noxious oxygen. Food Cosmet. Toxicol. *8*:93 (1970).
3. F. E. Hemphill, M. L. Kaeberle, and W. B. Buck, Lead suppression of mouse resistance to Salmonella typhimurium. Science *172*:1031 (1971).
4. H. E. Ganther, C. Goudie, M. L. Sunde, M. J. Kopecky, P. Wagner, Sang-Hwan Oh, and W. G. Hoekstra, Selenium: Relation to decreased toxicity of methylmercury added to diets containing tuna. Science *175*:1122 (1972).
5. R. C. Shank, J. E. Gordon, G. N. Wogan, A. Nondasuta, and B. Subhamani, Dietary aflatoxins and human liver cancer. III. Field survey of rural Thai families for ingested aflatoxins. Food Cosmet. Toxicol. *10*:71–84 (1972).
6. I. E. Liener (ed.). Toxic constituents of plant foodstuffs. Academic Press, New York (1969).
7. I. Gontzea and P. Sutzescu, Natural antinutritive substances in foodstuffs and forages. S. Karger, New York (1968).
8. N. Sapeika, Food pharmacology. Charles C Thomas, Springfield, Ill. (1969).
9. D. G. Crosby (symposium coordinator), Natural food toxicants. J. Agric. Food Chem. *17*:413–538 (1968).
10. A. A. Forsyth, British poisonous plants. Ministry of Agriculture, Fisheries and Food, Bull. No. 161. Her Majesty's Stationery Office, London (1968).
11. J. M. Kingsbury, Poisonous plants of the United States and Canada. Prentice-Hall, Englewood Cliffs, N.J. (1964).
12. W. N. Aldridge (ed.), Mechanisms of toxicity. Br. Med. Bull. *25*:219–309. (1969).

1 David W. Fassett

NITRATES
AND
NITRITES*

Probably the earliest account of the toxic effects of excessive amounts
of naturally occurring nitrates in foods or feeds was given in 1895 when
Mayo[1] described three episodes of fatal poisoning in cattle. The symptoms and circumstances were similar: The animals showed tremors, diuresis, collapse, and cyanosis, and in all cases they had been feeding on
cornstalks shown by chemical analyses to contain extraordinary
amounts (25% by dry weight) of potassium nitrate. Crystals were visible to the naked eye, and the stalks had the typical taste of nitrates.

The explanation for the high nitrate concentration was felt to be the
presence of large amounts of nitrates due to manure accumulation in
the soil where the corn was grown. Subsequently, the symptoms were
reproduced by oral dosing of cattle with doses of potassium nitrate at
about 1.3 g/kg. Although methemoglobin formation was not clearly
understood at the time, particular mention was made of the dark color
of the blood. Nitrites as well as nitrates were detected in the blood,
bile, and other tissues. It was shown that bile and blood could rapidly
convert some of the nitrates to nitrites *in vitro*, although neither was
found in the stomach at autopsy, probably indicating rapid absorption.

Thus, this remarkable study pointed to the now well-recognized elements in the acute toxicity of plant nitrates to livestock, namely, the

* Literature reviewed through January 1972.

large increase in nitrates in some plants with high nitrogen fertilization and the reduction of nitrate to nitrite in the rumen,[2] resulting in methemoglobin formation from absorption of the nitrite ion. Many episodes have since been described.

High concentrations of nitrates in well waters have also caused poisoning in both livestock and humans, especially children.[3-7] The conversion of nitrates in spinach to nitrites by bacterial action has caused cyanosis in children[8]; the accidental use of excessive amounts of nitrate-nitrite mixtures in meats has caused similar problems.[9] The ability of nitrites to react with secondary amines to form potentially carcinogenic nitrosamines *in vivo* has led to a number of studies of the possibility of a nitrite-induced carcinogenic hazard.[10]

An attempt will be made to review some of the more important facts regarding the chemistry of nitrates and nitrites, their occurrence and origin in nature and in foods, and the conditions under which toxic effects may occur and to suggest the need for further study or controls.

CHEMISTRY AND ANALYTICAL METHODS

Nitrogen is the smallest atom in Group V A of the periodic table and has five valence electrons. Because of its small size, the nucleus exerts a strong force on the electron, making it difficult to oxidize to an ionic state. It does not readily accept electrons to form an independent negative ion. Nearly all of its valence states are therefore the result of its sharing one or more pairs of electrons with other atoms. Its valence state can vary from minus three in the case of ammonia (NH_3), to plus three in the case of nitrites ($NaNO_2$), or plus five in the case of nitrates ($NaNO_3$).

Nitric acid (HNO_3) is one of the strongest acids and can act as a powerful oxidizing agent. The reaction products can be very complex, e.g., $Fe + HNO_3 \rightarrow NO, NH_3, N_2, N_2O, NO_2$. On the other hand, nitrous acid (HNO_2) is a very weak acid ($K = 4.5 \times 10^{-4}$ at 25 °C) and is unstable. Nitrate ions are very soluble in water; they are flat, symmetrical molecules existing in three resonance states. Nitrites are usually water-soluble and fairly stable. The nitrite ion is nonlinear and probably exists as a resonance hybrid. Nitrate ions in acid solution can react with either aromatic or aliphatic carbon atoms to form nitro compounds, e.g.,

$$HO-\langle\bigcirc\rangle + HNO_3 \rightarrow HO-\langle\bigcirc\rangle-NO_2 + H_2O$$

$$R_3CH + HNO_3 \rightarrow R_3CNO_2 + H_2O$$

Nitrite reactions are somewhat more complex. Nitrites react with primary amines to form the alcohol and nitrogen gas, e.g.,

$$R-N\begin{array}{c}H\\\\H\end{array} + HO-N=O \rightarrow R-N-N=O \rightarrow$$

$$R-(N=N)-OH \rightarrow ROH + N_2$$

The reaction with secondary amines leads to nitrosamines, e.g.,

$$\begin{array}{c}R\\\\R_1\end{array}N-H + HO-N=O \rightarrow \begin{array}{c}R\\\\R_1\end{array}N-N=O + H_2O$$

These are neutral materials with only a slight water solubility. The same type of reaction proceeds with amides or ureas. Tertiary aliphatic amines may, in some cases, also react with nitrites.[11,12]

Aromatic primary amines react with nitrites to form diazonium salts, e.g.,

$$\langle\bigcirc\rangle-NH_2 + 3HCl + NaNO_2 \xrightarrow{0\ °C}$$

$$\langle\bigcirc\rangle-N_2Cl + NaCl + HCl + 2H_2O$$

The ability to form diazonium salts with aromatic primary amines is a most important feature of many types of analytical methods for nitrates, nitrites, or aromatic amines.

The reaction of nitrites with aromatic secondary amines is similar to that with aliphatic secondary amines, and various aromatic nitrosamines can be formed. Aromatic tertiary amines react with nitrites to form nitroso compounds in the aromatic nucleus, e.g.,

$$\langle\bigcirc\rangle-N(CH_3)_2 \xrightarrow[NaNO_2]{HCl-H_2O} O=N-\langle\bigcirc\rangle-N(CH_3)_2$$

Dimethylaniline   *p*-Nitrosodimethylaniline

It is apparent from this brief review of nitrate–nitrite chemistry that there exists an enormous variety of possible chemical reactions with either living or nonliving matter. The wide variety of valence states and the ubiquitous nature of some of the enzymes involved in the nitrogen cycle make it necessary to have the most thorough understanding of chemical and biochemical factors in any considerations of toxic effects.

A variety of methods exists for determination of nitrate and nitrite content of water, foods, and soil. The analytical problems are generally simpler in the case of water than in foods or biological samples. Methods for water and wastewater are given in the monographs on standard methods.[13,14] One of the oldest and most widely used methods is based on the formation of a yellow color when the NO_3^- ion is reacted with phenoldisulfonic acid. Similarly, the reaction of nitrate ion with chromotropic acid or brucine gives rise to colored products that can be used as a basis for determination. Direct measurement of absorption by NO_3^- in the ultraviolet at 220 nm has also been used.

Since nitrite ions may interfere in some of these methods, oxidation by permanganate may be used to convert any NO_2^- to NO_3^-. Reduction of nitrate to nitrite followed by diazotization with sulfanilamide or sulfanilic acid, and coupling with 1-naphthylamine or similar compounds, has been extensively evaluated and appears particularly useful in food analyses.[13-18] The use of cadmium metal columns for reduction appears to be especially useful, and the reduction methods have been extensively tested with foods.[15] Nitrite can also be determined directly by diazotization and coupling and the ratio of nitrites to nitrates found by difference. Nitrates in meats can also be determined by reaction of the nitrate ion with m-xylenol.[13] Nitrites in meats can be determined directly by diazotization, etc.

The use of nitrate-specific ion electrodes appears promising, and nitrate analyses in spinach and beets has been carried out by their use.[19,20]

The methods for preparing different foods for analyses is of special importance, e.g., determination in milk can be improved by special methods of removing fat and protein.[21] Carbohydrates may interfere in some instances,[22] and other problems of this sort may occur.[23,24] Very little work appears to have been done on analyses specifically for metabolic studies in mammals; the methods used are generally an adaptation of some of those used with foods or meats.

The development of methods for nitrosamines in foods is in an early state. The U.S. Food and Drug Administration (FDA) studied this problem intensively and has published methods that appear promising for dimethyl nitrosamine in fish. These involve digestion by methanolic KOH, distillation, and final determination and identification by gas chromatography and mass spectrometry.[25,26] Some methods have used qualitative identification by thin-layer chromatography (TLC).[27,28]

Other methods involve isolation of the nitrosamines by TLC and photolytic decomposition to nitrites followed by diazotization and coupling.

It is evident from this review of analytical methods that, although many choices are available, a high degree of competence is necessary with very careful attention to details, particularly in food or tissue analyses where interference may be severe. Nitrosamine analysis is especially difficult because of the very minute quantities that appear to be present and because of the possibility of artificially producing such compounds from precursors during the analytical processes.

ORIGIN AND OCCURRENCE IN THE ENVIRONMENT

In order to understand the factors influencing the nitrate–nitrite content of foods, some consideration needs to be given to the sources and movement of nitrogen and its compounds in the environment. The origin of the nitrogen used in biological reactions is thought to be principally atmospheric N_2. However, a major portion of the earth's nitrogen is probably contained in its fundamental rocks.[29,30] Although much of the nitrogen in rocks may be unavailable, it may provide a larger proportion of the nitrate in waters than has been supposed in the past.[31]

The formation of nitrate–nitrite compounds in the atmosphere is not clearly understood. On a global basis nitrous oxide (N_2O) and nitric oxide (NO) are said to be biological in origin.[32] Some atmospheric ammonia may also be of biological origin, but the levels are low (0–15 $\mu g/m^3$). The most abundant oxide of nitrogen in the atmosphere is N_2O, the concentrations being about 500–1200 $\mu g/m^3$.[33] Combustion of fossil fuels generates principally NO, which is subsequently oxidized to NO_2. The details of the photolytic cycle of the nitrogen oxides have become available as the result of air pollution studies in recent years.[32,34]

The levels of nitrates in particulate matter analyzed in 96 air-pollution sampling stations on a biweekly basis from 1960–1965 were quite low, with a mean of 2.6 $\mu g/m^3$.[35] It has been estimated that lightning contributes some 60,000 tons/day as HNO_3 or HNO_2, although this amount seems relatively small compared to the amounts involved in biological effects.[30,36]

In a review of nitrogen compounds in natural water, Feth[30] discusses the evidence of nitrates, nitrites, and ammonia found in precipitation. In general, the amount of ammonia delivered to earth in rain or snow is twice that of nitrate. In one European study NH_3-N equalled 0.5–4.2 tons/mi² /yr (calculated as NO_3^-), compared with 0.2–2.7 tons/mi² /yr for NO_3-N. A 17-yr study in Canada indicated that $NO_3^- + NO_2^-$ accounted for some 30-35% of the total nitrogen in rain and snow. The total N reaching the land averaged about 2 tons/mi^2/yr of equivalent NO_3^- (about 7 lb/acre/yr), similar to the higher levels in the European study.

Few studies have been made of the levels of NO_2^- in rain and snow, but the amounts appear very small, perhaps only 1–5% of the NO_3^- content. In these studies some uncertainties have been expressed as to the possibilities of microbiological conversion of one nitrogen species to another in the sampling process.

In addition to the direct addition of nitrogen compounds to the soil and water by precipitation, there are a number of complex and close interrelationships affecting soil and water levels. These include: the direct addition of fertilizer (NH_3, urea, and nitrates) in agriculture; the fixation of atmospheric nitrogen by microorganisms and legumes, resulting in the formation of organic plant N; the microbial decomposition of nitrogenous compounds in plants and man's sewage and wastes, generating ammonia, nitrites, and nitrates; and the geochemical leaching of nitrate into ground water.[59-61]

The amount of nitrogen biologically converted to ammonia and ultimately into nitrates is large compared to that from direct precipitation, e.g., 40–200 lb N/acre/yr compared to 7 lb/acre/yr. It is now known that N_2 fixation is achieved by an enzyme system called nitrogenase, which is distributed among a number of apparently unrelated organisms or plant microorganism symbionts. Hardy and Burns[37] define it as a multiprotein complex containing nonheme iron, labile sulfide, and molybdenum, and as one that catalyzes the reduction of N_2 and a number of nitriles and alkynes (triple-bonded carbon compounds), the generation of hydrogen, and the concomitant hydrolysis of ATP.

The microbial oxidation of soil ammonia derived from decay processes or from added NH_3 is accomplished in two stages by soil organisms with remarkable specificity. *Nitrosomonas* and related genera convert NH_3 to NO_2^-, while *Nitrobacter* and related genera oxidize NO_2^- to NO_3^-.[38,39] Many plants readily absorb the leachable NO_3^- ion and then reduce it to nitrite by nitrate reductase enzymes.[40] These are molybdo-iron-flavoproteins. Many heterotrophic microorganisms also carry out such reactions, e.g., *E. coli, Proteus, Pseudomonas.* Further reduction by nitrite reductases occurs with the formation of hydroxylamine or NH_3. Some plants do not use absorbed nitrate but convert it to ammonia in the roots. Finally, some organisms can carry out so-called denitrifying processes, producing volatile compounds from nitrate, e.g., N_2O, NO, and N_2.

Since the report in 1964[8] of cyanosis in infants from spinach, there has been renewed interest in the nitrate–nitrite content of plants and soils and of the various factors influencing concentrations of these compounds. Several reviews and articles on this subject have appeared recently.[16,18,29,41–50]

Keeney[29] has summarized some of the factors known to affect the nitrate content of plants. The factors related to the plant itself are the species, variety, plant part, and stage of maturity. Those environmental factors causing an increase in nitrate include drought; high temperature; shading or cloudiness; time of day; deficiencies in certain nutrients (e.g., P, K, and Ca); excessive soil N from manure, legume residues, and fertilizer; and, finally, plant damage from insects or weed control chemicals.

Comparison of the levels of nitrates in vegetables in 1964 with a similar study made in 1907 by Richardson[51] shows a generally similar pattern in spite of the shift from manure to extensive use of chemical fertilizers.[29,42,52] Certain vegetables tend to have higher levels (e.g., spinach, beets, radishes, and lettuce), but a wide variability is common both between and within species.

There is little doubt that certain fertilization practices will generally increase the nitrate level in plants, but the magnitude of the increase is not necessarily related to the level of fertilization. In a careful quantitative study of this aspect, Brown and Smith[53] conclude that the effects were more noticeable in early maturing species. Fertilization rates greater than 50 lb N/acre seem necessary to show significant effects on NO_3^--N.

Phillips[42] has recently reviewed the nitrate–nitrite content of foods, with particular reference to the question of prepared infant foods. Normally, fresh spinach contains virtually no or very low nitrite. Storage at room temperature showed a loss of NO_3^- and an increase in NO_2^- in the first 4 days; then both NO_3^- and NO_2^- decreased in the next 3 days. Refrigeration delayed, but did not prevent, nitrite production. However, when kept frozen, nitrite-N concentration was only 1 ppm or less up to 5 months. Another study was made to determine whether nitrite would increase in partly eaten jars of commercial baby foods on storage. Ten classes of foods stored 7 days under refrigeration after partial use showed no increase in NO_2^--N.

Phillips also reports a study of the effects of increased levels of fertilization (zero, 95 lb N/acre, and 185 lb N/acre). Although fertilization increased the nitrate level, the amount of increase was not proportional to the level of fertilization. Some conversion of NO_3^- to NO_2^- occurred after storage of spinach, with elevated NO_3^- at 2 days at room temperature, but the amounts converted were small. No nitrite production is found during commercial canning processes. Phillips concludes that conversion of nitrate to nitrite before ingestion is the principal hazard and that conversion in the gastrointestinal tract is not well documented in humans. Furthermore, it appears that the conversion is probable only with nitrate-rich unprocessed spinach.

Studies on nitrate accumulation by Barker *et al.* and Peck *et al.*[54,55] give results for spinach and beets similar to those described previously. The dose rates of nitrogen were between 0–400 lb N/acre. Two or three types of N carriers were used as well as three types of spinach and one of beets. The nitrate increase did not appear to be linearly related to the dose of N applied. The response was proportionately greater at the lower levels. More NO_3^- accumulated in spinach leaves when the fertilizer was applied by broadcasting before planting than when applied later as a side-dressing. The type of N carrier (e.g., NH_4NO_3, KNO_3, or urea) made a significant difference in the case of side-dressing technics but not when broadcast.

Lee[56] has summarized in tabular form the results of a number of studies on vegetable nitrates and also of nitrates in water supplies. Although the general trend toward higher levels in certain vegetables (e.g., beets, spinach, radishes, lettuce) can be seen, the actual variations are so large that evaluation of the effect of various agricultural practices could be seen only by specially designed experiments. Lee expresses the opinion that attempts to control nitrate by the monitoring of food plant levels would present formidable difficulties. Little could be found in the literature on the possibility of breeding low NO_3^- strains of various vegetables, although it is evident from the work of Barker *et al.*[54,55] that under carefully standardized conditions varietal effects are very significant.

Inheritance of nitrate reductase in corn (*Zea mays* L.) has recently been studied by Warner *et al.*[57], who used two inbred lines of maize. Both enzyme synthesis and decay rates are factors determining the level of nitrate reductase activity in plants and can be shown to be inheritable qualities. Warner suggests that since nitrate reductase is a substrate-inducible enzyme, it is presumably under regulation by inducers and repressors; therefore, the rate of synthesis of this enzyme may be related to a regulator gene.[58] Nitrate reductase activity is not the only factor determining the nitrate level in plants, but it would seem that genetic investigations along these lines might ultimately be helpful in relation to the question of plant nitrate levels.

The discussion thus far has been concerned with atmospheric and soil nitrogen sources and with certain biochemical factors related to nitrate levels in plants. It is evident that plant nitrate levels are influenced not only by agricultural practices and inherent plant biochemical processes, but also by other complex interrelationships among soil chemistry, microbiology, and geochemical factors. There are a number of reviews of this aspect of the problem,[29,30,36,41,43,53,56] and no attempt will be made to discuss this in detail. The small, stable, and highly soluble nitrate ion is capable of moving readily with water in soil and tends to move downward to the water table as well as upward to plants. Surface runoff may remove considerable quantities of nitrate at certain times of the year.[36,59] The nitrite ion can also move readily but is generally less stable than nitrate.

Studies of soil cores in areas repeatedly fertilized by natural or artificial fertilization reveal that the peak NO_3^--N concentration may be found 5–10 ft under the surface.[41] Keeney[29] suggests that in areas of slow movement of percolate waters, the high NO_3^- levels in some aquifers may reflect the onset of farming many years previously. The potential hazard of locating shallow wells near feedlot areas or heavily fertilized areas is obvious. It is of interest that nitrate levels in ponds are often low, especially if algae or water plants are present; conversely, some river waters are high in nitrates.[60,61]

METABOLISM AND TOXIC EFFECTS IN MAN AND ANIMALS

Our knowledge of the toxic effects of large doses of nitrate ion in humans comes mainly from its long use in medicine and from its accidental ingestion in place of Epsom or other salts. Its diuretic effect was described in the seventeenth century, and it was used for this purpose until recent times as the K or NH_4 salt in oral doses of over 1 g/ day. The mechanism of the diuretic effect of KNO_3 is relatively simple, the NO_3^- ion being readily absorbed and excreted rapidly and completely in the urine. The nitrate ion has a tissue distribution similar to that of chloride, but its reabsorption in the renal tubule appears very much less, leading to sodium excretion and extracellular dehydration.[62]

The IV injection of 41 mEq/kg $NaNO_3$ (or 20 mEq/kg orally) produced no apparent toxic effect in dogs and no lowering of blood pressure; renal plasma flow and glomerular filtration were increased, and up to 90% of the nitrate was excreted in the urine.[63] Very little nitrite was found in the urine. Accidental ingestion of about 8–15 g or more of sodium or potassium nitrate is fatal in adults, the symptoms coming on rapidly and consisting of severe abdominal pain, bloody stools and urine, weakness, and collapse. Autopsy shows principally a severe gastroenteritis. Continued therapeutic doses not infrequently cause dyspepsia and also mental depression, headache, and weakness somewhat similar to thiocyanate, Br^-, or I^-.[62] Methemoglobin formation generally does not appear to be a part of the toxic action of nitrates as they have been encountered in medicine or accidentally.

Nitrites are considerably more toxic. They have two principal effects: relaxation of vascular and other smooth muscles and formation of methemoglobin. These properties are shared by various nitrate or nitrous esters, but the latter usually have a more rapid onset of vasodilation. The therapeutic dose of $NaNO_2$ is about 0.03–0.12 g orally for vasodilation in adults. The exact lethal dose in humans is not known but is estimated to be about 1 g in adults.[64] In lower doses the symptoms are flushing of the face and extremities, gastrointestinal discomfort, and headache; in larger toxic doses cyanosis, nausea, vomiting, abdominal pain, and collapse occur.

The metabolism of nitrites is poorly understood in humans. Sollman[62] states that 60% or more disappears in the body. $NaNO_2$ is used as an antidote in cyanide poisoning in doses of about 300 mg IV.[64] Other than for vasodilation, it does not appear to exert severe toxic effects under these conditions, in which it is used purposely to produce methemoglobin. Oser[65] states that man excretes about 0.5 g/day of NO_3^- in the urine and that NO_2^- is normally absent.

In the case of ruminants, considerable information is available on the metabolism of nitrates. It is generally recognized that nitrate toxicity in ruminants depends on the ability of the rumen flora to reduce NO_3^- to NO_2^-. Wang *et al.*[66] made a detailed study of nitrate metabolism (using $K^{15}NO_3$) in cattle with permanent rumen fistulas. The conversion of NO_3^- to NO_2^- and NH_4^+ in the rumen was followed and correlated with blood and urine levels as well as with methemoglobin formation. The findings emphasize the rapidity of conversion with maximum levels of NH_4^+ and NO_2^- reached in the rumen in 3 h. The doses needed to produce 15% methemoglobin were relatively large (100 g KNO_3/day); several days were required to reach this level. The maximum conversion of hemoglobin to methemoglobin occurred at the same time as the maximum level of NO_2^- in the rumen.

Plasma NO_3^- persisted much longer than the elevated methemoglobin, indicating that NO_2^- (and probably $NO_3^- + NH_4^+$) was probably being absorbed directly into the blood from the rumen. Urinary excretion reached a peak at 4 h after dosing, with the $NO_3^- - NO_2^-$ peaks being higher than urea or ammonia fractions. *In vitro* studies of the binding of $K^{15}NO_2$ to the hemin of methemoglobin showed the binding to be very strong, withstanding displacement by an acetone–HCl solution. Wright and Davison[50] conducted experiments with cows fed 0, 100, and 150 mg NO_3^--N/kg/day for 6–12 months and obtained data on the levels in milk and meat. The control values for NO_3^- nitrogen in milk were 1.1 μg/ml and for meat 0.2 μg/g. Although some increase could be seen in both meat and milk, the levels in treated animals were far below current standards for meat and water (only 4.5 μg/ml in milk and 2.5 μg/g in meat at the 150 mg/kg dose). It was concluded that the contribution to human nitrate intake from this source was negligible. Land and Virtanen[67] fed ^{15}N-labeled ammonium nitrate to cows and found that ^{15}N could be seen in milk protein as early as 1 h after feeding.

It seems probable from the somewhat inadequate data on humans and monogastric animals, plus the more satisfactory information on ruminants, that both NO_3^- and NO_2^- are probably rapidly absorbed directly through the wall of the stomach. The rapid excretion of NO_3^- in the urine appears to account for the lack of toxicity under normal conditions.

Chronic feeding studies adequate by present-day standards for predicting the hazard to man have yet to be reported, although the studies on rats are reasonably comprehensive.[68] Rats tolerate 1% of $NaNO_3$ in the diet for 2 yr with no effects and 5% with only slight growth depression. Dogs show no adverse effects at 2% $NaNO_3$ in the diet for 105–125 days. The no-effect level appears to be about 500 mg/kg/day from these studies.

In the case of $NaNO_2$ given to rats in drinking water, the no-effect level appears to be less than 100 mg/kg/day, since some shortening of life span and a slight growth inhibition were noted. However, remarkably few toxic effects were seen; there was no effect on fertility, and carcinogenic effects were not seen.

There have apparently been very few experimental human studies in which foods containing high nitrates have been fed to infants or adults. A study by Kübler[69] shows that infants tolerated a daily intake for a week of about 16–21 mg/kg/day of NO_3^- from spinach with no signs of methemoglobin formation, diuresis, or any other toxic effects. The spinach used contained 680 ppm NO_3^- in the prepared vegetable.

Since the report by Hölscher and Natzschka[8] of two cases of methemoglobinemia from spinach, 14 additional cases have been reported.[48] Phillips[41] has published a comprehensive review of recent studies of these cases and of other related investigations.[44–47] The problem appears to arise only with nitrate-rich unprocessed spinach, and the conversion to nitrite occurs before ingestion. The reduction to nitrite is, in all probability, brought about by nitrate reductases in common organisms and possibly by plant enzymes. Commercial processing does not appear to result in nitrite buildup.

The well-known hazard of high levels of nitrates in water supplies continues to receive attention. Winton et al.[70] and Lee[56] have recently reviewed various clinical reports and epidemiologic studies. Although such cases are not frequent, the wide publicity given to the problem of methemoglobin formation in infants and in cattle has not prevented the continued reporting of cases in various parts of the world.

Winton et al.[70] have attempted to evaluate the adequacy of the U.S. standard of 45 mg of NO_3^- ion/liter of water (equivalent to 10 ppm NO_3^--N). From the summaries by Sattelmacher[71] and Simon et al.[47] it can be concluded that a small number of cases (3–4%) apparently occur at or possibly below this limit. Most cases, however, occur with waters containing well over 100 mg/liter. There are obvious problems in studying these cases, such as the relative rarity of the cases, the lack of methemoglobin and water NO_3^- or NO_2^- data, the use of other cyanosis-producing drugs, the occurrence of congenital methemoglobinemia, and, finally, delays in analyses allowing microbiological growth to occur.

By making certain assumptions regarding the amount of NO_2^- needed to convert 1 g of hemoglobin, a hypothetical NO_3^- dose in mg/kg of body weight necessary to produce 10% methemoglobin was calculated. The average dose calculated for various ages was about 2 mg NO_3^-/kg (assuming complete conversion to NO_2^-).

A study[70] was also made in California and Illinois of over a hundred infants aged less than 2 weeks to 6 months; water and dietary intakes were recorded and methemoglobin levels were determined. Five of the infants were estimated to have a daily intake of 10–15 mg NO_3/kg, and three of these had slightly elevated methemoglobin (5.3% compared to a normal range of 0–2.9%). Switching these infants to low-nitrate water caused a lowering of methemoglobin. No toxic symptoms whatever were seen. The importance of excessive boiling of water in raising NO_3^- levels was demonstrated. The authors conclude that further work may be needed to clarify the adequacy of the present NO_3^- standards for water, but they do not recommend that they be raised on the basis of present evidence.

A recent study by Petukhov and Ivanov[72] compares two groups of children aged 12–14: One group of 39 used water containing 105 mg/liter of NO_3^-, and another group of 20 used water containing only 8 mg/liter of NO_3^-. Observations were made of simple reaction times to light and sound before and after school lessons. Increases in reaction times occurred in both groups after lessons, but the high NO_3^- group had a slightly but significantly greater increase.

Ten children from the low-nitrate group and eleven from the high group were tested for methemoglobin levels. The low group had a mean of 0.75% and the high a mean of 5.30%. These figures are consistent with the levels given by Winton *et al.*,[70] although more data could easily have altered the results.

In any consideration of the significance of water nitrates on infant health, the nature and amount of the microorganisms present may be of great importance in determining nitrate reductase activity and nitrite levels. The same is of course true for the microbial content of foods being diluted or prepared with water. The variation in climate and water intake may be of great importance in determining dose as well as the details of formula and food preparation.

There continues to be active work in clarifying the role of nitrates in animal feeds and drinking water. Studies have appeared on turkeys and chickens,[73,74] swine and sheep,[75] and steers.[76] Davison[77] reviews the question of "sublethal nitrate poisoning" and concludes that cattle and sheep forages and rations containing less than about 2% nitrate are not likely to cause vitamin A deficiency, poor growth, low milk production, or thyroid disturbances. Studies on turkeys show high mortality at nitrate levels of about 4,000 ppm but very little effect at 1,500 ppm. Some delayed growth may occur down to 660 ppm, however.[74] The effects were thought to be due to NO_3^- rather than to Na.

Brief mention should be made of the use of $NaNO_3$ and $NaNO_2$ in certain types of preserved meat and fish products at maximum levels of 500 and 200 ppm, respectively. Bacterial reduction of nitrate in these products causes the formation of nitric oxide, hemoglobin, or myoglobin, and results in a comparatively stable red or pink color. Outbreaks of poisoning from the accidental incorporation of excessive amounts of nitrate-nitrite mixtures in meat products have occurred.[9] Two of the 10 cases described by Orgeron *et al.*[9] were in children 2 and 3 yr old and followed the eating of wieners containing over 5,000 ppm of nitrite.

Because of continued interest in the control of botulism, there has been renewed attention to the mechanism and efficacy of the use of nitrate and nitrite additives. Pivnick *et al.*[78] conclude that the main value of nitrite in stabilizing canned, cured shelf-stable meats comes from its ability to aid in preventing growth from spores that survive heat processing and germinate during storage.

The large amount of work now being conducted on the nitrosamine class of experimental carcinogens has led to many studies on the possibility of the *in vivo* synthesis of these compounds from secondary amines, present in the diet or in the body, and nitrites in the food or water or generated under certain conditions in the gut. (See Chapter 23 and a review by Wolf and Wasserman.[79])

Magee[80] has recently reviewed this subject especially in regard to the evidence for the presence of nitrosamines in food or feeds and the possibility of their being active in humans. No proof has yet been produced that they act as carcinogens in humans, but their high potency in many different species makes this a possibility. The levels demonstrated in most foods are extremely low, generally on the order of a few ppb, which puts a strain on most analytical methods. Magee concludes that the possible hazard to man of exposure to very low concentrations of carcinogenic nitrosamines is difficult to assess in the absence of reliable data on dose–response relationships at low levels.

INTAKE BY MAN

Any estimate of the daily intake of nitrates and nitrites by man is subject to great uncertainty, since, except for studies on infants,[70] few attempts have been made in this direction. The lack of metabolic data adequate by current standards makes it difficult to construct any sort of balance study.

It is probable that respiratory intake can be neglected; nitrates in suspended particulate matter amount to only 2 or 3 $\mu g/m^3$. If 15 m^3 is assumed to be the daily respiratory volume, the total daily inhaled nitrate would be only 45 μg. Intake via water might be assumed to be 50 mg/day. The nitrate intake in a 100-g portion of a processed canned meat might be 50 mg, and a 100-g portion of a high-nitrate spinach might equal 200 mg. The nitrite intake under normal circumstances would be extremely low except for processed meat. In the case above, the 100-g meat portion would contribute 20 mg NO_2^-. The total nitrate intake in this example would then be 300 mg and the nitrite intake about 20 mg.

Considering the toxicology of these substances, the margin of safety in adults seems generally adequate for either nitrites or nitrates. The acceptable daily intake for nitrates suggested by the World Health Organization (WHO)[81] is 5 mg/kg in addition to naturally occurring nitrates, and that for nitrites 0.4 mg/kg.

CONCLUSIONS AND SUGGESTED RESEARCH

The principal toxic agent is nitrite, and the infant is especially susceptible for various reasons. Care in processing, storing, and handling high-nitrate vegetables is essential. However, the record of use of several hundred million jars of beets and spinach sold in North America in the past 20 yr with virtually no evidence of injury is reassuring.[42]

The relationship of nitrates and nitrites in soil, vegetation, and water is much better understood than formerly, and it should be possible by careful use of fertilizer to obtain the needed production with a minimum of disturbance to the environment. There is little evidence that today's vegetables have more nitrate than in 1907, when manure was the principal fertilizer. The application of modern genetic research to produce varieties with lower nitrate content would seem feasible but may not be necessary at present.

There is a lack of good data using modern methods on the absorption, distribution, metabolism, and excretion of nitrites and nitrates in humans; furthermore, the nitrate–nitrite balance in man is not well defined. It would seem desirable to reexamine the role of nitrate–nitrite preservation of meats and fish with respect to mechanisms, dosage rates, conditions of processing and effectiveness in control of botulism.

REFERENCES

1. N. S. Mayo, Cattle poisoning by potassium nitrate. Kans. Agric. Exp. Stn. Bull. *49*, Manhattan, Kans. (1895).
2. P. K. McIlwain and I. A. Schipper, Toxicity of nitrate nitrogen to cattle. J. Am. Vet. Med. Assoc. *142*:502 (1963).
3. H. H. Comly, Cyanosis in infants caused by nitrates in well water. J. Am. Med. Assoc. *129*:112 (1945).
4. E. H. W. J. Burden, The toxicology of nitrates and nitrites with particular reference to the potability of water supplies. Analyst *86*:429 (1961).
5. D. G. Steyn, The problem of methaemoglobinaemia in man with special reference to poisoning with nitrates and nitrites in infants and children. Publ. No. 11, University of Pretoria, Pretoria, Union of South Africa (1960).
6. G. Walton, Survey of literature relating to infant methemoglobinemia due to nitrate-contaminated water. Am. J. Public Health *41*:986 (1951).
7. U.S. Public Health Service drinking water standards, p. 47 (1962).
8. P. M. Hölscher and J. Natzschka, Methämoglobinämie bei jungen Säuglingen durch nitrithaltigen Spinat. Dtsch. Med. Wochenschr. *89*:1751 (1964).
9. J. D. Orgeron, J. D. Martin, C. T. Caraway, R. M. Martine, and G. H. Hauser, Methemoglobinemia from eating meat with high nitrite content. U.S. Public Health Rep. *72*:189 (1957).
10. H. Druckrey, D. Steinhoff, H. Beuthner, H. Schneider, and P. Klärner, Prufung von Nitrit auf chronisch toxische Wirkung an Ratten. Arzneimittel-Forsch. *13*: 320 (1963).
11. G. E. Heim, The reaction of tertiary amines with nitrous acid. J. Chem. Ed. *40*:181 (1963).
12. W. Fiddler, J. W. Pensabene, R. C. Doerr, and A. E. Wasserman, Formation of

N-nitrosodimethylamine from naturally occurring ammonium compounds and tertiary amines. Nature 236:307 (1972).

13. American Public Health Association standard methods for examination of water and wastewater. 13th ed. American Public Health Association, New York (1971).

14. Methods of analysis. 11th ed. Association of Official Analytical Chemists, Washington, D.C. (1970).

15. L. Kamm, D. F. Bray, and D. E. Coffin, Assessment of the naphthylazo-naphthylamine method for the determination of nitrate and nitrite. J. Assoc. Off. Anal. Chem. 51:140 (1968).

16. L. Kamm, G. G. McKeown, and D. M. Smith, New colorimetric method for the determination of the nitrate and nitrite content of baby foods. J. Assoc. Off. Anal. Chem. 48:892 (1965).

17. M. J. Follett and P. W. Ratcliff, Determination of nitrite and nitrate in meat products. J. Sci. Food Agric. 14:138 (1963).

18. A. Adriaanse and J. E. Robbers, Determination of nitrite and nitrate in some horticultural and meat products and in samples of soil. J. Sci. Food Agric. 20: 321 (1969).

19. P. Voogt, Die Bestimmung von Nitrat im Spinat mittels einer nitratselektiven Elektrode. Dtsch. Lebensm. Rundschau 65:196 (1969).

20. B. D. McCaslin, W. T. Franklin, and M. A. Dillon, Rapid determination of nitrate nitrogen in sugarbeets with the specific ion electrode. J. Am. Soc. Sugar Beet Technol. 16:64 (1970).

21. P. B. Manning, S. T. Coulter, and R. Jenness, Determination of nitrate and nitrite in milk and dry milk products. J. Dairy Sci. 51:1725 (1968).

22. R. D. Miller, Determination of nitrate nitrogen in sugarbeet petioles and soils with 2-6-dimethyl phenol. J. Am. Soc. Sugar Beet Technol. 15:504 (1969).

23. E. Mehnert, Eine Methode zur Bestimmung des Nitratgehaltes in Rüben. Arch. Exp. Veterinaermed. 22:851 (1968).

24. E. Mehnert, Eine Methode zur quantitativen Bestimmung von Nitrat und Nitrit in Futtermitteln, Tränkwasser und Mageninhalten. Arch. Exp. Veterinaermed. 21:1191 (1967).

25. J. W. Howard, T. Fazio, and J. O. Watts, Extraction and gas chromatographic determination of n-nitrosodimethylamine in smoked fish: Application to smoked nitrite-treated chub. J. Assoc. Off. Anal. Chem. 53:269 (1970).

26. T. Fazio, J. N. Damico, J. W. Howard, R. H. White, and J. O. Watts, Gas chromatographic determination and mass spectrometric confirmation of n-nitrosodimethylamine in smoke-processed marine fish. J. Anal. Food Chem. 19:250 (1971).

27. L. Hedler and P. Marquardt, Occurrence of diethylnitrosamine in some samples of food. Food Cosmet. Toxicol. 6:341 (1968).

28. M. J. H. Keybets, E. H. Groot, and G. H. M. Keller, Air investigation into the possible presence of nitrosamines in nitrite-bearing spinach. Food Cosmet. Toxicol. 8:167 (1970).

29. D. R. Keeney, Nitrates in plants and waters. J. Milk Food Technol. 33:425 (1970).

30. J. H. Feth, Nitrogen compounds in natural water—A review. Water Resour. Res. 2:41 (1966).

31. P. M. Chalk and D. R. Keeney, Nitrate and ammonium contents of Wisconsin limestones. Nature 229:42 (1971).

32. Air quality criteria for nitrogen oxides. Environmental Protection Agency, AP-84 (1971).
33. H. J. M. Bowen, Trace elements in biochemistry. Academic Press, New York (1966).
34. Air quality criteria for photochemical oxidants. Environmental Protection Agency, AP-63 (1970).
35. Air quality criteria for particulate matter. National Air Pollution Control Administration, AP-49 (1969).
36. K. M. Mackenthun and W. M. Ingram, Biological associated problems in fresh water environments. Federal Water Pollution Control Administration, U.S. Department of the Interior (1967).
37. R. W. F. Hardy and R. C. Burns, Biological nitrogen fixation. Annu. Rev. Biochem. *37*:331 (1968).
38. J. S. Fruton and S. Simmonds, General biochemistry. 2nd ed. Wiley, New York, (1958).
39. H. W. Doelle, Bacterial metabolism. Academic Press, New York (1969).
40. L. Beevers and R. H. Hageman. Nitrate reduction in higher plants. Ann. Rev. Plant Physiol. *20*:495 (1969).
41. G. E. Smith, Nitrate pollution of water supplies, pp. 273–287. In Trace substances in environmental health. III., D. D. Hemphill (ed.). University of Missouri, Columbia, Mo. (1969).
42. W. E. J. Phillips, Naturally occurring nitrate and nitrite in foods in relation to infant methaemoglobinaemia. Food Cosmet. Toxicol. *9*:219 (1971).
43. J. J. Hanway, J. B. Herrick, T. L. Willrich, P. C. Bennett, and J. T. McCall, The nitrate problems. Spec. Rep. No. 34, Iowa State University, Ames, Iowa (August 1963).
44. W. Schuphan, Der Nitratgehalt von Spinat (*Spinacia oleracea* L.) in Beziehung zur Methämoglobinämie der Säuglinge. Z. Ernaehr. Wiss. *6*:207 (1965).
45. W. Schuphan, Bildung von Nitrat und Nitrit im pflanzlichen Stoffwechsel. Nutr. Diet. *11*:120 (1967).
46. C. Simon, Nitrite poisoning from spinach. Lancet, *1*:872 (1966).
47. C. Simon, H. Manzke, H. Kay, and G. Mrowetz, Über Vorkommen, Pathogenese und Möglichkeiten zur Prophylaxe der durch Nitrit verursachten Methämoglobinämie. Z. Kinderheilkd. *91*:124 (1964).
48. A. Sinios and W. Wodsak, Die Spinatvergiftung des Säuglings. Dtsch. Med. Wochschr. *90*:1856 (1965).
49. U. S. Department of Agriculture, The effect of soils and fertilizers on the nutritional quality of plants. Agric. Inf. Bull. 299. Washington, D.C. (1965).
50. M. J. Wright and K. L. Davison, Nitrate accumulation in crops and nitrate poisoning in animals, p. 197. In Advances in agronomy 16, A. G. Norman (ed.). Academic Press, New York (1964).
51. W. D. Richardson, Nitrates in vegetable foods, in cured meats and elsewhere. J. Am. Chem. Soc. *29*:1757 (1907).
52. W. A. Jackson, J. S. Steel and V. R. Boswell, Nitrates in edible vegetables and vegetable products. Am. Soc. Hortic. Sci. *90*:349 (1967).
53. J. R. Brown and G. E. Smith, Nitrate accumulation in vegetable crops as influenced by soil fertility practices. Res. Bull. 920, University of Missouri, Columbia, Mo. (April 1967).
54. A. V. Barker, N. H. Peck, and G. E. MacDonald, Nitrate accumulation in vegetables. I. Spinach grown in upland soils. Agron. J. *63*:126 (1971).

55. N. H. Peck, A. V. Barker, G. E. MacDonald, and R. S. Shallenberger, Nitrate accumulation in vegetables. II. Table beets grown in upland soils. Agron. J. *63*: 130 (1971).

56. D. H. K. Lee, Nitrates, nitrites and methemoglobinemia. Environmental review no. 2. National Institute of Environmental Health Sciences, U.S. Department of Health, Education, and Welfare (1970).

57. R. L. Warner, R. H. Hageman, J. W. Dudley, and R. J. Lambert, Inheritance of nitrate reductase activity in *Zea Mays* L. Proc. Nat. Acad. Sci. *62*:785 (1969).

58. J. A. Pateman and D. J. Cove, Regulation of nitrate reduction in *Aspergillus nidulans*. Nature *215*:1234 (1967).

59. J. D. Hem, Study and interpretation of the chemical characteristics of natural water. 2nd ed., Geological Survey Water Supply Paper 1473 (1970).

60. W. H. Durum, Monitoring program of the U.S. Geological Survey with special reference to nitrate. National Academy of Sciences–National Research Council–National Academy of Engineering. (Talk on Nov. 17, 1970)

61. M. Goldberg, Sources of nitrogen in water supplies. Agricultural practices and water quality, Willrich and Smith (eds.). Iowa State University Press, Ames, Iowa (1970).

62. T. Sollman, A manual of pharmacology. 8th ed. W. B. Saunders, Philadelphia (1957).

63. E. P. Hiatt and I. Greene, Distribution, excretion and metabolism of the nitrate ion administered intravenously as $NaNO_3$. Fed. Proc. *11*:69 (1952).

64. M. N. Gleason, R. E. Gosselin, H. C. Hodge, and R. P. Smith, Clinical toxicology of commercial products. 3rd ed. Williams & Wilkins, Baltimore (1969).

65. P. B. Hawk, Physiological chemistry. 14th ed. B. L. Oser (ed.). McGraw-Hill, New York (1965).

66. L. C. Wang, J. Garcia-Rivera, and R. H. Burris, Metabolism of nitrate by cattle. Biochem. J. *81*:237 (1961).

67. H. Land and A. I. Virtanen, Ammonium salts as nitrogen source in the synthesis of protein by the ruminant. Acta Chem. Scand. *13*:489 (1959).

68. World Health Organization , Evaluation of the toxicity of a number of antimicrobials and antioxidants, pp. 69–75. Tech. Rep. No. 228 (1962).

69. W. Kübler, Die Bedeutung des Nitratgehaltes von Gemüse in der Ernährung des Säuglings. Z. Kinderheilkd. *81*:405 (1958).

70. E. F. Winton, R. G. Tardiff, and L. J. McCabe, Nitrate in drinking water. J. Am. Water Works Assoc. *63*:95 (1971).

71. P. G. Sattelmacher, Methemoglobinemia from nitrates in drinking water. Schriftenr. Ver. Wasser Boden Lufthyg. No. 21 (1962).

72. N. I. Petukhov and A. V. Ivanov, Investigation of certain psychophysiological reactions in children suffering from methemoglobinemia due to nitrates in water. Hyg. Sanit. *35*:29 (1970).

73. L. E. Marrett and M. L. Sunde, The use of turkey poults and chickens as test animals for nitrate and nitrite toxicity. Poult. Sci. *47*:511 (1968).

74. A. W. Adams, J. L. West, and A. J. Kahrs, Some effects on turkeys of nitrate in the drinking water. Poult. Sci. *48*:1222 (1969).

75. R. W. Seerley, R. J. Emerick, L. B. Embry, and O. E. Olson, Effect of nitrate or nitrite administered continuously in drinking water for swine and sheep. J. Anim. Sci. *24*:1014 (1965).

76. D. T. Buchman, R. L. Shirley, and G. B. Killinger, Nitrate and ammonia in rumen of steers fed millet. Q. J. Fla. Acad. Sci. *31*:143 (1968).

77. K. L. Davison, Sublethal nitrate poisoning—is it really a problem? Feed Age *16*:23 (1966).

78. H. Pivnick, M. A. Johnston, C. Thacker, and R. Loynes, Effect of nitrite on destruction and germination of *Clostridium botulinum* and putrefactive anaerobes 3679 and 3679h in meat and in buffer. Can. Inst. Food Technol. J. *3:* 103 (1970).

79. I. A. Wolf and A. E. Wasserman, Nitrates, nitrites and nitrosamines. Science *177*:15 (1972).

80. P. N. Magee, Toxicity of nitrosamines: Their possible human health hazards. Food Cosmet. Toxicol. *9*:207 (1971).

81. World Health Organization, Specifications for the identity and purity of food additives and their toxicological evaluation: Food colours and some antimicrobials and antioxidants, p. 25. Tech. Rep. No. 309 (1965).

2 George R. Meneely

TOXIC EFFECTS OF DIETARY SODIUM CHLORIDE AND THE PROTECTIVE EFFECT OF POTASSIUM*

INTRODUCTION

Sodium chloride is naturally present in nearly all living things and, therefore, has always been a component of food. By the beginning of recorded history, the human use of sodium chloride added to the diet as a condiment was well established. How it came to be so is entirely speculative. There is some evidence that use of salt is habit-forming in the same sense that tobacco is, but there certainly is no doubt that people accustomed to its use have fought wars to possess a source of it, and numberless men have risked death to smuggle it. There are parts of the ancient world where superficial excrescences of salt occur naturally, and the process of obtaining it by evaporation of saline waters is only a procedure copied by man from nature in areas where it occurs spontaneously on the shores of dead seas. The antiseptic properties of brine must have been noticed early by man. The use of salt to preserve foods that otherwise would decay seems a reasonable pathway by which early man may have developed his taste for it.

The elemental composition of sodium chloride was learned at the turn of the nineteenth century. Scheele discovered chlorine in 1774 but

* Literature reviewed to March 14, 1972.

thought it contained oxygen; Davy named it in 1810, recognizing that it was an element. He had isolated sodium by electrolysis in 1807. By the middle of the nineteenth century there were reports of disturbances of sodium balance in disease states, especially in cholera in which depletion of sodium is a striking feature. Physiologists were fascinated by sodium chloride in the latter half of the nineteenth century. Extensive speculations on the relation of the salt content of the herbivorous diet compared with the diet of the carnivores led to the theory, attributed to von Bunge, that herbivorous animals are compelled to go to salt licks to obtain extra sodium chloride to balance the high intake of potassium characteristic of herbivorous diet. It had been established by 1840 that the sodium chloride content of the natural herbivorous and carnivorous diets was more or less the same and that the difference between the two diets lay in the much higher potassium content of the former. The concept that sodium chloride is required to protect against high dietary potassium seems quite fallacious now. Indeed, the reverse is probably the case. As will be seen in the discussion of potassium in the diet, there is good animal and human experimental evidence that extra potassium exerts a protective effect on the toxic effects of excess sodium chloride ingestion.

SOURCES OF DIETARY SODIUM

Sodium is widespread in nature. It is the most abundant of the alkali elements and the seventh element in amount in the crust of the earth. It is highly reactive and never found free. In living organisms it occurs in manifold combinations, and it is erroneous to think of it as occurring always as the chloride, although frequently it is so expressed in chemical analyses. Sodium enters the body in five ways:

First, there is sodium in nearly all drinking water, quite a lot in certain areas, and, where water softeners are used, two atoms of sodium are added for every atom of calcium or magnesium exchanged. If the water supply contains as much as 25 mg of sodium per 100 ml, and if an intake of water in food and drink is taken to be 2 liters, the sodium intake will be as high as 500 mg per day. In Galveston, Texas, the municipal water supply contains 34 mg per 100 ml, and in Crandal, Texas, it contains 170 mg per 100 ml. The latter is rarely drunk, but it is used for cooking. The high sodium content of Galveston drinking water is well known to the medical profession as a problem in patients with congestive heart failure.

Second, sodium occurs naturally in all foods, although in many the content is very low; for example, fresh peas contain only 0.9 mg of sodium per 100 g.

The third pathway is via food processing, during which a great deal of sodium, usually in the form of sodium chloride, may be added. For example, canned peas, even with the liquor poured off, contain 230 mg of sodium per 100 g. Expressed as sodium chloride, this is 580 mg. Even the conventional freezing process uses sodium chloride so that frozen peas contain 100 mg per 100 g. A point worth noting (see also the discussion of potassium) is that, at the same time the sodium is added, the potassium is depleted. Fresh peas contain 380 mg of potassium per 100 g, while in canned peas drained of the liquor the potassium is reduced to 180 mg; in frozen peas it is reduced to 160 mg.

The fourth pathway is addition of salt in the cooking process within the home. It is highly variable from household to household, as is the matter of the disposition of the cooking water. It appears probable that the old custom of saving all or almost all cooking waters as *pot-au-feu* or pot liquor is vanishing in the United States. Generally, in the preparation of vegetables, salted water is brought to a boil and raw or frozen vegetables added. At the end of the cooking period, the vegetables are drained, the cooking water being discarded. The net effect is a further addition of sodium and a further depletion of potassium.

The fifth pathway is addition of common salt to food at the table. Again there is great individual variation, apparently dependent upon individual taste for salt. Dahl observed that patients on diets containing up to 250 mg of salt per day immediately noticed the addition of 1 g per day, whereas among subjects eating 10–20 g per day the addition of 5 or even 10 g might go unnoticed. On the other hand, Dahl found it easy to alter individual taste for salt, much easier than for some other well-recognized tastes.

HUMAN REQUIREMENTS FOR SODIUM

There are only a limited number of studies on the human requirement for sodium. It has long been recognized as essential to life. Estimates of the daily requirement have ranged as high as 15 g (as sodium chloride) per day, but clearly 5 g is ample and 1 g per day is more probably correct. Many studies have shown that humans with normal kidney function maintain salt balance easily on daily intakes below 1 g. Dahl thinks 4–8 mEq/day of sodium in the period of rapid growth during the first year of life would be a generous allowance. Foman thought 7–8 mEq/day advisable. This is less than 0.5 g of NaCl *per diem*. Dahl feels the requirements for healthy adults is similar.

SODIUM CHLORIDE AND HYPERTENSION

Hypertensive Effects of Dietary Salt in Man

That sodium chloride might have harmful effects if eaten in excess was suspected long before any objective evidence on the subject existed. Widespread use and familiarity with salt led most, however, to the assumption that it was a harmless substance. The earliest association of salt with human hypertension is thought by Chapman, in the Bell Symposium, to be the work of Ambard and Beaujard in 1904. Benefit in a disease state by restriction of an element in the diet does not, of course, establish it as having a causal relation to the disease. Therapeutic restriction of salt fell in and out of favor throughout the first four decades of this century, but the merit of salt restriction in controlling edema in congestive heart failure certainly was firmly established by the fourth decade. The association with hypertension proved more subtle. The effect of salt restriction in human hypertension, however, is now very well documented. In general, patients so treated fall into one of three categories: Some experience a return of the blood pressure to normal levels; some experience a reduction in blood pressure but not to normal; and some show no fall in blood pressure at all. Again, speaking generally, the longer the duration of the hypertension and the more severe its manifestations, the less likely is a completely favorable response. The success of the natriuretic agents in controlling hypertension further documents the association of human hypertension and dietary sodium chloride. Dahl found in experimental animals that, irrespective of the method used to produce the hypertension, the clinical course tended to be mild on low NaCl intakes while it was severe and rapidly progressive to death on high salt intakes. He holds the opinion that the same pattern obtains for man.

It has not proved easy to demonstrate a causal relation between sodium chloride intake and human hypertension. Suspicion of such a relationship was strong by 1951 when Braun–Menendez commented, at the Bell Symposium in Minneapolis, that whatever the experimental method for producing hypertension, increased salt intake facilitated the development of hypertension and salt restriction prevented it. Selye *et al.* and Knowlton *et al.* found hypertension could be produced by desoxy-corticosterone acetate with the addition of extra sodium chloride. With hypertonic saline as the sole source of liquid, Lenel, Katz, and Rodbard produced hypertension in the chicken; Sapirstein, Brandt, and Drury in the rat; and Fukuda in the rabbit.

Hypertensive Effects of Dietary Salt in Rats

In 1951 the author and his colleagues began experiments that showed that chronic ingestion of excess sodium chloride as the sole variable in an otherwise wholesome diet reliably produced hypertension in the rat that appeared to duplicate human hypertension clinically and morphologically.

Various levels of sodium chloride were investigated, but attention focused finally on three ranges as most revealing and most realistically related to the human problem. The first range, the "control" level, was from 0.15 to 2.0%. Over this range only minor differences in growth rate were found, and animals eating such diets never became hypertensive. The second range of interest was 2.8–5.6%, which represented a moderate excess of sodium chloride. Finally, 7.0–9.8% sodium chloride in the diet represented a high level of excess salt. It may seem that these levels are out of the range of human consumption, but this is not the case. These levels may be compared on a percentage of nutriment basis: In the purified rat diet 2.8% sodium chloride corresponds to 14 g of sodium chloride daily in an ordinary diet for man. The equivalent human intake in g per day may be obtained by multiplying the rat diet percent composition by five. Thus the control (0.15–2.0%) level corresponds roughly to 0.75–10 g of NaCl daily for man. The "moderate" excess range (2.8–5.6%) corresponds to 14–28 g per day and is frankly hypertensigenic and life-shortening. Finally, the "high" level of excess salt (7.0–9.8%), equivalent to 35–49 g daily, has its counterpart in man in only a few parts of the world, most notably northern Japan. It is drastically hypertensigenic in the rat and in the Japanese.

At all levels of salt feeding the rats evidenced growth and good development, but at levels above the control there were successive decrements in growth. These persisted throughout the life of the animal. The water consumption (and urine production) was proportional to the dietary sodium chloride content. This association of water drinking, urine formation, and salt intake is well known, the earliest observation being recorded in Pliny's *Natural History*. It was, for example, commented on by Thoreau who wrote in Walden: "Finally, as for salt, that grossest of groceries . . . if I did without it altogether, I should probably drink the less water." Consistent and reproducible blood pressure observations were obtained in early experiments about the ninth month, at which time hypertension was well established in animals eating above the control levels of salt.

It is of considerable interest to note that, although the mean blood pressure of each group was successively higher and essentially proportional to the sodium chloride content of the diet, there was a very considerable scatter of individual values. The mean systolic blood pressure at control levels of salt was approximately 122 mmHg. At the lower level of excess salt feeding (2.8%), the mean of the systolic blood pressures had risen to about 130. Yet there were individuals in this group who had pressures as high as 160 mmHg and others as low as 114. By the same token, at a high level of salt feeding (9.8%), the mean systolic blood pressure for the whole group of animals had risen to 152 mmHg, but there were rats with pressures as high as 205 and one rat with a pressure of only 125.

It is further of considerable interest that those animals lying significantly above or significantly below the means of their group tended to maintain this relative position throughout life. Thus, it is evident that even in fairly homogenous experimental material such as the male Sprague–Dawley rat there are substantial differences in susceptibility to hypertension induced by this means. One could reliably predict that those animals that had the higher levels of hypertension for their group were the more likely to show severe electrocardiographic changes later in life and also to show serum cholesterol elevation. Conversely, those that had the lower pressures were less likely to evidence severe electrocardiographic changes and less likely to manifest abnormally high cholesterol. The time relations of the blood pressure change was such that, at high levels of excess salt feeding, the blood pressure rose rapidly to high levels, while at lower levels of excess salt feeding the blood pressure rose less rapidly to intermediate hypertensive levels.

Among the hypertensive animals, specific abnormalities of the electrocardiogram were observed that were closely similar to those seen in humans with hypertension, namely, a high incidence of T wave abnormalities, S–T segment abnormalities, left axis deviation, left ventricular strain pattern, and prolonged duration of the QRS complex. On the other hand, arrhythmia and P–R interval abnormalities occurred only in low incidence.

Serum cholesterol levels tended to increase with increasing dietary sodium chloride. There was a strong positive correlation between serum cholesterol and the observed level of the blood pressure.

Perhaps the most sensitive index of the adverse effects of sodium chloride upon these rats was the survival data. No significant difference in survival was seen between control animals and those eating the lower levels of high salt (2.8–5.6%) until the seventeenth month of the experiment. If 10 days for a rat is equivalent to 1 yr for man, for human beings, this would correspond roughly to age 51. Thereafter the difference increased. The median duration of life for rats eating 5.6% sodium chloride was many months less than that of controls. In the case of the higher levels of high salt feeding, for example, 8.4%, there was an 8-month difference between the median duration of survival in the high-salt rats and the controls. If one were to translate this figure to man, this would be equivalent to a difference in the median duration of life of about 32 yr. Repeated experiments have shown that the slopes of the survival curves were associated with the level of dietary salt and were identical in comparable experiments.

One experiment of special interest was performed on a small number of elderly rats made available through the courtesy of Dr. Kenneth Kohlstaedt of Eli Lilly and Company. This colony of 26 male rats, nearly 2 yr in age, had been maintained previously on a chow diet. When placed on test diets containing 5.6 and 9.8% sodium chloride, they gradually became hypertensive, but it is important to note that the levels of elevated blood pressure attained were always less than was the case with young rats who ate the same ration for the same length of time. While sodium chloride did indeed have a hypertensigenic effect when started late in life, the effect was not nearly so great as when started early in life.

In young female rats fed corresponding levels of increased sodium chloride, the level of blood pressure obtained was never as high as that for the male rats.

Each animal that died was autopsied, the organs were weighed, and tissue sections were obtained for microscopic examination. The weight of the kidneys and the weight of the heart increased in proportion to the sodium chloride in the diet and, of course, to the level of blood pressure, which was also proportional to the salt in the diet. The findings in the adrenals were less consistent: At high levels of salt feeding there was a significant increase in adrenal weight, but the variability was considerable and there was only a general trend for the adrenals to increase in weight as sodium chloride increased. The characteristic alteration noted in the microscopic examination of the tissues among animals with severe hypertension was a diffuse disease involving especially the arterioles and small arteries. In the kidney this was manifest by relatively bloodless enlarged glomeruli with swelling and vacuolation of both endothelium and epithelium and large amounts of sudanophilic lipid. The tubules were dilated, and the epithelium was hyperplastic and swollen with lipid and hyaline droplets. The small arteries and arterioles showed fatty degeneration of muscle cells and often underwent smudgy eosinophilic necrosis. Similar arteriolar lesions were found in other viscera, particularly the pancreas and the testes. The late Dr. Ernest Goodpasture examined the tissues of all of the rats from Experiment I and drew particular attention to the apparent similarity between the morphological lesion seen at the high levels of high salt feeding and that seen in human malignant hypertension. He further found that when arteriolar lesions were prominent in the kidneys they were also always present in the testes. Since the testes of rats are readily available for biopsy, this suggested to him the possibility that one might follow serially the development of the morphological lesion. In rats that exhibited the clinical course of benign essential hypertension, there was a lack of striking anatomical alteration in the microscopic sections, as is true with humans. In fact, with ordinary hematoxylin and eosin stains, the several pathologists who examined these tissues were unable to find any consistent differences between these animals and the controls.

Epidemiological Observations

It is worthwhile to examine why the picture of chronic sodium chloride toxicity is so clear in animal experimental work and so blurry in human studies. Dahl has assembled an impressive body of evidence by examining the salt intake in *different* populations. The association of hypertension and salt intake is overwhelming. In contrast, studies *within* populations have largely been unconvincing. There are several factors that probably account for this latter finding. In any given region there tends to be an average level of salt intake with considerable variation about this mean but, in most instances, not a sufficient spread among a sufficient number of individuals to reveal the hypertensigenic salt effect in the presence of other variables. Of these, the most notable is the probable role of heredity, which we will discuss below, but there are also a number of ways of acquiring hypertension, especially in association with diseases of the kidney. In one investigation in Nashville, Tennessee (unpublished), some 3,000 individuals were queried concerning salt intake, and their blood pressures were measured. Three findings germane to the thesis of this report emerged. First, the distribution of observed blood pressures was not wide, due, it was thought, to the youth of the population studied (potential military draftees). Further, when hypertension was found in this group, it was almost always possible to elicit a history of kidney disease from the individual manifesting it. Finally, from a random sample of 24-hr urine collections it was abundantly apparent that there was no correlation between the amount of salt these individuals thought they were eating and the amount actually consumed. Another field study of a local population by this author and his colleagues gave equally indeterminate results. It is evident that a local population with a relatively low mobility comes to consume about the same amount of salt by reason of common local custom and identical sources of food. There will always be a few individuals distributed well away from the mean but apparently not enough to bring out the hypertensigenic effect of salt from among the other variables. On the other hand, as Dahl has so clearly shown, when different populations with widely differing salt-eating habits are investigated, the effect is abundantly evident.

Genetic Factors

It has long been known that there was a familial factor in hypertension, although it has not been clear whether the higher incidence of hypertension among the offspring of hypertensives was purely hereditary or in some way acquired in childhood. The reports of Brest and Moyer, of Schroeder, of Thomas, of Platt, of Pickering, and of many others in this connection are well known. It now appears that Dahl has resolved the problem. He interbred rats that developed high hypertension on increased salt intake and also interbred those that developed little or no elevation of blood pressure on high salt diets. By repeating this procedure, it proved possible to develop two distinct strains of rats, one extremely sensitive to increased salt intake and the other extremely resistant to it. It thus appears reasonable to believe that the toxic effect of chronic excess sodium chloride eating in man is conditional and depends upon his hereditary material. Given the appropriate hereditary proclivity and given a salt intake in excess of normal requirement, the result will be hypertension. Other recent work by Louis, Tabei, and Spector suggests that in hereditary hypertension in rats there may be two different sets of autosomal alleles, only one of which is sodium dependent.

DIETARY INTERACTIONS BETWEEN POTASSIUM AND SODIUM

Throughout nature, potassium is the principal intracellular cation. It therefore is present in all foods. There have been parts of the world where potassium salts have been used as a condiment. Lapicque found natives of Africa extracting the ash of certain plants (lixiviation) to make a condiment used somewhat like common salt. Many potassium salts, however, have a bitter disagreeable taste (salt of wormwood = potassium carbonate), and their use as condiments has never been widespread. Since potassium is so widespread in nature, it is extremely difficult to make an animal (or a normal human being) potassium deficient, and there is no evidence that normal man or animals ever eat an excessive amount of it. In disease states in man, however, excess and deficiency conditions of potassium exist. The former are usually associated with impaired renal function. One cannot increase total body potassium in normal subjects by feeding extra potassium, as the author and his colleagues found some years ago. On the other hand, in kidney disease serious states of potassium intoxication occur frequently as a clinical problem. Hyperkalemia (excessive potassium in the blood) may occur, but the electrocardiogram is a more sensitive indicator, both of excess and of deficit. There is about 20 times as much potassium in the cellular fluid as in the extracellular, and the electrocardiogram reflects changed intracellular energetics due to potassium deficit or excess before changes in plasma potassium level are detectable. Potassium deficiency occurs as a clinical problem usually as an iatrogenic disorder following administration of diuretics or the mineralocorticoid steroids. Alimentary tract loss of potassium in mucus colitis and certain rare tumors, and renal losses in certain uncommon renal disorders, also can induce potassium deficit. While exogenous hyperkalemic states are hard to induce, and probably impossible by mouth in the presence of normal kidneys, endogenous hyperkalemia readily occurs among individuals with borderline kidney function when disease or injury destroys large numbers of cells, releasing the high concentration of intracellular potassium into the extracellular compartment from which a moderately impaired kidney may be unable to drain it rapidly enough to avoid potassium intoxication.

Animal Experiments

In animal experiments it is easy to demonstrate a protective action of extra potassium against the toxic effects of chronic excessive dietary sodium chloride. The addition of extra potassium chloride to rat diets high in sodium chloride increased the median duration of life by 7 or 8 months. The concurrent blood-pressure observations were of special interest. As previously stated, at moderate levels of excess salt feeding, a moderate hypertension developed. When extra potassium chloride was added to a diet containing 5.6% sodium chloride, there was no change in the hypertensigenic action of the extra sodium chloride, but there was a tremendous improvement in survival. The median duration of life was increased by 7 months, and yet throughout life the blood pressure persisted at intermediate levels, just as in animals who received no extra potassium. In contrast to this, at levels of excess salt feeding, which ordinarily produced high levels of hypertension, the extra potassium chloride had the effect of ameliorating the hypertensigenic action of sodium chloride so that only moderate hypertension developed. Again, a dramatic increase in the median duration of life of approximately 8 months was observed.

It was evident from these data that there were at least two kinds of hypertension in the animals eating excessive amounts of salt. The first was a moderate hypertension from moderate levels of excess salt feeding, which was not significantly altered by the addition of extra potassium chloride; the second was a high hypertension associated with high levels of extra salt feeding, which was held to intermediate levels by the addition of extra potassium chloride. It was probably significant that the total body sodium of the moderate salt-eating animals was essentially the same as that of controls, whereas in animals eating high levels of excess sodium chloride there was a significant increase in total body sodium. Further, upon the addition of potassium chloride to each of these diets, no significant effect upon total body sodium was observed at moderate levels of sodium chloride increase, whereas at high levels of sodium chloride feeding with extra potassium, the total body sodium stayed within normal limits. It is of interest to note that the rats of Louis *et al.* showed increased excretion of sodium and an amelioration of hypertension with increased dietary potassium.

Man

The above observations shed light upon the puzzling situation with regard to human beings and dietary sodium and potassium. It is evident that there were five quite different categories of rats, and there should probably be at least five corresponding categories of man. First, there were those with optimal sodium and potassium intake who lived a long life and did not develop hypertension. Second, there were those with moderately increased sodium intake and normal potassium intake. These animals developed a moderate hypertension and exhibited a shortened life span but did not have any significant alteration in total body sodium content. Third, there were those with moderately excessive sodium intake and extra potassium intake. These animals were distinguishable from the second category only in that they survived significantly longer. Fourth, there were those with a highly excessive sodium chloride intake and a normal potassium intake. These animals developed a severe hypertension, their life span was greatly shortened, and their total body sodium was significantly elevated. In the fifth category were those rats with a highly excessive sodium chloride intake and an increased potassium intake. This group was characterized by the development of a moderate hypertension, a substantial prolongation of life when compared with animals eating the same amount of sodium chloride but without the supplemental potassium chloride, and a total body sodium that remained within normal limits.

If these data were transferable directly to man, it would account for the fact that some hypertensive patients exhibit a fall in blood pressure when extra potassium chloride is provided and others do not. One could hardly expect potassium to produce a fall in blood pressure unless the individual (a) had a hypertension corresponding to the high salt intake hypertension of the rat and (b) was not already receiving a sufficient amount of potassium. Further, the benefit of extra potassium fed to an individual eating an intermediate level of high salt could be detected, so far as one is able to determine, only by observing a prolongation of life. This is obviously impossible in the individual. The protective effect of extra potassium in diets high in sodium chloride has been confirmed in animals by Dahl. Some most interesting human studies by Sasaki confirm the effect in man. Kempner's "rice" diet has long been known to be effective in hypertension, but it should more properly be called a "rice–fruit" diet and is not only low in sodium but is high in potassium.

SALT CONSUMPTION IN HUMAN DIETS

The consumption of a food for humans is only of academic interest until it is consumed; from that time forward it is of biological significance to the consumer and those concerned with his well-being. As a practical matter, sodium does not occur naturally in potential foodstuffs at levels that could be toxic. Sodium is unique in that it is the only element naturally occurring in foods that is intentionally altered enormously by man. The human requirement for it seems, on generous estimate, to be only 8 mEq/day or less (equivalent to less than 0.5 g of NaCl), but in preserving, processing, cooking, and at table this level of sodium is manipulated upward by a factor of 10 or 20 and sometimes far more. On the face of it, this makes little sense and has to be attributed to custom, "taste," or, as Kaunitz and others think, habituation. The same food-processing steps that augment sodium tend also to deplete potassium. There is no doubt that excess sodium is poisonous for many species of animal, that potassium exerts a protective effect, that there is a hereditary component in individual susceptibility to the hypertensigenic effect of salt, and that young animals are more sensitive than older ones. There is incontrovertible evidence that excess salt raises blood pressure in some humans, that salt restriction lowers blood pressure in some hypertensive patients, and that extra potassium is beneficial in some hypertensives. Beyond these solidly established facts, the human data are less clear cut, but the weight of the evidence supports the transfer of the implications of the animal observations to man. Certainly if any newly proposed ingredient of diet or medicament evidenced such noxious effects in animal experiments, authorities would be compelled to view its promiscuous exhibition with grave alarm.

The use and abuse of salt is inextricably entwined with the food habits and customs of most people of a Western culture. There is good evidence it is noxious. Can anything be done about it? Certainly investigations of it should be pressed, but meanwhile, perhaps Tobian's advice should be given greater consideration: "An alteration of the amounts of sodium and potassium in the diet of populations susceptible to hypertension may be the most practical way to decrease the incidence of the disease." We suggested this some years ago when Robert Tucker tested the acceptability of sodium chloride–potassium chloride mixtures as condiments and found that mixtures up to 50–50 were tolerated; with lower fractions of KCl, the mixtures often were not detectably different from ordinary table salt (see Ball and Meneely, 1957). The idea was that such a mix would concurrently diminish sodium intake while augmenting that of potassium. More recently Frank and Mickelson have explored this possibility, and they too find it promising. Such a mixture is surely in the right direction, but more research is required before one can say with assurance that this is the solution of the problem of excessive sodium chloride consumption for all of the human race.

BIBLIOGRAPHY

F. M. Allen, Arterial hypertension. J. Am. Med. Assoc. 74:652 (1920).

F. M. Allen, J. W. Mitchell, and J. W. Sherrill, The treatment of combined diabetes and nephritis. J. Am. Med. Assoc. 75:444 (1920).

F. M. Allen, Treatment of arterial hypertension. Med. Clin. North Am. 6:475 (1922).

F. M. Allen, Treatment of kidney diseases and high blood pressure. Morristown, N.J., The Psychiatric Institute (1925).

F. M. Allen and J. W. Sherrill, The treatment of arterial hypertension. J. Metabol. Res. 2:429 (1922).

L. Ambard and E. Beaujard, Causes de l'hypertension arterielle. Arch. Gen. Med. 1:520 (1904).

C. O. T. Ball and G. R. Meneely, Observations on dietary sodium chloride. J. Am. Diet. Assoc. 33:366 (1957).

E. T. Bell (ed.), Hypertension. A symposium. University of Minnesota Press, Minneapolis (1951).

R. S. Berghoff and A. S. Geraci, The influence of sodium chloride on blood pressure. Ill. Med. J. *56*:395 (1929).

A. N. Brest and J. H. Moyer, The etiology and therapy of essential hypertension. A review. J. S. C. Med. Assoc. *56*:171 (1960).

G. von Bunge, Lehrbuch der physiologischen und pathologischen Chemie. 3rd. ed., Verlag von F. C. W. Vogel, Leipzig (1894).

L. K. Dahl, Medical progress. Salt intake and salt need. New Engl. J. Med. *258*:1152, 1205 (1958).

L. K. Dahl, Possible role of salt intake in development of essential hypertension. Essential hypertension, an international symposium. Springer Verlag, Heidelberg (1960).

L. K. Dahl, Studies on the role of salt and genetics in hypertension. Acad. Med. N.J. Bull. *10*:269 (1964).

L. K. Dahl, Salt in processed baby foods (guest editorial). Am. J. Clin. Nutr. *21*:787 (1968).

L. K. Dahl, Salt and hypertension. Am. J. Clin. Nutr. *25*:231–244 (1972).

L. K. Dahl, M. Heine, G. Leitl, and L. Tassinari, Hypertension and death from consumption of processed baby foods by rats. Proc. Soc. Exp. Biol. Med. *133*:1405 (1970).

L. K. Dahl, M. Heine, and L. Tassinari, Effects of chronic excess salt ingestion. Evidence that genetic factors play an important role in susceptibility to experimental hypertension. J. Exp. Med. *115*:1173 (1962).

L. K. Dahl, M. Heine, and L. Tassinari, Effects of chronic excess salt ingestion, vascular reactivity in two strains of rats with opposite genetics susceptibility to experimental hypertension. Circulation, Supp. II *29, 30*:11 (1964).

L. K. Dahl, M. Heine, and L. Tassinari, Effects of chronic excess salt ingestion. Further demonstration that genetic factors influence the development of hypertension: Evidence from experimental hypertension due to cortisone and to adrenal regeneration. J. Exp. Med. *122*:533 (1965).

L. K. Dahl and R. A. Love, Evidence for relationship between sodium (chloride) intake and human essential hypertension. Am. Med. Assoc. Arch. Intern. Med., *94*:525 (1954).

L. K. Dahl and R. A. Love, Etiological role of sodium chloride intake in essential hypertension in humans. J. Am. Med. Assoc. *164*:397 (1957).

L. K. Dahl and E. Schackow, Effects of chronic excess salt ingestion: Experimental hypertension in the rat. Can. Med. Assoc. J. *90*:155 (1964).

L. K. Dahl, L. Silver, and R. W. Christie, The role of salt in the fall of blood pressure accompanying reduction in obesity. New Engl. J. Med. *258*:1186 (1958).

L. K. Dahl, L. Silver, R. W. Christie, and J. Genest, Adrenocortical function after prolonged salt restriction in hypertension. Nature *185*:110 (1960).

V. P. Dole, L. K. Dahl, G. C. Cotzias, H. A. Eder, and M. E. Krebs, Dietary treatment of hypertension. Clinical and metabolic studies of patients on the rice-fruit diet. J. Clin. Invest. *29*:1189 (1950).

V. P. Dole, L. K. Dahl, G. C. Cotzias, D. D. Dziewiatkowski, and C. Harris, Dietary treatment of hypertension. II. Sodium depletion as related to the therapeutic effect. J. Clin. Invest. *30*:584 (1951).

G. L. Eskew, Salt, the fifth element. J. G. Ferguson and Associates, Chicago (1948).

S. L. Fomon, Infant nutrition. Saunders, Philadelphia (1967).

R. L. Frank and O. Mickelsen, Sodium–potassium chloride mixtures as table salt. Am. J. Clin. Nutr. 22:464 (1969).

T. Fukuda, L'hypertension par le sel chez les lapins et les relations avec la glande surrenale. Union Med. Can. 80:1278 (1951).

T. Fukuda, Investigation on hypertension in farm villages in Akita Prefecture. J. Chiba Med. Soc. (Japan.) 29:490 (1954).

A. Grollman and T. R. Harrison, Effect of rigid sodium restriction on blood pressure and survival of hypertensive rats. Proc. Soc. Exp. Biol. Med. 60:52 (1945).

A. R. Holmberg, Nomads of the long bow: The Siriono of eastern Bolivia. Smithsonian Institution, Institute of Social Anthropology, Publ. No. 10. U.S. Government Printing Office, Washington, D.C. (1950).

E. Hughes, Studies in administration and finance. University of Manchester Press, Manchester (1934).

S. V. Humphries, A study of hypertension in the Bahamas. S. Afr. Med. J. 31:694 (1957).

L. C. Isaacson, M. Modlin, and W. P. V. Jackson, Sodium intake and hypertension. (letter to the editor). Lancet 1:946 (1963).

E. Jones, Essays in applied psycho-analysis, Vol. 2. Hogarth Press, London (1951).

H. Kaunitz, Causes and consequences of salt consumption. Nature, 178:1141 (1956).

S. Kaneta, K. Ishiguro, S. Kobayashi, and E. Takahashi, An epidemiological study on nutrition and cerebrovascular lesions in Tohoku area of Japan. Tohoku J. Exp. Med. 83:398 (1964).

W. Kempner, Treatment of kidney disease and hypertensive vascular disease with rice diet. N.C. Med. J. 5:125 (1944).

W. Kempner, Treatment of hypertensive vascular disease with rice diet. Am. J. Med. 4:545 (1948).

A. I. Knowlton, E. N. Loeb, H. C. Stoerk, and B. C. Seegal, Desoxycorticosterone acetate: Potentiation of its activity by sodium chloride. J. Exp. Med. 85:187 (1947).

L. Lapicque, Documents ethnographiques sur l'alimentation minerale. Anthropologie 7:35 (1896).

J. Lemley-Stone, W. J. Darby, G. R. Meneely, Effect of dietary sodium: Potassium ratio on body content of sodium and potassium in rats. Am. J. Cardiol. 8:748 (1961).

R. Lenel, L. N. Katz, and S. Rodbard, Arterial hypertension in chicken. Am. J. Physiol. 152:557 (1948).

W. J. Louis, R. Tabei, and S. Spector, Effects of sodium intake on inherited hypertension in the rat. Lancet, p. 1283 (December 11, 1971).

J. McDonough and C. M. Wilhelmj, The effect of excess salt intake on human blood pressure. Am. J. Dig. Dis. 21:180 (1954).

G. R. Meneely, Salt. Am. J. Med. 16:1 (1954).

G. R. Meneely and C. O. T. Ball, Experimental epidemiology of chronic sodium chloride toxicity and protective effect of potassium chloride. Am. J. Med. 25:713 (1958).

G. R. Meneely, C. O. T. Ball, and J. B. Youmans, Chronic sodium chloride toxicity: Protective effect of added potassium chloride. Ann. Intern. Med. 47:263 (1957).

G. R. Meneely and L. K. Dahl, Electrolytes in hypertension: The effects of sodium chloride. The evidence from animal and human studies. Med. Clin. North Am. 45:271 (1961).

G. R. Meneely, J. Lemley-Stone, and W. J. Darby, Changes in body sodium of rats fed sodium and potassium chloride. In Seminar on the role of salt in cardiovascular hypertension, M. J. Fregly (ed.). Am. J. Cardiol. *8*:527 (1961).

G. R. Meneely, R. G. Tucker, and W. J. Darby, Chronic sodium chloride toxicity in albino rat. 1. Growth on a purified diet containing various levels of sodium chloride. J. Nutr. *48*:489 (1952).

G. R. Meneely, R. G. Tucker, W. J. Darby, and S. H. Auerbach, Chronic sodium chloride toxicity in albino rat. II. Occurrence of hypertension and syndrome of edema and renal failure. J. Exp. Med. *98*:71 (1953).

G. R. Meneely, R. G. Tucker, W. J. Darby, and S. H. Auerbach, Chronic sodium chloride toxicity: Hypertension, renal and vascular lesions. Ann. Intern. Med. *39*:991 (1953).

National Research Council, Subcommittee on Safety and Suitability of M S G and Other Substances in Baby Foods, Food Protection Committee, Food and Nutrition Board. Safety and suitability of salt for use in baby foods. National Academy of Sciences, Washington, D.C. (1970).

O. Paul, (discussion of) G. R. Meneely, The experimental epidemiology of sodium chloride toxicity in the rat, p. 248. In The epidemiology of hypertension—Proceedings of an internal symposium, J. Stamler, R. Stamler, and T. N. Pullman (eds.). Grune & Stratton, New York (1967).

G. W. Pickering, High blood pressure. Grune & Stratton, New York (1955).

W. W. Priddle, Observations on the management of hypertension. Can. Med. Assoc. J. *25*:5 (1931).

W. W. Priddle, Hypertension: Sodium and potassium studies. Can. Med. Assoc. J. *86*:1 (1962).

W. W. Priddle, Sodium, potassium ratios and essential hypertension. Nutr. Rev. *20*:195 (1962).

R. Platt, The nature of essential hypertension. Lancet *2*:55 (1959).

W. D. Reid and J. H. Laragh, Sodium and potassium intake, blood pressure, and pressor response to angiotensin. Proc. Soc. Exp. Biol. Med. *120*:26 (1965).

L. A. Sapirstein, W. L. Brandt, and D. R. Drury, Production of hypertension in rat by substituting hypertonic sodium chloride solutions for drinking water. Proc. Soc. Exp. Biol. Med. *73*:82 (1950).

N. Sasaki, On the geographic distribution of salt concentration in "miso" and its relation to the death rate from apoplexy in Japan. Med. Biol. (Japan.) *38*:187 (1956).

N. Sasaki, High blood pressure and the salt intake of the Japanese. Jap. Heart J. *3*:313 (1962).

N. Sasaki, The relationship of salt intake to hypertension in the Japanese. Geriatrics *19*:735 (1964).

N. Sasaki, J. Takeda, S. Fukushi, T. Mitsuhashi, H. Ukai, E. Saito, A. Ono, and T. Kawagishi, Some problems of salt intake, especially its relation to the apoplexy or hypertension in Japan. Medicine (Japan.) *15*:101 (1958).

H. A. Schroeder, Hypertensive diseases: Causes and control. Lea & Febiger, Philadelphia (1953).

H. Selye, C. E. Hall, and E. M. Rowley, Malignant hypertension produced by treatment with desoxycorticosterone acetate and sodium chloride. Can. Med. Assoc. J. *49*:88 (1943).

J. R. Smith, Salt. Nutr. Rev. *11*:33 (1953).

W. R. Smith, Salt: Ancient history and religious symbolism. Encyclopaedia Britannica, 11th ed., *24*:87 (1911).

S. Suzuki, T. Tezuka, S. Oshima, T. Kuga, K. Yamakawa, and S. Nagamine, Nutritional survey on the essential hypertension in Tohoku (east-northern area). Jap. J. Nutr. *17*:159 (1959).

Sodium and potassium analyses of foods and waters. Fifth List. Mead Johnson & Co., Evansville, Ind. (Oct. 1947).

E. Takahashi, An epidemiological approach to the relation between diet and cerebrovascular lesions and arteriosclerotic heart disease. Tohoku J. Exp. Med. *77*:239 (1962).

C. B. Thomas, Familial patterns in hypertension and coronary heart disease. Circulation *20*:25 (1959).

W. H. Thompson and I. McQuarrie, Effects of various salts on carbohydrate metabolism and blood pressure in diabetic children. Proc. Soc. Exp. Biol. Med. *31*:907 (1933–1934).

L. Tobian, Interrelationship of electrolytes, juxtaglomerular cells and hypertension. Physiol. Rev. *40*:280 (1960).

R. G. Tucker, C. O. T. Ball, W. J. Darby, W. R. Early, R. C. Kory, J. B. Youmans, and G. R. Meneely, Chronic sodium chloride toxicity in albino rat. III. Maturity characteristics, survivorship and organ weights. J. Gerontol. *12*:182 (1957).

3 E. J. Underwood

TRACE ELEMENTS*

INTRODUCTION

Trace elements occur in all foods as natural or inherent components of
plant and animal tissues and fluids. They may also be present as a result
of accidental contamination or of deliberate addition. Accidental contamination arises from exposure to atmospheric dust and fumes, from
the use of pesticides, fumigants, feed additives, and fertilizers, and from
contact with metals in food processing and cooking. Deliberate additives occur either through direct incorporation of trace elements into
particular foods to improve nutritive value, or indirectly through their
presence in pigments, gels, stabilizers, and preservatives designed to
improve the color, keeping quality, or physical properties of the food.

A high proportion of total daily trace element intakes by man comes
normally from their natural presence as inherent components of foods
and beverages. Substantial quantities of various trace elements, far exceeding those normally present in the diet, may also be ingested or
inhaled by workers in certain industries where such industrial exposure
is not adequately controlled. Acute intoxications of this nature lie
properly within the field of industrial toxicology and receive little consideration in this review. However, smaller quantities of some trace

* Literature reviewed to March 1972.

43

elements are continuously being injected into the environment and enter the food chain as a consequence of technological developments and the increasing industrialization and motorization of urban communities. It is therefore difficult or impossible to determine what are "natural" and what are "contaminated" levels in modern foods.

The only characteristic that the trace elements have in common is that they are present or exert activity in plant and animal tissues in low concentrations, relative to the major mineral elements. At present only 10 trace elements—iron, copper, manganese, zinc, cobalt, iodine, molybdenum, selenium, chromium, and tin—are unequivocally established as essential elements in mammalian nutrition. Nickel and vanadium are probably essential also. Certain other elements, notably bromine, fluorine, silicon, arsenic, barium, and strontium, can be beneficial under some conditions, but no vital metabolic function has yet been found for them. Silicon and fluorine have now been shown to be dietary essentials for the rat. A further 20–30 trace elements occur more or less regularly in foods and animal tissues in variable concentrations. It is not known if they are merely adventitious contaminants reflecting the contact of the organism with its environment or whether they serve some useful, as yet undefined, purpose.

Some of the trace elements, such as arsenic, lead, cadmium, and mercury are frequently classified as toxic elements because their toxicity to man and animals is relatively high and their biological activity is largely confined to toxic reactions. However, all the trace elements can be toxic if consumed in large-enough quantities or for long-enough periods. With some, such as fluorine in man and copper in sheep, the margins between beneficial and toxic intakes are quite small. Furthermore, the toxicity of a particular element can be greatly influenced by the extent to which other elements or compounds affecting its absorption, excretion, or metabolism are present in the diet. Interactions of this type are of such importance with some elements, notably iron, copper, molybdenum, and zinc, that there is no single maximum "safe" level in foods, or no single minimum toxic level. There is a series of such levels, depending upon the chemical form, the duration and continuity of intake of the element, and the nature of the rest of the diet, including the amounts and proportions of various other elements and organic compounds. These facts should constantly be borne in mind in any consideration of the toxic potential of trace elements occurring in foods.

Modern urbanized man enjoys a considerable degree of protection against deficiencies or toxicities arising from the wide variations that have been demonstrated in the trace element content of individual foods,[1-11] because he is at the end of the food chain. Most human dietaries contain a great variety of types of foods obtained from ever-widening geographical sources. Trace-element abnormalities due to local soil and climate influences and varietal differences in one area tend therefore to be counterbalanced by the consumption of a proportion of foods from other areas not so affected. In addition, modern agricultural techniques militate against the presence of abnormally low or excessively high trace-element concentrations in foods by defining the areas naturally low or high in those elements and by devising means of overcoming such abnormalities. Techniques aimed at improving the productivity of crops and stock usually result in the elimination of the extremes in the food products raised and sold, because plants and animals with abnormally low or high concentrations of trace elements in their tissues either die or fail to thrive. It is mainly for these reasons that "area" problems involving trace-element problems are much less prominent in man than they are in farm animals.[12] Several North American studies of total diets[13,14] and of school lunches[15,16] testify to the relatively small (twofold or less) variation in the total content of most trace elements.

ALUMINUM

There is no conclusive evidence that aluminum performs any vital function in plants or animals. It is present in low and highly variable concentrations in foods of plant origin and in even lower concentrations in foods of animal origins. A range of vegetables for human consumption was reported to contain 0.5–5.0 ppm Al.[2] The edible fresh portions of berries and stone fruits were later found to contain 2–4 ppm Al, and citrus and stone fruits usually less than 0.1–0.2 ppm.[1] The variability from sample to sample was higher for aluminum than for the other elements studied, probably as a result of ease of contamination from dust. Cow's milk normally contains very little aluminum (0.4–0.8 mg/liter), and muscle and organ meats 0.2–0.6 ppm Al on the fresh basis. Much higher levels can occur in the lungs through accumulation from inhaled atmospheric dust.

Normal adult North American diets apparently supply widely varying amounts of aluminum. Thus Zook and Lehmann,[13] in their study of total diets supplying 4,200 cal/day, observe a 14-fold range from as low as 3.8 to as high as 51.6 mg Al/day, with a mean of 24.6 mg/day. An even wider range in the aluminum content of school lunches has been reported.[15] The amount per lunch varied from <0.6 to 44.3 mg, with a mean of 8.3 mg Al. How far this extreme variation reflects comparable variations in the original foods composing the diets, or how far it results from variable contamination with aluminum during preparation and cooking or from the water supply, cannot readily be answered. However, this aluminum is very poorly absorbed and appears mostly in the feces.[17,18] Contamination with aluminum from aluminum vessels used domestically and in food processing and from the use of aluminum sulfate baking powders is normally small, and because of poor absorption does not constitute an appreciable health hazard.[19,20] Ten times the amounts likely to be ingested in these ways can be tolerated by man without ill effects. Still larger intakes may induce gastrointestinal irritation and produce rickets by interfering with phosphate absorption.[21]

ARSENIC

Arsenic poisoning in man invariably results from the accidental or deliberate (suicidal or homicidal) ingestion of inorganic or organic arsenic compounds, usually compounds such as calcium or lead arsenate or copper acetoarsanate used as pesticides or rodenticides. Toxic reactions from small amounts of arsenic present in ordinary uncontaminated foods and beverages are apparently unknown, except in certain localized areas considered later. Most human foods contain less than 0.5 ppm and rarely exceed 1 ppm As on the fresh basis.[22] This applies to fruits, vegetables, cereal products, meats, and dairy products. Foods of marine origin, especially crustacea, are normally much higher in arsenic. Many species of sea fish contain 2–8 ppm, oysters 3–10 ppm, and mussels, shrimps, and prawns from 42 to 174 ppm As.[22,23] Fish and crustacea from fresh water usually contain much lower concentrations than those just cited.

Arsenic is not readily absorbed by plants from soils, even when the levels in the soils have been raised by continued use of arsenical sprays, but surface contamination of fruits and vegetables with spray residues can raise their arsenic concentrations well above the 0.5 ppm level of As common in such materials. Such residues can readily be removed by washing. The replacement of arsenical pesticides and weedicides with various organic compounds, free from arsenic, has reduced this form of contamination in recent years.

The amount of arsenic ingested in human diets is greatly influenced by the proportion of seafoods consumed. According to Schroeder and Balassa,[22] a typical U.S. adult diet supplies about 0.9 mg As/day. This represents an overall concentration close to 1 ppm on the dry basis. Diets unusually rich in seafoods would clearly supply much more. The maximum long-term intake compatible with health and well-being in man cannot be given with any accuracy because variation in individual susceptibility is high and because the chemical form of the arsenic greatly affects toxicity. Thus orchardists have been found to ingest as much as 6.8 mg As/day without signs of intoxication, due presumably to the prior oxidation of the arsenic from the trivalent to the less toxic pentavalent form. By contrast, 30 mg of As_2O_3 have been found to be fatal.[24] Rats have been fed diets supplemented with 50 ppm As as As_2O_3 without any toxic effects, whereas at 200 ppm a significant growth depression was observed.[25]

The relative toxicity of different forms of arsenic can be explained, in part, by the fact that the more toxic trivalent compounds, including arsenic trioxide, are retained in the tissues in greater amounts and are excreted more slowly than the less toxic. Arsenic in the forms in which it ordinarily occurs in foods, including the organically bound arsenic of shrimp, is well absorbed and rapidly eliminated, mainly in the urine. Arsenic trioxide is also well absorbed but more of it is retained in the tissues in man and in rats.[26] The arsenic of organic compounds, such as arsanilic acid used as growth stimulants in the rations of pigs and poultry, is also well absorbed, disappears rapidly from the tissues, and is excreted mostly in the feces.[27] Arsenic in such pentavalent forms, when fed to these species in the recommended proportions, does not therefore accumulate continuously to excessive concentrations (Table 1).

TABLE 1 Arsenic Deposition in Chickens and Turkeys Fed Arsenicals in Recommended Doses[a]

Feed Supplement	Arsenic Added to Feed (ppm As)	Level in Fresh Liver (ppm As)	Level in Fresh Muscle (ppm As)
Chickens			
Arsanilic acid (0.01%)	34	1.1	—
3-nitro-4-hydroxyphenyl-arsonic acid (0.005%)	14	1.3	—
Turkeys			
None	—	0.04	0.03
Arsanilic acid (0.01%)	26	0.76	0.31
Dodecylamine p-chlorophenyl-arsonate (0.01%)	13.4	1.0	0.24

[a]Calculated from data of Frost *et al.,* Agric. Food Chem. *3*:235 (1955).

The retained arsenic has a predilection for keratin, so that the concentration in hair and fingernails is higher than in other tissues and can reach very high levels where arsenic intakes are well above normal. The arsenic content of human hair is therefore of value in the diagnosis of arsenic poisoning or alleged arsenic poisoning. Using a very sensitive neutron activation technique on over 1,000 samples from living subjects, Smith[28,29] obtained the results for arsenic content of hair set out in Table 2. This worker contends that hair samples showing an As concentration greater than 3 ppm should always engender suspicion of arsenic poisoning; those with 2–3 ppm require further examination; and those with less than 2 ppm should not be dismissed where arsenic poisoning is suspected. The highest value (74 ppm As) recorded was established as due to abnormal exposure to arsenic.

The symptoms of acute arsenic poisoning by the oral route—nausea, vomiting, diarrhea, burning of the mouth and throat, and severe abdominal pains—have frequently been described. Chronic exposure to smaller toxic doses results in weakness, prostration, and muscular aching, with few gastrointestinal symptoms. Skin and mucosal changes usually develop, together with a peripheral neuropathy and linear pigmentations in the fingernails.[24] Symptoms of headache, drowsiness, confusion, and convulsions are seen in both acute and chronic arsenic intoxication. The biochemical basis for these symptoms is presumed to be an inhibition by arsenite of a wide variety of enzyme systems. Enzymes containing active thiol groups are effectively inhibited through combination of arsenic with these groups.[30] Conclusive evidence that arsenic is carcinogenic in man is lacking,[31] and experiments with rats and mice indicate that arsenites are remarkably free from carcinogenicity.[32] High levels of arsenic can induce goiter in rats,[25] and reports of an arsenic–thyroid antagonism in man have appeared.[33] A high incidence of goiter, with deaf-mutism, occurs in the Styrian Alps, the home of the arsenic eaters, and in the Cordoba Province of Argentina, where chronic arsenic poisoning is endemic. Arsenic concentrations in the drinking water of this

TABLE 2   Arsenic Content of Human Hair[a]

Description	As (ppm)
Mean	0.81
Median	0.51
Range	0.03–74
95% samples	<2
99% samples	<4.5

[a]From Smith.[28]

latter region as high as 1.4 mg/liter have been reported.[33] This concentration is 10–100 times higher than that of most natural waters as consumed by man.

IRON

Iron absorption in normal healthy humans is regulated so efficiently in accordance with body iron needs that intakes from natural foods of sufficient magnitude to produce toxic effects are inconceivable. The disease hemochromatosis is characterized by excessive deposits of iron in almost all the body tissues, especially in the liver and pancreas. Enlargement of the liver, liver insufficiency, pigmentation of the skin, diabetes mellitus, and often cardiac failure also occur. This rare idiopathic disease does not result from excessive intakes of iron from the food. It arises primarily from an inherited inborn error of metabolism and must be distinguished from iron overload of dietary origin. In some patients hemochromatosis occurs following prolonged intakes of medicinal iron or repeated blood transfusions (transfusional siderosis). Hemochromatosis can also occur in some alcoholics associated with high dietary intakes of iron, probably due to the relatively high iron content of many alcoholic beverages. Hemochromatosis has been observed in malnourished Bantus in South Africa (Bantu siderosis) as a consequence of long-term iron overload.[34] The native diet may supply more than 200 mg iron daily due to gross contamination from iron cooking vessels and to a high consumption of Kaffir beer, which has been reported to contain from 15 to 120 mg Fe/liter.[34] Iron intakes of this magnitude are 10–20 times greater than those obtained from ordinary mixed diets free from major sources of contamination.

Rich sources of iron are the organ meats (liver, kidney, and heart), egg yolk, dried legumes, cocoa, cane molasses, shellfish, and various wines. Liver may contain several thousand parts per million. Poor sources include milk and milk products, white sugar, white flour and bread (unenriched), potatoes, and most fresh fruit.[35] Boiling can reduce the levels of iron in vegetables by as much as 20%.[36] The iron content of flour is also much lower than that of the original whole grain, due to removal of the iron-rich germ and branny layers in the milling process. In a study of North American wheats and flours, the mean iron content of the whole grain was found to be 43 ppm and that of the flour (72% extraction) 10.5 ppm Fe.[37]

Overall dietary iron intakes vary appreciably with the amounts and proportions of iron-rich and iron-low foods and beverages consumed.

With normal men and postmenopausal women there is little reason for concern that these intakes may be too low or too high for health and well-being. With women during their fertile period the position is more precarious. Intakes can be deficient or marginal, especially as food iron consumption may be declining due to a progressive fall in total calorie intake and to reduced opportunities for iron contamination as a result of improved cleanliness in food handling and declining use of iron cooking vessels. Some form of iron supplementation may therefore be necessary for such women, or food fortification with iron, as in the "enriched" flour adopted in some countries, may be desirable. The chances of deleterious excess of iron arising from such practices are negligible at present levels of fortification, i.e., 16.5 mg/lb flour. (The safety of substantially higher levels of iron fortification cannot be assumed.)

COPPER

In all animals the continued ingestion of copper in excess of requirements leads to some accumulation in the tissues, especially in the liver. The extent of such accumulation and the tolerance to high copper intakes varies greatly among species. Rats are extremely tolerant. In one experiment with this species, dietary copper levels of 200 ppm were reached before liver copper retention became marked,[38] and in another experiment normal growth and health were maintained on diets containing 500 ppm Cu, or about 200 times normal, despite a 14-fold increase in liver copper.[39] Similarly, pigs reveal no signs of toxicity on diets supplemented with copper sulfate at the rate of 250 ppm Cu and may, in fact, show a growth stimulation, provided that these diets supply adequate amounts of zinc and iron, two of the elements with which copper interacts at the absorptive level.[40,41] Complete protection against copper toxicosis can be achieved at even higher copper intakes of 450, 600, and 750 ppm Cu if the zinc and iron intakes are sufficiently high. If they are not, a severe copper toxicosis develops, characterized by a marked depression in feed intake and growth rate, anemia, and jaundice; greatly elevated levels of liver and serum copper and of serum aspartate aminotransferase (A A T) activity are also observed.[40,41]

In contrast to pigs, sheep are very susceptible to chronic copper poisoning and can, in some circumstances, develop very high liver copper concentrations of 1,000 ppm Cu, or more, on the dry, fat-free basis, at dietary copper levels of only 10–15 ppm.[42] These circumstances may be the consumption of plants containing hepatotoxic alkaloids that cause liver damage or of plants exceptionally low in molybdenum

(0.1–0.2 ppm Mo or less), so that the overall Cu:Mo dietary ratio is very high. Molybdenum, in the presence of sufficient inorganic sulfate, is a copper antagonist that inhibits copper retention.[43] Providing supplementary molybdate to maintain a more "normal" Cu:Mo dietary ratio is highly effective in reducing both the liver copper levels and the mortality from the disease. The mortality from this manifestation of chronic copper poisoning in sheep, arising from a hemolytic crisis due to a more or less sudden release of copper into the blood from the high liver-copper stores, is associated with hemoglobinemia, hemoglobinuria, and usually with icterus.[42] In areas where the molybdenum content of the herbage is naturally higher, or where alkaloid-containing plants are absent, copper intakes of 10–15 ppm are harmless, and the disease "yellows" or hemolytic jaundice is unknown. The toxicity of a particular dietary level of copper is thus influenced by the ratio of this amount of copper to the amounts of molybdenum and inorganic sulfate present in the diet.

Little is known about the minimum levels of dietary copper capable of inducing chronic copper poisoning in man or of the influence of the other dietary components considered in the preceding paragraphs. If it is assumed that the human organism handles copper as do the other two monogastric species, rats and pigs, for which considerable data are available, a very wide margin of safety exists between normal intakes from the food and water supply and those likely to induce signs of chronic copper poisoning. A total dietary concentration of 200 ppm Cu on the dry basis could probably be tolerated by man for prolonged periods. This is more than 20 times the concentration normally present in human dietaries.

The copper content of leafy plants consumed as food rarely exceeds 25 ppm and usually lies between 10 and 15 ppm of the dry matter. The application of copper-containing fertilizers or sprays does not result in a very marked increase in the copper content of plant tissues, as can occur with other elements such as iodine or cobalt following comparable treatment with those elements. Whole cereal grains normally contain 4–6 ppm Cu and white flour and bread 1–2 ppm.[37] Nuts, dried legumes, dried vine and stone fruits, and cocoa may contain 20–40 ppm Cu. Crustacea and shellfish, especially oysters, and the organ meats (liver and kidney) can carry copper concentrations as high as 200–400 ppm on the dry basis,[6] but these latter food items normally comprise a very small proportion of the total diet.

Public health measures in most countries now effectively control the use of copper compounds once favored for the coloring and preserving of foods, and copper compounds are not now so prominent among available fungicides, insecticides, and anthelmintics as they were several decades ago. However, copper finds widespread use in brass and copper water pipes and domestic utensils, which could provide a significant source of contamination. It has been claimed that some soft domestic waters, with their capacity to corrode metallic copper, could raise human copper intakes by as much as 1.4 mg/day, whereas hard waters would reduce this source of copper to 0.5 mg/day, or less.[44] The former figure represents a very substantial addition to the 2–5 mg Cu/day ingested normally by human adults,[45] but it is unlikely to be harmful if the human species is as tolerant of copper as are the rat and the pig.

The only significant example of copper toxicity in man, apart from cases of extreme industrial exposure, is the rare idiopathic disorder known as hepatolenticular degeneration or Wilson's disease. This disorder of copper metabolism is inherited as an autosomal recessive trait and is associated with excessive accumulations of copper in the liver and later in the brain, which lead to hepatic cirrhosis and to necrosis and sclerosis of the corpus striatum.[46] Wilson's disease was previously progressive and fatal within a few years after the appearance of clinical signs. It can now be arrested by the administration of chelating agents that mobilize copper from the tissues and promote its excretion in the urine. The most valuable of these agents is penicillamine. The precise nature of the primary biochemical defect or defects in Wilson's disease is not known, although there appears to be an increased rate of absorption of copper from the gastrointestinal tract. Biliary obstruction to copper excretion is also probably important, because the markedly elevated hepatic copper pool is not accompanied by increased bile copper concentrations.[47] The disease is not related in any way to unusually high copper intakes from the food.

MOLYBDENUM

Molybdenum merits some attention in a review on toxicants in foods because of the severe molybdenosis occurring naturally in cattle grazing certain pastures in several countries.[6] These pastures usually contain 20–100 ppm Mo on the dry basis and induce scouring (diarrhea) varying from a mild form to a severe debilitating condition resulting in death. Sheep are much less affected and horses not at all. The disease can be controlled by massive oral treatment with copper sulfate or by intravenous injections of smaller quantities of this compound. Scouring can occur in cattle at much lower (5 ppm Mo) dietary concentrations of molybdenum than those just cited where the pastures are abnormally low in copper. In these circumstances the molybdenosis can be controlled simply by restoring the copper content of the affected pastures to normal levels.

All other species have a much greater tolerance to high molybdenum intakes than cattle. Levels of 1,000 ppm Mo in the diet induced no ill effects when fed to pigs over a period of 3 months.[48] Young rats grew normally at intakes of sodium molybdate equivalent to 500–1,000 ppm Mo when the diet was supplemented with copper sulfate to provide the very high total level of 277 ppm Cu. Growth was depressed at those levels of molybdenum on the unsupplemented diet containing 77 ppm Cu.[49] The significance of the Cu:Mo dietary ratio to molybdenum toxicity is illustrated by the results of another experiment with rats in which as little as 80 ppm Mo inhibited growth and induced some mortality on a Cu-deficient diet but had no such effects when the copper content of this diet was raised to 35 ppm.[50] Diarrhea is not a conspicuous feature of molybdenosis in rats or other laboratory species as it is in cattle. Marked loss of body weight, anorexia, and anemia, due to the Mo-induced copper deficiency, are the main toxic manifestations in these species.

Extrapolation from the results obtained with other monogastric species suggests strongly that molybdenum toxicity in man is impossible from the molybdenum occurring naturally in ordinary foods and dietaries. In one study the leguminous seeds varied from 0.2 to 4.7 ppm Mo and the cereal grains from 0.12 to 1.14 ppm.[51] In a later investigation of North American wheats and flours, the whole grain samples ranged from 0.30 to 0.66 ppm Mo, with a mean of 0.48 ppm. The white flours made from these wheats averaged 0.25 ppm Mo.[37] Milk is usually low in molybdenum but is extremely susceptible to differences in dietary intakes of the element. On ordinary rations cows produce milk containing 20–30 μg Mo/liter (approximately 0.15–0.23 ppm of the dry matter).[52] These levels can be raised severalfold by supplementing the cow's diet with molybdate.[52,53] The concentrations of molybdenum in liver and kidney are similarly responsive to high Mo intakes by the animal, especially if the inorganic sulfate and protein status of the diet is low. These organ meats usually contain 2–4 ppm Mo on the dry basis, which is about 10 times the levels common in muscle meats and other animal organs.[6] On the basis of very limited data, total dietary intakes of molybdenum by adults approximate 0.1 mg Mo/day, or about 0.13 ppm of the dry diet.[17] The above findings indicate a wide margin of safety for this element.

COBALT

Cobalt has a low order of toxicity in all species studied. Daily doses of 3 mg/kg body weight, which approximate 150 ppm Co in the diet (or some 1,000 times normal levels), can be tolerated by sheep for many weeks without harmful effects.[54] With doses of 4 mg/kg body weight, or higher, appetite and body weight are severely depressed; the animals become anemic and some die. Rats and other species, other than the adult ruminant, fed very large amounts of cobalt salts develop a true polycythemia, accompanied by hyperplasia of the bone marrow, reticulocytosis, and increased blood volume.[55] The condition can be enhanced or suppressed by various means that do not act in the same way in all species.[46]

The oral intakes of cobalt necessary to produce significant polycythemia are many times greater than those that could conceivably be obtained from normal foods and beverages. They approximate 200–250 ppm Co of the total diet. The green, leafy vegetables are the richest and the most variable sources of cobalt in human dietaries, and dairy products and refined cereals are among the lowest. Typical values are: spinach, 0.4–0.6; cabbage and lettuce, 0.2; corn (maize) seed, 0.01; and white flour 0.003 ppm Co on the dry basis. Even the higher values are less than 1% of the levels required to produce polycythemia or any other signs of toxicity. The significance of cobalt in human health and nutrition is apparently confined to its presence as a component of vitamin B_{12}.

Cobalt has been incriminated as the precipitating factor in several epidemics of severe cardiac failure in heavy beer drinkers. Cobalt was suspected because of the high incidence of polycythemia, thyroid epithelial hyperplasia, and colloid depletion noted in the fatalities, in addition to the congestive heart failure.[56] Cobalt salts had been added to the beer to improve its foaming qualities at concentrations of 1.2–1.5 ppm Co. At such concentrations the consumption of 24 pints daily would supply only about 8 mg of cobalt sulfate. This is well below the amount that can be taken with impunity by normal individuals. In fact, up to 300 mg daily of cobalt salts have been used therapeutically without cardiotoxic effects. It seems that high cobalt and high alcohol intakes are both necessary to induce the distinctive cardiomyopathy, plus a third factor, which has been suggested as low dietary protein[57] or thiamine deficiency.[58] A satisfactory biochemical explanation of the syndrome has not yet appeared.

NICKEL

Nickel has a low toxicity when orally ingested, due in part to poor absorption. Acid foods take up the element from nickel vessels, but it is poorly absorbed and causes no detectable damage.[59,60] On the other hand, exposed workers in nickel refineries exhibit a high incidence of respiratory tract neoplasia and dermatitis,[61,62] and nickel has been implicated as a pulmonary carcinogen in tobacco smoke.[63]

Levels of dietary nickel of 250, 500, and even 1,000 ppm have no effect on growth rate or reproduction and induce no signs of toxicity in rats and monkeys after 3–6 months of continuous feeding.[59,60] Intakes of 1,100 and 1,600 ppm Ni, as the acetate, appear to have no adverse effects on adult mice. The former level results in reduced growth and food consumption in young female mice but not in similar young males.[64] The mode of action of nickel in affecting growth and food consumption at these high levels is unknown, although it seems likely, from comparable experiments on nickel toxicity in chicks, that nitrogen retention, as well as feed intake, is depressed.[65]

The levels of nickel necessary to induce signs of toxicity in experimental animals are far greater than those that could be obtained from normal human dietaries. Human adults consuming a good mixed diet ingest approximately 0.3–0.6 mg Ni/day.[66,67,68] At a total daily drymatter intake of 800 g, this represents an overall dietary concentration of 0.4–0.8 ppm Ni. Fruits, tubers, and grains have been reported to contain 0.15–0.35 ppm Ni, compared with 10 times these concentrations in green leafy vegetables and with consistently lower levels in meats, eggs, and dairy products.[68] There is some evidence that tea (7.6 ppm) and oysters (6.0 ppm on the dry basis) are exceptionally rich in nickel,[68] but more extensive and systematic analyses are necessary to establish the relative values of different foods as sources of this element. There is no evidence to suggest that such analyses would reveal nickel concentrations in any common foods that could possibly incriminate food nickel as a potential toxicant.

ZINC

A wide margin of safety exists between normal intakes of zinc from foods and those likely to produce deleterious effects in man, if the results of experiments with other monogastric animals can safely be extrapolated to the human species. Dietary zinc intakes of 0.25%, or 2,500 ppm Zn, have no discernible effects on rats whether ingested as

the metal, chloride, or carbonate.[69] Intakes of 5,000 or 10,000 ppm
Zn, as the carbonate, produce severe anemia in young rats in addition
to subnormal growth, anorexia, and, at the higher rate, heavy mortality.[70] Pigs similarly suffer no ill effects from diets containing 1,000
ppm Zn, either as the sulfate or the carbonate. At higher levels,
amounting to 4,000 and 8,000 ppm, growth and appetite are depressed; arthritis, internal hemorrhages, and anemia develop; and
mortality is high.[71] The anemia is of the hypochromic, microcytic
type and is accompanied by subnormal levels of copper, iron, catalase, and cytochrome oxidase in the liver and other tissues.[6] These
changes can largely be prevented by supplements of copper and iron.
It appears therefore that the anemia of zinc toxicity in the rat and the
pig results from induced copper and iron deficiencies brought about
through an interference, by the high zinc intakes, with the absorption
and utilization of these metals. The growth depression that character-
izes zinc toxicity is due largely, but not entirely, to reduced food consumption, perhaps as a result of the unpalatability of the high-Zn
diets.[72]

Normal adult diets supply 12–15 mg Zn/day,[73] which gives an overall zinc concentration of 15–20 ppm of the dry matter. Wheat germ and
bran (40–120 ppm) and oysters, which may contain 1,000 ppm Zn, are
among the richest sources of this element; white sugar, pome, and citrus
fruits are among the lowest (less than 1 ppm of fresh edible portion).
Whole cereal grains typically contain 25–40 ppm Zn and white flour
6–8 ppm.[37,73] Opportunities for contamination of foods with zinc are
decreasing due to a declining use of galvanized iron pipes and containers
and to greater cleanliness and more hygienic food handling and processing practices. The problem of zinc in human health and nutrition is
much more likely to be related to inadequate or marginal intakes than
to the very remote possibility of toxic intakes from ordinary foods or
beverages. However, cases of zinc poisoning in humans due to the prolonged consumption of water from galvanized pipes and vessels have
been reported.[74,75] Where the water contained the abnormally high zinc
content of 40 ppm Zn, the symptoms observed in two adults included
irritability, stiffness and pain in the muscles of the back and neck, loss
of appetite, and some nausea.[75]

MANGANESE

Manganese resembles iron and zinc in having a low order of toxicity in
mammals and birds. The growth of rats is unaffected by dietary man-

ganese intakes as high as 1,000–2,000 ppm although larger amounts interfere with phosphorus retention.[76,77] Hens tolerate 1,000 ppm Mn without ill effects,[76,77] but pigs are less tolerant, since 500 ppm retards growth and depresses appetite.[78] The adverse effects of excess manganese on growth are mainly a reflection of depressed appetite. High manganese intakes are known to depress hemoglobin formation and the concentrations of iron in the blood serum, liver, kidney, and spleen of several species. The depressing effects that occur in mature rabbits and baby pigs fed diets containing 1,250 and 2,000 ppm Mn are prevented when these diets are supplemented with iron at a level of 400 ppm Fe.[79] The minimum level of dietary manganese capable of interfering with iron absorption and of depressing hemoglobin formation in those species may be as low as 50–125 ppm.[79] Whether these findings can be applied to man is unknown, but they suggest that the dietary ratio of manganese to iron could have some significance in considering possible toxic effects from manganese in foods.

Manganese toxicity in man arising from excessive intakes of this element in foods has never been reported and is virtually impossible, except where industrial contamination has occurred, as discussed later. The average concentrations of manganese in common foods range from 20–30 ppm in nuts, cereals, and leafy vegetables (fresh basis) to as low as 0.2–0.5 ppm in meats, fish, and dairy products.[80,81] The only dietary items exceptionally rich in manganese are tea and cloves.[81] One cup of tea has been reported to contain 0.30[82] to 1.3 mg Mn,[81] compared with very much lower amounts in a cup of coffee. Total dietary manganese intakes by adult man vary from about 2 to about 8 mg Mn/day,[66,67,81,82] depending upon the amounts and proportions of unrefined cereals, green leafy vegetables, nuts, and tea consumed. These estimates represent an overall manganese concentration in the dietary dry matter of some 3–12 ppm. Such concentrations are very much lower than those shown to induce signs of toxicity in other animal species. Furthermore, the human body has an extremely efficient homeostatic control mechanism regulating the levels of manganese in the tissues through controlled excretion via the bile, the pancreatic juice, and the intestinal wall.[83,84]

Chronic manganese poisoning occurs among miners following prolonged working with manganese ores. In this case excess manganese enters the body, mainly as oxide dust via the lungs and also via the gastrointestinal tract from the contaminated environment.[85] The lungs apparently serve as a depot from which the manganese is continuously absorbed. The disease is characterized by a severe psychiatric disorder (locura manganica) resembling schizophrenia, followed by a permanently crippling neurological disorder clinically similar to paralysis agitans or Parkinson's disease.

SELENIUM

Both selenium deficiency and selenium toxicity occur naturally in animals in widely separated parts of the earth.[6] The natural selenium content of animal feeds thus varies extremely widely, from concentrations too low to concentrations too high to sustain satisfactory growth, health, and fertility in animals. There is little evidence that the human populations living in the affected areas are similarly affected by selenium deficiency or toxicity. The difference between man and his domestic animals in susceptibility to chronic selenium poisoning is unlikely to be associated with a higher tolerance in the human species, since species differences in tolerance to selenium appear to be small. The absence of the more obvious signs of chronic selenosis in man in seleniferous areas more probably arises from two facts: The first of these is the wide geographical source of many of the foods composing modern human dietaries; in this way the food comes from a variety of soil types, resulting in a wide range of selenium concentrations. In the second place, most of these foods, unlike animal feeds, are subject to modification by processing and cooking. For instance, white flour and other refined products made from seleniferous wheat are lower in selenium than is the original whole grain, due to some concentration and loss in the branny layers during milling.[86] Values ranging from 0.25 to 1.0 ppm Se have actually been recorded for white bread from seleniferous districts.[87,88] Most garden vegetables, especially cabbage, are capable of taking up significant amounts of selenium from seleniferous soils, but the inedible portions, such as the peel of potatoes, contain the highest concentrations.[89] In addition, much of the selenium in such vegetables is discarded with the water during cooking.[90] Little is known of the extent to which the selenium in meat is lost during cooking, but some loss seems certain.

The minimum dietary level at which selenium will accumulate in the tissues of animals and ultimately produce signs of toxicity is generally accepted as 3–4 ppm of the dry diet. This can tentatively be taken as the minimum toxic or the maximum safe level for man, although the nature of the rest of the diet, particularly its protein and sulfate contents, can greatly influence toxicity. Thus 10 ppm Se in a 10% protein diet is highly toxic to rats, whereas 10 ppm Se in a 20% protein diet has no adverse effects.[91] Increasing levels of sulfate up to 0.87% of a sulfate-free diet similarly progressively decrease the growth inhibition induced in young rats by 10 ppm Se, as selenite or selenate.[92] However, inorganic sulfate is much less effective in protecting against organic forms of selenium, such as occur largely in foods, than against inorganic forms. The toxicity of selenium is also affected by the level of arsenic consumed. In rats, 5 ppm As in the drinking water completely prevents signs of selenosis,[93] and arsenic in some forms can alleviate selenium poisoning in pigs, dogs, chicks, and cattle. It is probable that the arsenic acts by increasing selenium excretion via the bile and decreasing retention in the tissues.[94,95]

Chronic selenium poisoning is characterized in all animals by a marked reduction in food intake and growth and by anemia. In the rat and the dog, a microcytic hypochromic anemia of progressive severity develops and the liver becomes necrotic, cyrrhotic, and hemorrhagic in varying degrees. Hair is lost from the mane and tail of horses; the body of pigs and the hoofs become sore and distorted, often with sloughing. Stiffness and lameness, due to erosion of the joints of the long bones and atrophy of the heart ("dish-rag" heart), also commonly occur. These manifestations of chronic selenium toxicity normally appear after a few weeks on diets containing 5–10 ppm Se. At selenium intakes of 15–20 ppm signs of toxicity may appear within a few days, and death usually results.

The mechanism of selenium toxicity is not well understood. At toxic intakes selenium concentrations in the blood and tissues rise steadily until levels as high as 5–7 ppm in liver, kidneys and 1–2 ppm in the muscles are reached. Beyond these tissue levels, which are many times normal, excretion begins to keep pace with absorption, so that selenium is not continuously cumulative in the body. It has long been assumed that selenium replaces sulfur in sulfur-containing compounds and that it occurs predominantly in the tissues as selenocystine and selenomethionine in both protein-bound and -free forms. This concept has now been challenged and the suggestion made that the selenium-containing compounds associated with fractions containing cystine or methionine merely consist of selenite bound to the sulfur compounds.[96] It seems likely that this selenite inhibits a number of enzyme systems. *In vitro* studies of tissues to which selenite and selenate have been added indicate a general inhibition of dehydrogenating enzymes and of urease and point to the removal of sulfhydryl groups essential to oxidative processes as possible biochemical sites of the toxic effects of selenium.[97] The liver succinic dehydrogenase levels of rats fed seleniferous diets are reduced below normal and can be maintained at normal levels by appropriate intakes of arsenic.[98] How far such changes are basically responsible for the toxic manifestations of selenium is unknown.

It is difficult to visualize any normal human dietaries, composed of foods grown or raised on normal soils, containing 3–4 ppm Se, the level suggested as the maximum safe level. Little appears to be known of normal or typical overall human dietary selenium concentrations. From a consideration of relatively limited data for a range of individual foods, this would be expected to be highly variable but usually less than one tenth of the "safe" level indicated above. Commercial whole wheat grain from different countries has been reported to average from as low as 0.007 to as high as 1.3 ppm Se.[99] The white flour and bread made from such wheats would be appreciably lower, as mentioned earlier. Milk and eggs from "normal" areas averaged 0.05–0.07 ppm and 0.4–0.5 ppm Se on the dry basis, respectively, compared with approximately one tenth of these concentrations in these foods obtained from known selenium-low areas.[100] Muscle and organ meats similarly vary widely in selenium concentrations. The kidney is the highest in selenium of the body tissues. Kidney cortex can contain 4–8 ppm Se on the dry basis, even in normal healthy animals. Muscle meats from such animals typically contain 0.5 ppm or less, with somewhat higher concentrations common in heart and liver. The possibility of undesirable or dangerously high levels of selenium appearing in the edible tissues of animals treated with selenium salts to prevent selenium deficiency in selenium-low areas appears remote, so long as the animals are treated at recommended rates.[101,102,103] Selenium supplementation of feeds for this purpose is at present illegal in the United States because of fears of high tissue levels. No such ban exists in New Zealand or Australia.

Epidemiological studies with children and some studies with experimental animals have provided indications that above-normal intakes of selenium during the developmental period of the teeth increase the incidence of caries.[100] The results reported would be more convincing if the actual selenium intakes of the children in the different groups had been measured. More evidence is needed before the caries-enhancing effect of selenium is fully established and its mode of action understood.

Selenium acquired a reputation as a carcinogen from early studies with rats. These reports were severely criticized by Frost,[104] and they received little support from later investigations.[105] Furthermore, limited epidemiological evidence suggests that selenium may be a possible protective agent against human cancer.[106] The whole question of selenium and cancer, as well as of selenium and dental caries, clearly requires further critical investigation before selenium can unequivocally be linked with these public health problems.

LEAD

Biological interest in lead has largely been confined to its toxic properties as an industrial hazard to man and animals. In recent years chronic human exposures to lead have changed in origin and have probably increased in magnitude. Exposure from lead in water pipes, food containers, paints, and insecticides has decreased. This has been compensated, or more than compensated, however, by increased exposure to lead from cigarette smoking and cosmetics and especially from motor vehicle exhausts in highly motorized urban communities. The latter source of lead arises from direct inhalation and indirectly through deposition on soils and plants along highways and in urban areas.[107-109]

Most human foods contain less than 1 ppm Pb when uncontaminated. Cow's milk normally contains 0.02-0.08 ppm Pb[110,111] and muscle meats approximately 0.1 ppm. The only animal tissues with substantially higher lead concentrations are the bones. Lead has a marked affinity for bone, and levels between 5 and 20 ppm on the fresh basis have been reported.[18] Very little is known of the natural levels of lead in foods of plant origin, but these must be quite low because average intakes from the food by adult man have been variously estimated to range from 0.22 to 0.4 mg Pb/day. This approximates 0.3 to 0.5 ppm of the dry diet.[112,113,114] In addition, smaller amounts of lead are ingested with the drinking water and are inhaled from the atmosphere and from cigarette smoke. Patterson[113] gives these additional daily lead intakes as 0.01 mg from the water supply, 0.026 mg from urban air, 0.01 mg from rural air, and 0.024 mg from cigarette smoke for individuals smoking 30 cigarettes per day.

It is doubtful that lead intakes of the magnitude mentioned in the preceding paragraph could lead to harmful accumulations in the tissues. Food lead is poorly absorbed in man (to the extent of about 5%) and is excreted mainly in the feces.[18,113] The lead that is absorbed enters the blood and reaches the bones and soft tissues, including the liver, from which it is gradually excreted via the bile into the small intestine and then eliminated in the feces. Up to certain intakes, lead excretion virtually keeps pace with ingestion so that retention is negligible. Critical levels of intake, above which significant lead retention occurs in man, cannot be given with any accuracy. Cantarrow and Trumper,[110] in their classical monograph on lead poisoning, give the lower limits of safety in man as 0.2–2.0 mg Pb/day. Under U.S. environmental conditions lead concentrations in the tissues (notably the aorta, bones, kidney, liver, and lungs) increase with age.[114] These findings indicate that excretion is not quite keeping pace with intakes from all sources, resulting in a small retention over time. There is no evidence that tissue lead accumulations of this small magnitude are either harmful or harmless to man. Similar tissue lead concentrations, brought about by the consumption of water containing 5 ppm Pb as lead acetate, were nontoxic to rats as judged by the length of the life span, although some loss of hair and body weight was evident.[115] On the other hand, toxic intakes of lead can come from the consumption of illicitly distilled (moonshine) whiskey and of fruit juices stored in lead-glazed earthenware pottery. In one such case the juice was reported to contain no less than 157 ppm Pb, compared with the maximum allowed by the U.S. Food and Drug Administration of 7 ppm.

Acute lead intoxication is manifested by abdominal colic, encephalopathy, myelopathy, peripheral neuropathy, and anemia and is accompanied by increased urinary excretion of porphyrins and of delta-aminolevulinic acid (ALA). The anemia is hypochromic, and microcytic; it is rarely severe (resembling the anemia of thalassemia) and is characterized by the presence of large numbers of erythrocytes with basophilic stippling.[24] The anemia is probably enhanced by a lead inhibition of heme synthesis. A significant correlation has been demonstrated between the levels of urinary ALA and urinary lead in children (see Figure 1). Determination of urinary ALA has been suggested as a screening procedure for the detection of early lead exposure in asymptomatic children.[116] More recently it has been demonstrated that erythrocyte δ-aminolevulinic acid dehydrase (ALA-D) is more accurate and more sensitive than ALA in urine as an indicator of the amount of circulating lead, particularly at blood lead levels below 40 μg/100 ml.[117] A close negative correlation between the concentration of lead in blood, and the logarithm of erythrocyte ALA-D was found for 159 persons, with blood lead levels ranging from 5 to 95 μg/100 ml.

Little is known of the biochemical effects, if any, of the smaller tissue lead concentrations characteristic of "normal" motorized, urban man. Certain ATPases are sensitive to small concentration of lead, and lead strongly inhibits lipoamide dehydrogenase, an enzyme crucial to cellular oxidation.[118] Lead has also been shown to bind to the specific subcellular constituents, metallothionein and liver RNA,[118] and to accumulate as a lead–protein complex within intranuclear inclusion bodies.

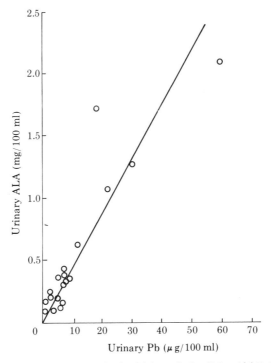

FIGURE 1 Relation between urinary levels of delta-aminolevulinic acid (ALA) and of lead in children. (From Davis and Andelman.[116])

isolated from the kidneys of lead-poisoned rats.[119] The significance of these findings to the whole question of modern exposure to lead from the food and the physical environment remains to be evaluated.

TIN

Data on the tin content of foods obtained by modern acceptable methods of analysis are exceedingly meager. Mean daily intakes of tin by U.S. adults have been variously reported to range from 1.5 mg[17] and 3.5 mg[120] to 17 mg.[18] Analytical discrepancies may account for part of these differences, but variations in the amounts and proportions of different food and beverage items comprising the total diet are also important. Thus Schroeder *et al.*[120] calculate that a diet composed largely of fresh meats, cereals, and vegetables, which usually contain less than 1 ppm Sn, would supply only 1 mg Sn/day, whereas a diet that included substantial amounts of canned vegetables, fruit juices, and fish could supply as much as 38 mg/day. The introduction of lacquered cans and the crimping of the tops, thus allowing little contact of food with the solder, have reduced the amount of contamination of canned foods from tin plate. Storage of canned food, even in lacquered cans, can nevertheless result in some accumulation of tin, presumably due to corrosion starting from defects in the lacquer.[112] Relatively high concentrations of tin have been reported in oily fish in uncoated cans.[120]

Convincing evidence of human poisoning from tin in canned or other foods is difficult to find. A few instances have been reported where tin to the amount 2,000–3,000 ppm was found in the food,[121] but the possibility of bacterial poisoning cannot be completely excluded in these cases. Ingested tin is very poorly absorbed and is excreted mostly in the feces, with little or no accumulation with age in any human tissue other than the lungs.[120] Mean tissue concentrations of tin are significantly higher in North American individuals than in European, Asian, and African, suggesting that the former are exposed to more tin than the latter groups. There is no evidence, however, that such concentrations are harmful or promote any toxic reactions. Mice and rats given 5 ppm Sn, as stannous ions, in the drinking water from weaning to natural death grew normally, and the life span of mice of both sexes and of male rats was unaffected. However, female rats showed a reduced longevity; an increased incidence of fatty degeneration of the liver and of vacuolar changes in the renal tubules was apparent in both sexes.[32,115] These findings indicate that tin has a very low order of toxicity, but far more information is required on the maximum long-term intakes compatible with health and well-being and on the normal levels of tin in human foods and dietaries. The importance of the latter has been highlighted by the recent findings of Schwarz et al.,[122] indicating that tin must now be considered an essential element in mammalian nutrition.

CADMIUM

Few systematic analyses of the cadmium content of human foods and dietaries have been carried out. This is unfortunate because this metal has specific toxic effects on the male and female reproductive organs in rats and other experimental animals. It also has important interactions with several other elements, especially zinc, copper, and iron. Daily intakes of cadmium by human adults have been estimated as 0.2–0.5 mg, with considerable variation according to sources and types of food.[73] These estimates now appear to be much too high. For instance, a mean total cadmium content 0.013 mg was recently reported for school lunches served to sixth-grade children in 300 U.S. schools.[15] The total dietary cadmium intakes of institutionalized children (age 9–12 yr) in 28 U.S. cities were found to average 0.092 mg/day, with a range of 0.032–0.158 mg/day.[123]

Oysters are exceptionally rich in cadmium, as they are in zinc. Levels of 3–4 ppm have been recorded, compared with levels one tenth or one hundredth of these in most other foods.[73] Appreciable amounts of cadmium may also be obtained from the air and the water supply. Soft water remaining overnight in galvanized or black polythene pipes can take up 0.15 to 1.1 μg Cd/liter, although total intakes from these sources were calculated to supply no more than 1–2 μg/Cd/day.[124] The cadmium level in the air of 28 U.S. cities was shown to range from undetectable to as high as 0.06 μg Cd/m^3.[125]

Whether cadmium intakes from the food, air, and water supply of the magnitude outlined above present any long-term hazards to human health is at present a matter of conjecture. Factory workers exposed to cadmium oxide dust and fumes develop higher cadmium concentrations in the liver and kidney than normal individuals not so exposed. The workers excrete more cadmium in the urine, together with a low molecular weight protein and, subsequently, may develop emphysema. Acute high-level exposures may cause a severe, acute, or even fatal pneumonitis. Outbreaks of acute cadmium poisoning, accompanied by nausea, vomiting, diarrhea, and prostration, have been reported from the consumption of jellies and ices containing 15–530 ppm Cd derived from cadmium-plated trays and vessels and from the consumption of lemonade containing 100 ppm Cd that had been in contact for some hours with cadmium-plated vessels.[126] It was concluded that 15 ppm is necessary to produce mild symptoms of cadmium poisoning in man. The addition of 45 ppm Cd to the food of rats for a period of 6 months caused only slight toxic symptoms.[127] Such toxic intakes are many times greater than those that could conceivably be derived from normal foods and beverages.

A progressively increasing incidence of systolic hypertension develops in rats exposed to 5 ppm Cd in the drinking water from the time of weaning.[128] The rats must be constantly exposed to the cadmium for 1 yr or more and must have accumulated considerable quantities of cadmium in their kidneys if hypertension is to appear and to be sustained. The pathological changes associated with cadmium hypertension in rats, including renal arterial and arteriolar lesions and glomerular changes, are indistinguishable from those accompanying benign hypertension from other causes.[129] The mechanism of action of the cadmium is not understood, and the relationship, if any, between this condition and "essential" human hypertension remains obscure. Some hypertensive patients exhibit a higher than normal urinary excretion of a range of metals, especially cadmium, and carry significantly higher renal cadmium concentrations and a higher Cd : Zn ratio in their tissues than similar normotensive individuals.[130,131] Others do not, however.[132,133] Epidemiological evidence obtained by Carroll[125] appeared to further implicate cadmium as a factor associated with human hypertension. This worker found the average concentration of cadmium in the air of 28 U.S. cities to be markedly positively correlated with the death rates from hypertension and arteriosclerotic heart disease. A later epidemiological study in 77 midwestern U.S. cities shows no apparent correlation between the cadmium content of dustfall and cardiovascular death rates in urban areas.[134] In a study of postmortem material, Morgan[132] found no significant differences in kidney or liver cadmium levels between a control group and two groups of patients characterized by hypertensive cardiovascular disease or by ischemic cardiac or cerebrovascular disease. Hammer *et al.*[133] were also unable to demonstrate increased renal cadmium in patients dying with hypertension. Furthermore, hypertension is an uncommon sign of chronic or acute cadmium poisoning in man. It is clear therefore that cadmium cannot unequivocally be incriminated as a causal factor in human hypertension and cardiovascular diseases. The whole question of the relationship to human health of cadmium in the environment is well reviewed by Friberg[135] and by Fassett.[136]

Consideration of the remarkable highly selective effects of injected cadmium on the reproductive organs of animals, and their amelioration by zinc and by selenium (see Underwood[6]) lies outside the scope of this review on toxicants occurring naturally in foods. However, it is appropriate to mention that part of the toxic effects of ingested cadmium relates to the metabolic antagonism between this element and zinc. Signs of zinc deficiency can be accentuated by high intakes of cadmium, and the toxic effects of high cadmium intakes can be ameliorated by increasing the zinc status of the diet. These findings imply a competition between zinc and cadmium for protein-binding sites for transport across the intestinal wall, and probably for the zinc metallo-enzymes. They also illustrate the principle, stressed earlier in this chapter, that the toxicity of a particular dietary level of an element is influenced by the dietary levels of other elements with which it interacts. In this case it is clear that the Cd : Zn dietary ratio, as well as actual gross intakes, must be considered in studies of possible cadmium toxicities.

MERCURY

Mercury occurs widely in the biosphere and has long been known as a toxic element presenting occupational hazards associated with both ingestion and inhalation. It has no known essential function in living organisms. Mercury poisoning has been prominent at times among goldsmiths and mirror makers, and the expression "mad as a hatter" derives from the symptoms shown by workers in the treatment of furs and felts with mercuric nitrate. Typical manifestations of such subacute mercury poisoning may be salivation, stomatitis, and diarrhea—or they may be primarily neurological, with Parkinsonian tremors, vertigo, irritability, moodiness, and depression.[24] Oral ingestion of as little as 100 mg of mercuric chloride produces toxic symptoms, and 500 mg are almost always fatal unless immediate treatment is instituted.[24]

More than 30 years ago Stock[137] reported levels of 0.005–0.035 ppm Hg in fruits, vegetables, cereal grains, meats, and dairy products, with higher levels (0.020–0.18 ppm) in fish. The average intake of mercury from food was estimated to be only 0.5 μg/day. Subsequently, a higher estimate of 20 μg Hg/day was given.[138] These levels of intake have been substantially confirmed by recent studies using neutron activation techniques for total mercury[139,140,141] and gas chromatography for methylmercury.[142] Thus, Westöö[143] analyzed homogenates of 12 fish-free Swedish diets and found their total mercury content to range from 4 to 20 (mean 11) μg Hg/day. In a later more extensive study of Swedish diets,[144] the mercury content was found to range from 1.0 to 30.6 (mean 5.6) μg Hg/day. The importance of the fish content is evident from the fact that 90 of the diets that contained no fish averaged only 3.5 μg Hg/day, whereas the 55 diets containing fish of any kind averaged 9.0 μg Hg/day.

The increasing amounts of mercury being injected into the environment have evoked considerable public health concern in some countries and have stimulated studies of the amounts and chemical forms of mercury in foods and water supplies.[141,145] The mercury comes from the burning of coal, from the use of organic mercury compounds as pesticides and fungicides in agriculture and industry, and from certain chemical industries. The pulp and paper industries, where mercurial compounds are used as antisliming agents, and the alkali industry, where mercury cells are used to separate chlorine from brine solutions, can be major sources of pollution. Particular interest has centered upon the levels of methylated forms of mercury, such as methylmercury $(CH_3 \cdot Hg^+)$ and dimethylmercury $(CH_3 \cdot Hg \cdot CH_3)$. These compounds are more hazardous than inorganic forms of the element because they are retained in the tissues for longer periods and have a more specific effect upon the central nervous system.[146]

Methylated mercury compounds enter the food chain through the activity of microorganisms that have the ability to methylate the mercury present in industrial wastes.[147] The mercury in fish from polluted waters occurs almost entirely as methylmercury.[148] Methylated mercury compounds may also enter the food chain through their use in the protective treatment of grain. When birds were fed for 4 weeks on wheat treated with methylmercury dicyandiamide, 8 ppm of mercury was found in the eggs and liver and 4 ppm in the muscle tissue. These are remarkably high levels in comparison with the negligible concentrations found in control birds.[149]

The decrease in the methylmercury content of foods of animal origin in Sweden since methoxyethyl mercury was substituted for methylmercury as a seed disinfectant is illustrated in Figure 2.[150] Prior to this,

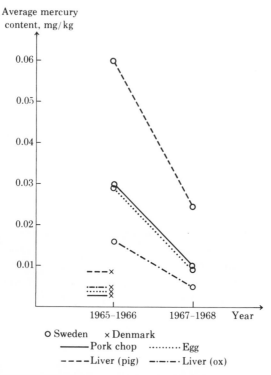

FIGURE 2 Decrease of methylmercury content of animal foods in Sweden, due to changes in seed disinfection. (From Westöö.[150])

considerable amounts of mercury were found in the tissues of seed-eating birds and their predators and even in small rodents; these cases were associated with lethal and sublethal mercury poisoning in Swedish wildlife.[151]

The maximum acceptable overall dietary concentration of mercury is at present arbitrarily set at 0.05 ppm.[152] This level could readily be exceeded where the diet contains contaminated staples such as bread, meat, and fish.[141] In an investigation of Canadian foods, concentrations ranging from 0.005 to 0.075 ppm Hg were found in a variety of substances not directly exposed to mercury at any time. Concentrations of 1 ppm Hg were found in specimens from Hg-contaminated areas. In Canada and the United States the maximum permissible level of mercury in fish has been placed at 0.5 ppm. Although there is considerable evidence that man-made mercury pollution of freshwater rivers and lakes can greatly increase the mercury levels in freshwater fish, recent evidence suggests that such pollution of the oceans has not significantly increased the mercury levels in wide-ranging ocean fish.[153] The mercury levels of museum specimens of seven tuna caught 62–93 yr ago (0.26–0.64 ppm wet weight) were found to be in the same range as those found in five specimens caught recently (0.13–0.48).

The maximum dietary intakes of total mercury or methylmercury compatible with long-term human health and well-being cannot yet be given with any confidence. Individual variability in tolerance is high, and a great deal has still to be learned about the possible modifying influence on Hg toxicity of other elements in the diet. For instance, recent evidence indicates that the toxicity of methylmercury to rats and to Japanese quail can be decreased by increasing the selenium content of the diet.[154] Completely satisfactory diagnostic criteria for incipient or preclinical mercury poisoning are also lacking. The critical urinary mercury concentration, above which mercury poisoning can be suspected, was placed by Monier-Williams[112] at 0.1–0.2 μg/ml, but a range of 0.001–0.133 μg Hg/ml was later observed in 46 normal human subjects.[155] The readiness with which the hair and nails acquire mercury from the environment has excited interest in the diagnostic possibilities of these structures. The head hair of normal individuals in Scotland with no known exposure to mercury was found to approximate 5–8 ppm Hg.[155,156] Much higher levels, averaging 32 ppm, were found in the head hair of dental assistants exposed to mercury amalgams, and up to 98 ppm Hg was found in a group of industrial workers with mercury contamination of their laboratory. Comparable mercury levels in hair from normal and from exposed individuals have been reported from Japan.[157] Lower hair-mercury levels, ranging from 0.2 to 6.0 ppm, were obtained

for Canadian controls, compared with 5–10 ppm in individuals with
occupational exposure to mercury.[141] Extremely high head-hair levels
ranging from 186 to 2,436 ppm Hg were observed in the members of a
family affected with mercury poisoning from the consumption of pork
contaminated from treated grain. It was estimated that "early symptoms
of mercury toxicity correspond to hair concentrations of about 150
ppm Hg, depending on the individual's tolerance."

Goldwater[158] contends that measurements of Hg levels in hair, urine,
blood, and saliva are of limited value in predicting incipient poisoning.
On the other hand, the expert group that made an evaluation of the
risks from methylmercury in fish[145] states that, "because of the accumulation of methylmercury in the blood cells, the level of methylmercury or Hg in this fraction is the best available index of the degree of
exposure." The group states further that the level in whole blood and in
hair may also be used. Clinically manifest poisoning of adults sensitive
to methylmercury, according to this group, "may occur at a level in
whole blood down to 0.2 μg Hg/g, which level seems to be reached on
exposure to about 0.3 mg Hg as methyl mercury/day, or about 4 μg
Hg/kg body-weight/day." If, as the group believes, a factor of 10 gives
a sufficient margin of safety, the acceptable level in whole blood would
be 0.02 μg Hg/g, corresponding to about 0.04 μg/g in the blood cells
and about 6 μg/g in the hair.

It must be emphasized that the above estimates are based on knowledge that is incomplete. They may therefore need to be revised as more
information is obtained on the levels and forms of mercury in foods, on
their relationship with other elements with which they may interact,
and on the maximum long-term mercury intakes from all sources that
can be considered tolerable by man and animals.

Whatever future investigations may disclose, there can be no doubt,
on the basis of existing evidence, that mercury discharge into the environment must be kept at the lowest possible level. The toxic effects on
man of such discharge was dramatically illustrated during the early
1950's when some 50 persons out of more than 100 affected in Japan
died of the strange "Minamata disease." The deaths were shown to be
caused by the consumption of mercury-contaminated fish and shellfish
from Minimata Bay, which had received large amounts of methylmercury in the waste effluents from a plastics factory.[159]

CHROMIUM

Since 1959, when Schwarz and Mertz[160] showed that trivalent chromium increases the glucose tolerance of rats subsisting on certain diets,

interest in chromium has centered more upon its physiological than its toxicological role in human nutrition. Acute toxicity studies, with rats given chromium (III) intravenously, established the lethal dose for 50% of the animals at about 1 mg/100 g body weight.[161] Oral administration of excessive levels of chromate (50 ppm Cr) is associated with growth depression and liver and kidney damage in experimental animals.[162] Chronic exposure to chromate dust has been correlated with increased incidence of lung cancer in man.[163] Hexavalent chromium is much more toxic than the trivalent form. Trivalent chromium produced no increase in the incidence of tumors, but appeared to protect female rats from lung infection, when fed to mice and rats from weaning to natural death at levels of 2 ppm or 5 ppm.[164,165] There was little evidence of chromium accumulation in the tissues at those levels of intake.

Although information is rather meager and there is reason to suspect some of the published data on the chromium content of foods because of analytical inadequacies, it is probable that a wide margin of safety exists between the amounts of the element ordinarily ingested from the food and water supply and inhaled from the atmosphere and those likely to induce deleterious effects. Some years ago chromium concentrations in vegetable tissues were reported to range from 0.01 to 1 ppm, with the levels in most foods of plant origin lying between 0.1 and 0.5 ppm.[166] These values are of the same order as those observed in more recent studies of a rather heterogeneous range of tissues and human foods.[167,168] However, DDT and certain therapeutic preparations were found to be surprisingly high in chromium.[167]

Reported dietary chromium intakes by man are highly variable. In two studies with diabetics and old people, in which some responses in glucose tolerance to chromium supplementation were obtained,[169,170] the daily intake was estimated to be as low as 50 μg Cr/day. In another study, an institutional diet was shown to provide about 80 μg Cr/day.[168] These intakes are very much lower than those reported for two adults by Tipton *et al.*,[17] namely, 330 and 400 μg Cr/day, in a comprehensive study of trace elements in diets and excreta. Some of these variations reflect differences in the intakes of refined carbohydrates, notably white flour and white sugar, which are very low in chromium; analytical errors, however, are also certainly involved.

Much more information and more reliable data are clearly necessary on the factors affecting the movement of chromium in the food chain from the soil, through plants and animals, to man. Such information is likely to be of far more interest to the possibilities of inadequate or marginal intakes of chromium by vulnerable sections of the population, particularly women suffering repeated pregnancies and old people, than to the remote possibilities of toxic or harmful intakes from the food and water supply. Orally administered trivalent chromium is poorly absorbed (to the extent of about 1% or less) and appears mostly in the feces, regardless of dose and dietary chromium.[161,171,172] Hexavalent chromium is better absorbed than trivalent,[162] which perhaps accounts for its higher toxicity. Unlike most other trace elements, the levels of chromium in human tissues, other than the lungs, decline with age.[168] This does not suggest harmful or potentially harmful intakes from ordinary diets. Questions of possible inadequate dietary intakes, the function of chromium as a cofactor with insulin, and the chemical forms of chromium in foods, particularly as the glucose-tolerance factor (GTF), lie outside the scope of this text. These aspects are discussed elsewhere by Mertz[173] and by Underwood.[6]

FLUORINE

Human populations obtain widely varying quantities of fluorine from the food, the water supply, and the atmosphere, depending upon location. Except in areas directly associated with industrial sources of pollution (such as aluminum and superphosphate works, steel mills, and enamel factories), fluorine concentrations in the air are very low and do not constitute a significant source of this element to man.[174] Fluoride intakes from surface waters as used for drinking and cooking in most communities are also low, since such waters generally contain 0.2 ppm F or less.[174] Where the population is dependent upon the waters of deep wells and artesian bores, fluoride intakes from this source may be much higher and may induce signs of endemic fluorosis in animals and man as described later. Fluoride concentrations of 4–8 ppm are common in such areas, while in certain parts of India[175] and South Africa [176] concentrations of 20 ppm or even 50 ppm F occur.

Food is the major source of fluorine in individuals not exposed to industrial contamination or to naturally or artificially fluorided water. Very few foods other than sea fish contain more than 1–2 ppm F (dry basis), and most of them contain less than 0.5 ppm.[177] Plants have a limited capacity to absorb fluorine from the soil, even when fluoride-containing fertilizers, such as superphosphate, are applied.[178] The tea plant and the camellia are exceptions in this respect, and concentrations of 100 ppm F or more are common in those species.[179,180] Sea fish and fish products are also much higher in fluorine than most other foods. Concentrations between 5 and 10 ppm F have been reported.[177]

Normal North American diets, which include little tea, contribute 0.3–0.5 mg F daily,[181] approximately 80% of which is absorbed.[174,182]

Where artificially fluorided water is consumed, the amount obtained from the food would be appreciably higher because of the use of such water in cooking. The consumption of 1,500 ml/day of water containing 1 ppm F provides 1.5 mg F, or substantially more than is normally ingested with the food. The consumption of tea containing 100 ppm F, two thirds or more of which passes into the infusion, can increase total dietary fluoride intakes in some communities by 1 mg or more daily even when the water is not fluoridated artificially.[180] In communities where tea is commonly consumed in large amounts by children as well as by adults, and where the water is artificially fluoridated, it is obvious that total dietary fluoride intakes would be substantially greater than the 0.3–0.5 mg estimated for normal North American diets.

Tolerance levels of dietary fluorine are difficult to define because they vary greatly with the age and species of the animal, the chemical form, duration, and continuity of the fluorine ingested, and the nature of the whole diet. The significance of these factors to chronic fluorine toxicity is now well established for most laboratory and domestic animals[6] but is less well known for man. In all species, protection against potentially toxic intakes of fluoride is achieved for prolonged periods of time by two physiological mechanisms acting concurrently. These are (a) a rise in urinary excretion of fluorine, which follows directly upon increased intakes but reaches a maximum that cannot be surpassed, and (b) deposition of retained fluorine in the skeleton—a process that initially proceeds rapidly and then more slowly as the fluorine levels in the bones rise, until a stage of saturation is reached. Beyond this point, "flooding" of the soft tissues with fluorine occurs, plasma fluoride levels rise, and metabolic breakdown occurs.

The level of fluoride below which all ingested fluoride is excreted in man (and therefore is not retained in the bones) must be very low indeed, if any such level exists. Fluorine normally accumulates with age in human bones, even where intakes from the food and water supply are very small. The capacity of the skeleton to sequester fluoride without serious pathological change is so great that such normal accumulations are not necessarily harmful but in some circumstances (e.g., in osteoporosis in middle-age and older women) may actually be beneficial. Hodge and Smith[183] distinguish three stages in this process: bone fluorosis or chemical fluorosis, bone mottling, and abnormal bone. Bone fluoridation alone is characteristic of bones containing less than 2,500 ppm F; bone mottling occurs in bones containing 2,500–5,000 ppm F; and abnormal bones, with gross abnormalities and an enlarged, heavy, chalk white appearance, are characteristic of bones with fluoride levels above 5,000–6,000 ppm. A daily intake of 2 ppm F in the diet for 50 yr results in chemical fluorosis only (i.e., with no bone mottling or other abnormalities), while a continuous intake of 8 ppm in the diet for 35 yr has been estimated to be necessary before the critical levels of 6,000 ppm F in the bones are attained.[184] Prolonged intakes of 10 ppm of dietary fluorine for many years can result in symptomatic skeletal fluorosis in man.[183] Shortt and co-workers[185] have reported upon an endemic fluorosis area in India where the drinking water contains such high fluoride concentrations. Mottling of the teeth of children occurs initially with no other ill effects; at about 30 yr of age, however, pain and stiffness of the spine and joints develop until the whole spine becomes one continuous column of bone, with excessive calcification of tendons and ligaments and the presence of exostoses. In advanced cases the victims exhibit a definite cachexia, loss of appetite, and emaciation, usually followed by death. These manifestations are very similar to the severe forms of industrial skeletal fluorosis in man.

Endemic dental fluorosis or mottled enamel from the consumption of naturally fluoridated waters has been reported from many countries.[6] Mottled teeth are characterized by chalk white patches with a secondary infiltration of yellow to brown staining. The enamel is structurally weak and sometimes there is a loss of enamel accompanied by "pitting," which gives the tooth surface a corroded appearance. In its mild forms mottled enamel is cosmetically undesirable but has little public health significance. Studies in the United States (see Hodge and Smith[183]) indicate that the incidence of mottled enamel in children consuming water containing 1 ppm F is negligible; at 2–3 ppm F the mottling is "very mild"; and at 5–6 ppm F "moderate" mottling can be expected. It should be stressed that these conclusions necessarily apply only to North America where the climate is temperate and where extremely little tea is consumed. The mottled enamel potential of drinking water of a given fluoride concentration clearly depends upon the amount of the water consumed daily and upon the amount of fluoride contributed by the rest of the diet. In tropical and subtropical areas where larger quantities are normally consumed daily, or in communities where the consumption of tea and marine fish is high (as in many parts of England), the "safe" levels of fluoride in the drinking water might well be lower than those quoted above.

IODINE

Iodine occurs ubiquitously in the biosphere in low and highly variable concentrations. The air contributes insignificant quantities of iodine to human intakes, except where it is polluted from the combustion of fossil fuels or organic matter.[186] The iodine content of most fresh, ground waters is similarly low, unless it is contaminated with human or animal wastes.[187] Foods provide by far the major source of iodine in human dietaries in both goitrous and nongoitrous areas. Foods of both plant and animal origin are so extremely susceptible to variations in environmental iodine that they are difficult to classify as sources of iodine. Such a classification has been attempted by Vought and London,[188] based on data obtained in the United States in 1964. These data are presented in Table 3 but probably need modification in the light of various developments affecting the levels of iodine in bread and dairy products to be described later. Sea fish and shellfish, as a food class, are particularly rich in iodine and their oils are even higher.[189] The edible flesh of sea fish can contain 300–3,000 ppb I on the fresh basis, compared with only 30–40 ppb for freshwater fish. Marine plants, especially seaweed, are uniquely high in iodine. The concentration varies with the species and the season of the year but values as high as 0.4–0.6%, or 4,000,000–6,000,000 ppb on the dry basis, are common.[190]

Direct determinations of total human dietary intakes of iodine, employing acceptable modern methods of analysis, are few. In 1964 the average daily intake in the Maryland suburbs of Washington, D.C., was directly measured at 395 μg I,[188] and in 1969 the estimated daily average for the continental United States ranged from 238 μg in the northeastern states to 738 μg in the Southwest.[191] A higher median intake (465 μg I/day), with a range of 270–870 μg, was subsequently estimated for the Maryland suburbs by Vought.[187] It appears that there is an upward trend in iodide consumption in the United States and that average intakes are two- to sevenfold greater than the 100 μg I/day generally be-

TABLE 3 Iodine Content of Composites of Food Categories[a]

Food Category	Number of Samples	Iodine (μg/wet kg)	
		Mean ± S.E.	Median
Sea foods	7	660 ± 180	540
Vegetables	13	320 ± 100	280
Meat products	12	260 ± 70	175
Eggs	11	260 ± 80	145
Dairy products	18	130 ± 10	139
Bread and cereal	18	100 ± 20	105
Fruits	18	40 ± 20	18

[a]From Vought and London.[188]

lieved to be adequate.[192] A recent consideration of iodine balance and excretion studies has led to the claim that a safe daily intake of iodine lies between a minimum of 50 μg and a maximum of 1,000 μg.[193] Wolff[194] has suggested that 2,000 μg I/day should be regarded as an excessive or potentially harmful level of intake.

Normal diets composed of natural foods are very unlikely to supply as much iodine as 2,000 μg/day, and 1,000 μg/day would be unusual, except when the diets are very high in marine fish. However, Vought[187] has drawn attention to the cumulative additions of this element from adventitious sources, notably bread, salt, vitamin preparations, iodine-containing medications, and coloring matters. These additions to "normal" supplies, if continued, could invalidate the above conclusions. In addition, Connolly,[195] working in Tasmania, has shown that the use of iodophors as antiseptic agents in milking machines, storage vats, and bulk milk tankers leads to a marked increase in the iodine contents of milk, ice cream, and confections containing dairy products. The iodine concentration of milk from four areas where iodophors were not used was found to range from 1.3 to 2.3 μg/100 ml, compared with a range of 11.3–34.6 μg/100 ml in milk from five areas where this type of bactericidal agent was employed. The use of potassium iodate in place of bromate, as a dough conditioner or "improver" in bread making represents a further adventitious source of iodine to man. In Tasmania the level of iodine from iodate added to bread has been maintained at about 1 mg or less per lb of bread, and the mean daily intake of iodine from bread alone was estimated at 80–270 μg, depending upon the age and sex of the individual.[195] In the United States bread may contain as much as 4 mg I/lb, and it has been calculated that iodine intakes of individuals with a very high bread consumption could reach 1,000 μg/day.[193]

Fortuitous sources of iodine, such as those mentioned in the preceding paragraph, would obviously be of great value in areas naturally low in environmental iodine where simple goiter is endemic. A fall in goiter incidence to an acceptably low level in school children in Tasmania following the incorporation of iodate in bread has been reported by Clements et al.[196] There is also evidence from the same area of a concurrent marked increase in the incidence of thyrotoxicosis. The increase was mostly confined to women in the 40–80-yr age group, almost all of whom had preexisting goiter.[197] It seems that the thyroid gland of such individuals is particularly susceptible to relatively high iodine intakes and that dietary iodine levels that are safe in areas free from endemic goiter are not free of the risk of thyrotoxicosis (iodbasedow) in iodine-deficient populations.

The effect of iodine in producing thyrotoxicosis in some individuals, usually those with large nodular goiters, as described above, is not well understood. Other manifestations of iodide excess, including iodide goiter, are also poorly understood. Wolff[194] defines four degrees of iodide excess as follows:

1. Relatively low levels, which lead to temporary increases in the absolute iodine uptake by the thyroid and the formation of organic iodine, until such time as the thyroid is required to reduce iodide clearances;
2. a larger amount, which can inhibit iodine release from the thyrotoxic human thyroid or from thyroids in which iodine release has been accelerated by thyroid-stimulating hormone (TSH);
3. a slightly greater intake, which leads to inhibition of organic iodine formation and which probably causes iodide goiter (the so-called Wolff–Chaikoff effect); and
4. very high levels of iodide, which saturate the active transport mechanism for this anion. The acute pharmacological effects of iodide can usually be demonstrated before saturation becomes significant.

Iodide goiter or myxedema may arise either as a consequence of iodine therapy in amounts greatly in excess of the daily requirements for hormone biosynthesis or from such amounts occurring in diets high in seaweed. The former circumstances can occur particularly in asthmatic patients, since iodide is administered liberally in the treatment of asthma and other chronic lung diseases and also in patients with Grave's disease being treated with potassium iodide or Lugol's solution. Endemic iodide goiter is more important in the context of the present review because the excess iodine occurs naturally in the diets consumed. This type of goiter has been reported from the coastal regions of Hokkaido, the northern island of Japan.[198] The usual diets of the inhabitants of these districts contain a large quantity of seaweed that, as pointed out earlier, is outstandingly high in iodine. Iodine intake in some individuals reached the astonishing total of 50,000 to 80,000 μg/ day. Urinary excretion in five of the patients exhibiting clinical signs of goiter exceeded 20 mg/day. This is about 100 times higher than urinary iodine excretion in individuals consuming more conventional diets. Restriction of seaweed consumption induced a marked decrease in the size of the goiter and in urinary iodine excretion in a number of patients who accepted this dietary change.

REFERENCES

1. E. G. Zook and J. Lehmann, Mineral composition of fruits. J. Am. Diet. Assoc. *52*:225 (1968).
2. H. Hopkins and J. Eisen, Mineral elements in fresh vegetables from different geographic areas. J. Agric. Food Chem. *7*:633 (1959).
3. J. E. Greaves and C. T. Hirst, The mineral content of grain. J. Nutr. *1*:293 (1929).
4. P. J. Schaible, S. L. Bandemer, and J. A. Davidson, Manganese content of feedstuffs and its relation to poultry nutrition. Mich. Agric. Exp. Stn. Tech. Bull. No. 159 (1938).
5. E. J. Underwood, T. J. Robinson, and D. H. Curnow, The manganese content of Western Australia cereal grains and their by-products and of other poultry feeds. J. Agric. W. Aust. *24*:259 (1947).
6. E. J. Underwood, Trace elements in human and animal nutrition, 3rd ed. Academic Press, New York (1971).
7. I. J. B. Blom, Studies in mineral metabolism. XXIX. The iodine content of foodstuffs in relation to occurrence of endemic goitre in the Longkloof Valley. Onderstepoort J. Vet. Sci. Anim. Ind. *2*:139 (1934).
8. M. Kirchgessner, Wechselbeziehungen zwischen Spurenelementen in Futtermitteln und tierischen Substanzen sowie Abhängigkeitsverhältnisse zwischen einzelnen Elementen bei der Retention. V. Mitteilung: Die Wechselwirkungen zwischen verschiedenen Elementen in der coldstral und normalen Milch. VI. Mitteilung: Abhängigkeitsverhältnisse zwischen verschiedenen Spurenelementen bei der Retention. Z. Tierphysiol. Tierernähr. Futtermittelk. *14*:270, 278 (1959).
9. G. P. Gurevic, Increasing the iodine content of eggs by supplementary feeding of hens with seaweed and fishmeal. Vopr. Petaniya *18*:65 (1959); Nutr. Abstr. Rev. *30*:697 (1960).
10. O. H. M. Wilder, E. M. Bethke, and P. R. Record, The iodine content of hens' eggs as affected by the ration. J. Nutr. *6*:407 (1933).
11. A. B. Beck, The copper content of the liver and blood of some vertebrates. Aust. J. Zool. *4*:1 (1956).
12. E. J. Underwood, Geographical and geochemical relationships of trace elements to health and disease, p. 3. In Trace substances in environmental health, IV, D. D. Hemphill (ed.). University of Missouri Press, Columbia (1970).
13. E. G. Zook and J. Lehmann, Total diet study: Content of ten minerals—aluminum, calcium, phosphorus, sodium, potassium, boron, copper, iron, manganese, and magnesium. J. Assoc. Offic. Anal. Chem. *48*:850 (1965).
14. N. O. Price, G. E. Bunce, and R. W. Engel, Copper, manganese, and zinc balance in preadolescent girls. Am. J. Clin. Nutr. *23*:258 (1970).
15. E. W. Murphy, L. Page, and B. K. Watt, Major mineral elements in type A school lunches. J. Am. Diet. Assoc. *57*:239 (1970).
16. E. W. Murphy, B. K. Watt, and L. Page, Regional variations in vitamin and trace element content of type A school lunches, p. 194. In Trace substances in environmental health, IV, D. D. Hemphill (ed.). University of Missouri Press, Columbia (1970).
17. I. H. Tipton, P. L. Stewart, and P. G. Martin, Trace elements in diets and excreta. Health Phys. *12*:1683 (1966).

18. R. A. Kehoe, J. Cholak, and R. V. Storey, A spectrochemical study of the normal ranges of concentration of certain trace metals in biological materials. J. Nutr. *19*:579 (1940).

19. J. H. Burn, The physiological action of aluminum. Analyst *57*:428 (1932).

20. J. Wührer, Zur gesundheitlichen Beurteilung des Aluminiums, insbesondere im Aluminium Ess-, Trink- und Kochgeschirr. Arch. Hyg. *112*:198 (1934).

21. H. J. Deobald and C. A. Elvehjem, The effect of feeding high amounts of soluble iron and aluminum salts. Am. J. Physiol. *111*:118 (1958).

22. H. A. Schroeder and J. J. Balassa, Abnormal trace elements in man: Arsenic. J. Chron. Dis. *19*:85 (1966).

23. A. C. Chapman, On the presence of compounds of arsenic in marine crustaceans and shell fish. Analyst *51*:548 (1926).

24. I. L. Bennett and A. Heyman. In Principles of internal medicine, T. R. Harrison, R. D. Adams, I. L. Bennett, W. H. Resnik, G. W. Thorn, M. M. Wintrobe (eds.), p. 1405. Fifth Ed. McGraw-Hill, New York (1966).

25. G. R. Sharpless and M. Metzger, Arsenic and goiter. J. Nutr. *21*:341 (1941).

26. E. J. Coulson, R. E. Remington, and K. M. Lynch, Metabolism in the rat of the naturally occurring arsenic of shrimp as compared with arsenic trioxide. J. Nutr. *10*:255 (1935).

27. L. R. Overby and D. V. Frost, Nonavailability to the rat of the arsenic in tissues of swine fed arsanilic acid. Toxicol. Appl. Pharmacol. *4*:38 (1962).

28. H. Smith, The interpretation of the arsenic content of human hair. J. Forensic Sci. Soc. *4*:192 (1964).

29. H. Smith, The distribution of antimony, arsenic, copper and zinc in human tissue. J. Forensic Sci. Soc. *7*:97 (1967).

30. R. M. Johnstone, In Metabolic inhibitors, Vol. II, R. M. Hochster and J. H. Quastel (eds.). Academic Press, New York (1963).

31. D. V. Frost, Arsenicals in biology—Retrospect and prospect. Fed. Proc. *26*: 194 (1967).

32. H. A. Schroeder, M. Kanisawa, D. V. Frost, and M. Mitchener, Germanium, tin and arsenic in rats: Effects on growth, survival, pathological lesions and life span. J. Nutr. *96*:37 (1968).

33. M. Scott, The possible role of arsenic in the etiology of goiter, cretinism and endemic deaf-mutism. Trans. of the 3rd International Goitre Conference, p. 34. Berncliff Press, Portland, Oregon (1938).

34. R. A. MacDonald, B. J. P. Becker, and G. S. Picket, Iron and liver disease in South Africa. Arch. Intern. Med. *3*:315 (1963).

35. H. K. Stiebeling, The iron content of vegetables and fruit. U.S. Dep. Agric. Circ. No. 205 (1932).

36. O. E. Skeets, E. Frazier, and D. Dickins, Conservation of iron in vegetables by methods of preparation and cooking. Miss. Agric. Exp. Stn. Bull. No. 291 (1931).

37. C. P. Czerniejewski, C. W. Shank, W. G. Bechtel, and W. B. Bradley, The minerals of wheat flour and bread. Cereal Chem. *41*:65 (1964).

38. D. B. Milne and P. H. Weswig, Effect of supplementary copper on blood and liver copper-containing fractions in rats. J. Nutr. *95*:429 (1968).

39. R. Boyden, V. R. Potter, and C. A. Elvehjem, Effect of feeding high levels of copper to albino rats. J. Nutr. *15*:397 (1938).

40. N. F. Suttle and C. F. Mills, Studies of the toxicity of copper to pigs. 1. Ef-

fects of oral supplements of zinc and iron salts on the development of copper toxicosis. Br. J. Nutr. *20*:135 (1966).

41. N. F. Suttle and C. F. Mills, Studies of the toxicity of copper to pigs. 2. Effect of protein source and other dietary components on the response to high and moderate intakes of copper. Br. J. Nutr. *20*:149 (1966).

42. L. B. Bull, British Commonwealth Special Conference on Agriculture in Australia 1949, p. 300. Her Majesty's Stationery Office, London (1951).

43. A. T. Dick, Molybdenum in animal nutrition. Soil Sci. *81*:229 (1956).

44. H. A. Schroeder, A. P. Nason, I. H. Tipton, and J. J. Balassa, Essential trace elements in man: Copper. J. Chron. Dis. *19*:1007 (1966).

45. G. E. Cartwright and M. M. Wintrobe, Copper metabolism in normal subjects. Am. J. Clin. Nutr. *14*:224 (1964).

46. I. H. Scheinberg and I. Sternlieb, Wilson's disease. Ann. Rev. Med. *16*:119 (1965).

47. J. A. Bush, J. P. Mahoney, M. Markowitz, C. J. Gubler, G. E. Cartwright, and M. M. Wintrobe, Studies on copper metabolism. XVI. Radioactive copper studies in normal subjects and in patients with hepatolenticular degeneration. J. Clin. Invest. *34*:1766 (1955).

48. G. K. Davis, in Symposium on copper metabolism, W. D. McElroy and W. G. Glass (eds.). Johns Hopkins Press, Baltimore (1950).

49. J. B. Nielands, F. M. Strong, and C. A. Elvehjem, Molybdenum in the nutrition of the rat. J. Biol. Chem. *172*:431 (1948).

50. C. L. Comar, L. Singer, and G. K. Davis, Molybdenum metabolism and interrelationships with copper and phosphorus. J. Biol. Chem. *180*:913 (1949).

51. W. W. Westerfeld and D. A. Richert, Distribution of the xanthine oxidase factor (molybdenum) in foods. J. Nutr. *51*:85 (1953).

52. L. I. Hart, E. C. Owen, and R. Proudfoot, The influence of dietary molybdenum on the xanthine oxidase activity of the milk of ruminants. Br. J. Nutr. *21*:617 (1967).

53. J. G. Archibald, Molybdenum in cows' milk. J. Dairy Sci. *34*:1026 (1951).

54. D. E. Becker and S. E. Smith, The level of cobalt tolerance in yearling sheep. J. Anim. Sci. *10*:266 (1951).

55. W. C. Grant and W. S. Root, Fundamental stimulus for erythropoiesis. Physiol. Rev. *32*:499 (1952).

56. Epidemic cardiac failure in beer drinkers. Nutr. Rev. *26*:173 (1968).

57. C. S. Alexander, Cobalt and the heart. Ann. Intern. Med. *70*:411 (1969).

58. H. T. Grinvalsky and D. M. Fitch, A distinctive myocardiopathy occurring in Omaha, Nebraska: Pathological aspects. Ann. N.Y. Acad. Sci. *156*:544 (1969).

59. S. S. Phatak and V. N. Patwardhan, Toxicity of nickel. Indian J. Sci. Ind. Res. *9b*:70 (1950).

60. S. S. Phatak and V. N. Patwardhan, Accumulation of nickel in rats fed on nickel-containing diets and its elimination. Indian J. Sci. Ind. Res. *11b*:173 (1952).

61. G. A. Stephens, An important factor in the causation of industrial cancer. Med. Press *187*:216 (1933).

62. G. A. Stephens, Further observations regarding carbon monoxide gas as an important factor in the causation of industrial cancer. Med. Press *187*:283 (1933).

63. F. W. Sunderman and F. W. Sunderman, Jr., Nickel poisoning. XI. Implication of nickel as a pulmonary carcinogen in tobacco smoke. Am. J. Clin. Pathol. *35*:203 (1961).

64. C. W. Weber and B. L. Reid, Nickel toxicity in young growing mice. J. Anim. Sci. *28*:620 (1969).

65. C. W. Weber and B. L. Reid, Nickel toxicity in growing chicks. J. Nutr. *95*: 612 (1968).

66. N. L. Kent and R. A. McCance, The absorption and excretion of "minor" elements by man. I. Silver, gold, lithium, boron and vanadium. Biochem. J. *35*:837 (1941).

67. N. L. Kent and R. A. McCance, The absorption and excretion of "minor" elements by man. II. Cobalt, nickel, tin and manganese. Biochem. J. *35*:877 (1941).

68. H. A. Schroeder, J. J. Balassa, and I. H. Tipton, Abnormal trace elements in man: Nickel. J. Chron. Dis. *15*:51 (1961).

69. V. G. Heller, and A. D. Burk, Toxicity of zinc. J. Biol. Chem. *74*:85 (1927).

70. W. R. Sutton, and V. E. Nelson, Studies on zinc. Proc. Soc. Exp. Biol. Med. *36*:211 (1937).

71. M. F. Brink, D. E. Becker, S. W. Terrill, and A. H. Jensen, Zinc toxicity in the weanling pig. J. Anim. Sci. *18*:836 (1959).

72. D. R. Grant-Frost and E. J. Underwood, Zinc toxicity in the rat and its interrelation with copper. Aust. J. Exp. Biol. Med. Sci. *36*:339 (1958).

73. H. A. Schroeder, A. P. Nason, I. H. Tipton, and J. J. Balassa, Essential trace elements in man: Zinc. Relation to environmental cadmium. J. Chron. Dis. *20*:179 (1967).

74. Outbreaks of food poisoning due to zinc, 1942–1956. U.K. Min. Health Lab. Serv. Mon. Bull. (1957).

75. G. Lawrence, Zinc poisoning. Br. Med. J. *1*:582 (1958).

76. W. D. Gallup and L. C. Norris, The amount of manganese required to prevent porosis in the chick. Poult. Sci. *18*:76 (1939).

77. W. D. Gallup and L. C. Norris, The effect of a deficiency of manganese in the diet of the hen. Poult. Sci. *18*:83 (1939).

78. R. H. Grummer, O. G. Bentley, P. H. Phillips, and G. Bohstedt, The role of manganese in growth, reproduction, and lactation of swine. J. Anim. Sci. *9*: 170 (1950).

79. G. Matrone, R. H. Hartman, and A. J. Clawson, Studies of a manganese-iron antagonism in the nutrition of rabbits and baby pigs. J. Nutr. *67*:309 (1959).

80. W. H. Peterson and J. T. Skinner, Distribution of manganese in foods. J. Nutr. *4*:419 (1931).

81. H. A. Schroeder, J. J. Balassa, and I. H. Tipton, Essential trace elements in man: Manganese. A study in homeostasis. J. Chron. Dis. *19*:545 (1966).

82. B. B. North, J. M. Leichsenring, and L. M. Norris, Manganese metabolism in college women. J. Nutr. *72*:217 (1960).

83. P. S. Papavasiliou, S. T. Miller, and G. C. Cotzias, Role of liver in regulating distribution and excretion of manganese. Am. J. Physiol. *211*:211 (1966).

84. A. J. Bertinchamps, S. T. Miller, and G. C. Cotzias, Interdependence of routes excreting manganese. Am. J. Physiol. *211*:216 (1966).

85. G. C. Cotzias, Manganese in health and disease. Physiol. Rev. *38*:503 (1958).

86. A. L. Moxon, O. E. Olson, E. I. Whitehead, R. J. Hiomoe, and S. N. White,

Selenium distribution in milled seleniferous wheats. Cereal Chem. *20*:376 (1943).

87. M. I. Smith, K. W. Franke, and B. B. Westfall, The selenium problem in relation to public health. A preliminary survey to determine the possibility of selenium intoxication in the rural population living on seleniferous soil. U.S. Public Health Rep. *51*:1496 (1936).

88. M. I. Smith and B. B. Westfall, Further field studies on the selenium problem in relation to public health. U.S. Public Health Rep. *52*:1375 (1937).

89. J. W. Hamilton and O. A. Beath, Amount and chemical form of selenium in vegetable plants. J. Agric. Food Chem. *12*:371 (1964).

90. H. D. Anderson and A. L. Moxon, Isolation of glutathione and thionine from the blood of selenized steers. Proc. S. D. Acad. Sci. *21*:16 (1941).

91. M. I. Smith, The influence of diet on the chronic toxicity of selenium. U.S. Public Health Rep. *54*:1441 (1939).

92. A. W. Halverson and K. J. Monty, An effect of dietary sulfate on selenium poisoning in the rat. J. Nutr. *70*:100 (1960).

93. A. L. Moxon, The effect of arsenic on the toxicity of seleniferous grains. Science *88*:81 (1938).

94. O. A. Levander and C. A. Baumann, Selenium metabolism. V. Studies on the distribution of selenium in rats given arsenic. Toxicol. Appl. Pharmacol. *9*:98 (1966).

95. O. A. Levander and C. A. Baumann, Selenium metabolism. VI. Effect of arsenic on the excretion of selenium in the bile. Toxicol. Appl. Pharmacol. *9*:106 (1966).

96. L. M. Cummins and J. L. Martin, Are selenocystine and selenomethionine synthesized *in vivo* from sodium selenite in mammals? Biochemistry *6*:3162 (1967).

97. C. I. Wright, Effect of selenium on urease and arginase. J. Pharmacol. Exp. Ther. *68*:220 (1940).

98. H. L. Klug, A. L. Moxon, D. F. Peterson, and V. R. Potter, The *in vivo* inhibition of succinic dehydrogenase by selenium and its release by arsenic. Arch. Biochem. *28*:253 (1950).

99. P. Lindberg, Selenium determination in plant and animal material, and in water. Acta Vet. Scand. Suppl. 23 (1968).

100. D. M. Hadjimarkos, Selenium: A caries-enhancing trace element. Caries Res. *3*:14 (1969).

101. F. R. Cousins and I. M. Cairney, Selenium metabolism in sheep. Aust. J. Agric. Res. *12*:927 (1961).

102. K. A. Handreck and K. O. Godwin, Distribution in the sheep of selenium derived from ^{75}Se-labeled ruminal pellets. Aust. J. Agric. Res. *21*:71 (1970).

103. K. Ostadius and B. Aberg. Distribution of Se[75]-tagged sodium selenite in pigs. Acta Vet. Scand. *2*:60 (1961).

104. D. V. Frost. In Selenium in biomedicine, O. H. Muth (ed.). Avi, Westport, Conn. (1967).

105. J. R. Harr, J. F. Bone, I. J. Tinsley, P. H. Weswig, and R. S. Yamamoto. In Selenium in biomedicine, O. H. Muth (ed.). Avi, Westport, Conn. (1967).

106. R. J. Shamberger and D. V. Frost, Possible protective effect of selenium against human cancer. Can. Med. Assoc. J. *100*:682 (1969).

107. D. Purves, Contamination of urban garden soils with copper, boron and lead. Plant Soil *26*:380 (1967).

108. J. J. Connor, J. A. Erdman, J. D. Sims, and R. J. Ebens, Roadside effects on trace element content of some rocks, soils and plants of Missouri, p. 26. In Trace substances in environmental heatlh, IV, D. D. Hemphill (ed.). University of Missouri Press, Columbia (1970).

109. J. P. Creason, O. McNulty, L. T. Heiderscheit, D. H. Swanson, and R. W. Buechly, Roadside gradients in atmospheric concentrations of cadmium, lead and zinc, p. 129. In Trace substances in environmental health, V, D. D. Hemphill (ed.). University of Missouri Press, Columbia (1971).

110. A. Cantarrow and M. Trumper, Lead poisoning. Williams & Wilkins, Baltimore (1944).

111. G. K. Murthy, U. Rhea, and J. T. Peeler, Rubidium and lead content of market milk. J. Dairy Sci. *50*:651 (1967).

112. G. W. Monier-Williams, Trace elements in food. Chapman & Hall, London (1949).

113. C. C. Patterson, Contaminated and natural lead environments of man. Arch. Environ. Health *11*:344 (1965).

114. H. A. Schroeder, and I. H. Tipton, The human body burden of lead. Arch. Environ. Health *17*:965 (1968).

115. H. A. Schroeder and J. J. Balassa, Arsenic, germanium, tin and vanadium in mice: Effects on growth, survival, and tissue levels. J. Nutr. *92*:245 (1967).

116. J. R. Davis and S. L. Andelman, Urinary delta-aminolevulinic acid (ALA) levels in lead poisoning. Arch. Environ. Health *15*:53 (1967).

117. S. Hernberg, J. Nikkanen, G. Mellin, and H. Lilius, δ-Aminolevulinic acid dehydrase as a measure of lead exposure. Arch. Environ. Health *21*:140 (1970).

118. D. D. Ulmer and B. L. Vallee, Effects of lead on biochemical systems, p. 7. In Trace substances in environmental health, II, D. D. Hemphill (ed.). University of Missouri Press, Columbia (1968).

119. R. A. Goyer, Pathobiology of lead in the kidney, p. 342. In Trace substances in environmental health, IV, D. D. Hemphill (ed.). University of Missouri Press, Columbia (1970).

120. H. A. Schroeder, J. J. Balassa, and I. H. Tipton, Abnormal trace elements in man: Tin. J. Chron. Dis. *17*:483 (1964).

121. H. R. Kenwood and H. Kerr. Hygiene and public health. Lewis, London (1929).

122. K. Schwarz, K. B. Milne, and E. Vinyard, Growth effects of tin compounds in rats maintained in a trace element-controlled environment. Biochem. Biophys. Res. Comm. *40*:22 (1970).

123. G. K. Murthy, U. Rhea, and J. T. Peeler, Levels of antimony, cadmium, chromium, cobalt, manganese and zinc in institutional total diets. Environ. Sci. Tech. *5*:436 (1971).

124. H. A. Schroeder and J. J. Balassa, Abnormal trace elements in man: Cadmium. J. Chron. Dis. *14*:263 (1961).

125. R. E. Carroll, The relationship of cadmium in the air to cardiovascular disease death rates. J. Am. Med. Assoc. *198*:267 (1966).

126. S. Frant and I. Kleeman, Cadmium "food poisoning." J. Am. Med. Assoc. *117*:86 (1941).

127. O. G. Fitzhugh and F. H. Meiller, The chronic toxicity of cadmium. J. Pharmacol. Exp. Ther. *72*:15 (1941).

128. H. A. Schroeder, Cadmium hypertension in rats. Am. J. Physiol. *207*:62 (1964).

129. M. Kanisawa, and H. A. Schroeder, Renal arteriolar changes in hypertensive rats given cadmium in drinking water. Exp. Mol. Path. *10*:81 (1969).
130. H. M. Perry, Jr., Chelatin therapy in circulatory and sclerosing disease. Fed. Proc. *20*:254 (1961).
131. H. A. Schroeder, Cadmium as a factor in hypertension. J. Chron. Dis. *18*:647 (1965).
132. J. M. Morgan, Tissue cadmium concentration in man. Arch. Intern. Med. *123*: 405 (1969).
133. D. I. Hammer, J. F. Finklea, J. P. Creason, S. H. Sandifer, J. E. Keil, L. E. Priester, and J. F. Stara, Cadmium exposure and human health effects, p. 269. In Trace substances in environmental health, V, D. D. Hemphill (ed.). University of Missouri Press, Columbia (1971).
134. W. F. Hunt, Jr., C. Pinkerton, O. McNulty, and J. Creason, A study in trace element pollution of air in 77 midwestern cities, p. 56. In Trace substances in environmental health, IV, D. D. Hemphill (ed.). University of Missouri Press, Columbia (1970).
135. L. T. Friberg, M. Piscapor, and G. Nordberg, Cadmium in the environment, p. 166. Chemical Rubber Co., Cleveland, Ohio (1971).
136. D. W. Fassett. In Cadmium in metallic contaminants and human health, D. H. K. Lee (ed.). Academic Press, New York (1972).
137. A. Stock, Der Quecksilbergehalt des menschlichen Organismus. XXX. Mitteiling über Wirkung und Verbreitung des Quecksilbers. Biochem. Z. *304*:73 (1940).
138. O. S. Gibbs, H. Pond, and G. A. Hansmann, Toxicological studies on ammoniated mercury. J. Pharmacol. Exp. Ther. *72*:16 (1941).
139. C. Kellershohn, D. Comar, and C. Lopoce, Determination of the mercury content of human blood by activation analysis. J. Lab. Clin. Med. *66*:168 (1965).
140. H. Smith and J. Lenihan. In Methods in forensic science, A. S. Curry (ed.). Interscience, London (1964).
141. R. E. Jervis, D. Debrun, W. Le Page, and B. Tiefenbach, Mercury residues in Canadian foods, fish and wildlife. Department of Chemical Engineering and Applied Chemistry, University of Toronto, Toronto, Canada (1970).
142. G. Westöö, Determination of methyl-mercury salts in various kinds of biological material. Acta Chem. Scand. *22*:2277 (1968).
143. G. Westöö, Mercury in foodstuffs—Is there a great risk of poisoning? Vår föda, no. 4 (1965).
144. A. Norden, I. Dencker, and A. Schutz, Experiences from a food consumption survey based on the double-portion technique in the Dalby community in 1968–69. Näringsforskning *14*:40 (1970).
145. Methyl-mercury in fish. A toxicologic-epidemiologic evaluation of risks. Report from an expert group. Nord. Hygien. Tidskr. Suppl. 4 (1971).
146. L. Friberg, Studies on the metabolism of mercuric chloride and methyl mercury dicyandiamide. Arch. Ind. Health *20*:42 (1959).
147. S. Jensen and A. Jernelov, Biological methylation of mercury in aquatic organisms. Nature *223*:753 (1969).
148. G. Westöö, Determination of methylmercury compounds in foodstuffs. I. Methylmercury compounds in fish, identification and determination. Acta Chem. Scand. *20*:2131 (1966).
149. N. A. Smart and M. K. Lloyd, Mercury residues in eggs, flesh and livers of hens fed on wheat treated with methylmercury dicyandiamide. J. Sci. Food Agric. *14*:734 (1963).

150. G. Westöö, Methylmercury compounds in animal foods, p. 75. In Chemical fallout, M. W. Miller and G. C. Berg (eds.). Charles C Thomas, Springfield, Ill. (1969).

151. K. Borg, H. Wanntorp, K. Erne, and E. Hanko, Mercury poisoning in Swedish wildlife. J. Appl. Ecol. *3* (Suppl.):171 (1966).

152. Mercury contamination of man and his environment. Joint WHO/FAO/IAEA International Discussion, Amsterdam (1967).

153. G. E. Miller, P. M. Grant, R. Kishore, F. J. Steinkruger, F. S. Rowland, and V. P. Guinn, Mercury concentrations in museum specimens of tuna and swordfish. Science *175*:1121 (1972).

154. H. E. Ganther, C. Goudie, M. L. Sunde, M. J. Kopecky, P. Wagner, S.-H. Oh, and W. G. Hoekstra, Selenium: Relation to decreased toxicity of methylmercury added to diets containing tuna. Science *175*:1122 (1972).

155. R. A. Howie and H. Smith, Mercury in human tissue. J. Forensic Sci. Soc. *7*:90 (1967).

156. W. J. Rodger and H. Smith, Mercury absorption by fingerprint officers using "grey powder." J. Forensic Sci. Soc. *7*:86 (1967).

157. O. Hoshino et al. Cited by Jervis et al.[141] Eiseikagaku (J. Hyg. Chem.) *12*:94 (1966).

158. L. J. Goldwater, International Conference on Environmental Mercury Contamination. University of Michigan, Ann Arbor, Mich. (1970).

159. L. T. Kurland, S. N. Faro, and H. S. Siedler, Minamata disease. The outbreak of a neurologic disorder in Minimata, Japan, and its relationship to the ingestion of seafood contaminated by mercuric compounds. World Neurol. *1*:320 (1960).

160. K. Schwarz and W. Mertz, Chromium (III) and the glucose tolerance factor. Arch. Biochem. Biophys. *85*:292 (1959).

161. W. Mertz, E. E. Roginski, and R. C. Reba, Biological activity and fate of trace quantities of intravenous chromium (III) in the rat. Am. J. Physiol. *209*:489 (1965).

162. R. D. Mackenzie, R. U. Byerrum, C. F. Decker, C. A. Hoppert, and R. F. Langham, Chronic toxicity studies. II. Hexavalent and trivalent chromium administered in drinking water to rats. Arch. Ind. Health *18*:232 (1958).

163. H. P. Brinton, E. S. Fraiser, and A. L. Koven, Morbidity and mortality experience among chromate workers. U.S. Publ. Health Rep. *67*:835 (1952).

164. H. A. Schroeder, J. J. Balassa, and W. H. Winton, Jr., Chromium, lead, cadmium, nickel and titanium in mice: Effect on mortality, tumors and tissue levels. J. Nutr. *83*:239 (1964).

165. H. A. Schroeder, J. J. Balassa, and W. H. Winton, Jr., Chromium, cadmium and lead in rats: Effects on life span, tumors and tissue levels. J. Nutr. *86*:51 (1965).

166. L. D. Saint-Rat, The presence of chromium in vegetation. C.R. Acad. Sci. *277*:150 (1948).

167. J. P. Carter, A. Kattab, K. A. abd-al-Hadi, J. T. Davis, A. E. Gholmy, and V. N. Patwardhan, Chromium (III) in hypoglycemia and in impaired glucose utilization in Kwashiorkor. Am. J. Clin. Nutr. *21*:195 (1968).

168. H. A. Schroeder, J. J. Balassa, and I. H. Tipton, Abnormal trace elements in man: Chromium. J. Chron. Dis. *15*:941 (1962).

169. W. H. Glinsmann and W. Mertz, Effect of trivalent chromium on glucose tolerance. Metabolism *15*:510 (1966).

170. R. A. Levine, D. H. Streeten, and R. J. Doisy, Effects of oral chromium supple-

mentation on the glucose tolerance of elderly human subjects. Metabolism *17*:114 (1968).

171. R. M. Donaldson and R. F. Barreras, Intestinal absorption of trace quantities of chromium. J. Lab. Clin. Med. *68*:484 (1966).

172. W. J. Visek, I. B. Whitney, U. S. G. Kuhn, and C. L. Comar, Metabolism of Cr^{51} by animals as influenced by chemical state. Proc. Soc. Exp. Biol. Med. *84*:610 (1963).

173. W. Mertz, Chromium occurrence and function in biological systems. Physiol. Rev. *49*:163 (1969).

174. J. Cholak, Fluorides: A critical review. 1. The occurrence of fluoride in air, food, and water. J. Occup. Med. *1*:501 (1959).

175. C. G. Pandit, T. N. Raghavacheri, D. S. Rao, and V. Krishnamurti, Endemic fluorosis in south India. A study of the factors involved in the production of mottled enamel in children and severe bone manifestations in adults. Indian J. Med. Res. *28*:533 (1940).

176. T. Ockerse, Fluorine and dental caries in South Africa. In Dental caries and fluorine. Am. Assoc. Adv. Sci., Washington, D.C. (1946).

177. F. J. McClure, Fluorine in foods. Survey of recent data. U.S. Public Health Rep. *64*:1061 (1949).

178. E. B. Hart, P. H. Phillips, and G. Bohstedt, Relation of soil fertilization with superphosphates and rock phosphate to fluorine content of plants and drainage waters. Am. J. Public Health *24*:936 (1934).

179. M. P. Ham, and M. D. Smith, Fluoride studies related to the human diet. Can. J. Res., Sect. F *28*:277 (1950).

180. M. F. Harrison, Fluorine content of teas consumed in New Zealand. Br. J. Nutr. *3*:162 (1949).

181. F. J. McClure, Ingestion of fluoride and dental caries. Quantitative relations based on food and water requirements of children one to twelve years old. Am. J. Dis. Child. *66*:362 (1943).

182. W. Machle, E. W. Scott, and E. J. Largent, The absorption and excretion of fluorides. Part 1. The normal fluoride balance. J. Ind. Hyg. Toxicol. *24*:199 (1942).

183. H. C. Hodge and F. A. Smith. In Fluorine chemistry, Vol. 4, J. H. Simons (ed.). Academic Press, New York (1965).

184. F. M. McClure, H. G. McCann, and N. C. Leone, Excessive fluoride in water and bone chemistry. Comparison of two cases. U.S. Public Health Rep. *73*: 741 (1958).

185. H. E. Shortt, G. R. McRobert, T. W. Barnard, and A. S. M. Nayer, Endemic fluorosis in the Madras presidency. Indian J. Med. Res. *25*:553 (1937).

186. R. L. Vought, F. A. Brown, and W. T. London, Iodine in the environment. Arch. Environ. Health *20*:516 (1970).

187. R. L. Vought, Upward trend in iodide consumption in the United States. In Trace substances in environmental health, V, D. D. Hemphill (ed.). University of Missouri Press, Columbia (1971).

188. R. L. Vought and W. T. London, Dietary sources of iodine. Am. J. Clin. Nutr. *14*:186 (1964).

189. Iodine content of foods. Chilean Iodine Educ. Bur., London (1952).

190. Iodine and plant life. Chilean Iodine Educ. Bur., London (1950).

191. T. H. Oddie, D. A. Fisher, W. M. McConahey, and C. S. Thompson, Iodine intake in the United States: A reassessment. J. Clin. Endocrinol. *30*:659 (1970).

192. National Research Council, Food and Nutrition Board Recommended dietary allowances. 7th ed. National Academy of Sciences, Washington, D.C. (1968).

193. National Research Council, Food and Nutrition Board, Iodine nutriture in the United States, Summary of a Conference, October 1970. National Academy of Sciences, Washington, D.C. (1970).

194. J. Wolff, Iodide goiter and the pharmacologic effects of excess iodide. Am. J. Med. *47*:101 (1969).

195. R. J. Connolly, An increase in thyrotoxicosis in southern Tasmania after an increase in dietary iodine. Med. J. Aust. *1*:1268 (1971).

196. F. W. Clements, H. B. Gibson, and J. F. Howeler-Coy, Goitre prophylaxis by addition of potassium iodate to bread. Lancet *1*:489 (1970).

197. R. J. Connolly, G. I. Vidor, and J. C. Stewart, Increase in thyrotoxicosis in endemic goitre area after iodation of bread. Lancet *1*:500 (1970).

198. H. Suzuki, T. Higuchi, K. Sawa, S. Ohtaki, and Y. Horiuchi, "Endemic coast goiter" in Hokkaido, Japan. Acta Endocrinol. *50*:161 (1965).

4 C. L. Comar and J. H. Rust

NATURAL RADIOACTIVITY IN THE BIOSPHERE AND FOODSTUFFS*

Although it is known that large amounts of radioactivity deposited in the body can produce harm, no evidence exists of deleterious effects from the amounts of radioactive materials that occur naturally in the diet and in the body. This does not mean that no such effects occur, but they have not been, and possibly cannot be, observed, and it is obvious that there is no interference with the ability of the human population to develop and progress. For this reason, and because of difficulties of measurement of such small amounts, relatively few data have been accumulated. Within recent years, however, there has been the added incentive of needing to know more about the natural background of radiation to permit assessment of the effects of artificial radioactivity, i.e., the man-

---

* For a more detailed coverage, the reader is referred to three important recent publications:

1. National Research Council Committee on Food Protection, *Radionuclides in Foods*, National Academy of Sciences, Washington, D.C. ISBN 0-309-02113-8 (1973).
2. National Research Council Advisory Committee on the Biological Effects of Ionizing Radiations, *The Effects on Populations of Exposure to Low Levels of Ionizing Radiation*, National Academy of Sciences, Washington, D.C. (1972).
3. United Nations Scientific Committee on the Effects of Atomic Radiation, *Ionizing Radiation: Levels and Effects*, Vol. 1 and 2, Suppl. No. 25 (A/8725) (1972).

made additions arising from nuclear weapons tests and expanded peace-time uses of atomic energy. Because of the persistence of some forms of artificial radioactivity, it may in the future become less useful to delineate natural radioactivity and more meaningful to consider the total radiation dose to which the population is committed.

A vast amount of data on the levels, behavior, and implications of artificial radioactivity is available in the literature[1-3]; therefore, these matters will not be treated in detail here, except for mention of radiation dosages. The reports of the United Nations Scientific Committee on the Effects of Atomic Radiation[1] present a detailed and comprehensive coverage of radiation exposure to the human population from all sources. The general references[1-9] listed in the bibliography will serve to document all statements made that do not carry specific citations.

Since the discovery of polonium and radium in the late nineteenth century, over 40 naturally occurring radionuclides have been identified and characterized. Most are elements of high atomic weight, with atomic numbers greater than 81; they fall into three distinct series, each of which begins with a very long-lived radionuclide and ends with a stable isotope of lead. These are known as the uranium series, the thorium series, and the actinium series; a listing is presented in Table 1.

Also in existence are a few naturally occurring radionuclides that are not members of these series (Table 2). Some of them have half-lives sufficiently long to have enabled them to exist from the time of formation of the earth's crust. On the other hand, others must be produced continuously. The latter are formed by nuclear reactions between components of cosmic radiation and stable nuclei. Carbon-14 is formed by the action of neutrons upon the nitrogen of the atmosphere; tritium (^{3}H) is formed by several different reactions. Other radionuclides, known to be formed naturally from the interaction of cosmic-ray neutrons with the atmosphere, include ^{7}Be, ^{22}Na, ^{32}P, ^{33}P, and ^{35}S. Of the radionuclides listed in Table 2, tritium, ^{14}C, and ^{40}K are of greatest biological interest. Carbon-14 and especially tritium have received increased attention in recent times, because their natural equilibrium levels have been and probably will continue to be significantly increased by man's use of nuclear energy.

NATURAL RADIOACTIVITY IN THE EARTH'S CRUST AND LOWER ATMOSPHERE

Naturally occurring radioactive elements are widely distributed throughout the earth's crust. The more important of these radionuclides are

TABLE 1 Naturally Occurring Radioactive Nuclides of the Uranium, Thorium, and Actinium Series[15]

Element	Symbol	Common Name	Older Generic Symbol	Major Type of Radiation[a]	Half-Life
Uranium series					
Uranium	^{238}U	Uranium I	U₁	α, γ, e^-	4.5×10^9 yr
Thorium	^{234}Th	Uranium X₁	UX₁	β^-, γ, e^-	24.1 days
Protactinium	^{234}Pa	Uranium X₂	UX₂	β^-, γ	1.17 min
Uranium	^{234}U	Uranium II	U II	α, γ, e^-	2.5×10^5 yr
Thorium	^{230}Th	Ionium	Io	α, γ, e^-	8.0×10^4 yr
Radium	^{226}Ra	Radium		α, γ, e^-	1.6×10^3 yr
Radon	^{222}Rn	Radon	Em	α, γ	3.82 days
Polonium	^{218}Po	Radium A	RaA	α	3.05 min
Lead	^{214}Pb	Radium B	RaB	β^-, γ, e^-	26.8 min
Bismuth	^{214}Bi	Radium C	RaC	α, β^-, γ	19.7 min
Polonium	^{214}Po	Radium C'	RaC'	α, γ	1.6×10^{-4} s
Thallium	^{210}Tl	Radium C''	RaC''	β^-, γ, e^-	1.32 min
Lead	^{210}Pb	Radium D	RaD	$\alpha, \beta^-, \gamma, e^-$	20.4 yr
Bismuth	^{210}Bi	Radium E	RaE	α, β^-, γ	5.0 days
Polonium	^{210}Po	Radium F	RaF	α, γ	138 days
Lead	^{206}Pb	Radium G	RaG	None	Stable
Thorium series					
Thorium	^{232}Th	Thorium		α, γ, e^-	1.41×10^{10} yr
Radium	^{228}Ra	Mesothorium I	MsTh₁	β^-, e^-	6.7 yr
Actinium	^{228}Ac	Mesothorium II	MsTh₂	β^-, γ, e^-	6.13 h
Thorium	^{228}Th	Radiothorium	RdTh	α, γ, e^-	1.90 yr

Element	Isotope	Historical name	Abbr.	Emissions	Half-life
Radium	^{224}Ra	Thorium X	ThX	α, γ, e^-	3.64 days
Radon	^{220}Rn	Thoron	Tn	α, γ	55.3 s
Polonium	^{216}Po	Thorium A	ThA	α	0.145 s
Lead	^{212}Pb	Thorium B	ThB	β^-, e^-, γ	10.6 h
Bismuth	^{212}Bi	Thorium C	ThC	$\alpha, \beta^-, \gamma, e^-$	60.6 min
Polonium	^{212}Po	Thorium C	ThC'	α	3×10^{-7} s
Thallium	^{208}Tl	Thorium C	ThC''	β^-, γ, e^-	3.1 min
Lead	^{209}Pb	Thorium D	ThD	None	Stable
Actinium series					
Uranium	^{235}U	Actinouranium	AcU	α, γ	7.1×10^8 yr
Thorium	^{231}Th	Uranium Y	UY	β^-, γ, e^-	255 h
Protactinium	^{231}Pa	Protactinium	Pa	α, γ, e^-	3.25×10^4 yr
Actinium	^{227}Ac	Actinium	Ac	$\alpha, \beta^-, e^-, \gamma$	21.6 yr
Thorium	^{227}Th	Radioactinium	RdAc	α, γ, e^-	18.2 days
Francium	^{223}Fr	Actinium K	Fr	β^-, e^-, γ	22 min
Radium	^{223}Ra	Actinium X	AcX	α, γ, e^-	11.44 days
Radon	^{219}Rn	Actinon	An	α, γ, e^-	4.0 s
Polonium	^{215}Po	Actinium A	AcA	α	1.78×10^{-3} s
Lead	^{211}Pb	Actinium B	AcB	β^-, γ	36.1 min
Astatine	^{219}At	Astatine		α	0.9 min
Bismuth	^{211}Bi	Actinium C	AcC	α, γ, e^-	2.16 min
Polonium	^{211}Po	Actinium C'	AcC'	α, γ	0.5 s
Thallium	^{207}Tl	Actinium C''	AcC''	β^-, γ	4.79 min
Lead	^{207}Pb	Actinium D	AcD	None	Stable

^{a} α—alpha-particle emission; β^-—negatron (beta-particle) emission; γ—gamma-ray emission; e^-—electron emission.

TABLE 2   Some Naturally Occurring Nonseries Radioactive Nuclides[15]

Element	Symbol	Major Type of Radiation[a]	Half-Life
Formed with earth's crust			
Potassium	^{40}K	β^+, β^-, γ	1.3×10^9 yr
Vanadium	^{50}V	β^-, γ, χ	6×10^{14} yr
Rubidium	^{87}Rb	β^-	4.8×10^{10} yr
Indium	^{115}In	β^-	6×10^{14} yr
Lanthanum	^{138}La	β^-, γ, χ	1.1×10^{11} yr
Samarium	^{147}Sm	α	1.05×10^{11} yr
Lutecium	^{176}Lu	β^-, e^-, γ	2.2×10^{10} yr
Produced continuously			
Tritium	^{3}H	β^-	12.3 yr
Beryllium	^{7}Be	γ	54 days
Beryllium	^{10}Be	β^-	2.5×10^6 yr
Carbon	^{14}C	β^-	5,730 yr
Sodium	^{22}Na	β^+, γ	2.6 yr
Silicon	^{32}Si	β^-	650 yr
Phosphorus	^{32}P	β^-	14.3 days
Phosphorus	^{33}P	β^-	24.4 days
Sulfur	^{35}S	β^-	88 days
Chlorine	^{36}Cl	β^+, β^-, γ	3.1×10^5 yr

[a] β^-—negatron or beta particle; β^+—positron; γ—gamma ray; e^-—electron; χ—x rays

TABLE 3   Some Mean Values for Radium, Thorium, and Potassium-40[a] Content in Various Rocks and in Soil[1 a]

Type of Rock	^{226}Ra (g/g $\times 10^{12}$)	^{232}Th (g/g $\times 10^6$)	^{40}K (g/g $\times 10^2$)
Igneous or plutonic rocks			
Acidic rocks (>65% SiO_2)			
granite	3.1	20	0.04
granodiorite	2.7	18	0.03
Intermediate rocks (65–55% SiO_2)			
diorite	1.4	6	0.02
Basic rocks (<55% SiO_2)			
gabbro	0.9	5	0.008
basalt	1.0	9	0.015
peridotite	0.5	3	0.009
Sedimentary rocks			
sandstones	0.7	6	0.01
shales	1.1	10	0.03
limestones	0.4	1.3	0.003
alum shales	60.0	1.5	0.04
Soil			
United States, type unspecified	0.09–0.8	—	0.001–0.04

[a] Potassium-40 levels calculated for K values.

long-lived ^{238}U and ^{232}Th; their shorter-lived daughter products ^{226}Ra and ^{228}Ra; ^{40}K; and the cosmic-ray-produced nuclides.

Natural radionuclides, such as ^{40}K, ^{228}Ra, and ^{232}Th, are generally found to be more concentrated in acidic rocks (e.g., granites and grano-diorite) than in basic rocks (e.g., gabbro, basalt, and peridotite) (Table 3). Limestone and sandstones are generally low in radionuclide content, but certain shales may be more radioactive, especially those containing organic matter. Marine sediments appear to contain more radioactivity than do nonmarine or estuarine deposits. In various countries, there are large local deposits of uranium ore and monazite, the principal thorium-bearing mineral.

Potassium, relatively abundant in nature, contains 0.0118% radio-active ^{40}K. The potassium content of soils is estimated to range from about 10^{-3} to 3×10^{-2} g K/g soil, which represents 1–30 pCi ^{40}K/g soil.*

Radium-226, one of the daughter products of ^{238}U, has been found to vary between 0.09 and 0.8 pCi/g soil in the United States. Where-ever there are uranium or thorium minerals in soil, their respective short-lived gaseous daughter products, ^{222}Rn and ^{220}Rn, accumulate in soil and rocks. They diffuse into the air at a variable rate, depending upon many factors of soil and climatic conditions. Although these gaseous radionuclides can deliver a radiation dose directly to the lungs and other tissues, they do not make a significant contribution via the food chain.

The concentration of ^{210}Pb, the long-lived decay product of ^{222}Rn, and its daughter ^{210}Po, should be low in the troposphere because of removal by precipitation. In contrast, ^{14}C, which is produced in the at-mosphere, is incorporated into all living things on earth. Experimental determinations of the specific activities† of natural ^{14}C in the biosphere have ranged from 12.9 to 15.3 disintegrations/min/g of carbon. Tritium

---

*Amounts of radioactive material are expressed in units related to the curie (Ci), where 1 Ci represents an amount of a radionuclide that undergoes 3.7×10^{10} disintegrations/sec.

> 1 curie (Ci) = 1,000 millicuries (mCi)
> 1 millicurie (mCi) = 1,000 microcuries (μCi)
> 1 microcurie (μCi) = 10^6 picocuries (pCi)

†Specific activity—The measured radioactivity of a given radionuclide per unit (usu-ally in metric weight) of a specific chemical compound or tissue; or, the measured radioactivity per unit of mass, or atomic number, of the same stable element; or, the measured radioactivity per mass, or atomic number, of a stable element that is closely related biochemically or chemically. The amount of radioactivity is usually expressed in curies or fractions of curies.

also is continuously produced in the atmosphere and enters the biosphere. The tritium content of molecular hydrogen in the troposphere of the middle-latitude regions of the northern hemisphere in 1949–1951 was about 30 pCi/g hydrogen. Nuclear weapons tests have added both ^{14}C and ^{3}H to the atmosphere.

The other radionuclides produced in the atmosphere (Table 2) are present in much lower amounts and contribute no significant radiation dose by ingestion to the human population.

NATURAL RADIOACTIVITY IN WATER

The natural radioactivity in various types of water is highly variable, depending upon origin and treatment. Certain natural springs in areas of high soil levels of uranium and thorium have high levels of radioactivity originating from these elements.

Public water supplies are of interest as a possible source of radioactivity for the population. Table 4 presents some data on the concentrations of ^{226}Ra and ^{222}Rn in various public water supplies. Drinking water supplies may also contain ^{232}Th and its decay products. In a comparison of well waters from Illinois, it was found that ^{226}Ra concentrations ranged from 3 to 36 pCi/liter, whereas ^{228}Ra ranged from 0.9 to 7.9 pCi/liter. Table 5 presents some values for concentrations of ^{238}U, ^{226}Ra, and ^{222}Rn in various natural waters and springs. Spring waters may have high concentrations of ^{222}Rn, but, since this radionuclide has only a

TABLE 4   Radium-226 and Radon-222 in Public Water Supplies[1b]

Location	^{226}Ra (pCi/liter)	^{222}Rn (pCi/liter)
Austria (Bad Gastein)	0.6	–
Germany	0.03–0.3	≤220
Sweden	0.2–1	–
U.K.		
ground and surface water	≤0.7	≤200
Cornish waters	≤2.4	≤3,000
Devon waters	–	≤13,000
United States		
tap water	≤0.2	–
deep sandstone well	≤37	–
surface water	<0.2	–
U.S.S.R., fresh water	1	–

TABLE 5 Uranium-238, Radium-226, and Radon-222 in Natural Waters and Springs[1b]

Location	^{238}U (pCi/liter)	^{226}Ra (pCi/liter)	^{222}Rn (pCi/liter)
Austria, springs	⩽4	–	⩽10^5
France, springs	–	⩽139	⩽10^5
Germany			
river water	–	0.07–0.8	–
springs	–	0.07–18	⩽10^3
Japan, springs	⩽0.3	–	⩽7×10^5
Lebanon, springs	–	–	⩽6×10^3
U.K.			
river water	–	0.01	0.2–0.3
springs	–	⩽12	⩽7×10^2
United States			
river water	0.005–0.01	0.03	–
lake water	1.7	–	–
groundwater	⩽40	⩽22	–
springs	–	–	⩽3×10^5
U.S.S.R., springs and			
brooks	⩽3	–	–

mean life in the body of about 1 h, the resulting radiation dose is small.

The levels of natural radioactivity in seawater in terms of pCi/liter are about as follows: ^{40}K, 300; ^{87}Rb, 3; uranium series, 3; ^3H, 0.6–3.

NATURAL RADIOACTIVITY IN FOODSTUFFS

Natural radioactivity in soil and water reaches man by way of the food chain. There is little or no information on the routes and mechanisms of the transfer of naturally occurring radionuclides through the various links of the food chain. Knowledge is limited almost entirely to a few observations of concentrations of some of these substances in various food products.

Data are available on the total alpha-particle activity of foods; values vary from less than 1 to 1.7×10^4 pCi/kg food. In general, values are low for milk products, fruits, and vegetables but high for cereals and nuts. Total intakes vary according to proportions of various food components that are eaten; however, it has been estimated that an adequate Western diet is not likely to contain less than 2–5 pCi of alpha activity/day. This is not deemed to be a serious hazard.

RADIUM-226 AND ITS DESCENDANTS

Radium-226 reaches man largely by way of foodstuffs, except for a very few regions in the world where the drinking water has unusually high levels. Because ^{226}Ra is a divalent cation, it follows calcium metabolically and tends to concentrate in the bones. Measurements of total body burdens of ^{226}Ra in human bones from New York City, San Francisco, and San Juan have been estimated at 35 pCi, 30 pCi, and 19 pCi of alpha particles, respectively. A value of 30 pCi ^{226}Ra has been suggested as typical of the body burden in areas of normal intakes. The concentration of ^{226}Ra in human bones is independent of age or sex but is governed by the intake; the total body burden increases with growth of the skeleton. The estimated whole-body and bone dose from ^{226}Ra and decay products is 0.5 and 0.6 mrad/yr, respectively.

The average total intake of ^{226}Ra varies little within the United States (Table 6). About 75% is derived from foods of plant origin and the remainder largely from animal products (Table 7).

Radon-222, the first descendant of ^{226}Ra, is a noble gaseous element with a short half-life (3.8 days). Only a small amount is ingested as such in food and water. The principal source of ^{222}Rn in the body is from the decay of consumed ^{226}Ra that has been trapped in the bone crystals. Therefore, the alpha-ray exposure due to this isotope is largely delivered to the cells lining the bone and to the bone marrow. A small amount reaches the lungs and is expired; some is dissolved in body lipids. The whole-body dose to man from ^{222}Rn is estimated to be 0.3 mrad/yr.

Lead-210 and ^{210}Po, in equilibrium, have been found in certain ani-

TABLE 6   Average Amount of Radium-226 in the Diet in Several Cities, 1964–1967[11]

Location	pCi/kg of Diet
Boston, Massachusetts	0.52
Palmer, Alaska	0.54
Chicago, Illinois	0.58
Idaho Falls, Idaho	0.58
Seattle, Washington	0.61
Denver, Colorado	0.61
Cleveland, Ohio	0.62
Burlington, Vermont	0.62
Honolulu, Hawaii	0.64
Wilmington, Delaware	0.70
Pittsburgh, Pennsylvania	0.73

TABLE 7   Radium-226 in Foodstuffs in U.S. Diet, 1963[1b]

Food	New York City (pCi/yr)	Chicago (pCi/yr)	San Francisco (pCi/yr)
Milk	51	46	46
Cereal, whole grain, and bakery products	206	277	187
Eggs, meat, poultry, and fish	141	134	102
Vegetables	263	181	161
Fruits	177	102	110
Water	6	10	4
TOTAL	844	750	610

mal foods, plants (grasses), and in some seafoods that are consumed directly by man. It is most likely that these isotopes are not, because of the relatively long half-lives of several of their lineal precursors, derived from metabolized or ingested ^{226}Ra but are ingested directly by the plant or sea animal. The whole-body dose from ^{210}Po is estimated to be 0.3 mrad/yr; the bone dose is estimated to be 2 mrad/yr.

Values for the ^{226}Ra content of foodstuffs collected in New York City, Chicago, and San Francisco are given in Table 7. It was estimated that the average daily intake of ^{226}Ra from all foodstuffs, including water, in these three cities in 1962 was about 2.3, 2.1, and 1.7 pCi, respectively. Studies of infant diets in New York City suggest that the intake by infants during their first year of life would be about 0.6 pCi/day, of which about one third comes from milk and one half from cereals. The ^{226}Ra contents of a wide variety of foods in Germany have been reported to range from 0.1 to 6 pCi/kg, which is in general agreement with the data of Table 7 for the United States.

RADIUM-228 AND ITS DESCENDANTS

No evidence has been found for the presence in foodstuffs of ^{232}Th, the long-lived parent of the thorium chain; nevertheless, ^{228}Th, a daughter in the series, has been found. Since the metabolic uptake of thorium is known to be poor, it is postulated that ^{228}Ra, a continuously produced daughter of ^{232}Th, is taken up metabolically, and within the biological system ^{228}Th and other daughters are produced. The average ratio of ^{228}Th/^{226}Ra in bone ash has been found to vary between 0.25 and 0.4. An average body burden of 10 pCi ^{228}Th has been suggested.

POTASSIUM-40

As mentioned earlier, ^{40}K is present as a constant percentage (0.0118%) of all potassium. The ^{40}K content of food and the relative contribution of various foods to the dietary ^{40}K can thereby be estimated from data on total potassium. The ^{40}K intake for the United States has been estimated to be about 2,300 pCi/day. The whole-body dose from ^{40}K is estimated to be 17 mrad/yr.*

CARBON-14

The amount of ^{14}C has markedly increased in the biosphere because of fission and fusion thermonuclear testing (Table 8). Because of the long half-life of ^{14}C and the fact that man-made additions are of the order of natural levels, it is necessary to take into account the actual levels (nat-

TABLE 8   Percent Increase in the Carbon-14 of the Tropospheric Air of the Northern Hemisphere[1d,1e]

Year	Percent over Pretest Values
1956	5
1957	11
1958	16
1959	24
1960	23
1961	25
1962	30
1963	65
1964	92
1965	90
1966	78
1967	65

*Definitions of commonly used ionizing radiation are:

Roentgen (R)—The unit for measurement of ionizing radiation in air. It is equal to 2.58 × 10^{-4} coulomb/kg air, or about 83 ergs/g air.

Absorbed dose (rad)—The unit for measurement of ionizing radiation in any medium, excluding air. It is equal to 0.01 joule/kg matter, or about 100 ergs/g tissue.

Roentgen equivalent, man (rem)—A unit of dose equivalence. It is equal to the rad multiplied by a quality factor (sometimes called relative biological effectiveness) and any other modifying factor or factors.

ural plus artificial) when attempting any correlations from the late 1950's on.

Atmospheric ^{14}C is almost exclusively in the form of carbon dioxide and is utilized by plants in photosynthesis to become incorporated in all living things. There seems to be little geographic variation in the concentrations of ^{14}C over the United States. Little attention has been given to metabolic patterns of ^{14}C in foodstuffs because, essentially, the specific activity of ^{14}C in foods, and even in the population (except for lag times of up to a year), will be the same as that existing in the atmosphere. The specific activity of tropospheric carbon dioxide is estimated to have been about 14.5 disintegrations/min/g carbon (6.6 pCi/g) before nuclear testing.

HYDROGEN-3 (TRITIUM)

The primary interest in tritium is in connection with the amounts that may be produced from the nuclear power industry and added to those already present from natural production processes and the testing of atomic weapons. A rough idea of the comparative amounts can be gained from the following[5,9]:

Natural production	4–8 MCi/yr
Production from nuclear testing to date	1,700 MCi
Estimated production in a free-world nuclear power economy in the year 2000	15 MCi/yr

By about the year 1990 the levels in the biosphere from each source will be roughly equal, assuming no further testing, the continued development of nuclear power as presently envisaged, and the release of all tritium generated. It is probable that improved technology can in the future reduce the contribution of the nuclear-power industry to the biosphere.

It is conventional to express tritium levels in terms of the number of hydrogen atoms in the sample; the term "tritium ratio" (formerly called tritium unit), defined as the number of tritium atoms per 10^{18} atoms of hydrogen, is a measure of specific activity. It presently is less than 100 (Table 9).

Three important principles govern the movement of tritium in the environment and the body burdens to be acquired by man: (a) Practi-

TABLE 9 Concentration of Tritium[a] in Precipitation and Estimated Body Burden in Ottawa, Canada[12]

Year	Tritium Ratios in Precipitation	Estimated Body Burden (pCi)
Natural level to 1952	5	700
1953	20	2,700
1954	130	17,000
1955	45	6,000
1956	140	19,000
1957	110	15,000
1958	800	110,000
1959	350	47,000
1960	140	19,000
1961	180	24,000
1962	900	120,000
1963	3,000	400,000
1964	1,600	200,000
1965	900	120,000
1966	500	67,000
1967	400	54,000
1968	200	27,000

[a] One tritium ratio in a liter of water is equal to 3.2 pCi.

cally all tritium, regardless of how or where it is released, ends up in the form of water as part of the hydrosphere; (b) the specific activities in the body water and tissues of man will essentially be the same as that in his foodstuffs and water or essentially the same as in the biosphere; (c) when tritium is released to the biosphere, its specific activity thereafter cannot increase; it can only be decreased by dilution with hydrogen.

An example of tritium concentration in precipitation and body burdens showing the effects of atomic testing is presented in Table 9. The amount of tritium in precipitation tends to be greater in higher latitudes and higher altitudes, as shown in Table 10. The average total-body exposure of man by tritium is less than 1 mrem/yr.

AREAS OF HIGH NATURAL RADIOACTIVITY

In some of the midwestern states concentrations of ^{226}Ra in drinking water reach 1–10 pCi/liter, which has led to levels of ^{226}Ra in bone three to four times higher than in "normal" areas. Radium activities in plants grown in certain areas of Brazil with high terrestrial radioactivi-

TABLE 10   Tritium Ratios in Precipitation in the
United States, 1963 Averages[13]

Location	Tritium Ratios
Palmer, Alaska	2,950
Menlo Park, California	480
Salt Lake City, Utah	3,670
Denver, Colorado	3,110
Albuquerque, New Mexico	1,870
Lincoln, Nebraska	2,280
Madison, Wisconsin	2,510
Bismarck, North Dakota	4,370
St. Louis, Missouri	1,560
Baton Rouge, Louisiana	830
Boston, Massachusetts	1,410
Washington, D.C.	1,130
Ocala, Florida	620
San Juan, Puerto Rico	240

ties contribute to concentrations of ^{226}Ra in teeth of inhabitants two to three times higher than those in "normal" areas. Skeletal levels of ^{226}Ra in these areas are probably similarly elevated. In Kerala State in India, where there are large monazite deposits, five samples of human bones analyzed showed average concentrations of radium higher by one order of magnitude than those from "normal" areas.

High concentrations of ^{210}Pb and ^{210}Po have been found in lichens and in caribou and reindeer meat in Arctic areas. Members of populations consuming these animal products have been shown to have tissue concentrations 8–10-fold higher than those found in the northern temperate zone.

IMPORTANCE TO MAN

A major interest is the relative contribution of natural radioactive materials to the radiation dosage received by the human population. The radiation dosages represent the combined effect of the extent of occurrence, the efficiency of transport through the food chain, and pattern of retention in the body. Table 11 presents a summary of radiation dosages from external and internal natural sources in "normal" areas. It should be noted that irradiation from internally deposited sources contributes about 22 mrad/yr out of a total of 100 mrad/yr. Of the internal emitters, ^{40}K is by far the most important, with lesser contributions

TABLE 11   Dose Rates Due to External and Internal Irradiation from Natural Sources in "Normal" Areas[1d]

Source of Irradiation	Dose Rates (mrad/yr)		
	Gonads	Cells Lining Bone Surface[a]	Bone Marrow
External irradiation			
Cosmic rays			
Ionizing component	28	28	28
Neutrons	0.7	0.7	0.7
Terrestrial radiation (including air)	50	50	50
Internal irradiation			
^{40}K	20	15	15
^{87}Rb	0.3	<0.3	<0.3
^{14}C	0.7	1.6	1.6
^{226}Ra	−	0.6	0.03
^{228}Ra	−	0.7	0.03
^{210}Po	0.3	2.1	0.3
^{222}Rn (dissolved in tissues)	0.3	0.3	0.3
TOTAL[b]	100	99	99
Percentages from alpha particles and			
neutrons	1.3	4.4	1.4

[a] The dose rates under this heading were actually calculated for the Haversian canals of bone. Doses to cells lining bone surfaces may be somewhat lower than those quoted here.

[b] Totals have been rounded off to two significant figures.

made by ^{87}Rb, ^{14}C, ^{226}Ra, ^{228}Ra, ^{210}Po, ^{222}Rn (plus decay products), and even lower contributions by those not listed, such as ^{3}H.

Table 12 gives the radiation-dose commitment from nuclear tests carried out before 1968. In comparing exposures from natural sources, it should be remembered that the values in Table 12 are total doses to be delivered over many years—up to the year 2000 for ^{14}C, for example (i.e., the dose commitment). The following estimates are given by Spiers[10] for the year 1963 for the radiation dose from fallout to cortical bone, in mrad/yr: ^{137}Cs, 2.0; ^{14}C, 0.3; ^{90}Sr (child), 11.6; ^{89}Sr (child), 10; external, 5; total, approximately 29.

SUMMARY

To recapitulate and to put into perspective the matter of human radiation exposure by those things that man ingests, we should compare the

TABLE 12 Dose Commitments from Nuclear Tests Carried Out before 1968[1e]

Source of Irradiation	Dose Commitments (mrad)		
	Gonads	Cells Lining Bone Surfaces	Bone Marrow
External irradiation			
Short-lived	23	23	23
^{137}Cs	23	23	23
Internal irradiation			
^{137}Cs	21	21	21
^{14}C[a]	13	16	13
^{90}Sr	–	130	64
^{89}Sr	–	<1	<1
TOTAL[b]	80	220	140

[a] Only the doses accumulated up to year 2000 are given for ^{14}C; the doses from the other nuclides will have essentially been delivered in full. The total dose commitment to the gonads and bone marrow due to the ^{14}C from tests up to the end of 1967 is about 180 mrad and that to cells lining bone surface is about 230 mrad.

[b] Totals have been rounded off to two significant figures.

radiation exposures received from various man-made and natural sources.[14] The external exposure of man from terrestrial sources has decreased slowly since his origin on earth. It presently ranges from 30 to about 115 mrem/yr in the United States, with an average of about 60. Cosmic rays have varied considerably over geologic time but have been relatively constant for the past 25,000 yr. They presently contribute from 30 to 130 mrem/yr to man's burden, depending upon his location on the earth. Exposures are higher in higher altitudes, and for the United States the average is about 45 mrem/yr. Since the appearance of man or man-like beings on earth, variations in his total natural radiation background have been more closely related to the place he lived than to changes in the amount of cosmic radiation.

The natural internal radiation exposure of man, at the present time, is contributed from various natural radionuclides. Potassium-40 contributes the greatest amount, i.e., about 17 mrem/yr to the whole body; ^{14}C about 1 mrem/yr; and tritium (^{3}H) less than 1 mrad/yr. The nuclides ^{210}Po, ^{222}Rn, ^{226}Ra, and ^{228}Ra contribute about 37 mrem/yr to the endostial cells and 6 mrem/yr to the whole body.

Nuclear weapons fallout had two peaks, one in 1959 and another in 1963. At those times, peak external-exposure levels in the middle latitudes of the northern hemisphere reached about 20 mrem/yr. By 1970 the exposure from fallout had declined to about 4 mrad/yr.

Medical use of radiation, largely in diagnostic procedures, has contributed in the past an average exposure of about 100 mrems/yr to the individual in the United States. The current contribution from the nuclear-power industry is substantially below an average of 1 mrad/yr to individuals in the entire U.S. population. Modern developments in reactor technology show promise that these levels need not be exceeded, even with the prospective increase in the number of power reactors. Other sources of radiation from occupational and miscellaneous activities such as television sets, jet aircraft flights, and luminous dial watches, do not contribute more than a few mrad/yr, at the most, to the population average.

In conclusion, radiation from ingested internal emitters (approximately 20–25 mrad/yr) is about 25% of the average natural background and about 10% of the average background plus medical and other sources in the United States. There is little that can be done to reduce the natural radiation exposures arising from dietary intakes without destroying the quality of the food. In any event, there is little question that the harm from radiation so avoided would be far outweighed by the deleterious effects of the manipulation of diets.

REFERENCES

1. United Nations Scientific Committee on the Effects of Atomic Radiation, Report, General Assembly, New York.
   a. 13th Session, Suppl. No. 17 A/3838 (1958).
   b. 17th Session, Suppl. No. 16 A/5216 (1962).
   c. 19th Session, Suppl. No. 14 A/5814 (1964).
   d. 21st Session, Suppl. No. 14 A/6314 (1966).
   e. 24th Session, Suppl. No. 13 A/7613 (1969).
2. R. S. Russell (ed.), Radioactivity and the human diet. Pergamon Press, London (1966).
3. National Research Council, Radionuclides in foods. National Academy of Sciences, Washington, D.C. (1962).
4. R. A. Dudley, Natural and artificial radiation background of man. In Low-level irradiation, A. M. Brues (ed.). American Association for the Advancement of Science, Washington, D.C. (1959).
5. D. G. Jacobs, Sources of tritium and its behavior upon release to the environment. TID-24635. U.S. Atomic Energy Commission, Division of Technical Information, Oak Ridge, Tenn. (1968).
6. J. A. S. Adams and W. M. Lowder (eds.), The natural radiation environment. University of Chicago Press, Chicago (1964).
7. S. Glasstone (ed.), Sourcebook on atomic energy. Van Nostrand, Princeton, N.J. (1958).
8. R. E. Lapp and H. L. Andrews, Nuclear radiation physics. Prentice-Hall, Englewood Cliffs, N.J. (1963).
9. H. T. Peterson, Jr., J. E. Martin, C. L. Weaver, and E. D. Harward, Environ-

mental tritium contamination from increasing utilization of nuclear energy sources. In Environmental contamination by radioactive materials. International Atomic Energy Agency, Vienna (1969).

10. F. W. Spiers, Radioisotopes in the human body: Physical and biological aspects. Academic Press, New York (1968).

11. B. Shleien, Evaluation of Radium-226 in total diet samples, 1964–June 1967, Radiol. Health Data Rep. *10*:547–549 (1969).

12. Quarterly Health Physics Reports of Atomic Energy of Canada, Ltd., 1953–1968.

13. G. L. Stewart and C. N. Hoffman, Tritium rainout over United States in 1962–1963. U.S. Geological Survey, Circ. No. 520 (1966).

14. P. G. Gustafson, Environmental radiation, past, present, and future. Inst. Electr. Electron. Eng. Trans. Nucl. Sci. *NS-19*:104–106 (1972).

15. C. M. Lederer, J. M. Hollander, and I. Perlman, Table of isotopes. 6th ed. Wiley, New York (1967).

5 Werner G. Jaffé

TOXIC PROTEINS AND PEPTIDES*

INTRODUCTION

If one considers the varied biological activities of many proteins and peptides such as enzymes, hormones, transport proteins, and antigens, it is not surprising that some members of this large group of substances should exhibit toxic actions in organisms other than those in which they had been produced. Indeed, several proteins—bacterial toxins, snake venoms, and plant toxins (ricin)—are among the most toxic agents known.

The proteins are essential constituents of nearly all foods. Therefore, a discrimination among the nutritional effects caused by amino acid deficiency or imbalance, poor digestibility, and toxic effects may be difficult. Moreover, additional factors, such as protein inhibition of digestive enzymes, may play an important if still unknown role in determining whether or not a certain protein can exert a harmful action.

Most animals have evolved detoxification mechanisms against the action of foreign proteins. In a certain sense the immunological defense mechanisms can be regarded as such, although they may lead to the opposite effect, i.e., hypersensitivity and allergic reactions. Another defense mechanism is gastrointestinal digestion. Although it serves the

*Literature reviewed to March 1970.

106

purpose of primarily transforming foods into components that can be absorbed through the intestinal wall, it simultaneously destroys the native structure of ingested proteins and peptides, abolishing their biochemical activities and possible toxicities.

Toxicity may be detected, therefore, in certain proteins or peptides existing in foods if they enter the body by other than the oral route or if they resist digestive destruction. They might possibly contain toxic constituents not destroyed by digestion, like selenium, or the proteinaceous substances might act in some way on the food product before it is ingested, as in the destruction of vitamins by certain enzymes.

The specific biological activity of practically all proteins is destroyed by heat, although considerable differences exist between proteins with respect to their rate of heat inactivation. Consequently, most food products, if properly prepared, can be consumed without harmful effect. Notable exceptions are some of the allergy-producing foods, which will be dealt with later on, and the selenoproteins.

The mode of action of most of the toxic proteins is still obscure. In some cases specific *in vitro* activities can be detected, and considerable efforts have been made to relate these to *in vivo* effects. Some of the better known groups of proteins with recognized toxic or antinutritional action are bacterial toxins, animal toxins, hemagglutinins, enzyme inhibitors, vitamin-binding proteins (avidin), vitamin-destroying enzymes, enzymes releasing toxic compounds, and selenium-containing proteins. Not all are discussed in this chapter. For further information on the other toxins the reader should refer to other chapters in this volume.

HEMAGGLUTININS

Hemagglutinins are proteins that have the interesting ability to clump or agglutinate red blood cells (RBC) in a fashion similar to antibodies. Moreover, like antibodies, they show a remarkable specificity in that they may act in high dilution on one kind of erythrocyte and not at all or only weakly on another. Each specific hemagglutinin is therefore clearly different from all others and must be studied individually; the results obtained with one kind cannot be applied to another without verification. Also, the chemical composition of different hemagglutinins may be quite different from one another, as discussed later in this chapter.

Hemagglutinins have been found mostly in plants. Because of the specificity of their action on RBC from different animals, Boyd and Shapleigh[1] have proposed the term *lectins* from the latin word *legere*, to choose. Plant hemagglutinins are sometimes referred to as phyto-hemagglutinins, frequently abbreviated simply as PHA.

A small number of similarly acting substances of animal origin have been studied from snails and fish eggs,[2] slugs,[3] sponges,[4] and others. The term *protectins* has been proposed to designate these compounds[5] because they are believed to confer protections against bacterial infection. Nothing is known about their possible toxic action in humans, and they will therefore not be treated further in this chapter.

Occurrence and Nature of Plant Hemagglutinins

Hemagglutinins have been found in a great number of plants and in different plant organs or parts.[6] The first to be recognized was the very toxic ricin from castor beans, which was described as early as 1889 by Stillmark in a paper that led to all later work in this field.[7] The most interesting group of lectins from the standpoint of nutrition is that found in legumes; this group was discovered in 1908 by Landsteiner and Raubitschek.[8]

Between 1890 and 1910 a remarkable number of outstanding research papers was published relating to phytohemagglutinins, including studies of their toxicity and specificity. This early work has been reviewed by Ford.[9] Later, interest in this group of substances declined until Boyd and Reguera[10] and Renkonen[11] discovered the existence of specific hemagglutinins for different human blood groups. In 1960 Nowell described their stimulating effect on mitosis of cultured human leucocytes.[12] Since then the number of papers published on different *in vitro* and *in vivo* effects of phytohemagglutinins has increased enormously and is still rising rapidly. The effects studied include stimulation of DNA, RNA, and protein synthesis in cell cultures[13]; effect on immunorepression[14]; protein–carbohydrate interaction[15]; their use in the investigation of the structure of specific receptor sites in erythrocytes and other cells[16]; and specific interaction with cancer cells.[17] Nevertheless, our knowledge of the toxicity of phytohemagglutinins and of the cause of their toxic action has advanced relatively little in the last 50 yr. Some review articles on the nutritional aspects of phytohemagglutinins have appeared recently.[18,19,20]

A number of edible fruits, seeds, or tubers contain agglutinins. Examples include potatoes,[21] bananas,[22] mangoes,[22] and wheat germ,[23] but nothing is known about their possible toxic action.

By far, however, the most studied group in this respect are the legumes. Many leguminous seeds contain other toxic factors, especially enzyme inhibitors, besides lectins. These different protein factors are not easily separated from each other, and the extraction and precipitation procedures used for fractionation of toxic seed extracts often will not yield pure products. It is important, therefore, that the different biochemical activities be simultaneously measured in such fractions in order to be able to draw valid conclusions on the relative importance of the hemagglutinins and any other toxicants that might be present. Unfortunately, interpretation of numerous published experiments is difficult, because this precaution has been disregarded.

As proteins, the phytohemagglutinins are heat labile. Normal cooking destroys their specific action. If the nutritional value of a plant product is not enhanced by cooking when tested in a nutritionally complete experimental diet, and if the presence of an agglutinin can be demonstrated in this product, it is safe to conclude that this specific agglutinin is nontoxic for the animal species used, at least at the concentration present in the test diet. Thus, the growth-promoting value of peas, lentils, and peanuts is not significantly improved by heat treatment. Indeed, the isolated hemagglutinin from peas did not exert a significant action on the growth of rats when 1% was included in a test diet.[24]

On the other hand, if the food value of a hemagglutinin-containing plant product is improved by heating, it cannot be concluded that this improvement is due to the destruction of the hemagglutinin. Other factors may be involved: destruction of enzyme inhibitors or heat improvement of the digestibility of proteins may enhance food value.

Still another problem exists in experimental work on toxic phytohemagglutinins. Because of the specificity of their action, standard tests with human or rabbit blood may fail to detect the hemagglutinating activity of some extracts or protein fractions. Therefore, before claims on the separation of agglutinating and nonagglutinating toxic factors are made, it is advisable that a thorough study on the possible hemagglutinating action of the fractions be undertaken with different blood types.

Legume Hemagglutinins

Soybean Hemagglutinin Heated soybeans cause better growth than raw soybeans when fed in an experimental diet to rats or chicks. This fact, known for over 50 yr, points to the existence of heat-labile, toxic factors in these beans. Indeed, it is well established that several enzyme inhibitors and hemagglutinins can be found in soybeans, but their respective effects on the nutritional value is still an object of discussion.

A phytohemagglutinin of the soybean has been studied extensively by Liener and his coworkers.[19] In 1953, Liener and Pallansch[25] isolated a protein from soybeans that agglutinated rabbit blood cells at high dilution. This particular hemagglutinin, although shown to be homogeneous by several criteria, is apparently only one of at least four hemagglutinins subsequently shown by chromatographic separation to be present in soybeans.[26] All of these proteins seem to be quite similar in composition and physicochemical properties. The amount of hemagglutinin present in soybean protein has been estimated by immunochemical methods to be about 3% by Liener and Rose.[27]

When isolated soybean agglutinin was injected into rats, the LD_{50} was found to be in the order of 50 mg/kg,[25] indicating a relatively high toxicity compared to that of the orally ingested agglutinin. Given in an experimental diet to rats at the level of 1%, the hemagglutinin depressed growth to about 75% of normal, but no lethal effect was observed.[28] The oral ingestion of raw soybeans or protein fractions prepared from them has never been demonstrated to have a lethal effect on any animal species tested. The isolated agglutinin was given by stomach tube to rats in the amount of 500 mg/kg without producing death of the animals.[27]

The low toxicity of the soybean agglutinin when given orally, as compared to its rather high toxicity when injected, is noteworthy, because the observations with other bean agglutinins are quite different. The LD_{50} of hemagglutinin of black bean (*Phaseolus vulgaris*)[29] when injected is similar to that of the soybean agglutinin. Diets containing raw beans or orally administered bean agglutinin cause loss of weight and death of the rats.[30] Different susceptibility to digestion could possibly account for the difference in oral toxicity of these hemagglutinins, since the soybean agglutinin is inactived *in vitro* by pepsin[31]; the bean agglutinin is relatively resistant to this enzyme,[32] and hemagglutinating action can be detected in the feces of rats after the ingestion of raw beans.[33] A portion of the soybean agglutinin may nevertheless withstand gastric digestion, which may thus account for its moderate oral toxicity. This aspect of the problem awaits further investigation.

Unheated soybean meal increases the animals' requirements for certain vitamins, minerals, and other nutrients, compared to heated soy protein. Although nothing is known about the exact nature of the responsible factors, their heat lability points to their proteinaceous nature. The hemagglutinin of kidney beans (*Phaseolus vulgaris*) reduces intestinal absorption and will be discussed later in this chapter. The soybean hemagglutinin may exert a similar effect when raw soybeans are fed to animals, but this point has not been investigated in any detail.

Rats fed a diet containing raw soybeans develop enlarged thyroid glands.[34] This effect may be destroyed by steaming the soybeans. The goitrogenic effect of soybeans is readily overcome by adding supplemental iodine to the diet.[35] Several workers have reported cases of goiter in human infants fed soy milk.[36,37] Fecal loss of thyroxine was observed in rats fed raw soybeans, which may be attributed to the fact that reabsorption of thyroxine from the gut, where it has been excreted via the bile, is inhibited.[38]

Reduced amino acid absorption through the intestinal wall can be observed in rats fed raw soybeans.[39] Low fat absorption due to the presence of raw soybean fractions in an experimental diet has likewise been described.[40] This effect may be related to the increased fecal excretion of bile acids in chicks fed a raw soybean diet.[41] Evidence for increased requirement for the fat-soluble vitamins A,[42] D,[43] and K,[44] in animals subsisting on a raw soybean diet has also been presented. For example, turkey poults suffered severe rickets when fed a soy-protein glucose ration, even though the diet contained normally adequate levels of vitamin D_3, calcium, and phosphorus. Growth and tibia ash were improved by an increase of vitamin D_3 or by the replacement of the unheated soybean protein by heated soybean meal.[43] Likewise, unheated soybean protein increased the vitamin D_2 requirement of baby pigs.[45] The enhanced requirement for vitamin K in chicks receiving unheated soybean meal[44] has been attributed to the use of trichlorethylene in the extraction procedure.[46] Vitamin B_{12} in amounts that support normal growth in animals on a control diet was insufficient when a diet containing unheated soymeal was fed.[47] Recent results seem to exclude the explanation that an impairment in absorption plays a role in producing a deficiency of this vitamin in rats fed unheated soybean flour, but the real cause is not clear.[48]

The reasons for the increased requirements for some nutrients in animals fed diets containing unheated soy protein remain to be elucidated. Although in some cases crude preparations of trypsin inhibitor have been found to decrease intestinal absorption,[39] the possibility exists that these inhibitor fractions may have also contained hemagglutinins and other proteins[49] that complicate the issue.

The existence of other unindentified, heat-labile, toxic factors in soybeans was suggested by Stead *et al.*[50] because they found that two of the protein fractions separated by chromatography on DEAE-cellulose were toxic when injected into rats. Only one of them, however, had significant hemagglutinating activity when tested with rabbit blood. After extraction of the soluble proteins from soy flour, the residue was still not capable of supporting normal growth if not submitted to heat treatment.[51] An unidentified growth-depressing factor can be released by papain digestion from extracted soybean meal.[52] The possible presence of a toxic peptide fraction from soybeans will be discussed later in this chapter.

No other foodstuff has been reported to produce as many antinutritional effects as the soybean.[53] Is this because this legume is exceptionally rich in different heat-labile toxicants or because no other foodstuff has been tested so thoroughly? If the latter alternative is indeed true, one might expect many more unrecognized toxicants in foods that have not received as much detailed study.

Other Bean Hemagglutinins   Hemagglutinins have been purified from extracts of black beans,[32] red beans,[30] yellow wax beans,[54] and other varieties of *Phaseolus vulgaris.*[55,56] In most cases, at least two different hemagglutinating factors were present and could be separated by electrophoresis or chromatography. Two hemagglutinins differing in molecular weight and amino acid composition were isolated from a particular variety of *P. vulgaris* grown in Sweden.[56] In general, most of the hemagglutinins isolated from different varieties of *P. vulgaris* have molecular weights ranging from 91,000 to 130,000; differences in isoelectric points, however, have been observed.[56]

The toxic properties of these purified preparations have been studied in only a few cases. Thus, Honavar *et al.* observed a marked inhibitory effect on the growth of rats fed a diet containing purified kidney-bean agglutinin at a level of 0.5%.[30] All animals died within 2 weeks of ingestion of this diet. An agglutinin isolated from black beans was likewise toxic when fed to rats or when injected into mice.[29] In the latter case, the LD_{50} was about 50 mg/kg. The black-bean agglutinin was found to be somewhat less toxic than that obtained from red kidney beans.[30]

Diets containing unheated, ground kidney beans cause loss of weight, and their ingestion usually results in death of the experimental animals. Food consumption is very low, and most of these animals have diarrhea. Balance studies have shown that overall digestibility and nitrogen retention are low in rats ingesting raw bean diets, compared with animals kept on a diet prepared with properly heated beans.[29] The extracted residue of the bean meal from which the hemagglutinin had been prepared retained part of the toxicity of the original material, since it reduced the growth of rats when added to a casein diet.[29]

The supplementation of a raw bean diet with predigested casein had no beneficial effect on growth and survival of rats, an observation that was interpreted to mean that the trypsin inhibitors present in the beans were not responsible for the toxic manifestations.[57] In similar experiments, diets prepared with bean varieties with strong hemagglutinating activity produced the effects already described (i.e., rapid weight loss and death of the rats), whereas diets containing nonhemagglutinating bean meals had no lethal action and permitted slow growth. The addition of predigested casein resulted in normal growth in the latter case but was without effect when used in a diet prepared with hemagglutinin-containing bean meal.[33]

Notwithstanding the evidence cited for the toxicity of the bean hemagglutinins, there are several claims for a partial separation of the toxic and hemagglutinating activities of beans[50,58,59] and for lack of correlation between toxic and hemagglutinating activities measured simultaneously in a number of different bean species and varieties.[60] These observations do not allow the conclusion that bean hemagglutinins are nontoxic, but they are consistent with the assumption that there may be present other unidentified heat-labile and toxic factors in raw beans.

Recent observations of differences between hemagglutinins from various bean varieties in specificity, heat resistance, and toxicity may help to explain some of these contradictory observations.[61] By the use of rabbit red blood cells (RBC) and trypsin-activated cow RBC, it is possible to distinguish four types of bean hemagglutinins, because the extracts of some bean samples agglutinate only one of these blood preparations, both of them, or none at all. Toxicity tested by IP injection of extracts into mice and by addition of the ground beans to experimental diets of rats was detected only in the bean varieties containing the hemagglutinins active with trypsin-activated cow RBC. Heating to 85 °C for several hours did not destroy the toxicity and the action on cow blood cells, but the action on rabbit blood cells disappeared. Cooking the soaked beans 1 h at 100 °C destroyed toxicity and hemagglutinating activity completely.

Treatment with proteolytic enzymes has been recommended for the reduction of the cooking time required for the preparation of beans.[62] Mixtures of ground beans with ground cereals are being used in infant feeding programs in order to raise the protein intake and to achieve an optimal proportion of these ingredients.[63] These mixtures are quite palatable after a relatively short cooking time at 90 °C. Too-short cooking of partially precooked bean flakes produced a serious outbreak of poisoning in Berlin.[64]

The toxicity of bean products will depend on the heat treatment they have received. Some of the intermediary stages of toxicity may not be easily detected. Before new bean products are used in industrial procedures or feeding programs, it is advisable that the heat treatment required for complete destruction of toxic factors be established by careful investigations.

Other Legume Hemagglutinins   Field beans or hyacinth beans (*Dolichos lablab*) are consumed in India, Africa, and some parts of South America. They show a degree of toxicity similar to that of kidney beans when fed to rats. A hemagglutinin obtained from these seeds produced loss of weight and death of rats when given in amounts of 1.5 or 2.5% in a casein diet. Necropsy revealed focal liver necrosis in these animals.[65]

Lima beans or double beans (*Phaseolus lunatus*) contain two blood-group-A-specific hemagglutinins.[66] A partly purified preparation of a lima-bean agglutinin reduced growth of rats when fed with a casein diet but did not produce death under these conditions. When injected into rats or mice, this preparation was lethal at a dose of 65 and 140 mg/kg, respectively, but a highly purified preparation was less toxic.[67]

Another anti-A-group-specific hemagglutinin has been isolated from the horse gram (*Dolichos biflorus*).[68] Rats fed with a diet containing horse gram showed greatly retarded growth and did not survive for more than 3 weeks,[69] but these effects were not observed when autoclaved material was used. A crude hemagglutinin preparation had a growth-retarding effect, but the purified hemagglutinin was innocuous when parenterally administered to rats or mice.[70]

Properties of Hemagglutinins

Degree of Toxicity   The experimental animal species used for testing, the route of administration, and even the age of the test animals may be responsible for different toxic effects. Hemagglutinin purified from kidney beans and added to a rat diet caused loss of weight and death,[30] but in similar experiments with chicks no lethal action was detected.[71] Rats or chicks fed diets prepared with unheated soybean meal as the only source of protein grow fairly well, although less than animals given heated soy meal; mice kept on a raw soy diet may lose weight,[72] as do calves fed a lightly cooked soy-flour milk replacer.[73] It has not been proved, however, that the factor causing body-weight loss in these cases is the soybean hemagglutinin.

Among the legume seeds that contain measurable amounts of hemagglutinins,[74] and that will show no or only a minimum improvement of food value after heating, are peas (*Pisum sativum*), red gram (*Cajanus cajan*), and lentils (*Lens culinaris*).[18] The different degrees of oral toxicity of soybean and kidney-bean agglutinins have been mentioned already. The most toxic hemagglutinins of the edible legumes are those of kidney beans and the field beans. In human diets prepared with well-cooked beans of either kind, no toxic effects have been observed. The uncooked beans are highly unpalatable.

Mode of Toxic Action of Hemagglutinins It seems likely that both the hemagglutinating and the toxic actions are related to the ability of these plant proteins to react with certain receptor groups of the membrane of the target cells.[17] Only those plant agglutinins capable of interaction with receptors of cells of certain animal species would be expected to be toxic for the corresponding animals. The cancerostatic action of several hemagglutinins (described below) may be an example of such a specific cell toxicity.

Interaction of hemagglutinins from kidney beans with the cells lining the gut has been postulated as an explanation for their oral toxicity.[29] The adsorption of bean agglutinin on the mucosal cells of rat intestine can be shown in *in vitro* experiments.[29] Their resistance to digestion in the animal is easily demonstrated by the hemagglutinating activity of extracts from feces of rats after they ingested a raw bean diet.[33] As mentioned, reduced intestinal nitrogen absorption can be observed in rats fed a raw bean diet.[29] Glucose absorption from a ligated intestinal loop is low, compared to the control animals previously given blackbean agglutinin by stomach tube.[75] Rats fed a bean diet may experience severe hypoglycemia, which could be caused by poor absorption of glucose.[77] Evidence for interference of raw beans with aminoacid absorption and for the reduced utilization of vitamin E in chicks[76] has been presented.[57] It has been mentioned above that raw soybeans may also interfere with the absorption of various nutrients.

The food intake of animals fed raw beans, soybeans, or field beans is impaired. This may be related to slow stomach emptying.

The fact that the different phytohemagglutinins react in a specific manner with different receptor groups existing on the surface of cells makes them valuable tools for the investigation of those groups and, at the same time, may offer a clue to their toxicity. The observation of receptor groups for lectins on cancer cells, their appearance during cancerous transformation in cell cultures,[78] and the anticancerous effect of various phytohemagglutinins merit special interest. Thus, Nungester and Van Halsema[79] found that bean extracts may interact with Flexner–Jabling carcinoma cells of rats; Steck and Wallach[17] found purified bean PHA to react with Ehrlich ascites carcinoma of mice. Concanavalin A, the agglutinin from the jack bean (*Canavalia ensiformis*), has a definite cancerostatic action in mice inoculated with a cancer-producing virus,[78] and the trypsin-treated lectin inhibits *in vivo* growth of cancer cells.[80] Ricin and abrin, the agglutinins from the castor bean and from the seeds of *Abrus precatorius,* respectively, suppress Ehrlich ascites tumor growth in mice[81]; the wheat-germ hemagglutinin reacts with some kinds of cancerous cells as well as with some normal cells.[82] The receptor groups of the cancer-cell surface may also exist on normal cells. It is, therefore, likely that some of the hemagglutinins may interact with some normal cells, resulting in a toxic effect, but this effect would be more difficult to prove experimentally than is the case with the cancer cells.

Chemical Properties   Until now most plant hemagglutinins obtained in pure form have been carbohydrate-containing proteins; the only exception is concanavalin A from the jack bean, which is free of sugars.[83] Only two plant hemagglutinins are known to contain sulfhydryl groups: the lima-bean agglutinin[84] and that of the meadow mushroom *Agarius campestris.*[85] Among the hemagglutinins obtained in pure form from edible legumes are soybean,[26] black beans,[32] wax bean,[54] lentil,[86] pea,[24] lima bean,[66] horse gram,[68] *Vicia cracca,*[87] and peanut.[88] In most of these seeds several hemagglutinins with very similar characteristics are present. The agglutinins from kidney beans[89] and from the jack bean[90] can be dissociated into subunits by urea.

The kidney-bean agglutinin is probably a lipid-containing protein, as is shown by the staining of the corresponding immunoprecipitates.[91] In two plant hemagglutinins, concanavalin A from the jack bean[92] and the agglutinin from lentils,[93] significant amounts of calcium and manganese exist as constituents essential for the activity. Many plant hemagglutinins are remarkably stable against the action of a great number of proteolytic enzymes.

Detection

Hemagglutinins are detected in the extracts of ground seeds prepared with physiological saline solution by their action in serial dilution on washed R B C. A microdilution test has been used in many of the recent papers on phytohemagglutinins.[87] A photometric method was proposed by Liener.[94] As all phytohemagglutinins are more or less specific, the choice of the right kind of blood cells is important. Treatment of the red cells with proteolytic enzymes often enhances the sensitivity of the assay. Pronase has been found to be well suited for this purpose in most cases.[95] For the soybean agglutinin, rabbit blood is the most satisfactory, but for the kidney-bean agglutinins, trypsin-activated cow blood and rabbit blood should be used, because some types of these agglutinins are detected by only one of these blood types and not by the other.[61] The agglutinins from horse gram (*Dolichos biflorus*) and from lima beans will agglutinate only human-group-A blood. Some agglutinins are active at low temperature but will not give a positive reaction at 37 °C.[74]

It should be remembered that a positive agglutination test does not necessarily distinguish between toxic and nontoxic hemagglutinins. The test is most useful for the detection of agglutinins in seed varieties or fractions suspected to be toxic. In special cases a distinction between toxic and nontoxic agglutinins may be possible, as has been mentioned for the kidney bean.

ALLERGENIC FOODS

Many people show more or less violent local or generalized reactions after ingestion of certain foods or contact with certain types of proteinaceous material, i.e., pollen, which does not produce harm in other persons. The nature of these allergic reactions is not yet fully understood, notwithstanding the tremendous amount of research devoted to the subject. Unlike effects from other food toxins, the intensity of this reaction will depend not so much on the quantity of the food ingested as on the sensitivity of the affected person. The allergens are, therefore, not toxic food constituents in the general sense, and the reason for the toxic action rests rather with the individual who has an altered reactivity (allergy). For this reason, allergens will be treated only very briefly here; the interested reader is referred to an extensive review by Mansmann in the first edition of this book[96] and to other recent review articles.[97,98,99]

Allergy is a rather common affliction. It has been estimated that about 20% of American schoolchildren suffer some kind of allergy.[100] Most foods have been reported to induce allergy in some people; exceptions are fats, pure sugar, and salt. Common causes of food allergy are grains, milk, eggs, fish, crustaceans, tomatoes, strawberries, nuts, chocolate, and many others. Milk allergy has been studied mostly in children. Diarrhea, abdominal pain, and vomiting are the most common symptoms.[101] Although the exact nature of the allergens in foods is generally unknown, they are probably mostly proteins.[102] In some cases, but not in all, heating to 120 °C for 30 min will abolish allergenicity.[103] The best way to avoid food allergies is the complete elimination of the offending product from the diet. Desensitization and the use of various specially developed drugs are other therapeutic measures sometimes used to alleviate the suffering of the allergic patient.

The allergic reaction is brought about by a certain type of antibody called reagins, but the reagin titer is not always correlated with the patient's sensitivity. There is considerable evidence for a hereditary factor in human allergy, although little is known about specific genetic factors that cause allergy in humans. While most organs can be involved in allergic reactions, the most commonly affected are the skin and the respiratory tract. The predominant characteristic of reagins is their ability to become fixed to the skin or to other tissues. A recently discovered class of immunoglobulin, IgE, appears to be the skin-sensitizing antibody in man.[104] By far the most commonly employed procedure for the detection of food allergens is the skin test, performed by superficial scarification or by intradermal injection of extracts of the suspected products, which will result in a wheal or flare reaction. Such other methods as the dietary history and elimination diets are also used for diagnostic purposes.

CELIAC DISEASE

Celiac disease is a malabsorption syndrome mostly seen in children but that can also be observed in adults. Although the exact cause is unknown, it is clearly related to the ingestion of wheat products and specifically of gluten.[105] Indeed, the complete elimination of gluten-containing foods from the patient's diet is the most important therapeutic measure, and relapse after ingestion of a test dose of gluten is an important diagnostic sign. In the celiac patient a normal food protein has a toxic effect, a situation similar to that for food allergies. In adults a gluten-sensitive enteropathy is often referred to as nontropical sprue, idiopathic steatorrhea, or adult celiac disease.

The mucosa of biopsy samples of the jejunum taken from celiac patients is flat, and the villi are small or absent.[106] Abnormally large amounts of fat are present in the stool, and the absorption of many other nutrients, such as amino acids, glucose, vitamins K, B_{12}, and others is impaired. Celiac disease may therefore lead to a state of advanced malnutrition. Not only wheat but also rye, barley, and oats may be harmful to patients with celiac disease, and milk also is often not well tolerated. A gluten-free diet must be observed, often for many years.[107] A secondary deficiency of the intestinal enzymes, disaccharidase and peptidase, has often been observed.[108] Gluten is not well digested,[109] and the oligopeptides derived from gluten may cause intestinal lesions.[110] When different peptides obtained through *in vitro* digestion of gluten are tested in celiac patients, important differences are observed in their ability to elicit the pathological signs characteristic of celiac disease.[111]

From immunological studies the absorption of antigenic derivatives of gluten into intestinal epithelium has been postulated.[112] A hereditary factor may be involved in the susceptibility to this syndrome.[113]

SELENIUM-CONTAINING PROTEINS

Selenium is abundant in some types of soil and is absorbed by most plants more or less efficiently. Thus it can accumulate in diverse foods. (See Chapters 3 and 7.) It may be incorporated into amino acids, replacing sulfur atoms, and these seleno–amino acids may then be incorporated into proteins. If the selenium concentration is high enough, these products may produce toxic effects. From dialysis experiments with extracts of wheat and other cereals, it was concluded many years ago that selenium may be present in protein-bound form.[114] Olson *et al.* showed that wheat with a high selenium content contains seleno-methionine in the gluten, but it contains no seleno-cystine.[115] The selenium in defatted sesame seeds is also present in the seed proteins,[116] and the major part of selenium in fish can be recovered in the protein fraction.[117]

The occurrence of selenium-containing proteins in edible plant products is of special significance when these materials are used for the preparation of protein isolates, because in this way the toxic selenium may inadvertently be concentrated. This possibility should be kept in mind when oilseed products are processed for high-protein foods, particularly since the seleno-proteins cannot be rendered harmless by heat processing.

ENZYMES

Because of their specific activity on biological compounds, some enzymes can produce toxic effects, but only very few are important in foods. They may act through the decomposition of such essential constituents as the vitamins, or they may liberate toxic compounds.

Among the first group, the thiamine-destroying enzymes, called thiaminases, may be mentioned. They have been found in bracken fern, *Pteridum aqualinum*,[118] which is sometimes eaten by horses or cattle, in fish, especially the carp,[119] and the sardine,[120] and in some crustaceans.[118]

A lipoxygenase that oxidizes and destroys carotene has been observed in soybeans.[121] Low blood values of vitamin A and carotene have been found in the liver and blood of calves fed a diet containing raw soybeans, but the importance of the lipoxygenase in causing these low vitamin blood levels has not been ascertained.[42]

Great amounts of urease are found in some legume seeds, notably in the jack bean (*Canavalia ensiformis*) and to a lesser degree in the soybean. This enzyme may produce toxic effects when ingested by animals[122] and is highly toxic when injected, because it will liberate ammonia from the blood urea. Its harmful action may be of importance only when urea is used in feed for cattle or sheep.

Several foods contain cyanogenetic glucosides. (See Chapter 14, p. 300.) Specific glucosidases that are frequently present in the same products release the highly toxic hydrocyanic acid from these compounds. This release is enhanced when the plant products are crushed and soaked in water.

Intestinal β-glucosidase may release the toxic methylazoxymethanol from the glucoside cycasin that exists in plants of the cycad family.[123] In these cases, the enzyme acts in releasing a toxic factor, and it is a matter of semantics whether or not one should call it toxic.

TOXIC PEPTIDES

Peptides are often not recognized in complex biological materials because they are lost in many of the fractionation procedures, especially if these include prolonged dialysis. This may be the reason only few toxic peptides have been identified in food products. In a recent study of the toxic principles of raw soybeans, Schingoethe *et al.*[72] observe that a fraction separated from a crude preparation of the soybean trypsin inhibitor had a growth-inhibitory activity when fed to mice. By its retardation on a Sephadex G-25 column and its passage through dialysis membranes the peptide nature of this product was indicated. The presence of at least eight positively charged peptides, one of which was a glycopeptide, could be shown by high-voltage electrophoresis.

A highly toxic cyclic peptide called islanditoxin has been isolated from so-called yellow rice, that is, rice infected with the mold *Penicillium islandicum*.[124] It contains β-aminophenylalanine, two molecules of serine, aminobutyric acid, and a dichlorinated proline. Islanditoxin is a highly toxic carcinogenic hepatoxin, but removal of the chlorine atoms gives a nontoxic product. Feeding of low amounts of rice infected with *P. islandicum* induces liver cirrhosis in experimental animals.

Collection of wild mushrooms for the purpose of eating them is a popular hobby not free of danger. Knowledge of the edible and inedible varieties should be an indispensable prerequisite, because mistakes may have a fatal outcome. By far the most common cause of mushroom poisoning is the ingestion of species belonging to the genus *Amanita,* which might be confused with the edible champignon. They contain a variety of very toxic peptides, the structure of which has been elucidated mostly by the work of Wieland and his collaborators.[125,126,127]

Two groups of peptides called phallotoxins and amatoxins can be distinguished. Phallotoxins are cyclic heptapeptides, and amatoxins are comprised of closely related cyclic octapeptides. Both have several unusual characteristics. There is a thioether formed between a L-cysteine and L-tryptophan in the phallotoxins, while in the amatoxins these two amino acids are united in a sulfoxide structure. The phallotoxins contain hydroxyamino acids derived from L-leucine, while the amatoxins contain derivatives of γ-hydroxyisoleucine.

The two groups of toxins show striking differences in their respective biological actions; amatoxins are much more toxic than the phallotoxins. Since both groups of peptides are present at approximately the same concentration in poisonous species of *Amanita,* the poisonous nature of these mushrooms must be attributed mainly to the amatoxins.

The organ affected by both groups of peptide toxins from mushrooms is the liver.[128] The toxins have been identified in liver extracts from fatal human cases of intoxication.[129] Phalloidin has a marked affinity for the microsomal fraction of the liver, as has been shown with labeled toxins.[130] It is interesting that phalloidin acts only if administered to the intact animal. It seems likely, therefore, that it is converted into an unknown toxic substance by some metabolic process.

The toxic action of amatoxins appears considerably later after ingestion than that of phallotoxins, and the nuclei are the part of the liver cell mostly affected.

Islanditoxin[123]

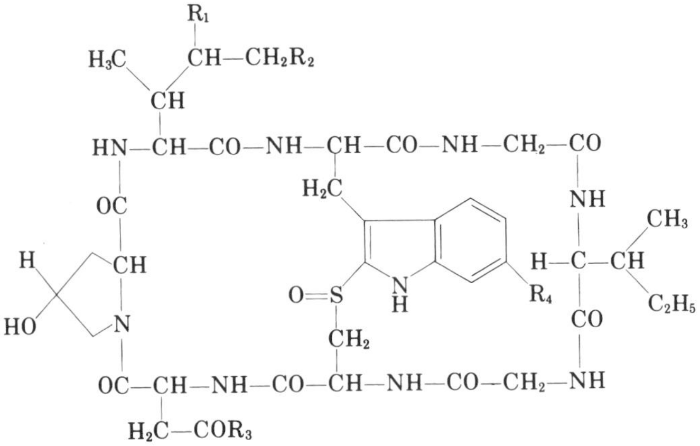

Amatoxins[125]

	R_1	R_2	R_3	R_4
α-Amanitin	OH	OH	NH_2	OH
β-Amanitin	OH	OH	OH	OH
γ-Amanitin	H	OH	NH_2	OH
Amanin	OH	OH	OH	H
Amanullin	H	H	NH_2	OH

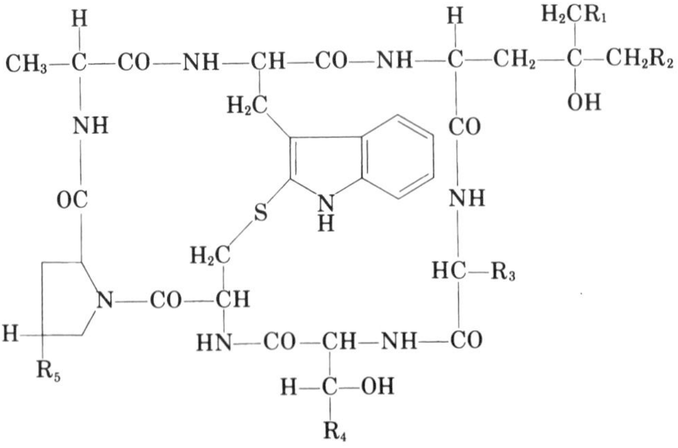

Phallotoxins[125]

	R_1	R_2	R_3	R_4	R_5
Phalloidin	OH	H	CH_3	CH_3	OH
Phalloin	H	H	CH_3	CH_3	OH
Phallisin	OH	OH	CH_3	CH_3	OH
Phallicidin	OH	H	$CH(CH_3)_2$	COOH	OH
Phallin B	H	H	$CH_2C_6H_5$	CH_3	H
(tentatively)					

Several other biologically active principles exist in mushrooms of the *Amanita* family, but they are not peptides and seem to be of little importance relative to toxicity. The poisonous *Amanita* mushrooms contain about 10–15 mg of both toxins per 100 g fresh weight. A single mushroom weighing 50 g may contain enough toxins to kill a man.

REFERENCES

1. W. Boyd and E. Shapleigh, Specific precipitating activity of plant agglutinins (lectins). Science *119*:419 (1954).
2. O. Prokop, G. Uhlenbruck, and W. Köhler, A new class of antibody-like substances having anti-blood group specifity. Vox Sang. *14*:321 (1961).
3. R. T. Pemberton, Haemagglutinins from the slug *Limax flavus*. Vox Sang. *18*: 74 (1970).
4. R. Y. Dodd, A. P. Maclennan, and D. C. Hawkins, Haemagglutinins from marine sponges. Vox Sang. *15*:386 (1968).
5. O. Prokop, G. Uhlenbruck, and W. Köhler, Protectine eine neue Klasse antikörperähnlicher Verbindungen. Dtsch. Gesundheitswes *23*:318 (1968).
6. J. Tobishka, Die Phythämagglutinine. Akademie Verlag, Berlin (1964).
7. H. Stillmark, Uber Ricin. Arch. Pharmakol. Inst. Dorpat *3*:59 (1889).
8. K. Landsteiner and H. Raubitschek, Beobachtungen über Hämolyse und Hämagglutination. Zent. Bakteriol. Parasitenkd. Abt. II Orig. *45*:660 (1908).
9. W. W. Ford, Plant poisons and their antibodies. Zent. Bakteriol. Parasitenkd. Abt. I Ref. *58*:129, 193 (1913).
10. W. C. Boyd and R. M. Reguera. Hemagglutinating substances for human cells in various plants. J. Immunol. *62*:333 (1949).
11. K. O. Renkonen. Studies on the hemagglutinins present in seeds of some representatives of the family of Leguminosae. Ann. Med. Exp. Fenn. (Helsinki) *26*:66 (1948).
12. P. Nowell, Phytohemagglutinin: An initiator of mitosis in cultures of normal human leucocytes. Cancer Res. *20*:462 (1960).
13. J. P. P. V. Monojardino and A. J. Mac Gillivray, RNA and histone metabolism in small lymphocytes stimulated by phytohemagglutinin. Exp. Cell Res. *60*: 1 (1970).
14. M. W. Elves, Suppression of antibody production by phytohaemagglutinin. Nature *213*:495 (1967).
15. E. E. Smith, Z. H. Gunja Smith, and I. J. Goldstein, Protein-carbohydrate interaction. Biochem. J. *107*:715 (1968).
16. M. Krüpe, Blutgruppen-spezifische pflanzliche Eiweisskörper (Phytagglutinine). Ferdinand Enke Verlag, Stuttgart (1956).
17. T. L. Steck and D. F. H. Wallach, The binding of kidney bean phytohemagglutinin by Ehrlich ascitis carcinoma. Arch. Biochem. Biophys. *97*:510 (1965).
18. I. E. Liener, Toxic factors in edible legumes and their elimination. Am. J. Clin. Nutr. *11*:281 (1962).
19. I. E. Liener, Seed hemagglutinins. Econ. Bot. *18*:27 (1964).
20. W. G. Jaffé, Hemagglutinins. In Toxic constituents of plant foodstuffs, I. E. Liener (ed.). Academic Press, New York (1969).

21. M. Krüpe and A. Ensgraber, Untersuchungen über die Natur der Phytoagglutinine in chemischer, immunochemischer und pflanzenphysiologischer Sicht III. Analytische Studien am Agglutinin aus der Kartoffelknolle (*Solanum tuberosum*). Behringwerk Mitt. *42*:48 (1962).

22. V. A. Tiggelmann-van Krugten, C. M. Ostendorf-Doyer, and W. A. Collier, Uber Haemagglutinin in Pflanzenextrakten. Antonie van Leuwenhoek J. Microbiol. Serol. *22*:289 (1956).

23. R. Liske and D. Franks, Specifity of the agglutinin in extracts of wheat germ. Nature *217*:860 (1968).

24. S. V. Hupriker and K. Sohonie, Haemagglutinins from Indian pulses II. Purification and properties of haemagglutinin fractions isolated from white pea (*Pisum sp.*). Enzymologia *28*:333 (1965).

25. I. E. Liener and M. J. Pallansch, Purification of a toxic substance from defatted soy bean flour. J. Biol. Chem. *197*:29 (1952).

26. H. Lis, C. Fridman, N. Sharon, and E. Katchalski, Multiple hemagglutinins in soybeans. Arch. Biochem. Biophys. *117*:301 (1966).

27. I. E. Liener and J. E. Rose, Soyin, a toxic protein from the soybean III. Immunochemical properties. Proc. Soc. Exp. Biol. Med. *83*:539 (1953).

28. I. E. Liener, Soyin, a toxic protein from the soybean I. Inhibitor of rat growth. J. Nutr. *49*:527 (1953).

29. W. G. Jaffé, Uber Phytotoxine und Bohnen, Arzneim. Forsch. *10*:1012 (1960).

30. P. M. Honavar, C. V. Shih, and I. E. Liener, The inhibition of growth of rats by purified hemagglutinin fractions isolated from *Phaseolus vulgaris*. J. Nutr. *77*:109 (1962).

31. I. E. Liener, Inactivation studies on the soybean hemagglutinin. J. Biol. Chem. *233*:401 (1958).

32. W. G. Jaffé and K. Hannig, Fractionation of proteins from kidney beans (*Phaseolus vulgaris*). Arch. Biochem. Biophys. *109*:80 (1965).

33. W. G. Jaffé and C. L. Vega Lette, Heat-labile growth inhibiting factors in beans (*Phaseolus vulgaris*). J. Nutr. *94*:203 (1968).

34. G. R. Sharpless, J. Pearsons, and G. S. Proto, Production of goiter in rats with raw and with treated soybean flour. J. Nutr. *17*:545 (1939).

35. R. J. Block, R. H. Marel, H. W. Howard, C. D. Bauer, and D. M. Anderson, The curative action of iodide on soybean goiter and the changes in the distribution of iodoamino acids in the serum and in thyroid gland digests. Arch. Biochem. Biophys. *93*:15 (1961).

36. J. I. Vanwyk, M. B. Arnold, J. Wynn, and F. Pepper, The effect of a soybean product on thyroid function in humans. Pediatrics *24*:752 (1959).

37. J. D. Hydowitz, Occurrence of goiter in an infant on a soy diet. N. Engl. J. Med. *262*:351 (1960).

38. R. N. Beck, Soy flour and fecal thyroxine loss in rats. Endocrinology *62*:587 (1958).

39. H. J. H. de Muelenaere, Studies on the digestion of soybeans. J. Nutr. *82*:197 (1964).

40. M. C. Nesheim, J. D. Garlich, and D. T. Hopkins, Studies on the effect of raw soybean meal on fat absorption in young chicks. J. Nutr. *78*:89 (1962).

41. J. A. Serafin and M. C. Nesheim, Influence of dietary heat-labile factors in soybean meal upon bile acid pools and turnover in the chick. J. Nutr. *100*:786 (1970).

42. J. C. Shaw, L. A. Moore, and J. F. Sykes, The effect of raw soybeans on blood

plasma carotene and vitamin A and liver vitamin A of calves. J. Dairy Sci. *34*: 176 (1951).

43. C. W. Carlson, H. C. Saxena, L. S. Jansen, and J. McGinnis, Rachitogenic activity of soybean fractions. J. Nutr. *82*:507 (1964).

44. S. L. Balloun and E. L. Johnson, Anticoagulant properties of unheated soybean meal in chick diets. Arch. Biochem. Biophys. *42*:355 (1953).

45. E. R. Miller, D. E. Ullrey, C. L. Zutaut, J. A. Hoefer, and R. L. Luecke, Comparison of casein and soy proteins upon mineral balance and vitamin D_2 requirements of the baby pig. J. Nutr. *85*:347 (1965).

46. P. Griminger, W. D. Morrison, and H. M. Scott, Effect of unheated soybean meal on blood coagulation of chicks. Poult. Sci. *35*:911 (1959).

47. R. Frolich, Relation between the quality of soybean oil meal and the requirements of vitamin B_{12} for chicks. Nature *173*:132 (1954).

48. S. Edelstein and K. Guggenheim, Causes of the increased requirement for vitamin B_{12} in rats subsisting on an unheated soybean flour diet. J. Nutr. *100*: 1377 (1970).

49. A. C. Eldridge, R. L. Anderson, and W. J. Wolf, Polyacrylamide-gel electrophoresis of soybean whey proteins and trypsin inhibitors. Arch. Biochem. Biophys. *115*:495 (1966).

50. R. H. Stead, H. J. H. de Muelenaere, and G. V. Quicke, Trypsin inhibition, haemagglutination and intraperitoneal toxicity of *Phaseolus vulgaris* and *Glycine max.* Arch. Biochem. Biophys. *113*:703 (1966).

51. A. Gertler, Y. Birk, and A. Bondi, A comparative study of the nutritional and physiological significance of pure soybean trypsin inhibitors and of ethanol-extracted soybean meals in chicks and rats. J. Nutr. *91*:358 (1967).

52. R. Borchers, Bound growth inhibitor in raw soybean meal. Proc. Soc. Exp. Biol. Med. *112*:84 (1963).

53. O. Mickelson and M. G. Yang, Naturally occurring toxicants in foods. Fed. Proc. *25*:104 (1966).

54. T. Takahashi, P. Ramachandramurthy, and I. E. Liener, Some physical and chemical properties of a phytohemagglutinin isolated from *Phaseolus vulgaris*. Biochim. Biophys. Acta *133*:123 (1967).

55. D. A. Rigas and E. E. Osgood, Purification and properties of the phytohemagglutinin of *Phaseolus vulgaris*. J. Biol. Chem. *212*:607 (1955).

56. K. Dahlgren, J. Porath, and K. Lindahl-Kiessling, On the purification of phytohemagglutinins from *Phaseolus vulgaris* seeds. Arch. Biochem. Biophys. *137*: 306 (1970).

57. W. G. Jaffé, Toxicity of raw kidney beans. Experientia *5*:81 (1949).

58. M. L. Kakade and R. J. Evans, Growth inhibition of rats fed navy bean fractions. J. Agric. Food Chem. *13*:470 (1965).

59. M. L. Kakade and R. J. Evans, Growth inhibition of rats fed navy beans. J. Nutr. *90*:191 (1966).

60. H. J. H. de Muelenaere, Toxicity and haemagglutinating activity of legumes. Nature *206*:827 (1965).

61. W. G. Jaffé and O. Brücher, Relación entre poder hemaglutinante y toxicidad en frijoles. II., Arch. Latinoam. Nutr. *22*:267 (1972).

62. B. S. Bhatia, L. A. Ramanathan, M. S. Prasad, and P. K. Vijayaraghavan, Use of papain in the preparation of quick cooking dehydrated pulses and beans. Food Tech. *21*:1395 (1967).

63. K. W. King, W. Fougère, J. Foucould, G. Dominique, and I. D. Beghin, Re-

sponse of pre-school children to high intake of Haitian cereal-bean mixtures. Arch. Latinoam. Nutr. *16*:53 (1966).

64. C. Griebel, Erkrankungen durch Bohnenflocken (*Phaseolus vulgaris*) und Platterbsen (*Lathyrus tingitanus L*). Z. Lebensm. Untersuch. Forsch. *90*:191 (1950).

65. R. S. Salgarkar and K. Sohonie, Haemagglutinins of field bean (*Dolichos lablab*): Part II—Effect of feeding field bean haemagglutinin A on rat growth. Ind. J. Biochem. *2*:197 (1965).

66. N. R. Gould and S. L. Scheinberg, Isolation and partial characterization of two anti-A hemagglutinins from *Phaseolus lunatus*. Arch. Biochem. Biophys. *137*:1 (1970).

67. A. L. Joshi, Studies in proteins of double bean (*P. lunatus*) with special reference to its hemagglutinins. Toxicon *10*:89 (1972).

68. M. E. Etzler and E. A. Kabat, Purification and characterization of a lectin (plant hemagglutinin) with blood group A specificity from *Dolichos biflorus*. Biochem. *9*:869 (1970).

69. P. K. Ray, Nutritive value of horse gram (*Dolichos biflorus*). I. Effect of feeding raw and treated seed flour on the growth of rats. J. Nutr. Diet. *6*:329 (1969).

70. L. D. Manage, Studies on nutritive value and hemagglutinins of horse gram, *Dolichos biflorus*. Ph.D. Thesis, University of Bombay (1969).

71. P. V. Wagh, D. F. Klaustermeier, P. E. Waibel, and I. E. Liener, Nutritive value of red kidney beans (*Phaseolus vulgaris*) for chicks. J. Nutr. *80*:191 (1963).

72. D. J. Schingoethe, S. D. Aust, and J. W. Thomas, Separation of a mouse growth inhibitor in soybean from trypsin inhibitors. J. Nutr. *100*:739 (1970).

73. B. M. Colvin and H. A. Ramsey, Soy flour in milk replacers for young calves. J. Dairy Sci. *51*:898 (1968).

74. S. V. Huprikar and K. Sohonie, Haemagglutinins in Indian pulses: Part I—Detection of haemagglutinins and effect of autoclaving and germination on haemagglutinin activity. J. Sci. Ind. Res. *20C*:82 (1961).

75. W. G. Jaffé and G. Camejo, La acción de una proteína tóxica aislada de caraotas negras (*Phaseolus vulgaris*) sobre la absorción intestinal en ratas. Acta Cient. Venez. *12*:59 (1961).

76. H. F. Hintz and D. E. Hogue, Kidney beans (*Phaseolus vulgaris*) and the effectiveness of vitamin E for prevention of muscular dystrophy in the chick. J. Nutr. *84*:283 (1964).

77. H. F. Hintz, D. E. Hogue, and L. Kroog, Toxicity of red kidney beans (*Phaseolus vulgaris*) in the rat. J. Nutr. *93*:77 (1967).

78. J. Shoham, M. Inbar, and L. Sachs, Differential toxicity on normal and transformed cells in vitro and inhibition of tumor development in vivo by concanavalin A. Nature *227*:1244 (1970).

79. W. J. Nungester and G. Van Halsema, Reaction of certain phytoagglutinins with Flexner Jabling carcinoma cells of the rat. Proc. Soc. Exp. Biol. Med. *83*:863 (1953).

80. M. M. Burger and K. D. Noonan, Restoration of normal growth by covering agglutinin sites on tumor cell surface. Nature *228*:512 (1970).

81. J. Y. Lin, K. Y. Tserng, C. C. Cheng, L. T. Lin, and T. C. Tung, Abrin and ricin: New antitumor substances. Nature *227*:292 (1970).

82. G. Uhlenbruck, W. Gielen, and G. I. Pardoe, On the specificity of lectins with a broad agglutination spectrum. V. Further investigations on the tumor characteristic agglutinin from wheat germ lipase. Z. Krebsforsch. *74*:171 (1970).

83. H. O. J. Olsen and I. E. Liener, Some physical and chemical properties of con-canavalin A, the phytohemagglutinin of the jack bean. Biochemistry 6:105 (1967).

84. N. R. Gould and S. L. Scheinberg, Involvement of sulfhydryl groups in the activity of anti A hemagglutinins of *Phaseolus lunatus*. Arch. Biochem. Biophys. *141*:607 (1970).

85. H. J. Sage and S. L. Connet, Studies on a hemagglutinin from the meadow mushroom. J. Biol. Chem. *244*:4713 (1969).

86. I. K. McGregor and H. J. Sage, Purification and properties of a phytohemag-glutinin from the lentil. Fed. Proc. *27*:428 (1968).

87. K. Asberg, H. Holmen, and J. Porath, A nonspecific phytohemagglutinin found in *Vicia cracca*. Biochim. Biophys. Acta *160*:116 (1968).

88. J. M. Dechary, G. L. Leonard, and S. Corkern, Purification and properties of a non-specific hemagglutinin from *Arachis hypogaea* (peanut). Lloydia *33*: 271 (1970).

89. D. Rigas and C. Head, The dissociation of phytohemagglutinin of *Phaseolus vulgaris L.* by 8,0M urea and the separation of the mitogenic from the erythro-agglutinating activity. Biochem. Biophys. Res. Commun. *34*:633 (1969).

90. M. O. J. Olson and I. E. Liener, The association and dissociation of concanav-alin A, the phytohemagglutinin of the jack bean. Biochemistry *3*:3801 (1967).

91. A. Palozzo and W. G. Jaffé, Immunoelectrophoretic studies with bean proteins. Phytochemistry *8*:1255 (1969).

92. J. Yariv, A. J. Kalb, and A. Levitzki, The interaction of concanavalin A with methyl-α-D-glucopyranoside. Biochim. Biophys. Acta *165*:303 (1968).

93. M. Tichú, G. Entlicher, J. Koštiř, and J. Kocourek, Studies on phytohemag-glutinins, IV. Isolation and characterization of a hemagglutinin from the lentil, *Lens esculenta*. Moench. Biochim. Biophys. Acta *221*:282 (1970).

94. I. E. Liener, The photometric determination of the hemagglutinating activity of soyin and crude soybean extracts. Arch. Biochem. Biophys. *54*:223 (1955).

95. G. Uhlenbruck, Uber die Verwendung von Pronase in der Blutgruppenfor-schung. Arztl. Lab. *15*:174, 236 (1969).

96. H. C. Mansmann, Jr., Foods as antigens and allergens. In Toxicants occurring naturally in foods. 1st ed. National Academy of Sciences, Washington, D.C. (1966).

97. E. Blumink, Food allergy: The chemical nature of substances eliciting symp-toms. World Rev. Nutr. *12*:505 (1970).

98. F. Perlman, Allergens. In Toxic constituents of plant foodstuffs, I. E. Liener (ed.). Academic Press, New York (1969).

99. H. J. Sanders, Allergy, a protective mechanism out of control. Chem. Eng. News *48* (20):84 (1970).

100. H. I. Arbeiter, How prevalent is allergy among United States school children. Clin. Pediatr. *6*:140 (1967).

101. J. W. Gerrard, M. C. Lubos, L. W. Hardy, B. A. Holmund, and D. Webster, Milk allergy: Clinical picture and familial incidence. Can. Med. Assoc. J. *97*: 780 (1967).

102. J. J. Engelfried, Study in food allergy: The relationship between the allergic activity and protein fractionization of selected foods. J. Allergy *11*:569 (1940).

103. F. Perlman, Food allergy and vegetable proteins. Food Technol. *20*:1438 (1966).

104. K. Ishizaka, T. Ishizaka, and M. M. Hornbrook, Physicochemical properties

of human reaginic antibody. IV. Presence of a unique immunoglobulin as a carrier of reaginic activity. J. Immunol. *97*:75 (1966).

105. H. A. Weijers and J. H. van de Kamer, Some considerations of celiac disease. Am. J. Clin. Nutr. *17*:51 (1965).

106. N. Madanagopelau, M. Shiner, and B. Rowe, Measurements of small intestine mucosa obtained by peroral biopsy. Am. J. Med. *38*:42 (1965).

107. W. Sheldon, Prognosis in early adult life of coeliac children treated with a gluten-free diet. Brit. Med. J. *2*:401 (1969).

108. F. Lifshitz, A. P. Klotz, and G. H. Holman, Intestinal disaccharidase deficiencies in gluten-sensitive enteropathy. Am. J. Dig. Dis. *10*:47 (1965).

109. A. P. Douglas, Digestion of gluten peptides by normal jejunal mucosa and by mucosa from patients with adult coeliac disease. Clin. Sci. *38*:11 (1970).

110. H. D. Bronstein, L. J. Haefner, and O. Kowlessar, Enzymatic digestion of gliadin: The effect of the resultant peptides in adult celiac disease. Clin. Chim. Acta *14*:141 (1966).

111. M. Messer, C. M. Anderson, and L. Hubbard, Studies on the mechanism of destruction of the toxic action of wheat gluten in coeliac disease by crude papain. Gut *5*:295 (1964).

112. G. B. Malik, W. C. Watson, D. Murray, and B. Cruickshank, Immunofluorescent antibody studies in idiopathic steatorrhea. Lancet 1127 (1964).

113. W. C. MacDonald, W. O. Dobbins, and C. E. Rubin, Studies of the familial nature of coeliac sprue using biopsy of the small intestine. N. Engl. J. Med. *272*:448 (1965).

114. K. W. Franke and E. P. Painter, Selenium in proteins from toxic foodstuffs I. Remarks on the occurrence and nature of selenium present in a number of foodstuffs or their derived products. Cereal Chem. *13*:67 (1936).

115. O. E. Olson, E. J. Novacek, E. J. Whitehead, and I. S. Palmer, Selenium in wheat. Phytochemistry *9*:1181 (1970).

116. W. G. Jaffé, J. F. Chávez, and M. C. Mondragón, Contenido de selenio en muestras de semillas de ajonjolí (*Sesamum indicum*) procedentes de varios países. Arch. Latinoam. Nutr. *19*:299 (1969).

117. G. Lunde, Analysis of arsenic and selenium in marine raw materials. J. Sci. Food Agric. *21*:242 (1970).

118. A. Fujita, Thiaminase. Adv. Enzymol. *15*:389 (1954).

119. R. G. Green, W. E. Carlson, and C. A. Evans, The inactivation of vitamin B_1 in diets containing whole fish. J. Nutr. *23*:165 (1942).

120. W. G. Jaffé, Uber den Nährwert von Frischfisch, Fischkonserven und Fischmehl. Z. Lebensm. Unters. Forsch. *113*:472 (1960).

121. J. B. Sumner and A. L. Dounce, Carotene oxidase. Enzymologia *7*:130 (1939).

122. E. T. Kornegay, E. R. Miller, and J. A. Hoefner, Urease toxicity in growing swine. Anim. Sci. *24*:51 (1965).

123. M. G. Yang and O. Mickelson, Cycads. In Toxic constituents of plant foodstuffs, I. E. Liener (ed.). Academic Press, New York (1969).

124. J. R. Bamburg, F. M. Strong, and E. B. Smaley, Toxins from moldy cereals. J. Agric. Food. Chem. *17*:443 (1969).

125. T. Wieland, The toxic peptides of *Amanita phalloides.* Fortsch. Chem. Org. Naturst. *25*:214 (1967).

126. T. Wieland, Poisonous principles of mushroom of the genus *Amanita.* Science *159*:946 (1968).

127. J. W. Hylin, Toxic peptides and amino acids in foods and feeds. J. Agric. Food Chem. *17*:492 (1969).

128. O. Wieland, Changes in liver metabolism induced by the poisons of *Amanita phalloides*. Clin. Chem. *11*:323 (1965).
129. S. K. Abul-Haj, R. A. Ewald, and L. Kazyak, Fatal mushroom poisoning. Report of a case confirmed by toxicological analysis of tissue. N. Engl. J. Med. *269*:223 (1963).
130. D. Rehbinder, G. Löffler, O. Wieland, and T. Wieland, Studien über den Mechanismus der Giftwirkung des Phalloidins mit radioaktiv markierten Giftstoffen, Z. Physiol. Chem. *331*:132 (1963).

NOTE

After this chapter was completed, two extensive review articles were published on the biochemistry of plant agglutinins by Nathan Sharon and Halina Lis: *Science 177*(4053):949 (1972) and *The Annual Review of Biochemistry* (1973).

6 A. E. Harper

AMINO ACIDS
OF NUTRITIONAL
IMPORTANCE*

It is questionable whether the amino acids that occur in food proteins, many of which are essential nutrients, should be classed as naturally occurring toxicants. Nevertheless, many nutrients cause adverse effects or even toxic reactions if they are consumed in unduly large amounts and, since such effects have been observed in animals consuming large amounts of individual amino acids, the probability that excessive intakes of amino acids may cause untoward reactions in man requires consideration. A few food proteins do contain disproportionate amounts of some amino acids, but these are the exception rather than the rule. However, now that most of the nutritionally important amino acids are available as pure chemicals, new uses for them are being explored. Besides being used as food supplements, some have been tested as therapeutic or pharmacologic agents and some as flavoring and sweetening substances. The use of amino acids for such purposes can result in consumption of greater quantities of individual amino acids than would ordinarily be consumed in foods; thus, questions concerning their safety logically arise.

*Literature reviewed to March 1971.

NUTRITIONAL REQUIREMENTS AND USUAL INTAKES OF AMINO ACIDS

Nineteen amino acids are the structural units of food proteins. Of these 19, 9 are nutritionally indispensable for man[1] : histidine, methionine, tryptophan, threonine, leucine, isoleucine, valine, phenylalanine, and lysine. Histidine is indispensable for the human infant,[2] and, although adults can be maintained in nitrogen equilibrium for 60 days without it,[3] there is no evidence that histidine is synthesized by mammals.[4,5] Cystine and tyrosine are termed semi-indispensable; they can be synthesized in the body only from methionine and phenylalanine, respectively, and reduce the need for these two indispensable amino acids when they are present in the diet. Eight other amino acids occur in proteins: arginine, alanine, aspartic acid, glutamic acid, glycine, proline, hydroxyproline, and serine. These can be synthesized by man and are, therefore, nutritionally dispensable. Aspartic acid and glutamic acid commonly occur as amides, asparagine, and glutamine; these derivatives are synthesized by the body and occur naturally in foodstuffs.

There are compilations of the amino acid content of many foodstuffs.[6,7,8] However, these rarely include information about asparagine or glutamine, as the amides are converted to free aspartic and glutamic acids during hydrolysis of samples for analysis. Methods for the analysis of amino acids are well standardized. Most of the early methods have been described by Block and Weiss[6] ; currently, proteins are analyzed for amino acids mainly by ion-exchange column chromatographic methods[9,10] but gas chromatographic methods show considerable promise.[11]

Estimates of the amounts of each of the indispensable amino acids required by human adults and young children are shown in Table 1, together with estimates of the amounts that would be ingested by a human adult consuming 2,800 kcal from food products of animal or cereal origin and by a child consuming 1,200 kcal. The sample subjects represent the 18–35-yr-old male and the 1–2-yr-old child in the table of recommended dietary allowances.[12] Values for the amino acid content[7] and composition of the foods[13] are from the U.S. Department of Agriculture (USDA) compilations, and the basis for calculation is explained in the footnotes. The values for a subject consuming a diet of lean round steak represent something closer to the upper limit of intake possible from natural foodstuffs than to a probable upper limit. For men, the values for the mixed diet and for wheat serve as reasonable indicators of usual amino acid consumption. For women, with generally much lower caloric intakes, the values would be proportionately less.

TABLE 1 Amino Acid Requirements of the Rat and Man, Tolerance of the Rat for Excessive Amounts of Individual Amino Acids, and Amounts of Amino Acids in Wheat and Meat Diets

Amino Acid	% of Diet Level Causing Adverse Effects in Rat[a]	Req. for Young Rat[b]	In 70% Casein Diet[c]	Requirement for Adult Human[d] (g/day)		Amount in 2,800 kcal of			Req. for 12-kg Child[h] (g/day), Age 1–2 yr	Amount in 1,200 kcal of	
				Male (70 kg)	Female (58 kg)	Whole Wheat[e] (g)	Mixed Diet[f] (g)	Round Steak[g] (g)		Whole Wheat[e] (g)	Round Steak[g] (g)
Methionine	1.5	0.5	2.3	0.55	0.46	1.8	2.9	11.4	0.41	0.73	4.6
Tryptophan	2	0.12	1.0	0.16	0.13	1.5	1.5	5.4	0.17	0.58	2.2
Histidine	2	0.26	2.1	—	—	2.4	2.5	13.4	0.3	0.95	5.3
Tyrosine	3	—	4.5	—	—	4.4	5.1	13.0	—	1.7	5.2
Cystine	3	—	0.3	—	—	2.6	1.7	5.8	—	1.0	2.3
Phenylalanine	4	0.9	4.1	0.85	0.70	5.8	5.3	15.8	1.20	2.3	6.3
Leucine	2.5	0.7	7.0	0.88	0.72	8.0	9.2	37.8	1.20	3.1	15.2
Isoleucine	5	0.55	4.7	0.66	0.55	5.3	6.3	24.2	0.78	2.0	9.5
Valine	5	0.55	5.2	0.75	0.62	5.5	6.7	21.4	0.84	2.2	8.5
Lysine	5	0.9	5.8	0.66	0.55	3.2	8.6	40.4	0.96	1.3	16.2

Threonine	5	0.5	3.2	0.46	0.38	3.4	5.3	20.4	0.56	1.3	8.2
Serine	4	–	4.6	–	–	5.5	–	16.1	–	2.2	6.4
Arginine	4	0.2	2.8	–	–	5.7	–	24.6	–	2.2	9.7
Glycine	4–5	–	1.4	–	–	7.3	–	23.7	–	2.8	9.4
Aspartic acid	5	–	5.2	–	–	6.5	–	35.8	–	2.5	14.3
Proline	5	–	8.3	–	–	12.4	–	19.0	–	4.8	7.5
Alanine	5	–	2.3	–	–	4.2	–	22.2	–	1.6	8.8
Glutamic acid	7	–	16.0	–	–	32.2	–	58.0	–	14.5	23.2
Protein	12–14	–	–	40	32	118	122	464	12	47	182

[a] Based on information compiled for rats fed a low-protein diet.[14]

[b] Rama Rao et al.[15]

[c] Assuming 16% N in casein, USDA Handbook No. 4.[7]

[d] Values from Food and Nutrition Board[19] based largely on Hegsted[16] and Burrill and Shuck[17] but with downward adjustments in requirements for methionine and tryptophan. Requirement for methionine = that for total S-containing amino acids; requirement for phenylalanine = that for total aromatic amino acids.

[e] Assuming 330 kcal/100 g and 14.0% protein, USDA Handbooks No. 8[13] and No. 4.[7]

[f] From Evaluation of Protein Nutrition.[18]

[g] Assuming broiled, lean = 189 kcal/100 g and 31.3% protein, USDA Handbook No. 4[7] adjusted for difference in protein content. Requirement for methionine = that for total S-containing amino acids; requirement for phenylalanine = that for total aromatic amino acids.

[h] Assuming requirement of 1 g protein/kg/day of the amino acid composition of cow's milk.[7] Requirement for methionine = that for total S-containing amino acids; requirement for phenylalanine = that for total aromatic amino acids.

EFFECTS OF EXCESSIVE INTAKES IN ANIMALS

Much of the information about adverse effects of excessive intakes of individual amino acids by animals has been reviewed recently,[14] as has the pharmacology of amino acids.[20] The first column of Table 1 gives a rough estimate of the percentage of each of the amino acids that has been observed to cause adverse effects in the young, growing rat fed a low-protein diet.The indispensable and, below them, the dispensable amino acids are each listed in order of increasing tolerance. Leucine has been listed lower in the sequence than would appear appropriate because the tolerance for leucine increases greatly as the protein content of the diet is increased, and because the rat adapts rapidly to a diet containing an excess of leucine.

Examination of Table 1 indicates that the indispensable and semi-indispensable amino acids are generally less well tolerated than the dispensable ones; amino acids entering into a variety of metabolic pathways and serving as precursors of a variety of biologically active substances tend to be less well tolerated than those with less complex metabolic interactions. Methionine, for example, is a source of methyl groups, a precursor of homocysteine, cysteine, taurine, and various other sulfur-containing compounds and of α-ketobutyrate. Tryptophan is a precursor of nicotinic acid via a series of reactions that can give rise to a dozen or more aromatic compounds. Tryptophan, histidine, and tyrosine all yield biogenic amines; tyrosine is a precursor of the hormones, thyroxine, and epinephrine. The growth of the rat is retarded by quantities of individual indispensable amino acids ranging from 3 or 4 to 10 times those required for maximum growth when the diet is low in protein. Large excesses of some amino acids will induce severe toxic reactions.

Methionine is the least well tolerated of the nutritionally important amino acids. About three times the amount required by the young rat causes some growth retardation when the protein content of the diet is low, and double this amount causes histopathologic changes in pancreatic, liver, and kidney cells and iron deposition in the spleen.[14] The adverse effects of methionine are alleviated by supplements of glycine or serine, the degree of alleviation depending upon both the amount of methionine in excess and the amounts of serine or glycine provided. Vitamin B_6 deficiency reduces the tolerance of the rat for methionine. Adult animals tolerate larger amounts of methionine than do younger animals. Thus, many factors can influence the tolerance of an animal for an amino acid.

The information in column 1 of Table 1 indicates that most, if not all, of the individual amino acids can cause some adverse effect if the quantity in a low-protein diet is sufficiently high. Alanine, which appears to be an exception, has not been tested in as large amounts as glutamic acid. For the most part, the adverse effects observed have been depressed food intake and growth, but methionine in excess, as indicated above, will produce histopathologic lesions, and tyrosine in excess will cause a specific toxicity syndrome in rats fed a low-protein diet.[14] The paws of rats fed more than 3% of tyrosine in a 6% casein diet become red and edematous, and a dark exudate accumulates around the rats' eyes. Higher quantities of tyrosine cause weight loss and considerable mortality. Histopathologic changes have been observed in skin, pancreas, liver, and testes. The tolerance of the rat for tyrosine increases as the protein content of the diet is increased, as the rat becomes older, and if the diet is supplemented with the amino acids in which it is limiting. Riboflavin or niacin deficiency increases the susceptibility of animals to tyrosine toxicity.

These observations on methionine and tyrosine indicate some of the difficulties encountered in trying to establish the tolerance of animals and human subjects for amino acids. In addition to the age of the subject and the adequacy of the diet with respect to protein and certain vitamins, the relative proportions of amino acids in the diet influence the susceptibility of an animal to an amino acid load. After a short period of adjustment, the rat will tolerate quite well a diet containing 70% casein, which provides 10 amino acids in quantities that would depress growth individually in a low-protein diet (Table 1, column 3). Adverse effects from excesses of individual amino acids also tend to become less severe with time unless the load is so great that a clear toxic reaction develops, suggesting that animals undergo various types of adaptations that increase their ability to tolerate amino acids in excess.

There are more specific factors that influence the tolerance of animals for particular amino acids.[14] The presence of extra glycine or serine in the diet increases the tolerance for methionine; the presence of extra methionine increases the tolerance for glycine, the presence of extra isoleucine and valine increases the tolerance for leucine; the presence of extra threonine and tryptophan increases the tolerance for tyrosine; the presence of extra arginine increases the tolerance for lysine. Other amino acid interactions may also be important, but these examples are sufficient to indicate some of the reasons why a high-protein intake increases the tolerance of the body for many individual amino acids.

A high-protein intake also stimulates metabolic responses that should increase the tolerance of an animal for excessive amounts of amino acids.[14] Large excesses of individual amino acids, with the exceptions of tryptophan and tyrosine, do not cause rapid elevations of the enzymes of amino acid catabolism, whereas in animals ingesting a high-protein diet the activities of many of the enzymes of amino acid catabolism increase substantially within a short time. A response of this type should facilitate the removal of excessive quantities of amino acids that are not needed for the synthesis of proteins and can be used only as a source of energy. Even in animals fed a low-protein diet containing as much as 3% tyrosine, the lesions recede as the animal matures and may disappear within 3–5 weeks. Tyrosine transaminase, one of the enzymes involved in tyrosine catabolism, is known to increase in activity in animals ingesting a diet that is high in tyrosine. Apparently, animals fed a low-protein diet also undergo a measure of adaptation that enables them to tolerate excesses of several of the amino acids, but the adaptive responses occur more slowly than in those fed an adequate diet.

It is instructive to view the tolerance for amino acids in relation to the amounts provided by proteins. Whole-egg proteins contain about 3.4% of methionine; a diet that provided 15% of protein all from eggs would, therefore, contain 0.5% of methionine. Few food proteins contain more methionine than this, making it difficult to devise a diet from natural foodstuffs that would be higher in methionine. Since the young rat will tolerate 1.5% methionine in a diet containing 9% of protein (10% casein), this level of methionine could be attained in such a diet only with a protein containing 16.7% of methionine, or almost five times the amount in whole-egg proteins. A diet containing 60% of egg proteins would provide 2.0% of methionine, but this would be in a diet with a well-balanced amino acid pattern; a 70% protein (casein) diet that provides 2.3% of methionine causes only transitory depressions of food intake and growth in the rat. The possibility of obtaining quantities of individual amino acids that would cause adverse effects in a diet composed of natural foods is, therefore, remote.

AMINO ACID IMBALANCES

Quite severe depressions in food intake occur not only when animals are fed diets containing surpluses of individual indispensable amino acids but also when they are fed diets in which the amino acid pattern has been unbalanced by the addition of various mixtures of indispensable amino acids, particularly mixtures of all but one of the indispensable amino acids.[14] The latter type of modification, with none of the individual amino acids provided in a quantity that by itself would cause adverse effects, has been termed an amino acid imbalance. In general, the effects of imbalances of amino acids are alleviated if the food intake of the animal can be stimulated. As with animals fed surpluses of individual amino acids, those fed imbalanced diets appear to undergo adaptation, and the adverse effects are usually transitory. Animals receiving diets that meet their requirements for all amino acids tolerate substantial amounts of unbalanced amino acid mixtures without showing ill effects.

One of the underlying assumptions of methods for evaluation of the nutritional quality of proteins is that amino acids present in the diet in excess of the amounts that can be used for protein synthesis are innocuous.[21,22] The direct relationship observed between Chemical Scores calculated from the amino acid composition of proteins and estimates of protein quality obtained using biological methods for a variety of proteins over a fairly wide range of intakes tends to support this assumption, indicating that disproportionate amounts of amino acids encountered naturally do not commonly result in adverse effects. Adverse effects observed experimentally are usually the result of amino acid disproportions greater than would be encountered in nature; these are severe only when the protein content of the diet is low or the disproportion is very great. Nevertheless, when homeostatic mechanisms for the regulation of blood and body-fluid amino acid concentrations are deficient or defective, as they may be in human subjects with genetic defects of amino acid metabolism, liver damage or severe malnutrition (conditions resembling those in animals artificially overloaded with amino acids) might be anticipated.

EXCESSIVE INTAKES BY HUMAN SUBJECTS

Man existing exclusively on a diet of lean meat would be ingesting many times the requirements for most amino acids but in a well-balanced pattern. Human subjects have subsisted on meat, with protein intakes of 100–140 g/day for a year, without evidence of adverse effects.[23] Healthy male volunteers, who consumed a purified diet in which 70% of the calories were from protein, also showed no obvious ill effects over a 15-day period.[24] Thus it is evident that normal man, like laboratory animals, can tolerate large intakes of amino acids in a well-balanced pattern. However, large intakes of protein or amino acids cause liver and kidney hypertrophy in animals,[25] suggesting that such a metabolic load does place a strain on regulatory mechanisms in these organs even though specific signs of toxicity are not evident. Observations indicating that the life span of animals ingesting a high-protein diet is shortened,[26] and that, in man, calcium losses may be increased by a high protein intake,[27,28] argue against consumption of excessive amounts of protein.

There have been few methodical studies of the tolerance of human subjects for individual amino acids. However, some information about effects of large intakes can be gleaned from experiments in which amino acids have been tested as potential therapeutic agents or for specific metabolic effects. Glycine has been used in the treatment of patients with muscular dystrophy,[29] methionine in the treatment of patients with liver disease,[30] and several amino acids have been tested for their effects in mental patients.[31] Little evidence of therapeutic value was obtained in these studies, but observations on the reactions of subjects following ingestion of large amounts of a few amino acids are reported. Arginine has been tested in man for its ability to lower blood ammonia concentration,[32,33] and arginine-HCl and lysine-HCl have been tested as adjuvants to diuretics.[34,35]

Glycine

There have been a number of nutritional studies and clinical trials in which large amounts of glycine have been fed to human subjects as part of a diet composed of free amino acids or as a potential therapeutic agent. In nutritional studies on adult human subjects, from 16 to 22 g glycine/day have been fed for 1–2 weeks as a component of several different diets providing 10 g N/day. No untoward effects were reported, and the subjects maintained nitrogen equilibrium.[36-38] There have been many studies in which single doses of glycine of 15–30 g have been administered to human subjects without adverse effects being observed generally, although some individuals reported nausea and mild vomiting.[39-41] In other studies in which 50 g glycine was administered in two doses daily or 38 g in a single dose, the results were similar.[42,43] Glycine has also been administered in amounts of from 5 to 40 g daily over long periods of time to 100 patients with a variety of diseases, mainly chronic.[44] Many of these received 30 g of glycine/day, some for as long as 1 yr while they were consuming their regular diets; no untoward or adverse effects were reported. Quantities of gelatin that provided about 15 g glycine have been administered to men for up to 47 days without evidence of gastric distress.[44] These observations indicate that quantities of glycine administered in single doses of 30 g or more can result in nausea and vomiting in a few subjects but are tolerated by most individuals for long periods of time. When the dose is divided and administered with or after meals, adverse effects have not been observed.

In clinical trials nine children (3–12 yr of age) with muscular disease were administered 10–15 g glycine/day over long periods of time; four children (3–8 yr of age) with strabismus were treated for at least 2 months while eating "a relatively high protein diet, the principal constituent being meat." Their clinical condition did not improve, but no adverse effects were reported.[45] In another trial, five children (8–13 yr of age) with muscular dystrophy received 10 g glycine daily with their regular diet for 3 months[46]; they showed little objective clinical improvement as judged from examination of muscle biopsy specimens, but no adverse effects of the treatment were described. Glycine as a therapeutic agent for muscular diseases has been tested in children in quantities as high as 30 g/day, in addition to that consumed in the diet; there was no evidence of adverse effects,[47] indicating that this amino acid is metabolized efficiently even when administered in large quantities.[48]

Besides being used as a potential therapeutic agent, glycine has also been used commonly as a source of nonspecific nitrogen in highly purified diets. Two series of studies, one on the protein requirements of infants and another on the amino acid requirements of children, have been reported, in which glycine was a substantial component of the diet. Snyderman et al.[49] used glycine or urea as diluents in a modified milk formula to maintain constant the nitrogen content of the diet of young infants while the amount of milk protein was gradually decreased. A baby girl was continued on the modified milk formulas for 3 months. During one continuous 20-day period she received 0.21 g of nitrogen/kg/day from protein and 0.59 g/kg/day from glycine. With her weight increasing from 3.0 to 3.5 kg during this time, she would have consumed 9.45 to 11.0 g of glycine/day. She received comparable amounts of glycine during an additional 15 days. Over the entire period of 35 days she gained weight normally except for one 5-day period when the amount of protein provided by the diet was only 1 g/kg/day. No untoward effects were reported. Another infant gained normally for about 1 month except for about 5 days when the amount of protein provided by the diet was only 0.91 g/kg/day. His glycine intake was 3 g/kg/day; thus, with a body weight of from 4.5 to somewhat above 5.0 kg he would have been consuming 13.5–15 g of glycine/day. No undesirable effects were reported.

The second series of studies by Nakagawa and associates[50–55] was undertaken to determine the indispensable amino acid requirements of young boys 10–12 yr old. In the initial study glycine was the sole source of nonspecific nitrogen, with only 1.6 of the 11–14 g of nitrogen consumed coming from indispensable amino acids patterned after the adult requirements. With the diet that provided 12.4 g of nitrogen from glycine, the subjects, weighing between 31 and 43 kg, would have been consuming 66 g of glycine/day. Two of three subjects came into nitrogen balance and maintained weight on this diet, but one lost weight owing to "poor appetite." No other adverse signs were reported. Subsequently, the nonspecific nitrogen source in the basal diet was modified to provide a mixture of four dispensable amino acids, but the daily allotment still provided 22.9 g of glycine; it was fed to 15 boys weighing from 23 to 45 kg for up to 23 days. No ill effects that could be related to glycine were reported. In subsequent studies of the requirements for various amino acids, daily glycine intake was reduced initially to 10.7 g and subsequently to 7.2 g and 6.0 g. In experiments of 15, 16, and 20 days with 28 subjects, 10–12 yr old, weighing from 20 to 40 kg, all subjects achieved positive nitrogen balance when the amino acid complement of the diet was complete. In the entire series of studies, some 36 boys were fed quantities of glycine ranging from 6.0 to 66 g/day. Only with the highest amount was there some indication of appetite depression, and no other adverse effects were mentioned by the authors. With 22.9 g glycine/day and a complete mixture of indispensable amino acids, nitrogen balance was positive and performance satisfactory. In the experiments of Snyderman et al.,[49] infants were fed from 9.5 to 15 g glycine for 20 days continuously with no ill effects reported.

Glutamic Acid

Monosodium glutamate (MSG) has long been used to enhance the flavor of foods and is commonly included in commercially processed foods in the United States in amounts of 0.1–0.6% by weight. It has been used as a source of nitrogen in highly purified diets in many experimental studies on human subjects and has been tested as a therapeutic agent in mental patients.

In 1968 a syndrome associated with eating Chinese food was reported.[56] It was described as a feeling of numbness over the back of the neck and back, weakness, and palpitation, lasting up to 2 h but leaving no aftereffects. Subsequently this response was shown to be due to the high content of glutamate in such foods. Studies of the effects of ingestion of specific pure compounds indicated that in susceptible individuals 3 g or less of MSG would reproduce the syndrome and that it was in all probability due to L-glutamic acid. In some individuals as much as 21 g MSG orally was without effect, but intravenous injection of 25–125 mg would produce symptoms. According to Schaumberg et al.,[57] prior ingestion of food, which delays absorption of the agent, will protect the most susceptible individual from the phenomenon. It appears that the syndrome occurs when the concentration of MSG in the blood exceeds a threshold level, which differs among individuals. This may occur from ingestion of a large oral dose on an empty stomach or from parenteral injection. No lasting adverse effects have been reported.

Concern about possible adverse effects from glutamate ingestion has been expressed because of the observations that subcutaneous injection of 4–8 g/kg of sodium L-glutamate into neonatal mice produced changes in the retina.[58,59] Other observations[59-61] showed that large parenteral or oral doses (0.5–4 g/kg of body weight) of MSG will produce neuropathologic, growth, and endocrine changes in neonatal mice. The doses used to produce these lesions were large, and still larger doses were required in older animals.

Many food proteins contain from 20 to 35% of glutamic acid; adults in the United States would therefore commonly consume 20 to 35 g/day of glutamic acid throughout life, with children consuming proportionately less, depending on their energy and protein intake. These quantities in the food are obviously innocuous. Diets used by Nakagawa *et al.*[50] in studies of the amino acid requirements of boys 10–12 yr of age provided 12.75 g/day of free glutamic acid.

In studies of possible therapeutic benefits of glutamate, MSG has been administered in doses as high as 45 g/day (in three divided doses) for 10 weeks to adults without adverse effects being reported.[62] However, in another study[63] 15-g doses were reported to evoke side-effects, while a dose of 10 g/day was tolerated. No serious untoward reactions were observed in patients 6–29 yr of age consuming 24 g of MSG/day (in three doses after meals) for 16 weeks.[64] In studies of long-term maintenance of infants by parenteral alimentation, protein hydrolysates providing from 80 to 300 mg of glutamate/kg body weight/day have been used successfully.[65-67]

Although large doses of MSG administered to neonatal animals with a slowly developing nervous system will produce retinal and neuropathological lesions, other species with more developed nervous systems are more resistant.[59] The observations on both children and adult man indicate that human tolerance for this amino acid is high.

Methionine

Methionine has been administered to 17 adult patients with liver disease in quantities of from 8 to 20 g/day in divided doses for 3–9 days.[30] In 7 patients with portal cirrhosis, neurological deterioration occurred in from 1 to 4 days after total doses of 11–46 g of methionine. Large amounts of either protein or amino acids can cause hepatic coma when the liver is damaged. In 10 patients who had not previously exhibited neurological complications, methionine was tolerated without evidence of neurological change; in one at 20 g/day for 3 days and in another at from 10 to 14 g/day for 9 days. In patients with liver disease, methionine tolerance was impaired, with blood methionine levels remaining elevated 4 h after the intravenous infusion of 6 g of methionine, whereas in 3 normal subjects, the blood methionine concentration had returned to normal by this time. Administration of chlortetracycline with methionine largely protected susceptible patients from neurological deterioration, suggesting that the intestinal flora may be involved in the toxic effects observed. From a review of earlier work and their own studies, Phear et al.[30] conclude that methionine was not beneficial, and could be deleterious, to human subjects with liver disease. However, they demonstrate that subjects without severe liver involvement could tolerate from 10 to 20 g of methionine for short periods without adverse effects. Methionine at 20 g/day for 7 days (but not at 15 g/day) also caused behavioral changes and some gastric distress in schizophrenic patients.[31]

Tryptophan

Adult patients tolerated oral doses of 20–50 mg of tryptophan/kg of body weight (1.5–3.5 g/day/70 kg) without untoward effects, but when it was administered with a monamine oxidase inhibitor, these quantities of tryptophan produced "intoxication," drowsiness, and hyperreflexia.[68] In schizophrenic patients 7–15 g of tryptophan was tolerated for up to a week if iproniazid was not administered at the same time; when iproniazid was also administered, behavioral changes— some quite startling—were observed.[31] When tryptophan is administered with an amine oxidase inhibitor, such as iproniazid, it can be highly toxic.[69] Patients with Parkinsonism tolerated 8–9 g of tryptophan or 100 mg of vitamin B_6 daily for several days without event, but rapid deterioration in their condition was observed when the two were administered together.[70] When 5–7 g of DL-tryptophan was administered with vitamin B_6 for 28 days to 41 patients with depression, no adverse effects were noted in the patients, although 19 of them also received a monamine oxidase inhibitor.[71] In fact, most of them showed as much improvement in their condition as others treated with electroconvulsive therapy.

Certain tryptophan metabolites have been examined as possible bladder carcinogens.[72,73] There is no direct evidence that tryptophan metabolites produce bladder cancer in man, but from animal studies evidence has accumulated suggesting that they may act as cocarcinogens in the presence of specific carcinogenic agents. In one study, elevated levels of tryptophan metabolites were detected in about half the bladder cancer patients.[72] (See Chapter 23.)

Histidine

Histidine has not been studied extensively, but schizophrenic patients tolerated 20 g/day for a week without evidence of distress.[31] In a recent study,[74] adult volunteers tolerated up to 32 g histidine/day for short periods. When scleroderma patients were given doses of histidine of from 8 to 64 g/day for 2 days, alternated with 2-day periods without histidine, their serum zinc concentration fell, and their taste acuity deteriorated.

Phenylalanine and Tyrosine

Phenylalanine and tyrosine, administered orally in doses of 20 g/day to mental patients, were not observed to exert adverse effects.[31] In patients with Parkinsonism and in controls, a single oral dose of 7 g of phenylalanine was cleared quite well from the blood without event in 4 h.[75]

Arginine

Arginine has been tested as a therapeutic agent for controlling blood ammonia concentration with variable success. Najarian and Harper[32] infused 15 patients having elevated blood ammonia with from 25 to 50 g of arginine hydrochloride per day and observed improved mental status and reduced blood ammonia concentrations. Fahey et al.[76] infused 29–39 g of arginine HCl in patients with liver disease for longer than 60–120 min without observing beneficial effects. In another study[33] patients with hepatic insufficiency were infused intravenously with 30 g of arginine·HCl daily without evidence of side effects or much beneficial effect from the treatment. Arginine·HCl has also been used as an adjuvant to diuretics in patients with edema.[34] Intravenous administration of up to 42 g of arginine·HCl daily for as long as 9 days proved to be "a safe and effective method of producing hyperchloremic acidosis and restoring responsiveness to mercurial diuretics in patients" with fluid retention.[34] Single infusions of 30 g of arginine·HCl have also been shown to induce insulin response in healthy women and to be well tolerated.[77] Arginine·HCl has been administered in amounts up to 25 g/day for 10 days to 9–12-yr-old children with cystic fibrosis[78]; it appeared to improve fat absorption without producing observable side effects.

Lysine

Lysine·HCl, like arginine·HCl, has been used as an adjuvant to mercurial diuretics in treating refractory edema.[35] From 10 to 40 g/day were administered orally in four doses for up to 6 days to patients with congestive heart failure. Abdominal cramps or diarrhea occurred occasionally with the higher amounts but disappeared when the dose was reduced. Oral administration of 300 mg of lysine·HCl/kg of body weight to a normal child produced no noticeable effects[79] but led to coma in a child with lysinemia, a genetic defect of lysine metabolism.

Leucine

Leucine, either orally or parenterally, is known to cause a severe hypoglycemic reaction in persons who are genetically susceptible.[80] This amino acid stimulates insulin production. However, 10 g leucine administered orally to adults is without effect,[81] and 14–20 g causes only a small depression in blood glucose concentration.[81,82]

Observations by Gopalan and his associates[83,84] indicate that the high-leucine content of certain low-protein cereal diets may contribute to the development of pellagra. They observed that oral administration of leucine (10 g/day for 5 days) to pellagrins or normal subjects depressed the ability of erythrocytes to synthesize pyridine nucleotides and that inclusion of leucine in a nonpellagragenic diet for pups converted it to one that caused pellagra. Further reduction of the leucine content of a maize diet prevented pellagra in pups. Hankes et al.,[85] in a study of pellagra in South Africa, also conclude that the high leucine content of maize depressed synthesis of nicotinamide adenine dinucleotide phosphate in the body.

An antagonism between leucine and isoleucine and valine has been demonstrated in rats in which a high-leucine intake apparently increases the requirements for isoleucine and valine.[14] In studies of the amino acid requirements of adults, Rose and Wixom[3] and Linkswiler et al.[86] observe that nausea and anorexia were more severe in subjects consuming isoleucine-deficient diets than in those consuming diets deficient in other amino acids. The leucine content of their basal amino acid mixture was high, raising the possibility that this antagonism may also occur in man.

FURTHER OBSERVATIONS

Snyderman *et al.*[87] have administered single loads of each of the individual indispensable amino acids to infants in amounts equivalent to 5 or more times the requirement. These studies have not been reported in detail, but in preliminary reports no mention has been made of adverse effects. Plasma amino acid patterns have been altered, with the amino acid administered being greatly elevated, while certain other amino acids, depending upon the one administered, were depressed. Chronic loading for 1-week periods gave evidence that the body adapted to a high-leucine intake and, after the adaptation period, cleared leucine from the blood rapidly.[88]

Intravenous loads of individual amino acids have been administered to adults in acute studies after an 8-h fast.[89] A single intravenous dose of 30 g of arginine, lysine, phenylalanine, leucine, valine, or histidine was tolerated without event. However, 30 g of methionine caused vomiting and febrile reactions; 22.5 g of threonine or 15 g of isoleucine in a single infusion caused febrile reactions and headaches or backaches; and tryptophan in excess of 5 g caused severe flushing. These side effects were not associated with the degree of stimulation of insulin production, which was greatest for arginine, lysine, leucine, and phenylalanine, all of which were innocuous.

It would be difficult, without elaborate and well-controlled experiments, to distinguish between effects of amino acid deficiencies and amino acid imbalance in human subjects consuming natural diets. However, in some studies in which amino acid supplements have been tested for their ability to improve low-protein diets consisting largely of cereal products, amino acid imbalances may have been created. Addition of mixtures of several amino acids, each in small amounts, decreased nitrogen retention in adult men consuming a rice diet[90] and in children consuming a vegetable-protein diet based on maize. Addition of 0.14–0.34% of methionine to the diet depressed nitrogen retention, and the addition of 0.2% of isoleucine was required to prevent the effect.[91] The depressed nitrogen retention was associated with anorexia (G. Arroyave, personal communication).

GENETIC EFFECTS

Information about effects of accumulations of individual amino acids in human subjects has been obtained from the study of genetic defects of amino acid metabolism in which the initial enzyme for degradation of an amino acid is lacking. The amino acid for which the catabolic enzyme is missing accumulates in body fluids even when the amount consumed is not excessive. Defects involving all of the indispensable and semi-indispensable amino acids, except threonine, have been described[92-95]; they commonly cause mental deficiency and neurologic disorders. Probably the best known and most common genetic defect of this type is phenylketonuria, in which the absence of phenylalanine hydroxylase results in mental deficiency, decreased pigmentation, diminished serotonin formation, and various other changes, all of which are associated with high phenylalanine concentrations in body fluids. Restriction of such patients to a low-phenylalanine diet results in improved growth, development, and mental ability.[96-98] This is essentially nutritional control of an endogenous amino acid toxicity.

SUMMARY AND CONCLUSIONS

In the main, in subjects receiving single doses of individual indispensable amino acids either orally or intravenously in amounts that exceed the requirement by 10-fold or more, the major adverse effect reported has been mild gastric distress. This was observed primarily when the amino acid was administered in a single large dose on an empty stomach. The dispensable amino acids arginine and glycine are well tolerated in large doses, as is glutamic acid, except for some individuals who are susceptible to a specific transitory syndrome produced by this amino acid when it is ingested in amounts of 3 g or more on an empty stomach. This syndrome is not observed when glutamic acid is ingested with food. There is evidence that doses of methionine, isoleucine, and threonine in excess of 10 times the requirement administered intravenously may cause nausea, febrile reactions, or headaches. There is also evidence that methionine, and probably other amino acids, should not be administered to patients with liver dysfunction in doses of 10 times the requirement; that tryptophan in comparable amounts can produce a flushing reaction; and that tryptophan and methionine administered in doses of this order to mental patients treated with monoamine oxidase inhibitors can produce disorientation. Few amino acids, with the exception of glycine, have been administered individually to human subjects in long-term studies, but the ordinary mixed diet of adults in the United States provides many amino acids in 5 to 10 times the required amounts.

Apart from the observations that leucine may occur in maize and re-

lated cereal grains at levels high enough to induce pellagra when tryptophan and niacin intakes are low, there is little evidence to suggest that
individual amino acids are present in foodstuffs in large enough quantities to cause adverse effects. Also, amounts of individual amino acids
great enough to cause untoward reactions could not rationally be used
as supplements to foodstuffs. The amounts of amino acids (2–5%) in
the diet found to cause adverse effects in a rat fed a low-protein diet
would represent intakes of from 10 to 25 g/day by an adult man consuming about 500 g of dry matter and 2,800 kcal/day. Even general fortification of the diet with specific amino acids would be unlikely to increase the intake of individual amino acids by more than 1–2 g/day, and
these should be only the amino acids that are in short supply in the diet.

The extent to which it is possible to create an amino acid imbalance
in human diets through the use of amino acid supplements is not clear,
but it is a possibility that deserves consideration. An amino acid supplement is of value only if the diet is primarily deficient in that amino
acid. A supplement of an amino acid, other than the one that is most
deficient in the diet, is at best innocuous and may, if the analogy to animal experiments is valid, depress food intake. This is likely to occur
only if the diet is low in protein and marginal in some indispensable
amino acids. Although such effects may not be serious in view of the
ability of animals to adapt to diets with amino acid imbalances, they
are certainly not desirable and can be avoided readily by ensuring that
any supplement provided makes the diet complete in all regards.

Only if individual amino acids were administered regularly as pharmacologic or therapeutic agents, or for some other purpose, would there
be much likelihood of approaching the amounts shown to cause adverse
effects in animal studies or in such human trials as have been conducted.
Even then, unless protein intake or total food intake was low or the subject was otherwise debilitated, amounts of amino acids administered
orally would have to be very large to cause more than mild adverse effects. Information currently available concerning long-term effects of
large intakes of most of the individual amino acids is far from satisfactory, but the studies that have been conducted provide a reasonable
guide to amounts that are tolerated over short periods.

REFERENCES

1. W. C. Rose, The amino acid requirements of adult man. Nutr. Abstr. Rev. *27*:
631–647 (1957).

2. L. E. Holt, Jr., Amino acid requirements of infants. Curr. Ther. Res. *9* (Suppl.):149 (1967).

3. W. C. Rose and R. L. Wixom, The amino acid requirements of man. XVI. The role of the nitrogen intake. J. Biol. Chem. *217*:997–1004 (1955).

4. E. S. Nasset, Essential amino acids and nitrogen balance. In Some aspects of amino acid supplementation, W. H. Cole (ed.). Rutgers University Press, New Brunswick, N.J. (1956).

5. Anonymous, Evidence for liver damage in subjects fed amino acid diets lacking arginine and histidine. Nutr. Rev. *28*:229–232 (1970).

6. R. J. Block and K. W. Weiss, Amino acid handbook: Methods and results of protein analysis. Charles C Thomas, Springfield, Ill., p. 384 (1956).

7. M. L. Orr and B. K. Watt, Amino acid content of foods. U.S. Dep. Agric. (ARS) Home Econ. Res. Rep. No. 4, Washington, D.C., p. 82 (1957).

8. FAO. Amino acids content of foods and biological data on proteins. Rome, p. 280 (1968).

9. W. H. Stein and S. Moore, The free amino acids of human blood plasma. J. Biol. Chem. *211*:915 (1954).

10. P. B. Hamilton, Ion exchange chromatography of amino acids—microdetermination of free amino acids in serum. Ann. N.Y. Acad. Sci. *102*:55–75 (1962).

11. D. Roach and C. W. Gehrke, The gas-liquid chromatography of amino acids. J. Chromatog. *43*:303–310 (1969).

12. NRC, Food and Nutrition Board, Recommended dietary allowances. Revised 1968. National Academy of Sciences, Washington, D.C., p. 101 (1968).

13. B. K. Watt and A. L. Merrill, Composition of foods. U.S. Dep. Agric. (ARS) Consum. Food Econ. Res. Div. Agric. Handb. No. 8. Rev. ed. Washington, D.C., p. 190 (1963).

14. A. E. Harper, N. J. Benevenga, and R. M. Wohlhueter, Effects of ingestion of disproportionate amounts of amino acids. Physiol. Rev. *50*:428–558 (1970).

15. P. B. Rama Rao, V. C. Metta, and B. C. Johnson, The amino acid composition and the nutritive value of proteins. I. Essential amino acid requirements of the growing rat. J. Nutr. *69*:387–391 (1959).

16. D. M. Hegsted, Variation in requirements of nutrients—amino acids. Fed. Proc. *22*:1424–1430 (1963).

17. L. M. Burrill and C. Shuck, Phenylalanine requirements with different levels of tyrosine. J. Nutr. *83*:202–208 (1964).

18. NRC, Food and Nutrition Board, Evaluation of protein nutrition. National Academy of Sciences, Washington, D.C., p. 61 (1959).

19. H. H. Williams and A. E. Harper, Evaluation of protein nutrition. 2nd ed. National Academy of Sciences, Washington, D.C. (in preparation).

20. M. D. Milne, Pharmacology of amino acids. Clin. Pharmacol. Ther. *9*:484–514 (1968).

21. R. J. Block and H. H. Mitchell, The correlation of the amino acid composition of proteins with their nutritive value. Nutr. Abstr. Rev. *16*:249–278 (1946–1947).

22. B. L. Oser, A method for integrating essential amino acid content in nutritional evaluation of protein. J. Am. Diet. Assoc. *27*:396–402 (1951).

23. W. S. McClellan and E. F. Dubois, Clinical calorimetry. XLV. Prolonged meat diets with a study of kidney function and ketosis. J. Biol. Chem. *87*:651–668 (1930).

24. D. H. Calloway and S. Margen, Human response to diets very high in protein. Fed. Proc. *27*:725Abs (1968).

25. T. Addis, L. L. MacKay, and E. M. McKay, The effect on the kidney of the long continued administration of diets containing an excess of certain food elements. I. Excess of protein and cystine. J. Biol. Chem. *71*:139–166 (1926).

26. M. H. Ross, Protein, calories and life expectancy. Fed. Proc. *18*:1190–1215 (1959).

27. S. Margen and D. H. Calloway, Effect of high protein intake on urinary calcium, magnesium and phosphorus. Fed. Proc. *27*:726Abs (1968).

28. W. E. Johnson, E. N. Alcantara, and H. Linkswiler, Effect of level of protein intake on urinary and fecal calcium and calcium retention of young adult males. J. Nutr. *100*:1425–1430 (1970).

29. M. Adams, M. H. Power, and W. M. Boothby, The influence of glycine on the excretion of creatine and creatinine. Am. J. Physiol. *111*:596–610 (1935).

30. E. A. Phear, B. Ruebner, S. Sherlock, and W. H. J. Summerskill, Methionine toxicity in liver disease and its prevention by chlortetracycline. Clin. Sci. *15*:93 (1956).

31. W. Pollin, P. V. Cardon, Jr., and S. S. Kety, Effects of amino acid feedings in schizophrenic patients treated with iproniazid. Science *133*:104 (1961).

32. J. S. Najarian and H. A. Harper, A clinical study of the effect of arginine on blood ammonia. Am. J. Med. *21*:832 (1956).

33. T. B. Reynolds, A. G. Redeker, and P. Davis, A controlled study of the effects of L-arginine on hepatic encephalopathy. Am. J. Med. *25*:359 (1958).

34. D. A. Ogden, L. Scherr, N. Spritz, A. L. Rubin, and E. H. Luckey, Management of resistant fluid retention states with intravenous L-arginine monohydrochloride in combination with mercurial diuretics. Am. Heart J. *61*:16 (1961).

35. R. P. Lasser, M. R. Schoenfeld, and C. K. Friedberg, L-lysine monohydrochloride: A clinical study of its action as a chloruretic acidifying adjuvant to mercurial diuretics. N. Engl. J. Med. *263*:728 (1960).

36. M. E. Swendseid, C. L. Harris, and S. G. Tuttle, The effect of sources of nonessential nitrogen on nitrogen balance in young animals. J. Nutr. *71*:105–108 (1960).

37. J. H. Watts, B. Tolbert, and W. L. Ruff, Nitrogen balances for young adult males fed two sources of nonessential nitrogen at two levels of total nitrogen intake. Metabolism *13*:172–180 (1964).

38. H. E. Clark, N. J. Yess, E. J. Vermillion, A. F. Goodwin, and E. T. Mertz, Effect of certain factors on nitrogen retention and lysine requirements of adult human subjects. III. Source of supplementary nitrogen. J. Nutr. *79*:131–139 (1963).

39. J. R. Gustafson, K. N. Campbell, B. M. Harris, and S. D. Malton, The use of glycine in the treatment of peripheral vascular disease. Surgery *25*:539–546 (1949).

40. A. T. Milhorat, F. Techner, and K. Thomas, Significance of creatine in progressive muscular dystrophy, and treatment of this disease with glycin. Proc. Soc. Exp. Biol. Med. *29*:609–611 (1932).

41. W. M. Boothby, Myasthenia gravis: Effect of treatment with glycine and ephedrine. Proc. Staff Meet. Mayo Clin. *9*:593–597 (1934).

42. D. L. Loriaux, S. Delena, and H. Brown, Glycine loading test in acute intermittent porphyria patients and their relatives. Metabolism *18*:860–866 (1969).

43. C. Reid, Blood and urine chemistry during the specific dynamic action of gly-

cine in normal subjects and in schizophrenics. J. Ment. Sci. *80*:379–396 (1934).

44. M. Adams, M. H. Power, and W. M. Boothby, The influence of glycine on the excretion of creatine and creatinine. Am. J. Physiol. *111*:596–610 (1935); Studies on the urine at hourly intervals after the administration of glycine. Am. J. Physiol. *118*:562–568 (1937).

45. C. J. Tripoli, W. M. McCord, and H. H. Beard, Muscular dystrophy, muscular atrophy, myasthenia gravis and strabismus. Clinical and biochemical studies of the effects of amino acid therapy. J. Am. Med. Assoc. *103*:1595–1600 (1934).

46. J. G. Reinhold, J. H. Clark, G. R. Kingsley, R. P. Custer, and J. W. McConnell, The effects of glycine (glycocoll) in muscular dystrophy. J. Am. Med. Assoc. *102*:261 (1934).

47. H. B. Mettel and Y. K. Slocum, Pseudohypertrophic muscular dystrophy. Preliminary report on the treatment of three cases with glycine. J. Pediatr. *3*:352 (1933).

48. H. Anfanger and R. M. Heavenrich, Amino acid tolerance tests in children. Am. J. Dis. Child. *77*:425 (1949).

49. S. E. Snyderman, L. H. Holt, Jr., J. Dancis, E. Roitman, A. Boyer, and M. E. Balis, "Unessential" nitrogen: A limiting factor for human growth. J. Nutr. *78*: 57–72 (1962).

50. I. Nakagawa, T. Takahashi, and T. Suzuki, Amino acid requirements of children. J. Nutr. *71*:176–181 (1960).

51. I. Nakagawa, T. Takahashi, and T. Suzuki, Amino acid requirements of children: Isoleucine and leucine. J. Nutr. *73*:186–190 (1961).

52. I. Nakagawa, T. Takahashi, and T. Suzuki, Amino acid requirements of children: Minimal needs of lysine and methionine based on nitrogen balance method. J. Nutr. *74*:401–407 (1961).

53. I. Nakagawa, T. Takahashi, T. Suzuki, and K. Kobayashi, Amino acid requirements of children: Minimal needs of threonine, valine and phenylalanine based on nitrogen balance method. J. Nutr. *77*:61–68 (1962).

54. I. Nakagawa, T. Takahashi, T. Suzuki, and K. Kobayashi, Amino acid requirements of children: Minimal needs of tryptophan, arginine and histidine based on nitrogen balance method. J. Nutr. *80*:305–310 (1963).

55. I. Nakagawa, T. Takahashi, T. Suzuki, and K. Kobayashi, Amino acid requirements of children: Nitrogen balance at the minimal level of essential amino acids. J. Nutr. *83*:115–118 (1964).

56. R. H. Kwok, Chinese restaurant syndrome. N. Engl. J. Med. *278*:796 (1968).

57. H. H. Schaumburg, R. Byck, R. Gerstl, and J. H. Mashman, Monosodium L-glutamate: Its pharmacology and role in the Chinese restaurant syndrome. Science *163*:826 (1969).

58. R. R. Lucas and J. P. Newhouse, The toxic effects of sodium glutamate on the inner layers of the retina. Am. Med. Assoc. Arch. Ophthalmol. *58*:193–201 (1957).

59. Anonymous, Monosodium glutamate—Studies on its possible effects on the central nervous system. Nutr. Rev. *28*:124–129 (1970).

60. J. W. Olney, Brain lesions, obesity and other disturbances in mice treated with monosodium glutamate. Science *164*:719 (1969).

61. J. W. Olney and L. G. Sharpe, Brain lesions in an infant rhesus monkey treated with monosodium glutamate. Science *166*:386 (1969).

62. W. A. Himwich and I. M. Peterson, Ingested sodium glutamate and plasma levels of glutamic acid. J. Appl. Physiol. *7*:196 (1954).

63. H. E. Himwich, K. Wolff, A. L. Hunsicker, and W. A. Himwich, Some behavioral effects associated with feeding sodium glutamate to patients with psychiatric disorders. J. Nerv. Ment. Disord. *121*:40 (1955).

64. H. G. Loeb and R. D. Tuddenham, Does glutamic acid administration influence mental function? Pediatrics *6*:72 (1950).

65. S. J. Dudrick, D. W. Wilmore, H. M. Vars, and J. E. Rhoads, Long-term total parenteral nutrition with growth, development, and positive nitrogen balance. Surgery *64*:134 (1968).

66. D. W. Wilmore and S. J. Dudrick, Growth and development of an infant receiving all nutrients exclusively by vein. J. Am. Med. Assoc. *203*:860 (1968).

67. R. M. Filler, A. J. Eraklis, V. G. Rubin, and J. B. Das, Long-term total parenteral nutrition in infants. N. Engl. J. Med. *281*:589 (1969).

68. J. A. Oates and A. Sjoerdsma, Neurologic effects of tryptophan in patients receiving a monoamine oxidase inhibitor. Neurology *10*:1076–1078 (1960).

69. J. V. Hodge, J. A. Oates, and A. Sjoerdsma, Reduction of the central effects of tryptophan by a decarboxylase inhibitor. Clin. Pharmacol. Ther. *5*:149–155 (1964).

70. C. D. Hall, E. A. Weiss, C. E. Morris, and A. J. Prange, Jr., Rapid deterioration in patients with Parkinsonism from tryptophan–pyridoxine administration. (In press.)

71. A. Coppen, D. M. Shaw, B. Herzberg, and R. Maggs, Tryptophan in the treatment of depression. Lancet *ii*:1178 (1967).

72. O. Yoshida, R. R. Brown, and G. T. Bryan, A possible role of urinary metabolites of tryptophan in the heterotropic recurrence of bladder cancer in man. Am. J. Clin. Nutr. *24*:848 (1971).

73. G. T. Bryan, The role of urinary tryptophan metabolites in the etiology of bladder cancer. Am. J. Clin. Nutr. *24*:841 (1971).

74. R. I. Henkin, H. R. Keiser, and D. Bronzert, Histidine dependent zinc loss, hypogeusia, anorexia and hyposmia. Gastroenterology (In press).

75. J. Braham, I. Sarova-Pinhas, M. Crispin, R. Golan, N. Levin, and A. Szeinberg. Oral phenylalanine and tyrosine tolerance tests in Parkinsonian patients. Br. Med. J., *2*:552 (1969).

76. J. L. Fahey, D. Nathans, and D. Rairigh, Effect of L-arginine on elevated blood ammonia levels in man. Am. J. Med. *23*:860 (1957).

77. T. J. Merimee, D. A. Lillicrap, and D. Rabinowitz, Effect of arginine on serum-levels of human growth hormone. Lancet *ii*:668 (1965).

78. C. C. Solomons, E. K. Cotton, R. Dubois, and M. Pinney, The use of buffered L-arginine in the treatment of cystic fibrosis. Pediatrics *47*:384 (1971).

79. J. P. Colombo, W. Bürgi, R. Richterich, and E. Rossi, Congential lysine intolerance with periodic ammonia intoxication: A defect in L-lysine degradation. Metabolism *16*:910–925 (1967).

80. A. M. DiGeorge, and V. H. Auerbach, Leucine-induced hypoglycemia: A review and speculations. Am. J. Med. Sci. *240*:792–801 (1960).

81. A. M. DiGeorge, V. H. Auerbach, and C. C. Mabry. Leucine-induced hypoglycemia III. The blood glucose depressant action of leucine in normal individuals. J. Pediatr. *63*:295–302 (1963).

82. S. S. Fajans, R. E. Knopf, J. C. Floyd, Jr., L. Power, and J. W. Conn, The experimental induction in man of sensitivity to leucine hypoglycemia. J. Clin. Invest. *42*:216–229 (1963).

83. C. Gopalan, Leucine and pellagra. Nutr. Rev. *26*:323–326 (1968).

84. C. Gopalan, Some recent studies in the nutrition research laboratories, Hyderabad. Am. J. Clin. Nutr. *23*:35 (1970).
85. L. V. Hankes, J. E. Leklem, R. R. Brown, and R. C. P. M. Mekel, Tryptophan metabolism in patients with pellagra: Problem of vitamin B_6 enzyme activity and feedback control of tryptophan pyrrolase enzyme. Am. J. Clin. Nutr. *24*: 730–739 (1971).
86. H. Linkswiler, H. M. Fox, and P. C. Fry, Availability to man of amino acids from foods. IV. Isoleucine from corn. J. Nutr. *72*:397–403 (1960).
87. S. E. Snyderman, L. E. Holt, Jr., P. M. Norton, and E. Roitman, Effect of high and low intakes of individual amino acids on the plasma aminogram. In Protein nutrition and free amino acid patterns, J. H. Leathem (ed.). Rutgers University Press, New Brunswick, N.J. (1968).
88. L. E. Holt, A symposium on the child, pp. 321–329. The John Hopkins Press, Baltimore (1967).
89. J. C. Floyd, Jr., S. S. Fajans, J. W. Conn, R. H. Knopf, and J. Rull, Stimulation of insulin secretion by amino acids. J. Clin. Invest. *45*:1487–1501 (1966).
90. J. M. Hundley, Lysine, threonine and other supplements to rice diets in man: Amino acid imbalance. Am. J. Clin. Nutr. *5*:316 (1957).
91. N. S. Scrimshaw, R. Bressani, M. Behar, and F. Viteri, Supplementation of cereal proteins with amino acids. I. Effect of amino acid supplementation of corn-masa at high levels of protein intake on the nitrogen retention of young children. II. Effect of amino acid supplementation of corn-masa at intermediate levels of protein intake on the nitrogen retention of young children. J. Nutr. *66*:485–514 (1958).
92. D. Y. Y. Hsia. In Inborn errors of metabolism. Yearbook Publishers, Chicago (1960).
93. J. B. Stanbury, J. B. Wyngaarden, and D. S. Fredrickson. The metabolic basis of inherited disease. McGraw-Hill, New York (1960).
94. Nyhan, W. L. (ed), Amino acid metabolism and genetic variation, McGraw-Hill, New York (1967).
95. M. D. Milne, Pharmacology of amino acids. Clin. Pharmacol. Ther. *9*:484–514 (1968).
96. H. K. Berry, B. S. Sutherland, B. Umbarger, and D. O'Grady, Treatment of phenylketonuria. Am. J. Dis. Child. *113*:2–5 (1967).
97. J. L. Kennedy, Jr., W. Wertelecki, L. Gates, B. P. Sperry, and V. M. Cass. The early treatment of phenylketonuria. Am. J. Dis. Child. *113*:16–21 (1967).
98. P. W. Berman, H. A. Waisman, and F. K. Graham, Intelligence in treated phenylketonuric children: A developmental study. Child Dev. *37*:731–747 (1966).

7 E. A. Bell

AMINONITRILES AND
AMINO ACIDS
NOT DERIVED
FROM PROTEINS*

Twenty amino acids are found in all living organisms as protein constituents, while certain others such as citrulline, homoserine, and ornithine are widely distributed as metabolic intermediates. Most of the other natural amino acids are of more limited distribution; however, some are restricted to a single family, genus, or even species.

Some of these "unusual" amino acids are close chemical analogs of various of the "usual" amino acids, so it is not surprising to find that certain of the "unusual" amino acids can act as antimetabolites when introduced into organisms to which they are normally foreign.

Several reviews on toxic amino acids, both natural and synthetic, have appeared in recent years.[1,2,3,4] These have dealt variously with the roles that such compounds play as antimetabolites in animals, plants, and microorganisms. The present account, however, will be limited to a consideration of those amino acids and related aminonitriles that, because of their presence in plants or plant products likely to be eaten by man, are a danger or potential danger to human health.

When the circumstantial evidence suggests that one particular food plant is responsible for a particular toxic syndrome, it may still be far from easy to identify with absolute certainty the toxic factor in that

* Literature reviewed through 1970.

153

plant. And even when a toxic factor has been isolated, it has not always been established that the concentration and toxicity of that toxin could account for the toxicity of the plant. A toxin may not be present at all stages of the plant's development or in all organs. Its concentration may vary with the plant's environment. It may occur in high concentration in one species and be absent from a close relative in the same genus. Experimental animals used to assay the toxicity of such compounds may be less (or more) sensitive to a toxin than man. Even when results indicate that relatively high concentrations of a compound are required to induce toxic symptoms in an animal, such results do not preclude the possibility that lower concentrations of the same compound may be injurious to man, particularly if supplied as part of the diet over a long period. Some of these difficulties are clearly illustrated in this chapter.

THE LATHYROGENS

Classical lathyrism is a neurological disease that is largely restricted at the present time to the subcontinent of India. The disease affects horses, cattle, and man and is caused by eating the seeds of *Lathyrus sativus,* or, less frequently, those of *L. cicera* and *L. clymenum.* Historical accounts of the disease are given in reviews by Selye[5] and Sharma.[6] Sarma and Padmanaban[7] give a more detailed report of the toxins that have been isolated from different *Lathyrus* species and also a list of those synthetic compounds that have also been termed *lathyrogens.*

In man, classical lathyrism is characterized by muscular weakness, irreversible paralysis of the legs, and, in extreme cases, death. Outbreaks of this disease are usually associated with periods of famine when large quantities of *Lathyrus* meal are eaten for want of other food. Under these circumstances, not only is the intake of the toxin abnormally high but any competitive effects that it may exercise are likely to be enhanced by the abnormally low concentrations of normal metabolites.

As a supplement to an otherwise adequate diet, foods made from seeds of *L. sativus* do not appear to produce ill effects, and such foods are widely used in India. The danger to both man and animals arises when all or a large proportion of the food supply consists of these seeds.

β-N-(γ-L-Glutamyl)aminopropionitrile

The first toxic compound to be identified in the seed of any species of *Lathyrus* was β-N-(γ-L-glutamyl)aminopropionitrile,

$$NCCH_2 CH_2 NHOCCH_2 CH_2 CH(NH_2)CO_2 H.$$

This compound was isolated from seeds of *L. odoratus* by Strong and co-workers[8,9] and from *L. pusillus* by Dupuy and Lee.[10] Dasler[11] subsequently showed that the physiologically active part of the molecule is the β-aminopropionitrile moiety.

This compound produces severe skeletal abnormalities when fed to young rats[8] and also aortic aneurysms in both rats and chicks.[12] These symptoms are quite unlike those seen in classical lathyrism, however, and Selye[5] suggests that as there are at least two distinct syndromes associated with eating *Lathyrus* seeds; the classical form should be referred to as neurolathyrism and the syndrome produced by β-aminopropionitrile as osteolathyrism.

β-Aminopropionitrile and certain other synthetic compounds that produce osteolathyrism[13] appear to exercise their toxic effects by interfering with the formation of cross linkages between the polypeptide chains in collagen[14] and elastin,[15] thereby weakening the bones and blood-vessel walls. While osteolathyrism resulting from the consumption of plant foods does not appear to be a health problem, it is of interest that there are several inherited disorders of collagen in man that resemble closely the osteolathyrism produced in experimental animals by β-aminopropionitrile.

L-α,γ-Diaminobutyric Acid

The second toxic compound to be identified in a species of *Lathyrus*, and the first shown to produce neurological effects, was L-α,γ-diaminobutyric acid, $H_2NCH_2CH_2CH(NH_2)CO_2H$, a lower homolog of ornithine that was isolated from the seeds of *L. latifolius* (the everlasting pea) by Ressler and co-workers[16] and established as the chief toxic principle of this seed. Seeds of *L. sylvestris*, which are highly toxic when eaten by rats, contain as much as 1.4%[16] or 2.7%[17] α,γ-diaminobutyric acid (as the monohydrochloride). An extensive survey[17] of seed from 158 species belonging to 39 families showed that the amino acid occurs most frequently in species of the Leguminosae and Cruciferae; concentrations are usually low, however.

L-α,γ-Diaminobutyric acid was found to produce tremors, convulsions, and death in rats.[16] O'Neal and co-workers[18] have shown that it acts as an inhibitor of the ornithine transcarbamylase of mammalian liver, disrupting the urea cycle and inducing ammonia toxicity. Although L-α,γ-diaminobutyric acid is neurotoxic, the convulsions characteristic of poisoning by this compound are quite unlike the paralytic symptoms associated with classical lathyrism.

A survey made of the free amino acids and related compounds in 49 species of *Lathyrus*[19,20] showed, however, that the genus could be divided readily into subgenera, the members of each subgenus being characterized by associations of ninhydrin-reacting compounds, which gave clearly recognizable "patterns" after chromatography and electrophoresis on paper. This comparative survey showed that γ-glutamyl-β-aminopropionitrile (the osteolathyrogen) was present in the seeds of 3 species, while L-α,γ-diaminobutyric acid was the principal free amino acid in the seeds of 12 other species. Neither γ-glutamyl-β-aminopropionitrile nor L-α,γ-diaminobutyric acid, however, was present in the seeds of *L. sativus, L. cicera,* or *L. clymenum,* those species implicated in human lathyrism. All 3 of these species did, however, belong to a third subgenus (containing 11 species), in which the seeds were characterized by the presence of high concentrations of two previously unknown amino acids. One of these amino acids was isolated from seeds of *L. cicera*[21] and *L. sativus*[22] and found to be L-homoarginine:

$$H_2 NC(:NH)NHCH_2 CH_2 CH_2 CH_2 CH(NH_2)CO_2 H.$$

This higher homolog of arginine was not found to be toxic to rats, however.[22,23] The other amino acid that was strongly acidic in nature was isolated independently by Rao and co-workers[24] and by Murti and co-workers[25] from seeds of *L. sativus* and shown to be the first of a new series of oxalyl amino acids, β-N-oxalyl-L-α,β-diaminopropionic acid:

$$HO_2 CCONHCH_2 CH(NH_2)CO_2 H.$$

This compound is formed by the transfer of the oxalyl moiety from oxalyl coenzyme-A specifically to the β-nitrogen of α,β-diaminopropionic acid.[26] It is accompanied in the plant by lower concentrations of α-N-oxalyl-L-α,β-diaminopropionic acid, which appears to be formed by a simple chemical rearrangement of the β-oxalyl isomer rather than enzymatically.[27] The toxicity of this α-oxalyl isomer has not been determined. β-N-Oxalyl-L-α,β-diaminopropionic acid (possibly containing traces of the α-isomer) has been shown to produce neurological symptoms in young birds,[28] young rats, guinea pigs, and dogs.[29] The compound proved toxic when injected intraperitoneally in dosages varying from 10–20 mg in day-old chicks, to 100 mg in a 12-day-old dog weighing 550 g. It acts as a powerful excitant of spinal interneurones in the cat[30] and in the brains cells of young rats.[31] It also produces typical paralysis of the hind legs when administered intrathecally to adult monkeys.[32] The toxin, however, is not active when administered intraperitoneally to adult birds or animals. Curtis and Watson suggest that this difference in toxicity to young and old animals may be due to the exclusion of the compound by a blood–brain barrier that is not fully developed in the young animal.[33] If, however, β-oxalyl-L-α,β-diaminopropionic acid does not readily cross a blood–brain barrier in adult animals under experimental conditions, then some doubt must remain as to whether this compound is in fact the cause of classical lathyrism. Other environmental causes or dietary constituents may of course influence the permeability of such a barrier to the neurotoxin, and IP injection of the oxalyl amino acid has, in fact been found to produce neurological effects in adult animals after they are first rendered acidotic with calcium chloride.[34]

A second neurotoxin, tentatively identified as N-β-D-glucopyranosyl-N-α-L-arabionosyl-α,β-diaminopropionitrile, has recently been isolated from seeds of *L. sativus* by Rukmini.[35,36] This compound has been isolated only in low yield (0.003%), and as the toxic dosage to day-old chicks was 50 mg/100 g body weight, it is not clear whether this compound is a factor in human lathyrism.

The γ-oxalyl derivative of diaminobutyric acid, γ-N-oxalyl-L-α,γ-diaminobutyric acid, $HO_2CCONHCH_2CH_2CH(NH_2)CO_2H$, has been found together with the α-isomer in 10 species of *Lathyrus*.[27] The γ-oxalyl derivative is neurotoxic in young chicks at a dosage of 30–35 mg/chick.[37]

The seeds containing this compound also contain β-N-oxalyl-α,β-diaminopropionic acid and high concentrations of free L-α-γ-diaminobutyric acid. Any effects of the oxalyl compounds in animals eating these seeds are likely to be overshadowed by or superimposed on those of L-α,γ-diaminobutyric acid.

Other unusual amino acids such as lathyrine,[38] γ-methylglutamic acid,[39] and γ-hydroxynorvaline[40] are also found in various species of *Lathyrus*, but little is known of their toxicity in animals.

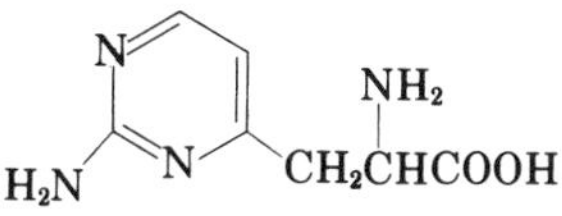

Lathyrine

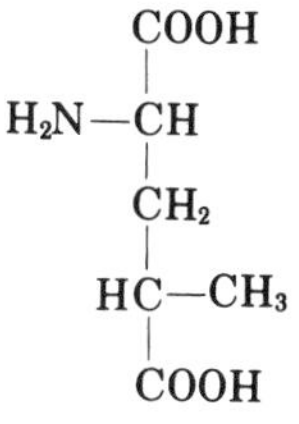

γ-Methyl-L-glutamic Acid

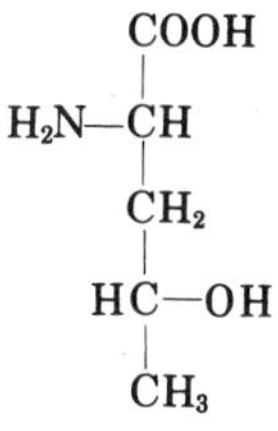

γ-Hydroxynorvaline

The distribution of known toxic compounds in the seeds of this genus is given in Table 1.

Detection of Toxins in Lathyrus Seeds

β-N-(γ-L-Glutamyl)aminopropionitrile gives a purple color with ninhydrin and can be identified from its R_f values after chromatography on paper.[8] Confirmation may be obtained by hydrolyzing the compound in acid solution and identifying the products of hydrolysis (glutamic acid and β-alanine) by chromatography or electrophoresis. Free β-aminopropionitrile gives a characteristic green spot when chromatograms are developed with ninhydrin, and it also yields β-alanine on hydrolysis.

α,γ-Diaminobutyric acid, β-N-oxalyl-α,β-diaminopropionic acid, and γ-N-oxalyl-α,γ-diaminobutyric acid may also be detected by paper chromatography, or on an amino acid analyzer,[16,17] but the most rapid and efficient method is high-voltage electrophoresis on paper at pH 3.6.[19,20,27]

β-Cyanoalanine and γ-Glutamyl-β-cyanoalanine

Ressler and co-workers[41,42,43] isolated from seeds of *Vicia sativa* (common vetch) the neurotoxin β-cyanoalanine, $NCCH_2 CH(NH_2)CO_2 H$, and its γ-glutamyl derivative and established these as the chief toxic principles of the seed. Earlier reports[44] indicated that *Lathyrus sativus* seeds from various localities in which lathyrism was common were sometimes contaminated with seeds of *V. sativa.* Moreover, ducks and monkeys fed seeds of *V. sativa* developed neurological symptoms, whereas the seeds of *L. sativus* were harmless.[44] This led to the suggestion that β-cyanoalanine might be a factor in human lathyrism. For that reason, this compound will be considered here under the general heading of the lathyrogens, although it is now generally believed that uncontaminated *L. sativus* seeds can cause lathyrism in man. The effects of β-cyanoalanine are convulsions, rigidity, prostration, and death when the compound is either injected into or fed to young or mature rats and chickens at toxic levels. The LD_{50} in young rats is 13.5 mg/100 g (subcutaneous).[45] Pyridoxal can delay and moderate the toxicity of a single injection of β-cyanoalanine.[45,46] Administration of β-cyanoalanine in the diet of rats results in the excretion of large amounts of cystathionine. β-Cyanoalanine inhibits rat liver cystathionase, the vitamin B_6-requiring enzyme that converts cystathionine to cystine[47]; the accumulation of cystathionine is the result of this enzyme inhibition.

Although it is unclear whether *Vicia sativa* is in any way concerned

TABLE 1   Distribution of Toxic Compounds in Various Species of *Lathyrus*

Species	Neurolathyrogens			Osteolathyrogen
	α,γ-Diaminobutyric Acid	N-γ-Oxalyl-α,γ-diaminobutyric Acid	N-β-Oxalyl-α,β-diaminopropionic Acid	γ-Glutamyl-β-aminopropionitrile
aurantius	++	—	—	—
luteus	++	—	—	—
laevigatus				
var. *aureus*	++	—	—	—
sylvestris	++	+	+	—
latifolius	++	+	+	—
heterophyllus	++	+	+	—
gorgoni	++	+	+	—
grandiflorus	++	+	+	—
cirrhosus	++	+	+	—
rotundifolius	++	+	+	—
tuberosus	++	+	+	—
multiflora	++	++	T	—
undulatus	++	++	T	—
setifolius	—	—	+++	—
alatus	—	—	++	—
articulatus	—	—	++	—
arvense	—	—	++	—
pannonicus	—	—	++	—
ochrus	—	—	++	—
clymenum[a]	—	—	++	—
sativus[a,b]	—	—	++	—
megallanicus	—	—	++	—
quadrimarginatus	—	—	T	—
cicera[a]	—	—	T	—
pseudocicera	—	—	T	—
tremolsianus	—	—	T	—
odoratus	—	—	—	+
hirsutus	—	—	—	+
pusillus	—	—	—	+
roseus	—	—	—	T

[a] Species implicated as the cause of classical lathyrism in man.

[b] Also contains N-β-D-glucopyranosyl-N-L-arabinosyl-α,β-diaminopropionitrile; nothing is known of the distribution of this compound in other species.

+ = 0.5–1% dry weight (approximately).
++ = 1–2% dry weight (approximately).
+++ = 2% dry weight (approximately).
T = trace.
— = not detected.

with lathyrism, the seeds of this plant have been frequently reported as contaminants of human foods. For that reason, the presence of β-cyanoalanine and its γ-glutamyl derivative in these seeds and in the seeds of a number of related species[42,48] is recorded in this survey.

Conclusions

Although there are still unanswered questions concerning the causes of human lathyrism, it is clear that the disease usually develops when the seeds of certain species of *Lathyrus* constitute a major part of the diet. All three species implicated in human lathyrism contain high concentrations of β-N-oxalyl-L-α,β-diaminopropionic acid in their seeds, and, although other factors may be involved, the presence of this compound is probably the main contributory factor in the disease. β-N-Oxalyl-L-α,β-diaminopropionic acid is also the principal free amino acid in the seeds of eight other species of *Lathyrus*[20] and two species of *Crotalaria*,[49] but as these plants are not of importance as food plants, the extent of their toxicity is not known.

Attempts have been made to remove the toxin(s) from *L. sativus* seeds by soaking them in water[50] and then draining off the water. Prolonged soaking in hot water removes the major part of the toxin(s), and such a method may be of practical application in areas where the seeds of this species are an important source of protein. Water extraction will of course also remove compounds such as the water-soluble vitamins, and the loss of these may lead to other nutritional problems. The best answer to human lathyrism, however, would seem to be the eventual replacement with other legumes of the three *Lathyrus* species concerned.

SELENO–AMINO ACIDS

The problem of selenium poisoning in man and animals has been extensively reviewed by Rosenfeld and Beath.[51] Selenium-rich soils are found in the United States, Ireland, Australia, Israel, and other parts of the world. One of the dangers to human (and animal) health is the use of food plants that may also become selenium-rich when grown on such soils. These authors showed, for example, that chronic selenium poisoning ("alkali disease") developed rapidly in hogs fed on corn containing 10 ppm of selenium, which occured in the form of selenium analogs of the sulfur amino acids of protein.

The selenium content of different plants growing on the same seleniferous soil may vary dramatically, however. Some plants known as selenium accumulator or indicator plants will grow only on selenium-rich soils and may accumulate up to 15,000 ppm of this element in their tissues.[51] Other species, called secondary selenium absorbers,[52] accumulate selenium when grown on seleniferous soils but grow equally well on normal soils. These secondary absorbers do not usually contain more than a few hundred ppm of selenium.[51] Where large concentrations of selenium occur in plants, the element is not found in the protein but in the form of low molecular weight compounds such as Se-methyl-selenocysteine. Peterson and Butler[53] have suggested that the synthesis of such compounds may be a detoxication mechanism that prevents the synthesis and incorporation of the selenium analogs of cystine and methionine into the plant protein. These accumulator plants are not a direct hazard to human health but have caused serious losses among grazing livestock. The third group of plants, into which virtually all human food plants fall, are the nonaccumulators. These are species that do not require selenium for their growth; indeed, their growth is inhibited if they absorb too much of the element. The concentration at which such inhibition occurs, however, may be well above the concentration at which plants become toxic to man, and herein lies the danger. The accumulator species may, however, play an indirect role in the toxicity of nonaccumulator species, because the accumulator species absorb inorganic selenium readily from the soil and convert it into soluble organic compounds, which, when returned to the soil, are readily absorbed by nonaccumulator plants. Crop plants grown in areas where selenium accumulators are growing or have grown may therefore be expected to contain higher concentrations of selenium than crops grown in other seleniferous areas.

In man the symptoms of selenium poisoning include dermatitis, fatigue, dizziness, and loss of hair and nails. In the United States,[54,55] and to a greater extent in Colombia,[51] many such cases have been traced to high concentrations of selenium in home-grown foods. The affected persons have recovered when placed on a selenium-free diet. An abnormally high incidence of gastrointestinal disturbances, icteroid discoloration of the skin,[56] and dental caries[57] have also been reported among people living in seleniferous areas of the United States.

Reports of acute poisoning in man by selenium-accumulating plants are all concerned with one species, *Lecythis ollaria* (monkey's coconut), belonging to the order Myrtales. *Lecythis ollaria* is a large tree that occurs widely in Central and South America, and its nuts have the reputation both in Brazil and Venezuela of causing loss of hair from the scalp and body when eaten. Kerdel-Vegas[58] describes nine cases of poisoning by the "coco de mono" nuts in Venezuela. The persons concerned were all strangers to the area and had either not been warned of the toxic nature of the nuts or had chosen to ignore the warnings. The least serious case involved a 12-yr-old boy who ate about seven nuts, which caused nausea and vomiting but no other ill effects. Other cases in which larger quantities had been eaten (15–80 nuts) were characterized by diarrhea, dizziness, and loss of hair (in some cases complete) from the scalp and also in some instances from the body. Fragility of the nails was also reported. The most serious case involved the death of a 2-yr-old boy.

In nonaccumulator crop plants it has now been shown[59,60] that selenium taken up by the plant is primarily incorporated into protein as L-seleno-methionine, $CH_3 SeCH_2 CH_2 CH(NH_2)CO_2 H$, or L-seleno-cystine, shown below:

$$SeCH_2 CH(NH_2)CO_2 H$$
$$|$$
$$SeCH_2 CH(NH_2)CO_2 H$$

In selenium accumulators, as previously mentioned, selenium is not incorporated into the protein but occurs in the form of soluble seleno-compounds of low molecular weight.[53,61] In *Lecythis ollaria* the toxic selenium compound is seleno-cystathionine,[62] $HO_2 CCH(NH_2)CH_2 CH_2 - SeCH_2 CH(NH_2)CO_2 H$. The effect of this compound in causing hair loss in man and experimental animals led to the suggestion[63] that the compound might be cytotoxic to the hair-follicle cell, and experiments have shown that it inhibits growth in mouse fibroblasts. Of various sulfur compounds added to fibroblast cultures inhibited with seleno-cystathionine, L-cystine proved to be most effective in reversing toxicity.[63]

For further information on selenium toxicity and selenium-containing compounds, see Chapters 3 and 5, respectively.

The principal causes of selenium toxicity in man are seleno-methionine and seleno-cystine, which are incorporated into the proteins of crop plants grown in seleniferous soils. Concentrations of selenium in these crops may reach levels of 20–30 ppm, which are several times greater than those that will induce selenium poisoning.[51] A high incidence of gastrointestinal disturbances, skin discoloration, and dental caries is found in populations living on seleniferous soils. In exceptional cases, acute selenium toxicity in man may be caused by eating the nuts of *Lecythis ollaria,* which contain seleno-cystathionine.

OTHER PLANT AMINO ACIDS THAT MAY BE TOXIC TO MAN

Canavanine

Canavanine, $H_2NC(:NH)NHOCH_2CH_2CH(NH_2)CO_2H$, a close chemical analog of arginine, is found in many species of the Papilionoideae (a subfamily of the Leguminosae) and may constitute more than 5% of the dry-seed weight of some species.

This amino acid acts as an antimetabolite to arginine in many organisms.[64] Tschiersch[65] showed that both the seed of *Canavalia ensiformis* and purified canavanine itself (at concentrations of 200 mg canavanine/kg mouse) are toxic when fed to mice.

The seeds of several wild species of *Canavalia* are reported to be toxic to man when eaten raw, but they are used by native peoples after cooking (Dr. J. Sauer, personal communication). Similarly, the seeds of a species of *Dioclea* (found in this laboratory to be rich in canavanine) are reported by Dr. D. H. Janzen (personal communication) to be eaten by the natives of Costa Rica after roasting. The hemagglutinating activity of *Canavalia ensiformis* seed is destroyed by heating, but the heated seed is still toxic to rats.[66] Preliminary experiments in this laboratory have shown that some but not all of the canavanine is destroyed or extracted when *Canavalia* seeds are roasted or boiled for periods of 15–45 min. It is possible, therefore, that this amino acid could produce toxic effects in man if canavanine-rich foods constituted a major part of the diet.

L-3,4-Dihydroxyphenylalanine (L-DOPA)

Low concentrations of L-3,4-dihydroxyphenylalanine (L-DOPA) are not uncommon in plants, but the pods of *Vicia faba* (the broad bean) contain as much as 0.25% of this amino acid either free or in the form of a β-glycoside.[67,68]

Kosower and Kosower[69] showed that reduced glutathione was lost from erythrocytes deficient in glucose-6-phosphate dehydrogenase (G6PD) when these were incubated in a medium containing L-DOPA. This observation led them to speculate that L-DOPA might be a factor in favism. (See Chapter 22.)

L-3,4-Dihydroxyphenylalanine (L-DOPA)

The recent interest in the use of L-DOPA in the treatment of Parkinson's disease[70] led to a re-investigation of this possibility, but no hemolytic effects were apparent when G6PD-deficient erythrocytes were exposed to high concentrations of L-DOPA *in vivo.*[71]

It is known, however, that L-DOPA may produce other undesirable side effects such as "nausea, vomiting and involuntary chewing movements" when administered orally in high dosage.[72]

At the present time the use of L-DOPA is limited by cost and availability, but the recent finding that seeds of various *Mucuna* species contain between 6 and 9% of free L-DOPA[73,74] may well make the amino acid itself, or plant extracts containing it, more widely available and the problem of toxicity a more serious one.

5-Hydroxy-L-tryptophan (5-HTP)

5-Hydroxy-L-tryptophan (5-HTP) is the precursor of 5-hydroxytryptamine (5-HT, Serotonin) a physiologically active amine in mammalian brain. Udenfriend and co-workers[75,76] have shown that 5-HTP (unlike 5-HT) can cross the blood–brain barrier and that 5-HTP when injected into dogs and rats can produce up to 10-fold increases in the level of 5-HT in the brain. Such increases of 5-HT produced "tremors, pupillary dilation, loss of light reflex, apparent blindness, salivation, marked hyperpnea and tachycardia."

HO—[indole ring]—CH$_2$CH(NH$_2$)COOH

L-5-Hydroxytryptophan (5-HTP)

The interrelationship between 5-HTP and L-DOPA is emphasized by reports of a case in which the Parkinson-like symptoms of chronic manganese poisoning that had been aggravated by treatment with L-DOPA were relieved with 5-HTP.[77] The latter amino acid has also given promising results in the treatment of Down's syndrome (Mongolism),[78] and produces an increase in rapid eye movement sleep in normal subjects.[79]

Like L-DOPA, 5-HTP is at present in short supply, but the discovery that the seeds of a West African legume (*Griffonia simplicifolia*) used in native medicine[80] contain 6–10% of free 5-HTP[81,82] may lead to the wider use of this potentially toxic, nonprotein amino acid and also to the explanation of some of the physiological effects ascribed to *Griffonia simplicifolia* by the peoples of West Africa.

α-Amino-β-Methylaminopropionic Acid

Various species of the cycads are used as human food and in medicine in different parts of the world. It is well known that some of these plants are extremely poisonous to man and to grazing animals and the presence of carcinogens in certain of them is discussed in Chapter 23. The carcinogenic glycosides that have been isolated from the cycads produce acute poisoning in experimental animals but there is no evidence that they produce the paralysis of the hind legs seen in cattle that have eaten leaves of *Zamia,* nor do they account for the high incidence of amyotrophic lateral sclerosis found among the peoples of Guam who use seeds of *Cycas circinalis* as a source of food starch.[83,84]

The seeds of *Cycas circinalis* do, however, contain an unusual amino acid L-α-amino-β-methylaminopropionic acid, $(H_3C)HNCH_2CH(NH_2)CO_2H$, that is neurotoxic in chicks and rats.[85,86]

This amino acid had not been found to produce permanent paralysis in experimental animals, nor are the concentrations of the free amino acid in the seeds of *Cycas circinalis* sufficiently high to account for neurological effects in man unless he is much more sensitive to this compound than are rats or chicks. Nevertheless, it has been found that L-α-amino-β-methylaminopropionic acid occurs in a bound form as well as in the free state in all species implicated as causes of paralysis in man and animals.[87] Like the neurotoxic agent of *Lathyrus sativus,* this new amino acid from *C. circinalis* is a β-*N*-substituted α,β-diaminopropionic acid, and it is possible that this compound may yet prove to be concerned in the toxicity of the cycads.

REFERENCES

1. V. V. S. Murti and T. R. Seshadri, Toxic amino acids of plants, Curr. Sci. *33*: 323 (1964).
2. B. Tschiersch, Toxische Aminosäuren. Pharmazie *21*:445 (1966).
3. L. Fowden, D. Lewis, and H. Tristram, Toxic amino acids: Their action as antimetabolites. Adv. Enzymol. *29*:89 (1967).
4. J. F. Thompson, C. J. Morris, and I. K. Smith, New naturally occurring amino acids. Ann. Rev. Biochem. *38*:137 (1969).
5. H. Selye, Lathyrism. Rev. Can. Biol. *16*:1 (1957).
6. D. N. Sharma, Lathyrism: The old and new concepts. J. Indian. Med. Assoc. *36*:299 (1961).
7. P. S. Sarma and G. Padmanaban, Lathyrogens. In Toxic constituents of plant foodstuffs, I. E. Liener (ed.). Academic Press, New York (1969).
8. G. F. McKay, J. J. Lalich, E. D. Schilling, and F. M. Strong, A crystalline

"lathyrus factor" from *Lathyrus odoratus*. Arch. Biochem. Biophys. *52*:313 (1954).

9. E. D. Schilling and F. M. Strong, Isolation, structure and synthesis of a lathyrus factor from *L. odoratus*. J. Am. Chem. Soc. *76*:2848 (1954).

10. H. P. Dupuy and J. G. Lee, The isolation of a material capable of producing experimental lathyrism. J. Am. Pharm. Assoc. Sci. Ed. *43*:61 (1954).

11. W. Dasler, Isolation of toxic crystals from sweet peas (*Lathyrus odoratus*). Science *120:*307 (1954).

12. T. E. Bachhuber, J. J. Lalich, E. D. Schilling, and F. M. Strong, Lathyrus factor activity of beta-aminopropionitrile. Fed. Proc. *14*:175 (1955).

13. C. I. Levene, Structural requirements for lathyrogenic agents. J. Exp. Med. *114*:295 (1961).

14. C. I. Levene, Studies on the mode of action of lathyrogenic compounds. J. Exp. Med. *116*:119 (1962).

15. B. L. O'Dell, D. F. Elsden, J. Thomas, S. M. Partridge, R. H. Smith, and R. Palmer, Inhibition of the biosynthesis of the cross-links in elastin by a lathyrogen. Nature *209*:401 (1966).

16. C. Ressler, P. A. Redstone, and R. H. Erenberg, Isolation and identification of a neuroactive factor from *Lathyrus latifolius*. Science *134*:188 (1961).

17. C. H. VanEtten and R. W. Miller, The neuroactive factor *alpha-gamma* diaminobutyric acid in angiosperm seeds. Econ. Bot. *17*:107 (1963).

18. R. M. O'Neal, C. Chen, C. S. Reynolds, S. K. Meghal, and R. E. Koeppe, The neurotoxicity of L-2,4-Diaminobutyric acid. Biochem. J. *106*:699 (1968).

19. E. A. Bell, Associations of ninhydrin-reacting compounds in seeds of 49 species of *Lathyrus*. Biochem. J. *83*:225 (1962).

20. E. A. Bell, Relevance of biochemical taxonomy to the problem of lathyrism. Nature, *203*:378 (1964).

21. E. A. Bell, The isolation of L-homoarginine from seeds of *Lathyrus cicera*. Biochem. J. *85*:91 (1962).

22. S. L. N. Rao, L. K. Ramachandran, and P. R. Adiga, The isolation and characterization of L-homoarginine from seeds of *Lathyrus sativus*. Biochemistry *2*: 298 (1963).

23. C. M. Stevens and J. A. Bush, New synthesis of α-amino-ϵ-guanidino-η-caproic acid (homoarginine) and its possible conversion *in vivo* into lysine. J. Biol. Chem. *183*:139 (1950).

24. S. L. N. Rao, P. R. Adiga, and P. S. Sarma, The isolation and characterization of β-N-oxalyl-L-α-β-diaminopropionic acid: A neurotoxin from seeds of *Lathyrus sativus*. Biochemistry *3*:432 (1964).

25. V. V. S. Murti, T. R. Seshadri, and T. A. Venkitasubramanian, Neurotoxic compounds of the seeds of *Lathyrus sativus*. Phytochemistry *3*:73 (1964).

26. K. Malathi, G. Padmanaban, and P. S. Sarma, Biosynthesis of β-N-oxalyl-L-α,β-diaminopropionic acid, the *Lathyrus sativus* neurotoxin. Phytochemistry *9*:1603 (1970).

27. E. A. Bell and J. P. O'Donovan, The isolation of α and γ-oxalyl derivatives of α,γ-diaminobutyric acid from seeds of *Lathyrus latifolius* and the detection of the α-oxalyl isomer of the neurotoxin α-amino-β-oxalylaminopropionic acid which occurs together with the neurotoxin in this and other species. Phytochemistry *5*:1211 (1966).

28. P. R. Adiga, S. L. N. Rao, and P. S. Sarma, Some structural features and neuro-

toxic action of a compound from *Lathyrus sativus* seeds. Curr. Sci. *32*:153 (1963).

29. S. L. N. Rao and P. S. Sarma, Neurotoxic action of β-*N*-oxalyl-L-α,β-diaminopropionic acid. Biochem. Pharmacol. *16*:218 (1967).

30. J. C. Watkins, D. R. Curtis, and T. J. Biscoe, Central effects of β-*N*-oxalyl-α,β-diaminopropionic acid and other lathyrus factors. Nature *211*:637 (1966).

31. P. S. Cheema, G. Padmanaban, and P. S. Sarma, Biochemical characterization of β-*N*-oxalyl-L-α,β-diaminopropionic acid, the *Lathyrus sativus* neurotoxin as an excitant amino acid. J. Neurochem. *17*:1295 (1970).

32. S. L. N. Rao, P. S. Sarma, K. S. Mani, T. R. Raghunatha Rao and S. Sriramachari, Experimental neurolathyrism in monkeys. Nature *214*:610 (1967).

33. D. R. Curtis and J. C. Watkins, The pharmacology of amino acids related to γ-aminobutyric acid. Pharmacol. Rev. *17*:347 (1965).

34. P. S. Cheema, G. Padmanaban, and P. S. Sarma, Neurotoxic action of β-*N*-oxalyl-L-α,β-diaminopropionic acid in acidotic adult rats. Indian J. Biochem. *6*: 146 (1969).

35. C. Rukmini, Isolation and purification of a new toxic factor from *Lathyrus sativus*. Indian J. Biochem. *5*:182 (1968).

36. C. Rukmini, Structure of the new toxin from *Lathyrus sativus*. Indian J. Chem. *7*:1062 (1969).

37. S. L. N. Rao and P. S. Sarma, Neurotoxic properties of *N*-substituted oxamic acids. Indian J. Biochem. *3*:57 (1966).

38. E. A. Bell and R. G. Foster. Structure of lathyrine (a new amino acid). Nature *194*:91 (1962).

39. J. Przybylska and F. M. Strong, Identification of γ-methylglutamic acid in *Lathyrus maritimus*. Phytochemistry *7*:471 (1968).

40. L. Fowden, Isolation of γ-hydroxynorvaline from *Lathyrus odoratus* seed. Nature *209*:807 (1966).

41. C. Ressler, Isolation and identification from common vetch of the neurotoxin β-cyano-L-alanine, a possible factor in neurolathyrism. J. Biol. Chem. *237*:733 (1962).

42. C. Ressler, S. N. Nigam, Y.-H. Giza and J. Nelson, Isolation and identification from common vetch of γ-L-glutamyl-β-cyano-L-alanine, a bound form of the neurotoxin β-cyano-L-alanine. J. Am. Chem. Soc. *85*:3311 (1963).

43. C. Ressler, S. N. Nigam, and Y.-H. Giza, Toxic principle in vetch. Isolation and identification of γ-L-glutamyl-L-β-cyanoalanine from common vetch seeds. Distribution in some legumes. J. Am. Chem. Soc. *91*:2758 (1969).

44. L. A. P. Anderson, A. Howard and J. L. Simonsen, Studies on lathyrism. Indian J. Med. Res. *12*:613 (1925).

45. C. Ressler, J. Nelson, and M. Pfeffer, Metabolism of β-cyanoalanine. Biochem. Pharmacol. *16*:2309 (1967).

46. C. Ressler, J. Nelson, and M. Pfeffer, A pyridoxal-β-cyanoalanine relation in the rat. Nature *203*:1286 (1964).

47. M. Pfeffer and C. Ressler, β-Cyanoalanine, an inhibitor of rat liver cystathionase. Biochem. Pharmacol. *16*:2299 (1967).

48. E. A. Bell and A. S. L. Tirimanna, Associations of amino acids and related compounds in the seeds of 47 species of *Vicia*: Their taxonomic and nutritional significance. Biochem. J. *97*:104 (1965).

49. E. A. Bell, Occurrence of the neurolathyrogen α-amino-β-oxalylaminopropionic acid in two species of *Crotalaria*. Nature *218*:197 (1968).
50. V. S. Mohan, V. Nagarajan, and C. Gopalan, Simple practical procedures for the removal of toxic factors in *Lathyrus sativus* (Khesari dhal). Indian J. Med. Res. *54*:410 (1966).
51. I. Rosenfeld and O. A. Beath, Selenium. Academic Press, New York (1964).
52. J. M. Kingsbury, Poisonous plants of the United States and Canada. Prentice-Hall, Englewood Cliffs, N.J. (1964).
53. P. J. Peterson and G. W. Butler, Significance of selenocystathionine in an Australian selenium-accumulating plant, *Neptunia amplexicaulis*. Nature *213*:599 (1967).
54. R. E. Lemley, Selenium poisoning in the human. A preliminary case report. J. Lancet *60*:528 (1940).
55. R. E. Lemley and M. P. Merryman, Selenium poisoning in the human. J. Lancet *61*:435 (1941).
56. M. I. Smith and B. B. Westfall, Further field studies on the selenium problem in relation to public health. U.S. Public Health Rep. *52*:1375 (1937).
57. D. M. Hadjimarkos, Effect of selenium on dental caries. Arch. Environ. Health *10*:893 (1965).
58. F. Kerdel-Vegas, Generalized hair loss due to the ingestion of "coco de mono" (*Lecythis ollaria*). J. Invest. Dermatol. *42*:91 (1964).
59. P. J. Peterson and G. W. Butler, The uptake and assimilation of selenite by higher plants. Aust. J. Biol. Sci. *15*:126 (1962).
60. A. Shrift, Aspects of selenium metabolism in higher plants. Ann. Rev. Plant Phys. *20*:475 (1969).
61. P. J. Peterson, Sulphur and selenium containing amino acids. Phytochemistry *9*:916 (1970).
62. F. Kerdel-Vegas, F. Wagner, P. B. Russell, N. H. Grant, H. E. Alburn, D. E. Clark, and J. A. Miller, Structure of the pharmacologically active factor in the seeds of *Lecythis ollaria*. Nature *205*:1186 (1965).
63. L. Arononow and F. Kerdel-Vegas, Seleno-cystathionine, a pharmacologically active factor in the seeds of *Lecythis ollaria*. Nature *205*:1185 (1965).
64. A. Meister, Biochemistry of the amino acids, vol. I. Academic Press, New York (1965).
65. B. Tschiersch, Zur Toxischen Wirkung der Jackbohne. Pharmazie *17*:621 (1962).
66. H. J. H. de Muelenaere, Toxicity and haemagglutinating activity of legumes. Nature *206*:827 (1965).
67. M. Guggenheim, Dioxyphenylalanine, eine neue Aminosäure aus *Vicia faba*. Z. Phys. Chem. *88*:276 (1913).
68. R. S. Andrews and J. B. Pridham, Structure of a DOPA glucoside from *Vicia faba*. Nature *205*:1213 (1965).
69. N. S. Kosower and E. M. Kosower, Does 3,4-dihydroxyphenylalanine play a part in favism. Nature *215*:285 (1965).
70. D. B. Calne and M. Sandler, L-Dopa and Parkinsonism. Nature *226*:21 (1970).
71. G. Gaetani, E. Salvidio, I. Pannacciulli, F. Ajmar, and G. Paravidino, Absence of haemolytic effects of L-dopa on transfused G-6PD-deficient erythrocytes. Experimentia *26*:785 (1970).
72. M. H. Van Woert and M. B. Bowers, The effect of L-dopa on monoamine metabolites in Parkinson's disease. Experimentia *26*:161 (1970).

73. E. A. Bell and D. H. Janzen, Medical and ecological considerations of L-DOPA and 5-HTP in Seeds. Nature *229*:136 (1971).
74. M. E. Daxenbichler, C. H. VanEtten, E. A. Hallinan, and F. R. Earle, Seeds as sources of L-dopa. J. Med. Chem. *14*:463 (1971).
75. S. Udenfriend, E. Titus, H. Weissbach, and R. E. Peterson, Biogenesis and metabolism of 5-hydroxyindole compounds. J. Biol. Chem. *219*:335 (1956).
76. S. Udenfriend, H. Weissbach, and D. F. Bogdanski, Increase in tissue serotonin following administration of its precursor 5-hydroxytryptophan. J. Biol. Chem. *224*:803 (1957).
77. I. Mena, J. Court, S. Fuenzalida, P. S. Papavasiliou, and G. C. Cotzias, Modification of chronic manganese poisoning. N. Engl. J. Med. *282*:5 (1970).
78. M. Bazelon, R. S. Paine, V. A. Cowie, P. Hunt, J. C. Houck, and D. Mahanand, Reversal of hypotonia in infants with Down's syndrome by administration of 5-hydroxytryptophan. Lancet *i*:1130 (1967).
79. R. J. Wyatt, Serotonin and sleep. In Serotonin now: Clinical implications of inhibiting its synthesis with parachlorophenylalanine. Ann. Intern. Med. *73*: 607 (1970).
80. F. R. Irvine, Woody plants of Ghana. Oxford University Press, London (1961).
81. E. A. Bell and L. E. Fellows, Free 5-hydroxytryptophan in plants. Nature *210*: 529 (1966).
82. L. E. Fellows and E. A. Bell, 5-Hydroxy-L-tryptophan, 5-hydroxy-tryptamine, and L-tryptophan-5-hydroxylase in *Griffonia simplicifolia*. Phytochemistry *9*:2389 (1970).
83. M. G. Whiting, Toxicity of cycads. Econ. Bot. *17*:271 (1963).
84. M. C. Yang and O. Michelsen, Cycads. In Toxic constitutents of foodstuffs, I. E. Liener (ed.). Academic Press, New York (1969).
85. A. Vega and E. A. Bell, α-Amino-β-methylaminopropionic acid, a new amino acid from seeds of *Cycas circinalis*. Phytochemistry *6*:759 (1967).
86. A. Vega, E. A. Bell and P. B. Nunn, The preparation of L- and D-α-amino-β-methylaminopropionic acids and the identification of the compound isolated from *Cycas circinalis* as the L-isomer. Phytochemistry *7*:1885 (1968).
87. S. F. Dossaji and E. A. Bell, Distribution of α-amino-β-methylaminopropionic acid in *Cycas*. Photochemistry *12*:143 (1973).

8 Walter Lovenberg

SOME VASO- AND PSYCHOACTIVE SUBSTANCES IN FOOD: AMINES, STIMULANTS, DEPRESSANTS, AND HALLUCINOGENS*

Our current generation is more concerned with using natural and synthetic chemical substances to alter the physiological and psychological state than any previous generation. Great benefits and hazards accompany our increased awareness of our ability to alter our state of being. Thus, hundreds of chemical compounds have been found to be useful therapeutic agents, and many of these were derived from natural products known to have beneficial effects on man's health. Conversely, many natural products are toxic or hazardous to man if consumed in large amounts or if consumed simultaneously with therapeutic agents.

Although man has used innumerable exotic concoctions throughout recorded history for psychotropic effects, this chapter will be limited largely to a discussion of psychoactive and vasoactive substances in commonly used food substances. The relationship between psychoactive and vasoactive substances lies in the probability that psychoactive substances exert their effect by altering neuronal transmission in the central nervous system, and that the normal neuronal transmitters are vasoactive substances in the periphery. In the current discussion stimulants and depressants are defined as substances that stimulate or depress the central nervous system.

* Literature reviewed to March 1972.

170

VASOACTIVE AMINES IN FOOD

It is known that certain naturally occurring phenethylamine derivatives (i.e., tyramine, dopamine, and norepinephrine) cause a very marked increase in blood pressure when administered intravenously to mammals.

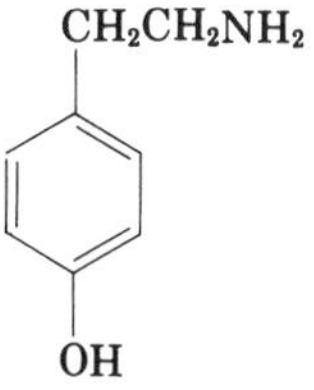

$CH_2CH_2NH_2$

OH

Tyramine

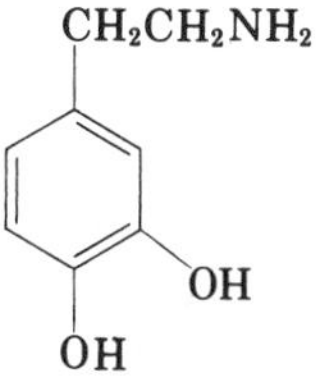

$CH_2CH_2NH_2$

OH
OH

Dopamine

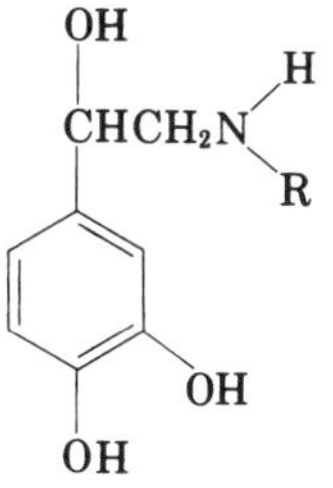

OH
$CHCH_2N\begin{smallmatrix}H\\R\end{smallmatrix}$

OH
OH

Epinephrine, $R = CH_3$
Norepinephrine, $R = H$

Serotonin (5-HT) and histamine are also strongly vasoactive compounds.[30] Investigations over the past decade make it clear that these amines are present in numerous foods. Amines are synthesized by certain plants or can arise from microbial contamination or fermentative processes. In general, however, animal products do not contain sufficient levels of endogenous amines to be of any concern.

Many bacteria have enzymes that catalyze the decarboxylation of a variety of amino acids.[29] It is therefore not surprising that aged or fermented food products that undergo limited proteolysis are known to contain many different amines. As early as 1877 Nencki[55] identified amylamine in putrefying meat. In 1903 Van Slyke and Hart[67] observed the presence of tyramine and probably putrescine in ripened cheddar cheese. In the next several years the presence of amines in cheeses was widely reported. Likewise, many amines were observed in putrefying meat.[5]

The finding of Waalkes *et al.*[68] in 1958 that bananas contain relatively large quantities of both serotonin and norepinephrine is of considerable interest, since in this case the amines were undoubtedly endogenous to a plant substance that is commonly used for food. Shortly thereafter, West[70] reported the presence of tryptamine in the tomato, and Udenfriend et al.[66] surveyed a number of fruits and vegetables and found amines to be rather widespread in normal food substances. Since that time several other edible plants have been reported to contain various amines, and the presence of amines in microbially contaminated and fermented foods has been re-established. The amine content of some commonly used plant food substances is shown in Table 1. This list is clearly incomplete and could be greatly expanded with a systematic examination. In addition to the foods given in Table 1, several other relevant reports have appeared. A whole series of phenylalkyl amines have been reported to be present in citrus fruits.[71] In addition to tyramine, these include N-methyltyramine, N,N-dimethyltyramine (hordinine), octopamine, synephrine, and feruloylputrescine. Tyramine and its mono- and di- N-methylated derivatives have also been found in sawa millet seeds.[60] It is likely that these tyramine derivatives are quite prevalent in a number of plant foods. In addition to amines Hodge et al.[37] have reported that broad beans contain rather large amounts of the amino acid dihydroxyphenylalanine (DOPA), which can be decarboxylated after consumption to form the pressor substance dopamine.

TABLE 1   Vasoactive Amines in Plant Foods

Plant Substance	Reference	Amine in μg/gm or μg/ml[a]				
		Serotonin	Tryptamine	Tyramine	Dopamine	Norepinephrine
Banana peel	66	50–100	0	65	700	122
Banana pulp	66	28	0	7	8	2
Plantain pulp	66	45	–	–	–	–
Tomato	66	12	4	4	0	0
Red plum	66	10	0–2	6	0	+
Red blue plum	66	8	2	–	–	–
Blue plum	66	0	5	–	–	–
Avocado	66	10	0	23	4–5	0
Potato	66	0	0	1	0	0.1–0.2
Spinach	66	0	0	1	0	0
Grape	66	0	0	0	0	0
Orange	66	0	0.1	10	0	+
Eggplant	66	0	0	–	–	–
Pineapple juice	16,27	25–35	–	–	–	–
Pineapple, ripe	27	20	–	–	–	–
Passion fruit	26	1–4	–	–	–	–
Pawpaw	26	1–2	–	–	–	–

[a] A dash means the food was not tested for this amine, 0 means that the level of the amine was below the detection threshold, and + indicates the material contained a trace of the amine.

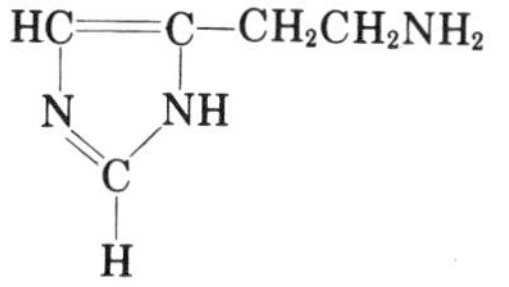

$$HC = C - CH_2CH_2NH_2$$

with ring: N, NH, C, H

Histamine

$$NH_2(CH_2)_nNH_2$$

Putrescine, $n = 4$
Cadeverine, $n = 5$

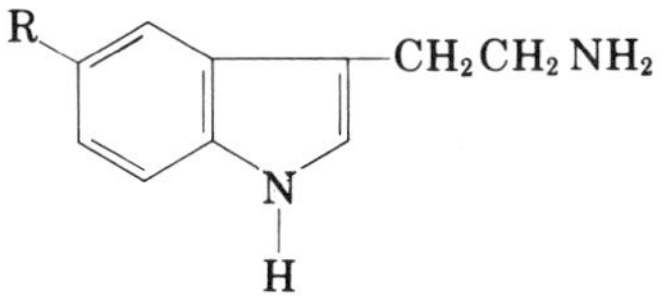

$$R - [indole ring] - CH_2CH_2NH_2$$

N
H

Tryptamine, R = H
Serotonin, R = OH

A finding of particular interest is that common tea contains significant amounts of 3,4-dimethoxyphenethylamine. This compound is also known as the "pink spot," because of its appearance on chromatograms of urinary extracts. It was originally identified in the urine of schizophrenic patients and has been the center of considerable controversy as to whether its excretion is unique to this disease or whether its formation *in vivo* contributes to the symptoms. It has been concluded that the presence of dimethoxyphenethylamine in urine is due to ingestion of plant foods such as tea and that it is not primarily related to schizophrenia.[63]

Food substances that have been prepared by a fermentative process, or have been exposed to microbial contamination during aging or storage, are likely to contain vasoactive amines. Table 2 lists a number of foods that have been shown to contain tyramine that is probably of microbial origin. Tyramine has been identified in food more often than other amines for several reasons. First, several organisms that are often present or used in the preparation of cheese and fermented food contain a very active tyrosine decarboxylase.[32] Second, there are sensitive, specific, and well-established assay procedures for measuring this amine.

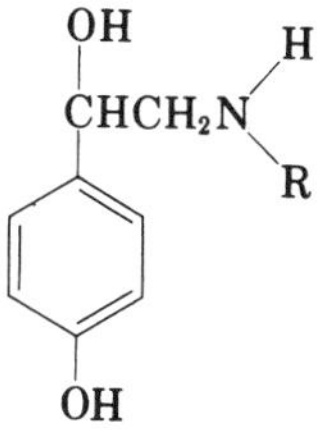

OH
$$CHCH_2N \begin{matrix} H \\ R \end{matrix}$$

OH

Octopamine, R = H
Synephrine, R = CH_3

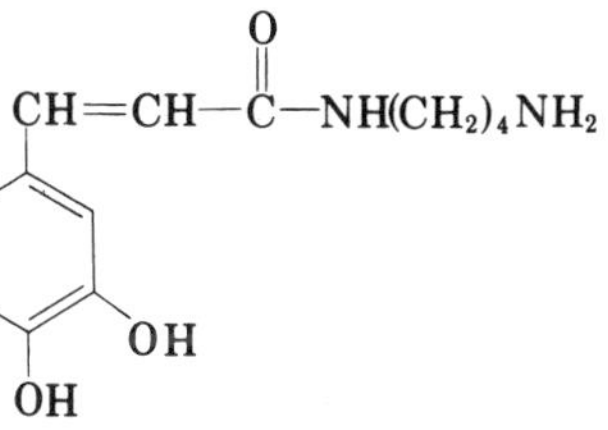

$$CH = CH - C(=O) - NH(CH_2)_4NH_2$$

OH
OH

Feruloylputrescine

TABLE 2   Foods Reported to Contain Tyramine of Probable Microbial Origin

Food Substance	Tyramine (μg/gm)	Reference
Cheese		
Cheddar	120–1,500	4,10,43,61
Camembert	20–2,000	4,43,61
Emmenthaler	225–1,000	4,43
Brie	0–200	43,61
Stilton blue	466–2,170	43,61
Processed	26–50	43,61
Gruyere	516	43
Gouda	20	61
Brick, natural	524	61
Mozzarella	410	61
Blue	30–250	61
Roquefort	27–520	61
Boursault	1,116	61
Parmesan	4–290	61
Romano	238	61
Provolone	38	61
Beer and ale	1.8–11.2	43,61
Wines	0–25	43,61
Marmite yeast and yeast extract	0–2,250	12,43,61
Fish		
Salted dried fish	0–470	61
Pickled herring	3,000	56
Meat		
Meat extracts	95–304	61
Beef liver (stored)	274	15
Chicken liver (stored)	100	36
Miscellaneous		
Soya	1.76	61

Finally, its relatively high content in certain foods, coupled with its great pressor activity in patients receiving monoamine oxidase inhibitors, has focused attention on foods that have precipitated hypertensive crises in such patients.

Since bacteria contain a variety of amino acid decarboxylases,[29,32] it is not surprising that many other amines have also been identified in food. Organisms that contain active histidine decarboxylases are also prevalent in foods,[32] although histamine is not widely reported in food substances. Blackwell et al.[12] found up to 2 mg of histamine per g of marmite, a concentrated yeast autolysate commonly used as a food in

Great Britain and Australia.[11] Alcoholic beverages such as wine and beer may contain significant amounts of histamine,[52,58] as do some other fermented foods such as sauerkraut[48] and chocolate.[51] It is also becoming apparent that fish may have rather high levels of histamine, depending on their exposure to bacterial contamination and on conditions of storage.[23] Other amines that have been reported in foods exposed to bacterial action include tryptamine,[4,43] phenylethylamine,[4,5,74] isoamylamine[13] and putrescine and cadaverine.[4,67] Recently, Harrison *et al.*[35] reported that the free total amine content of pork increases during an aging process. It is clear that these values, however, represented both amines and amino acids, reflecting both proteolysis and amine formation.

CLINICAL SIGNIFICANCE OF VASOACTIVE AMINES IN FOODS

The presence of amines in food is of concern to the physician for three reasons: (a) Amine metabolites in urine may lead to erroneous interpretation of certain clinical tests; (b) an amine-rich food is a distinct health hazard to an individual receiving a monoamine oxidase inhibitor; and (c) the amine may itself be toxic.

Amines are normally rapidly deaminated after they enter the body. Many tissues contain the enzyme monoamine oxidase. This mitochondrial enzyme catalyzes the oxidative deamination of most of the vasoactive amines, and it has only been since the introduction of inhibitors of this enzyme, as therapeutic agents, that the consumption of vasoactive amines has become a problem. During 1962 and 1963 a number of letters appeared in *The Lancet* reporting dangerous but unexplained side effects of the drug tranylcypromine. The physicians reported that patients taking this drug were subject to sporadic bouts of severe hypertension that were occasionally accompanied by intracerebral hemorrhage and death. These early observations have been reviewed by Blackwell *et al.*[13] In 1963 Blackwell[9] reported that this paroxysmal hypertension in several cases followed the ingestion of cheese meals. A number of letters in *The Lancet* confirming this correlation quickly followed. (See Blackwell *et al.*[13] for review.) The answer to this puzzle was already in the literature, since it was known that cheese contained tyramine and that tryamine was a strong pressor substance in subjects treated with monoamine oxidase inhibitors. Asatoor *et al.*[4] and Horwitz *et al.*[43] analyzed a number of cheeses for tyramine and found that this amine was prevalent in cheese, in some cases in very high concentrations (up to 2 mg/g). Under controlled hospital conditions, Horwitz *et al.*[43] examined the effect of tyramine and cheese on the blood pressure of a human subject before and after treatment with a monoamine oxidase inhibitor. This individual showed only minor response to either tyramine or cheese during the control period, but after inhibition of monoamine oxidase there was a marked blood pressure response to either tyramine or cheese. As little as 20 g of cheese resulted in a dangerous rise in blood pressure that had to be controlled by administration of phentolamine.

There are now numerous other reports of hypertensive crises in patients receiving monoamine oxidase inhibitors. Bethune et al.[8] reported that during 692 courses of monoamine oxidase inhibitor therapy, 8.4% of the patients experienced acute hypertensive crises, several of them in response to food known to contain tyramine. Although much remains to be learned about other amines in food as they relate to the individual receiving monoamine oxidase inhibitors, it now appears that tyramine is the major offender in precipitating hypertensive crises. It was recently suggested that aminoguanidine, a potent inhibitor of histaminase, a diamine oxidase,[6,75] may have therapeutic value. If this drug is prescribed, one should consider the possible potentiating effects of histamine-containing foods on the patients involved.

The biochemical hallmark of the diseases pheochromocytoma and malignant carcinoid is the elevated excretion of the metabolites of norepinephrine and serotonin, respectively. Measurement of these metabolites in urine provides simple diagnostic tests for these diseases. Consumption of several bananas results in sufficient amounts of norepinephrine metabolites in urine to give a positive test for pheochromocytoma.[20] Likewise, consumption of bananas and/or pineapple juice in sufficient quantities may result in a positive test for the carcinoid syndrome[16,19,20,27,28] in the absence of the disease. Medical personnel should therefore request that individuals being tested for these diseases refrain from serotonin- or norepinephrine-containing foods before undergoing such tests.

The direct toxic effects of vasoactive amines are somewhat more difficult to correlate. There is a high incidence of right-sided valvular heart lesions in a group of Africans who utilize plantains or bananas as a major food source.[28] Coincidentally, patients with the carcinoid syndrome who are also chronically exposed to excess serotonin because of the secretion of their tumors also have a high frequency of a similar type of heart disease.[62] While a direct correlation between serotonin and the above lesion has not been established, the similarity of the two situations makes such a relationship tenable. Another possible direct toxic effect of amines in foods may be headaches. It is known that the intravenous injection of as little as 1–2 mg of histamine may result in a headache,[42] although orally administered histamine is much less effective. Excess consumption of fermented beverages could cause a headache. Marmite, which contains up to 2.8 mg/g histamine,[11] could possibly cause headaches. The possible role of serotonin in migraine headache has been discussed broadly,[3,22] but the evidence is not yet clear that serotonin is directly related to this disease. It appears that histamine is responsible for some of the toxic effects seen in patients who have consumed contaminated fish.[24]

Because our knowledge of the vasoactive amine content of foods is still far from complete, and because microbial contamination can greatly alter amine levels, one must constantly be aware of potential interaction with various therapeutic agents.

PSYCHOACTIVE SUBSTANCES IN FOOD

It is generally thought that impulses in the central nervous system are transmitted from cell to cell by neurotransmitter substances. Among the compounds that serve as transmitters normally are norepinephrine, dopamine, serotonin, and possibly histamine. Although these amines are prevalent in common food substances, their ingestion has little or no effect on the central nervous system, since they do not penetrate the blood–brain barrier. The exact mechanism of how psychoactive compounds mediate their effect is not known, but it is likely that they interfere with the normal functioning of the neurotransmitters in specific areas of the central nervous system. Evidence for this type of action of a number of hallucinogenic alkaloids has recently been reviewed.[39]

There are innumerable toxic plant substances that exert some or all of their toxic effects on the central nervous system. Kingsbury[49] has extensively reviewed the toxic plants of North America. Man and animals generally select foods on the basis of nutritive value, availability, and lack of toxicity. Thus, many of the toxic plants cannot be considered typical foodstuffs. This review will be largely restricted to psychoactive substances present in commonly or intentionally used foods.

Table 3 summarizes the major types of psychoactive substances in food. It should be remembered that the effects of many psychoactive substances cannot be exclusively classified as stimulants, depressants, or hallucinogens, since the effects on the central nervous system are often dose-related.

TABLE 3 Some Examples of Psychoactive Substances in Plants That Can Be Used as Foods

Class of Compounds	Example	Food or Plant Source	Effect on Central Nervous System
Opiates	Morphine	Poppy	S[a] or H[b]
Tetrahydrocannabinols	Δ^9-THC	Hemp	S or H
Xanthines	Caffeine	Coffee	S
Tropane alkaloid	Scopolamine	Jimson weed	H or D[c]
	Dioscorine	Yams	D
	Atropine	Nightshade	S or D
Pyridines	Nicotine	Tobacco	S
Myristins	Myristicin	Nutmeg	H
Indoleamines	Psilocybin	Mexican mushroom	H
	Bufotenine	Cohoba snuff	H
Phenethylamines	Mescaline	Peyote cactus	H
Indole alkaloids	Lysergic acid amide	Morning glory seed	H
	Harmine	Caapi plant	H
	Ibogaine	Iboga plant	H

[a] S = stimulant.
[b] H = hallucinogen.
[c] D = depressant.

Stimulants

The most widely used food stimulants are the xanthines (caffeine, theophylline, and theobromine). Caffeine is present in coffee, tea, and cocoa.[14] These central-nervous-system stimulants are relatively nontoxic, and several grams of the pure compound may be consumed without adverse effect. It is estimated that a cup of coffee contains 100–150 mg of caffeine and that about 7 million kg of caffeine are consumed per year in the United States.[31] Caffeine is also present in the cola nuts (2%) and therefore is found in many of the common cola drinks.[2] A recent survey of cola-beverage manufacturers shows a range of caffeine content from 3.2 to 4.0 mg per fluid ounce (E. E. Lockhart, personal communication).

Scopolamine, one of the belladonna alkaloids, produces a central

Caffeine, R = R' = R'' = CH₃
Theobromine, R = H; R' = R'' = CH₃
Theophylline, R = R' = CH₃; R'' = H

stimulation when consumed in small doses, but causes hallucinations and is toxic in large doses. This alkaloid is found in Jimson weed and henbane, which have been consumed by members of the "drug culture" for its psychoactive effects. Several accidental poisonings have resulted.[47] A common custom in certain parts of the country is to graft tomato plants to the roots of the Jimson weed. Unless this is done correctly, the resulting tomatoes will contain significant amounts of atropine, a similar belladonna alkaloid; this has resulted in the poisoning of individuals.[39]

Nicotine, which is present in tobacco plants, is a central stimulant in low doses but is extremely toxic in larger doses; accidental poisoning has been reported from consumption of tobacco leaves.[49] A very powerful central-nervous-system stimulant, cicutoxin,[34] is present in the root of the water hemlock (*Cicuta maculata*). Eating even a small portion of the root of this plant results in convulsions and frequently death.[1] This plant, which is one of the most poisonous in this country, is also known by the names cowbane, poison parsnip, snakeroot, snakeweed, and wild carrot.

$$CH_3CH_2CH_2\overset{\displaystyle OH}{\underset{\displaystyle |}{C}}H(CH{=}CH)_3(C{\equiv}C)_2CH_2CH_2CH_2OH$$

Cicutoxin

Depressants

Depressants are considered to be compounds that decrease the activity of the central nervous system. Although many plants contain depressant substances, few have been used extensively. The most widely used drug that can be considered a central-nervous-system depressant is ethyl alcohol. This drug tends to be addictive and indeed alcoholism is one of

the major social problems of our times. Alcoholic beverages, however,
are a source of calories and are usually classed as foods.

A tropane alkaloid, dioscorine, was isolated from yams (*Dioscorea hispida*) in 1951,[59] and a similar alkaloid was isolated from a type of yam native to Nigeria in 1956.[7] Its pharmacologic properties differed from atropine, but it was reported to be a central-nervous-system depressant with an LD_{50} in mice of 65 mg/kg.[7] It is not clear from the literature whether yams contain toxic quantities of this alkaloid even if eaten in large quantities. If the toxicity in man is similar to that in the mouse, it would appear that it is unlikely that one could consume lethal amounts of the drug in yams.

Atropine is another tropane alkaloid that can cause intense central-nervous-system effects. The administration of 0.5–5 mg to man results in some central stimulation. Ten milligrams often results in hallucinations or severe central-nervous-system depression and may be lethal in children.[45] Both atropine and scopolamine can cause this toxicity; these are present in the leaves and fruit of purple nightshade, Jimson weed, and henbane. Death can occur in children eating as few as three berries from nightshade.

Bulbs of the camas lily, which grows in the Pacific Northwest, have been a food source of historical importance. A plant of similar appearance grows in the same area and is known as the death camas (*Zigadenus venenosus*). These plants appear to contain alkaloids that are strong depressants, and cases of accidental poisoning have been reported.[18]

Hallucinogens and Other Psychoactive Compounds

Many plants that are sometimes used for food contain substances that can greatly affect the psychological state of an individual. The effects produced by psychoactive compounds may vary from mild euphoria to hallucinations and psychotic behavior. The prevalent use of such hallucinogens and other psychoactive substances in society make this a subject of intense current interest. There are numerous books devoted entirely to this subject. *The Hallucinogens* by Hoffer and Osmond[39] is

Δ^1-Tetrahydrocannabinol

an excellent review. In the current discussion we can treat this subject only superficially.

For centuries the opiates (including morphine), which are derived largely from the poppy plant, have been smoked, injected, or eaten for their euphoric effects. These alkaloids are both physically and psychologically addictive and are posing an increasingly important social problem.

Another plant that has been consumed for centuries for its euphoric effect is the common hemp plant or marihuana. The leaves and dried flowering tops contain a group of tetrahydrocannabinols, of which the Δ^1-isomer (also called Δ^9) appears to be the major psychoactive component. This also is the active component of hashish.[54] The material is usually smoked, although the euphoric effects can be obtained by ingestion. These compounds do not appear to be physically addictive, but little is known of their overall toxicology.

It has also been reported recently[46] that catnip, long known to cause euphoric responses in cats, produces effects in man similar to those observed with marihuana. Unlike marihuana, however, the physiologically active compound in catnip oil is nepetalactone.[53]

Nepetalactone

Cocaine, an alkaloid present in the leaves of the coca plant, is a local anesthetic and a powerful central-nervous-system stimulant. The coca plant, *Erythroxylon coca*, grows in Peru and in Bolivia. Its leaves have been traditionally chewed by the Inca Indians for their euphoric effect and antifatigue properties. Although foods containing the compound are not available in this country, the drug is often used by opiate addicts for its central-nervous-system effect. Overdoses of cocaine cause hallucinations followed by severe central-nervous-system depression.[31]

A hallucinogenic food that is present in practically every home is nutmeg. The toxic nature of nutmeg has been known for centuries.[33] Nutmeg has been eaten in quantity (5–10 g) by women a number of times in an attempt to induce abortion. It appears to be ineffective as an abortifacient but usually produces unpleasant and toxic side effects. Nutmeg has also been used frequently by prison inmates who had previously used other psychoactive drugs.[69] The effects desired by these individuals were hallucinations and central-nervous-system stimulation. Consumption of 5–15 g of powdered nutmeg may result in euphoria, hallucinations, and a dreamlike feeling, followed by abdominal pain and, in some cases, depression and stupor. Myristicin (Chapter 20, p. 455), a compound that bears some structural relationship to mescaline and adrenochrome, has been isolated from nutmeg and is thought to be the active principle.[65] It is not clear whether this is the only active ingredient in nutmeg.

There are a number of plants that are eaten almost solely for their hallucinogenic effect. These plants were used mainly by primitive cultures in religious ceremonies, and only during the past 20 yr have they been important in Western cultures. The discovery of lysergic acid diethylamide (LSD) and its effects on man have aroused the interest of many individuals in the possibility of temporarily altering their mental state. Albert Hofmann, working on the chemical synthesis of alkaloids from the ergot fungus, made lysergic acid and, after preparing the diethylamide derivative, felt a strange dreamlike intoxication. He later consumed 250 μg of pure LSD and recorded the physiological and psychotropic effects, which were intense. LSD is not present in ergot fungi per se, although history records numerous instances of massive ergot poisoning due to fungus-infected grain. It is clear that some of the other alkaloids present in the ergot fungus have central as well as peripheral toxic effects.[50] LSD is one of the most potent psychoactive substances known; as little as 20 μg produces hallucinations. Although LSD is now illegal and considered dangerous with the possibility of long-lasting side effects, it is still widely used by members of the "drug cult." This group has experimented with numerous natural products for similar hallucinatory effects. In the early 1960's the hallucinatory effects of the ingestion of morning glory seeds (occasional contaminant of soybeans) became more widely known, and several cases of toxicity were reported.[44] The seeds of the morning glory or *ololiuqui* had been recognized as hallucinogenic by the Aztec Indians for centuries and used in their religious ceremonies. The active ingredient in these seeds appears to be lysergic acid amide[44]; the content is such that over 100 seeds are required for a psychotogenic effect.

The mechanism of action of LSD and related compounds is unknown, although they are known to be pharmacologic antagonists of serotonin. It is possible that they interfere with the normal role of serotonin in the brain. In this regard, many compounds that appear to be structurally related to serotonin also have marked central effects and produce hallucinations. L-Tryptophan, the normal dietary precursor of serotonin, can have marked central effects if administered in large doses to patients receiving monoamine oxidase inhibitors.[57] Patients under experimental conditions appeared and reported feeling intoxicated with ethanol. It is possible that the observed effects were due to the formation in the central nervous system of tryptamine, which could not be metabolized because of monoamine oxidase inhibition.

A number of species of mushrooms contain various indole compounds that are known to be hallucinogens. The most famous of these are the Mexican mushrooms *Psilocybe mexicana*. These mushrooms were used by the Mexican Indians for their hallucinatory effect in religious ceremonies. The active ingredients of these mushrooms are two tryptamine derivatives: psilocybin (*N,N*-dimethyl-4-hydroxytryptamine-*O*-phosphate) and psilocin (*N,N*-dimethyl-4-hydroxytryptamine). Several other indole-type alkaloids are also present.[39]

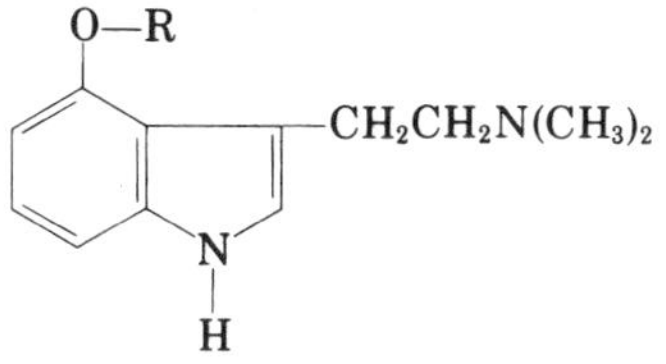

Psilocin, R=H
Psilocybin, R=PO₃H₂

Another type of mushroom, called fly agaric (*Amanita muscaria*), has been used in Siberia for years as a hallucinatory agent. The active components in this plant are: muscarine[17,72] (a cholinergic compound), bufotenine[73] (*N,N*-dimethyl-5-hydroxytryptamine), and toxic cyclic peptides.[72] (See Chapter 5, p. 120.) Of some 800 species of mushrooms studied in the United States, 53 are considered toxic. Although some contain hallucinatory indoles and muscarine, the nature of the toxin in many remains unidentified.[17]

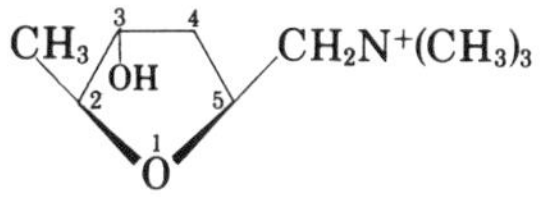

Muscarine

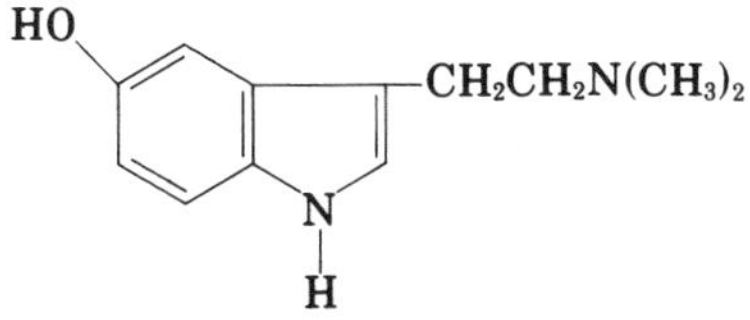

Bufotenine

The seeds of the leguminous shrub *Piptadenia peregrina* contain a hallucinogen. This plant is native to the West Indies and has been used for centuries to prepare cohoba snuff. The active ingredient of these seeds was identified as bufotenine.[64] Fish and Horning also identified this hallucinogen in other South American snuffs and disclosed the presence of *N,N*-dimethyltryptamine,[25] a fast but relatively short-acting hallucinogen. This and other *N,N*-dimethylindoles have been identified in a variety of South American plants from which hallucinatory snuffs and beverages were made.[38,40] There are also a number of alkaloids that may be formed from *N*-methyl-indolealkylamines known as the harmala alkaloids. These are also eaten in various plant materials for their hallucinogenic effects: Harmine is the major alkaloid in the caapi plant (*Banisteria caapi*), which is consumed for its psychic stimulatory power.[38] A somewhat more complex series of indole alkaloids is found in the roots of the African shrubs *Tabernanthe iboga*. The major alkaloid from this plant that is used for intoxicative purposes is ibogaine.[21]

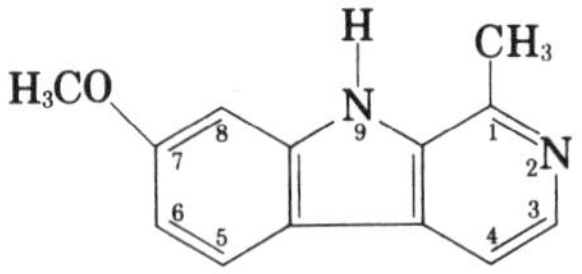

Harmine

One of the earliest psychoactive compounds to be identified was mescaline (2,4,5-trimethoxyphenylethylamine). This compound is found in the "mescal" buttons of the peyote cactus in Mexico, where it has been used for religious experiences by the Central American Indian for hundreds of years.[40] This is a good example, perhaps, of the potential importance of further studies on the presence of psychoactive compounds in food substances used by various peoples of the world. Many research programs have been built on these and other similar compounds in order to unravel the mysteries of the human mind and for treatment of mental disease.

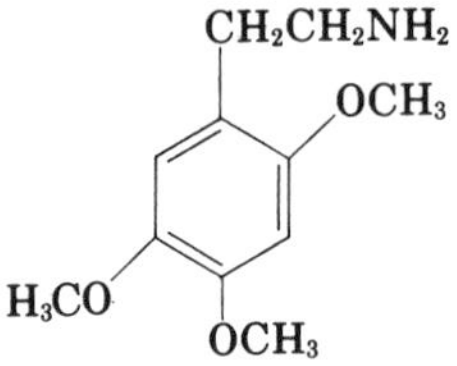

Mescaline

REFERENCES

1. E. F. L. J. Anet, B. Lythgoe, M. H. Silk, and S. Trippett, Oenanthotoxin and cicutoxin. Isolation and structure. J. Chem. Soc. 309 (1953).
2. Anonymous, Cola drinks. J. Am. Med. Assoc. *156*:1376 (1954).
3. M. Anthony, H. Hinterberger, and J. W. Lance, The possible relationship of serotonin to the migraine syndrome. Res. Clin. Stud. Headache *2*:29 (1969).
4. A. M. Asatoor, A. J. Levi, and M. D. Milne, Tranylcypromine and cheese. Lancet *2*:733 (1963).
5. G. Barger and G. S. Walpole, Isolation of the pressor principles of putrid meat. J. Physiol. *38*:343 (1909).
6. S. B. Baylin, M. A. Beaven, K. Engelman, and A. Sjoerdsma, Elevated histaminase activity in medullary carcinoma of the thyroid gland. N. Engl. J. Med. *283*:1239 (1970).
7. C. W. L. Bevan, J. L. Broadbent, and J. Hirst, A convulsant alkaloid of *Discorea dumetorum*. Nature *177*:935 (1953).
8. H. C. Bethune, R. H. Burrell, R. H. Culpan, and G. J. Ogg, Vascular crises associated with monoamine oxidase inhibitors. Am. J. Psychiatr. *121*:245 (1964).
9. B. Blackwell, Tranylcypromine. Lancet *2*:414 (1963).
10. B. Blackwell and L. A. Mabbitt, Tyramine in cheese related to hypertensive crises after monoamine-oxidase inhibition. Lancet *1*:938 (1965).
11. B. Blackwell, L. A. Mabbitt, and E. Marley, Histamine and tyramine content of yeast products. J. Food Sci. *34*:47 (1969).
12. B. Blackwell, E. Marley, and L. A. Mabbitt, Effects of yeast extract after monoamine-oxidase inhibition. Lancet *1*:940 (1965).
13. B. Blackwell, E. Marley, J. Price, and D. Taylor, Hypertensive interaction between monoamine oxidase inhibitors and foodstuffs. Br. J. Psychiatr. *113*:349 (1967).
14. F. R. Blood and G. G. Rudolph, Some naturally occurring stimulants and depressants, p. 62. In Toxicants occurring naturally in food. National Academy of Sciences, Washington, D.C. (1966).
15. A. A. Boulton, B. Cookson, and R. Paulton, Hypertensive crisis in a patient on MAOI antidepressants following a meal of beef liver. Can. Med. Assoc. J. *102*:1394 (1970).
16. D. W. Bruce, Carcinoid tumours and pineapples. J. Pharm. Pharmacol. *13*:256 (1961).
17. R. W. Buck, Mushroom toxins. A brief review of the literature. N. Engl. J. Med. *265*:681 (1961).
18. K. Cameron, Death Camus poisoning. Northwest Med. *51*:682 (1952).
19. M. A. Crawford, Excretion of 5-hydroxyindolylacetic acid in East Africans. Lancet *1*:352 (1962).
20. J. R. Crout and A. Sjoerdsma, The clinical and laboratory significance of serotonin and catecholamines in bananas. N. Engl. J. Med. *261*:23 (1959).
21. D. F. Downing, The chemistry of the psychotomimetic substances. Q. Rev. *16*:133 (1962).
22. Editorial Staff: Headache, tyramine, serotonin, and migraine. Nutr. Rev. *26*:40 (1968).
23. M. Ferencik: Formation of histamine during bacterial decarboxylation of histidine in the flesh of some marine fishes. J. Hyg. Epidemiol. Microbiol. Immunol. *14*:52 (1970).

24. M. Ferencik, V. L. Kramery, and J. Kriska, Fish poisoning caused by histamine. J. Hyg. Epidemiol. Microbiol. Immunol. 5:341 (1961).

25. M. S. Fish and E. C. Horning, Studies on hallucinogenic snuffs. J. Nerv. Ment. Dis. 124:33 (1956).

26. J. M. Foy and J. R. Parratt, A note on the presence of noradrenaline and 5-hydroxytryptamine in plantain (Musa sapientum, var. paradisiaca). J. Pharm. Pharmacol. 12:360 (1960).

27. J. M. Foy and J. R. Parratt: 5-Hydroxytryptamine in pineapples. J. Pharm. Pharmacol. 13:382 (1961).

28. J. M. Foy and J. R. Parratt, Urinary excretion of 5-hydroxyindolylacetic acid in West Africans. Lancet 1:942 (1962).

29. E. F. Gale, The bacterial amino acid decarboxylase. Adv. Enzymol. 6:1 (1946).

30. L. S. Goodman and A. Gilman, The pharmacological basis of therapeutics, p. 621. Macmillan, London (1970).

31. A. Goth, Medical pharmacology, p. 295, 335. C. V. Mosby, St. Louis (1968).

32. H. D. Graham, The safety of foods. Avi, Westport, Conn. (1968).

33. R. C. Green, Nutmeg poisoning. Va. Med. Mon. 86:586 (1959).

34. D. R. Haggerty and J. A. Conway, Report of poisoning by Cicuta maculata (water hemlock). N.Y. State Med. J. 36:1511 (1936).

35. D. L. Harrison, J. A. Bowers, L. L. Anderson, H. J. Tuma, and D. H. Kropf, Effect of aging on palatability and selected related characteristics of pork loin. J. Food Sci. 35:292 (1970).

36. D. L. Hedberg, M. W. Gordon, and B. C. Glueck, Six cases of hypertensive crises in patients on tranylcypromine after eating chicken livers. Am. J. Psychiatr. 122:933 (1966).

37. J. V. Hodge, E. R. Nye, and G. W. Emerson, Monoamine oxidase inhibitors, broad beans and hypertension. Lancet 1:1108 (1964).

38. F. A. Hochstein and A. M. Paradies, Alkaloids of Banisteria caapi and Prestonia amazonicum. J. Am. Chem. Soc. 79:5735 (1957).

39. A. Hoffer and H. Osmond, The hallucinogens, p. 211, 525. Academic Press, New York (1967).

40. A. Hofmann, Psychotomimetic agents, p. 169. In Drugs affecting the central nervous system, Vol. 2, A. Burger (ed.). Marcel Dekker, New York (1962).

41. B. Holmstedt and J. Lindgren, Chemical constituents and pharmacology of South American snuffs, p. 339. In Ethnopharmacologic search for psychoactive drugs, D. H. Efron (ed.). Public Health Service Publication, No. 1645 (1967).

42. B. T. Horton, The use of histamine in the treatment of specific type of head-aches. J. Am. Med. Assoc. 116:377 (1941).

43. D. Horwitz, W. Lovenberg, K. Engelman, and A. Sjoerdsma, Monoamine oxidase inhibitors, tyramine and cheese. J. Am. Med. Assoc. 188:1108 (1964).

44. A. L. Ingram, Morning glory seed reaction. J. Am. Med. Assoc. 190:1133 (1964).

45. I. R. Innes and M. Nickerson, Drugs inhibiting the action of acetylcholine on structures innervated by postganglionic parasympathetic nerves, p. 524. In The pharmacological basis of therapeutics. Goodman and Gilman (eds.). 4th Ed. MacMillan Co., London (1970).

46. B. Jackson and A. Reed, Catnip and alteration of consciousness. J. Am. Med. Assoc. 207:1349 (1969).

47. H. Jacooziner and H. W. Raybin, Briefs on accidental chemical poisonings in New York City. N.Y. State Med. J. 61:301 (1961).

48. W. Keil and H. Kutler, Zur Chemie und Pharmakologie vergorener Nahrungs-mittel. Arch. Exp. Pathol. Pharmakol. *175*:736 (1934).
49. J. M. Kingsbury, Poisonous plants of the United States and Canada, p. 287. Prentice-Hall, Englewood Cliffs, N.J. (1964).
50. M. B. Kreig, Green medicine. Rand McNally, Chicago (1964).
51. D. M. Krikler and B. Lewis, Dangers of natural foodstuffs. Lancet *1*:1166 (1965).
52. P. Marquardt, H. Schmidt, and M. Späth, Histamin in alkoholhaltigen Getränken. Arzneim. Forsch. *13*:1100 (1963).
53. S. M. McElvain and E. J. Eisenbraun, The constituents of the volatile oil of cat-nip. III. The strcuture of nepetalic acid and related compounds. J. Am. Chem. Soc., *77*:1599 (1955).
54. R. Mechoulam and Y. Gaoni, Recent advances in the chemistry of hashish. Prog. Chem. Org. Nat. Prod. *25*:175 (1967).
55. M. Nencki, Zur Kenntniss der Fäulnisprozesse. Berichte *10*:1032 (1877).
56. W. F. Nuessle, F. C. Norman, and H. E. Miller: Pickled herring and tranylcy-promine reaction. J. Am. Med. Assoc. *192*:726 (1965).
57. J. A. Oates and A. Sjoerdsma, Neurologic effects of tryptophan in patients re-ceiving a monoamine oxidase inhibitor. Neurology *10*:1076 (1960).
58. C. S. Ough, Measurement of histamine in California wines. J. Agric. Food Chem. *19*:241 (1971).
59. A. R. Pinder, An alkaloid of *Dioscorea hispida.* Dennst. Nature *168*:1090 (1951).
60. H. Sato, S. Sakamura, and Y. Obata, The isolation and characterization of *N*-methyl tyramine, tyramine and hordenine from sawa millet seed. Agric. Biol. Chem. *34*:1254 (1970).
61. N. P. Sen, Analysis and significance of tyramine in foods. J. Food Sci. *34*:22 (1969).
62. A. Sjoerdsma, Malignant carcinoid, p. 1447. In Cecil-Loeb textbook of medi-cine, P. B. Beeson and W. McDermott (eds.). 11th ed. W. B. Saunders, Philadel-phia (1963).
63. J. R. Stabenau, C. R. Creveling, and J. Daly, the "pink spot," 3,4 dimethoxy-phenylethylamine, common tea and schizophrenia. Am. J. Psychiatr. *127*:611 (1970).
64. V. L. Stromberg, Isolation of bufotenine from *Piptadenia peregrina.* J. Am. Chem. Soc. *76*:1707 (1954).
65. E. B. Truitt, Jr., E. Callaway, III, M. C. Braude, and J. C. Krantz, The pharma-cology of myristicin—A contribution to the psychopharmacology of nutmeg. J. Neuropsychiatr. *2*:205 (1961).
66. S. Udenfriend, W. Lovenberg, and A. Sjoerdsma, Physiologically active amines in common fruits and vegetables. Arch. Biochem. Biophys. *85*:487 (1959).
67. L. L. Van Slyke and E. B. Hart, The relation of carbon dioxide to proteolysis in the ripening of cheddar cheese. Am. Chem. J. *30*:   (1903).
68. T. P. Waalkes, A. Sjoerdsma, C. R. Creveling, H. Weissbach, and S. Udenfriend, Serotonin, norepinephrine and related compounds in bananas. Science *127*: 648 (1958).
69. G. Weiss, Hallucinogenic and narcotic-like effects of powdered myristica (nut-meg). Psychiatr. Q. *34*:346 (1960).
70. G. B. West, Tryptamines in tomatoes. J. Pharm. Pharmacol. *11*:319 (1959).

71. T. A. Wheaton and I. Steward, Biosynthesis of synephrine in citrus. Phyto-chemistry *8*:85 (1969).

72. T. Wieland, Poisonous principles of mushrooms of the genus *Amanita*. Science *159*:946 (1968).

73. T. Wieland, W. Motzel, and H. Merz, Über das Vorkommen von Bufotenin inn-gelben Knollenblätterpilz. Ann. Chem. *581*:10 (1953).

74. E. Winterstein and W. Bissegger, Zur Kenntnis der Bestandteile des Emmenthaler Kases. Z. Physiol. Chem. *47*:28 (1906).

75. E. A. Zeller, Diamine oxidases, p. 313. In The enzymes, Vol. 8, P. D. Boyer, H. Lardy, and K. Myrbäck (eds.). 2nd ed. Academic Press, New York (1963).

9 Fred H. Mattson

POTENTIAL
TOXICITY
OF FOOD
LIPIDS*

Fats and oils customarily consumed by humans have a long history of use. Consequently, it is not surprising that naturally occurring toxicants are either absent or are present at such low levels as to be of little practical significance. The potential for untoward adverse effects exists when there are departures from these established sources, or when new materials, either accidentally or intentionally, are introduced into the food chain. Because of this successful avoidance of toxic lipids, I mainly will point out potential rather than existing dangers.

ERUCIC ACID

Most plants of the order Rhoeadales of the family Cruciferae contain erucic acid[1,2] a 22-carbon mono-unsaturated fatty acid, *cis*-13-docosenoic acid:

$$CH_3(CH_2)_7HC=CH(CH_2)_{11}COOH$$

Erucic Acid

* Literature reviewed to April 1971.

The presence of this acid can be detected by standard gas–liquid chromatographic methods for the identification of the methyl esters of fatty acids. Suitable standards to establish relative retention times must be used; for example, on some polar liquid phases erucic and arachidonic acids have almost identical retention times. The two important edible oils in this family are obtained from the seeds of the rape, *Brassica napus* and *B. campestris,* and the mustard, *B. hirta* and *B. juncea.* Mustardseed oil contains about 20–40% of erucic acid. The level of this acid in the oil from the usual varieties of rape ranges from 20% to 55%. An important development of the selective breeding of these species of rape has been the successful propagation for commercial production of new varieties that contain little or no erucic acid; this acid is replaced by oleic acid.[3,4] The trivial name of one such variety is Canbra, a contraction derived from *Can*adian *Bra*ssica.

The worldwide production of rape- and mustardseed oils continues to increase, and these are now among the top six vegetable oils in tonnage. Although little is produced or consumed in the United States, rape is an important agricultural crop in Canada. Argentina, Mexico, China, India, Pakistan, Japan, and several European countries are other major producers and users of rape- and mustardseed oils, which are either consumed as such or, after partial hydrogenation, used as cooking oils, shortenings, and margarines.

Although these oils have a long history of consumption by humans, it is only within the past decade that they have been subjected to extensive, controlled biological investigation. Most of this work has been carried out in the Canadian Food and Drug Directorate Laboratories, in the laboratories of the French Ministry of Agriculture at Dijon, and in the Unilever Research Laboratories in the Netherlands. Because of its primary economic importance, most of these studies have employed rapeseed oil, but it is likely that the results also apply to mustardseed oil.

In 1960 Roine *et al.*[5] observed myocarditis in rats that had been fed 50–70% of their calories as rapeseed oil. This observation was subsequently confirmed in 2- and 12-month-old rats that were fed rapeseed oil as 15% by weight of the diet.[6] The changes in the heart muscle, observed by the French group and by the groups in Canada[7] and the Netherlands[8,9,10] all were similar. Weanling rats fed a diet high in rapeseed oil showed an accumulation of fat in the heart muscle within a single day. This deposition progressed and, between the third and seventh day on the diet, the lipid content of the heart was maximal, three to four times that in normal animals. At that time, the heart muscle was pallid and numerous fat droplets interspersed in the myocardium could be seen histologically. Similar compositional and histological changes occurred in the skeletal muscle.[9] The lipid that accumulated in the heart muscle, and probably also in the skeletal muscle, was mainly triglyceride with erucic acid constituting a large portion of the fatty acids.[7,11,12] Continuing the animals on these diets resulted in a decrease in the level of cardiac lipids; however, the control level was not attained. Although the fatty droplets in the heart muscle disappeared, this was followed by mononuclear cell infiltration and finally myocardial fibrosis.[9,10]

Accumulation of cardiac lipids was observed in hamsters,[8] minipigs, and squirrel monkeys[13] that were fed diets containing large amounts of rapeseed oil. Ducklings, while showing similar pathological changes, also developed hydropericardium and cirrhosis of the liver.[8,14] The striking abnormality in the guinea pig was marked enlargement of the spleen. From this and other changes, it appeared that rapeseed oil induced hemolytic anemia in this species.[8,15] Diets containing trierucin resulted in the same pathological changes in rats[9,16] and ducklings.[13] Thus, the primary responsible agent in rapeseed oil was concluded to be erucic acid. On the other hand, we have found that the feeding of completely hydrogenated rapeseed oil does not result in fatty infiltration of the heart. This may be due to the limited absorption of behenic acid, the saturated analog of erucic acid. Cetoleic acid, *cis*-11-docosenoic acid, of herring oil, like erucic acid, causes an

$$CH_3(CH_2)_9 HC=CH(CH_2)_9 COOH$$

Cetoleic Acid

accumulation of lipids in the myocardium of rats.[7]

The response of rats to rapeseed oil was found to be age dependent. Whereas the weanling rat showed massive fatty infiltration of the heart, there was only slight accumulation of lipids in the heart muscle, if the feeding of the oil was initiated when the animals were 2–3 months postweaning,[13] but there was mononuclear cell infiltration of the myocardium.[10]

A considerable intake of rapeseed oil was needed before these effects were seen. The minimum effective level for the weanling rat, which is a responsive experimental animal, was 10–20% of the calories.[7,9] Effects were seen in guinea pigs at 25% of the calories,[15] while in the duckling 30% of calories[14] was needed. Differences between laboratories in the minimum effective level may be due to the levels of erucic acid in the rapeseed oils that were used or to the level of saturated fatty acids in the diet. Other important variables, which may be responsible for these differences, are the strain of animal employed and the duration of the studies.

Since Canbra oil contains little or no erucic acid, the consumption of this fat even at high levels would not be expected to result in these pathological abnormalities. This expectation was confirmed in the Canadian[7] and Dutch[10] laboratories. However, the French group[5] fed Canbra oil as 15% by weight of the diet and found cardiac lesions, although these were less frequent and less severe than those that were seen in animals fed rapeseed oil. The opposing results obtained in these laboratories need to be resolved.

The feeding of diets containing a high level of rapeseed oil resulted in the suppression of the growth of rats,[6,17-23] pigs,[23] chickens,[24] turkeys,[25] mice, guinea pigs, hamsters, and ducklings.[8] A similar suppression of body-weight gain was seen in rats fed other fats to which erucic acid had been added.[26,27] Rats fed Canbra oil grew at a normal rate.[6,10,28] In these longer-term studies, the rats fed rapeseed oil showed only a slight elevation of total lipids in the heart, although appreciable amounts of erucic acid were present. The most striking pathological changes were fibrotic lesions in the cardiac muscle.[6,9]

Alexander and Mattson[29] demonstrated that the impaired growth of rats was due in part, to the consistency of diets that contain high levels of liquid oils. Support for this explanation seemd to be offered by the observation that the addition of saturated fatty acids to rapeseed oil corrected the impaired weight gain.[30,31] However, the addition of saturated fatty acids does more than alter the consistency of the diet. Thus, when saturated acids and *trans* double bonds were formed by partial hydrogenation of rapeseed oil without markedly reducing the level of erucic acid, there was a smaller accumulation of lipids in the cardiac muscle.[7] This improvement occurred in spite of the erucic acid level in the diet being essentially unchanged. Beare *et al.*[30] proposed that the improved growth of the animals receiving the supplemental saturated fat was due to palmitic acid. This was tested by Thomasson *et al.*[8] using various pure fatty acids. He found myristic and palmitic acids to be the most effective. The addition of saturated fatty acids to a diet containing toxic amounts of rapeseed oil prevented hemolytic anemia in guinea pigs.[15] This dietary modification corrected the impaired growth rate of ducklings, with the improvement proportional to the amount of palmitic acid added. The incidence and severity of hydropericardium and liver cirrhosis decreased also, but there was an increased fatty infiltration of the heart muscle.[15] The possibility that these observations were simply attributable to the ratio of unsaturated to saturated fatty acids in the diet was tested and found not to be the explanation.[11,15] The pathological changes in the heart took place only when erucic acid was present in the diet, but the mechanism by which saturated fatty acids mitigated these effects is unknown.

Rats that were fed diets high in rapeseed oil for their life span showed significantly greater degenerative changes in the liver and a higher incidence of kidney nephrosis than animals fed marine, animal, or other vegetable oils. In spite of these pathological changes, their life span was not shortened.[8,32,33] Rats fed rapeseed oil reproduced,[27] but the number and weight of the offspring were smaller.[34]

The mechanism responsible for the development of these abnormalities is not known. Erucic acid has been shown to be converted to oleic acid in the liver.[35,36] Whereas Carroll[37] offered evidence that this takes place at a slow rate, Bach *et al.*[38] attributed the accumulation of erucic acid to the overall conversion being lower, rather than to a difference in rate. On the other hand, Wagner *et al.*[39] reported the biological half-life of erucic acid to be the same as that of the usual dietary fatty acids. Mitochrondria isolated from the hearts of animals fed rapeseed oil showed a decreased ability to oxidize substrates such as glutamate, resulting in a decrease in the rate of ATP synthesis.[12] Similar changes were not observed in the liver. In heart muscle, an impairment in the conversion of erucate to oleate or in the ability to oxidize erucic acid could account for the accumulation of lipid in this organ. The hemolytic anemia observed in guinea pigs has been attributed to the accumulation of erucic and nervonic acids in the erythrocyte membrane, thus resulting in increased permeability of the cell.

$$CH_3(CH_2)_7 CH=CH(CH_2)_{13} COOH$$

Nervonic Acid

Erucic acid may be transferred in the food chain by animals that have in turn been fed diets containing rapeseed oil. Thus, following its feeding, this acid was found in the body fat of chickens,[24,40,41] turkeys,[25] and lambs[42] but not in the egg lipids of chickens.[43,44] Although erucate was found in the milk of rats,[34] it is unlikely that it would appear in the milk fat of ruminants; the hydrogenation system in the rumen probably would reduce any ingested erucic acid.

Although the consumption of diets containing rapeseed oil results in impaired growth and a variety of pathological changes in a number of different species of experimental animals, there are no reported cases of toxicity in humans. A natural protective mechanism is that the very young, who appear to be the most susceptible to this oil, probably are not exposed to it. In the case of the more mature, the minimum effective dose (probably about 20% of the calories) is in excess of the likely normal intake. On the other hand, the gross changes, such as a slight impairment in growth with no alteration in the life span, are such that a toxic effect in humans, even if present, would not be suspected.

In Canada it has been decided that although no harmful effects on humans have been attributed to the consumption of rapeseed oil, it is prudent to replace the conventional rapeseed with the varieties from which Canbra oil can be obtained. As a consequence, much Canbra oil was produced in 1971, and sufficient seed should be available for the entire crop in 1972.

BRANCHED-CHAIN FATTY ACIDS

Although an individual can normally metabolize branched-chain fatty acids, this is not true of those having Refsum's disease[45] (phytanic acid storage disease). Although only a limited number of cases have been reported, this disease deserves mention not only because it results from the consumption of a component of food but also because it is the first example of a genetic error in fatty-acid oxidation. For a thorough discussion, see the recent review by Steinberg.[46]

In Refsum's disease there is gross infiltration of many tissues with lipids that contain large amounts of phytanic acid, 3,7,11,15-tetra-methylhexadecanoic acid.[47]

$$\underset{\text{Phytanic Acid}}{CH_3CH(CH_2)_3CH(CH_2)_3CH(CH_2)_3CHCH_2COOH}$$

with CH_3 groups on positions as shown.

Whereas human plasma normally contains only trace amounts of this acid, phytanate constitutes from 5–30% of the plasma fatty acids of patients with Refsum's syndrome.[48,49] The accumulation of this acid with its resulting incorporation into myelin may be responsible for the neurological abnormalities that are characteristic of this disease.

Diets containing high levels of phytanic acid have been fed to a variety of experimental animals.[50-55] Although impaired growth and death were seen, neurological symptoms did not develop. An oral dose in humans of 9.5 g of phytol, which is converted in the body to phytanic acid, results in a small rise in the plasma phytanic acid level.[48] The failure by normal animals, including man, to develop the neurological syndrome is not attributable to poor absorption of phytanic acid or phytol; rather it is the result of a high capacity to oxidize phytanic acid.

The presence of a methyl group on the 3-position of phytanic acid blocks the normal pathway of beta-oxidation because dehydrogenation by L(+)-beta-hydroxyacyl-CoA dehydrogenase cannot take place. Studies by Steinberg, Avigan, and co-workers established the major pathway for the oxidation of phytanic acid in man and experimental animals.[54,56-60] The initial step was shown to be an alpha-oxidation in which phytanic acid was shortened by one carbon atom to yield pristanic acid, 2,6,10,14-tetramethylpentadecanoic acid:

$$\underset{\text{Pristanic Acid}}{CH_3\overset{\underset{\displaystyle |}{CH_3}}{C}H(CH_2)_3\overset{\underset{\displaystyle |}{CH_3}}{C}H(CH_2)_3\overset{\underset{\displaystyle |}{CH_3}}{C}H(CH_2)_3\overset{\underset{\displaystyle |}{CH_3}}{C}HCOOH}$$

The presence of a methyl substituent on position-2 does not block beta-oxidation, and pristanic acid was found to be oxidized by this pathway. The initial oxidation product was 4,8,12-trimethyltridecanoic acid and probably propionic acid. Beta-oxidation of the longer chain product yielded acetate plus 2,6,10-trimethylundecanoic acid. Based on the structure of the larger fragment formed at each oxidation step, the overall yield of products from phytanic acid appears to be one molecule of CO_2 (as the result of the alpha-oxidation step), three molecules each of propionic and acetic acids from the sequence of beta-oxidations, and the terminal fragment, 2-methylpropionic acid.

Although patients with Refsum's disease oxidize phytanate at only 5% of the normal rate, their ability to oxidize pristanic acid is not impeded. The enzyme defect is probably the first step in the metabolic pathway, namely, the conversion of phytanic acid to alpha-hydroxyphytanic acid.[60-66]

The parents or siblings of clinical cases accumulate phytanate but do not exhibit neurological disorders.[67,68] The 45-60% reduction in their ability to oxidize this acid,[69] as demonstrated in fibroblast cell culture, probably is the cause of the accumulation. Under normal dietary conditions the capacity of such individuals to oxidize phytanic acid is adequate to prevent the neurological syndrome. However, it is conceivable that an excessive intake of phytanate, or its precursors, could increase the level of stored acid to the point that such an individual would develop the clinical disease.

Phytol, 3,7,11,15-tetramethylhexadec-2-ene-1-ol, is a component of the chlorophyll molecule at a 1 : 1 molar ratio with the pyrrole ring to which it is bound. The body converts this alcohol to phytanic acid.[50,51,61,62,70,71] Free phytol is well absorbed by both normal human subjects and patients with Refsum's disease.[62] However, this alcohol as it occurs in chlorophyll is poorly—if at all—absorbed by such subjects or patients.[72]

Since man can neither synthesize phytanic acid nor absorb the phytol that is a component of the chlorophyll molecule, phytanic acid must be

$$\overset{\displaystyle CH_3}{|} \quad \overset{\displaystyle CH_3}{|} \quad \overset{\displaystyle CH_3}{|} \quad \overset{\displaystyle CH_3}{|}$$
$$CH_3CH(CH_2)_3CH(CH_2)_3CH(CH_2)_3C{=}CHCH_2OH$$

Phytol

derived, as such, from the diet, with the main sources being dairy products and ruminant fats.[73-75] It is likely that the phytanate in the tissues of these animals is formed from phytol, which is split from the dietary chlorophyll in the rumen. No more than trace amounts of phytanic acid and have been found in marine lipids[76-78] and in the few common foods that have been analyzed.[63] In two instances the daily intake of phytanic acid by man was estimated at 50–100 mg/day.[46,60] The large accumulation of phytanic acid in Refsum's disease is difficult to account for by the known dietary sources of this acid. Thus, there is the possibility that other dietary constituents, such as other branched chain fatty acids, may be precursors of this acid.

Diets from which dairy and ruminant fats have been excluded, so as to reduce the content of phytanic acid, have been fed to patients with Refsum's disease for periods of up to 4 yr.[63,79-81] The subjects showed a significant decrease in plasma phytanate level, and in a few instances there was some remission of the neurological complications. The decrease was the result of restricted intake, since the subjects showed no improvement in their ability to oxidize phytanic acid.[65]

CYCLOPROPENE ACIDS

Interest in the cyclopropene fatty acids has been stimulated primarily by their causing stored eggs to develop a pink or red color.[82] The occurrence of these acids in the human dietary, albeit at a very low level, merits their consideration here.

The cyclopropene fatty acids have the general structure:

$$\overset{\displaystyle CH_2}{\diagup \diagdown}$$
$$CH_3(CH_2)_7C{=}C(CH_2)_nCOOH$$

Cyclopropene Fatty Acids

In sterculic acid $n = 7$, whereas in malvalic acid $n = 6$. The presence of these acids is detected readily by the Halphen test,[83] which is claimed to be sensitive to a level of 0.001%.[84] A spectrophotometric adaptation of this test makes it particularly useful for determining low levels of these acids.[85] Total cyclopropene fatty acid content also can be determined by titration with hydrobromic acid[86]; the individual acids can be quantified by gas–liquid chromatography.[87] Because of the instability of these acids, special precautions must be taken in the application of these methods.

Eckey[88] has described the plants of the order Malvales that are sources, or potential sources, of oils containing cyclopropene acids. With only one exception, these acids have been found in the lipids of every plant of this order examined. The review article by Phelps[82] lists their concentration in a number of oils.

By far the most important edible oil containing cyclopropene acids is cottonseed oil, which is obtained from the seed of *Gossypium hirsutum.* The level of these acids in the crude oil ranges from 0.6 to 1.2%.[90] The one important edible fat of the order Malvales that does not contain malvalic or sterculic acid is cocoa butter, which is obtained from *Theobroma cocoa.* Kapok seed oil, from the seeds of either *Ciba pentandra* or *Bonbax malavaricum,* contains 10–14% of these acids. Crushing of kapok seeds is carried out in India, Ceylon, Japan, and Europe. It is likely that at least small amounts are used for edible purposes. Although it is not considered to be an edible oil, much of the experimental work has been done on the fat of *Sterculia foetida,* because it contains 70% or more of sterculic acid.[89]

The variation in the level of cyclopropene acids in cottonseed oil is due to differences in seed strains from which the oil was derived and to the subsequent processing of the oil.[90] The largest removal of these fatty acids is realized during the process of deodorization.[91] Thus, the total content of these acids in commercial cottonseed salad oils ranges from 0.1 to 0.5%,[6] levels considerably less than those of crude oils.[90] Hydrogenation of cyclopropene fatty acids destroys their ability to cause egg discoloration.[92] Sterculic and malvalic acids are found in the meal after processing cottonseeds to remove the oil; their level depends upon the amount of residual oil and is usually about 0.01% in meal obtained by modern commercial practices of extraction.[85]

Besides the effect on egg color, there have been only limited studies of cyclopropene fatty acids in other biological systems. Laying hens fed 250 mg of these acids per day ceased to lay. Normal laying was resumed in 12–32 days when these acids were removed from the diet.[93] Other abnormalities in the hen resulting from the consumption of high levels of these acids included retardation of comb development and enlargement of the gall bladder and liver.[94] Kapok seed oil, even when it constituted only 10% of the calories in the diet, caused a suppression of the growth of rats. At a level of 40% of the calories, all of the animals died within a few weeks.[95] *S. foetida* oil caused suppressed growth and at a caloric intake of about 10% resulted in death.[96] The consumption of diets containing 3% of *S. foetida* oil completely inhibited reproductive performance in female rats, but the males were not affected. In these studies there was retardation of follicular development and the uteri were smaller. By contrast, the appearance of the testes and epididymus and the production of sperm were normal.[97] Phelps[82] in his review reports that Braten and Shenstone have fed sterculic acid at levels up to 200 mg/kg body weight to mice. There was no apparent effect on the number of matings, fertility, or the mean litter size. The ability of cyclopropene fatty acids to accentuate the hepatotoxicity of other compounds is discussed in Chapter 23.

Cyclopropene acids can be carried in the food chain by the products of animals that are fed fats containing these acids. An appreciable portion of the ingested acids is deposited in the egg yolks of hens[93] and turkeys.[98] They are deposited in the body fat of laying hens[99] and probably also in broilers.

For many years it has been known that pigs fed a ration containing cottonseed meal produce a fat with a high melting point.[100] This is probably attributable to the effect of residual oil, with its accompanying cyclopropene acids, in the meal. Thus, when these acids were fed to animals, there was a decrease in the tissue levels of monounsaturated fatty acids and a corresponding increase in saturated fatty acids.[101-103] The increase in tissue saturated fatty acids could not be overcome by supplementing the diet with oleic or linoleic acid.[104]

Two mechanisms have been proposed for the inhibition by sterculic acid of the conversion of exogenous stearic acid to oleic acid. Raju and Reiser[105] and Johnson *et al.*[103] believe that sterculic acid directly inhibits the stearate desaturase enzyme. James *et al.*[106] and Gurr[107] have proposed that the inhibition is of the steroyl-CoA:ACP acyl transferase. The latter proposal is supported by the observation that, if sterculate and oleate are added to a culture of *Chlorella,* the conversion of the added oleate to linoleate is inhibited. However, if the *Chlorella* is first incubated with the oleate, so as to allow the acid to be incorporated into the cellular lipids, the subsequent addition of sterculate does not block the oleate to linoleate conversion. Neither of the mechanisms has been established with certainty and, as pointed out by Pande and Mead,[108] the problem is further complicated by the detergent effect of added stearoyl-CoA.

The long human experience with cottonseed oil as a dietary fat provides presumptive evidence that the consumption of low levels of cyclopropene fatty acids has no adverse effects. Whether the prolonged ingestion by humans of a fat containing higher amounts of these acids, such as are found in kapok seed oil, would be deleterious is unknown.

POLYUNSATURATED ACIDS

The effect that the composition of dietary fats can have on blood lipid levels and the association of an elevated blood cholesterol level with an increased incidence of coronary heart disease have led to recommendations that the dietary levels of saturated fatty acids should be decreased and polyunsaturated fatty acids increased. Whether a higher consumption of polyunsaturated fatty acids would have any effects, besides the desired lowering of blood cholesterol, is not known. The induction of a deficiency of vitamin E is one such possibility.[109]

Man's requirement for vitamin E has not been established with certainty. The only quantitative measurements are the extensive studies of Horwitt,[110-113] who also demonstrated that the need for vitamin E increased with increasing levels of unsaturated fatty acids. From the data in these experiments, Harris and Embree[114] have proposed that to avoid deficiency symptoms, the ratio, mg tocopherol to g polyunsaturated acids, should equal 0.6. From the same experiments, Jager[115] has concluded it is unlikely that a fixed ratio exists.

The only other controlled human study is that of Dayton *et al.*[116] For several years two groups of subjects received diets low or high in polyunsaturated acids. The men receiving the high level of unsaturated fats had higher plasma tocopherol levels and their erythrocytes showed a decreased susceptibility to hemolysis[117]; a deficiency of tocopherol results in increased erythrocyte fragility. This diet contained large amounts of vegetable oils and hence the intake of tocopherol, as well as unsaturated acids, was increased. (See Chapter 12, p. 267.)

An alternative basis to which the requirement for vitamin E can be related is the body weight in kg to the three quarter power.[118] Such a relationship indicates the basic requirements to be a function of the metabolic mass. This need apparently is increased by the level of unsaturated fat in the diet but more importantly by the level of unsaturated fatty acids in the body's tissues. The requirement relative to tissue unsaturated fatty acids depends also on the propensity of the particular fatty acid to undergo peroxidation.[113,119] Because of the interplay of these various tissue and dietary factors, it is unlikely that any single value can be used to express the vitamin E requirement.

It is the conclusion of the Food and Nutrition Board of the National Research Council[120] that the requirement of adults for vitamin E is from 10 to 30 IU per day, depending on whether the diet is low or high in polyunsataturated fatty acids. These levels of intake can be realized with presently available foodstuffs.

Perhaps it is fortunate that the vegetable oils recommended as a source of polyunsaturated acids in fat-modified diets are also the best sources of vitamin E.[121] This is not true of marine oils, which are rich in polyunsaturated fatty acids but contain little vitamin E.

The long-term feeding to humans of diets high in polyunsaturated fatty acids yielded an observation that is difficult to evaluate at the present time.[116] Although the subjects consuming this diet showed a significant decrease in acute atherosclerotic events, the overall death rate was not different from that of the control group. This was found to be due to a higher incidence of deaths due to carcinoma in the experimental group.[122] The significance of this observation is uncertain, since the excess cancer mortality was accounted for by men who had consumed the experimental diet for only a few days to a few months. It seems unlikely that the diet high in polyunsaturated fatty acids was responsible for the excess carcinoma mortality because this was not observed in the subjects who consumed the diet for several years. Similar types of studies employing fat-modified diets have been going on in four other centers. The combined experience from the five trials showed only a slight excess incidence of and mortality from malignant neoplasms in the experimental groups (high polyunsaturated diets), an excess that was well within chance.[123]

Although there is no direct evidence that a change to a diet high in polyunsaturated fatty acids results in any adverse effects, attention should be paid to possible harmful as well as beneficial effects. As Keys[124] has pointed out, no human population has customarily consumed diets high in polyunsaturated acids. This more cautious approach is reflected in the dietary recommendations of the Intersociety Committee of the American Heart Association.[125] Rather than emphasizing polyunsaturated fatty acids, the primary recommendation is to decrease the consumption of cholesterol and of saturated fatty acids, replacing these with monounsaturated acids and limiting the intake of polyunsaturated fatty acids to less than 10% of the calories.

OXIDIZED AND POLYMERIZED FAT

Oxidized and polymerized fats, although not naturally occurring, can be formed under conditions used in the preparation of foods. There is an extensive literature in this field. The reader is referred to the recent review by Artman[126] for a complete discussion of the chemical changes ensuing from the exposure of fats to atmospheric oxygen or heat, and of the resulting changes in biological value. There are two practical conditions under which significant changes in the composition of fats might take place. These are storage at room temperature and use in cooking.

The storage of fats, particularly those high in polyunsaturated fatty acids, in the presence of oxygen but in the absence of heat, can result in the formation of hydroperoxides. It is unlikely that fats containing any significant amounts of these would be consumed because the hydroperoxides readily break down to compounds that have strong and unpleasant flavors. Moreover, Andrews *et al.* [127] fed rats a fat with a peroxide value of 100 without adversely affecting the growth of the animals. Since a fat with a peroxide value considerably less than 10 is organoleptically unacceptable, room-temperature oxidation poses no health threat.

A number of studies of fats heated under laboratory conditions have been conducted. In many instances, the heating conditions were so specialized as to have little practical significance. In evaluating these experiments, it should be noted that deep-fat frying is normally at a temperature of 180 °C. Moreover, the evolution of water vapor from the food results in a steam-stripping of volatiles from the frying fat and in the formation of a barrier to the entrance of oxygen into fat. In spite of deviations from normal conditions of use, these studies have pointed to compounds that might be formed during the preparation of fried foods.

One such class of compounds is made up of the cyclic monomers, originally recognized in linseed oil that had been heated at 275 °C in the absence of oxygen. The cyclic monomers were isolated as a distillable fraction that would not form adducts with urea. [128] Small amounts of related materials have been shown to be present in used frying fats. Although these cyclic monomers are toxic when fed as an isolated concentrate, their level, even in abused frying fats, is not great enough to elicit any adverse effects. This has been demonstrated in growth, survival, and reproductive experiments with rats. [126] In these studies, fats that had been used in cooking for long periods, or until they were no longer suitable for use, were fed as the sole dietary fat. Except for a slight decrease in feed efficiency (attributable to poorly absorbed polymer), growth rate, survival, and the composition and appearance of the organs were normal. That no adverse effects were seen is probably attributable to the fact that little cyclic monomer is formed under normal-use conditions. Morever, only 30% of the oxidation products formed at elevated temperatures is absorbed. [129]

Artman [126] concluded that fats heated in the normal cooking processes are not harmful to people. Studies [130-132] carried out subsequent to those reviewed by him have supported his position.

HYDROPERICARDIUM-PRODUCING FACTORS

In the light of new evidence, accumulated since the earlier edition of this book, it seems unlikely that the hydropericardium-producing factors are naturally occurring. The structure of one of these was shown by single-crystal x-ray analysis to be 1,2,3,7,8,9-hexachlorodibenzo-*p*-dioxin[133]:

Hydropericardium-Producing Factor

Subsequently J. C. Wootton (personal communication) prepared a synthetic hexachlorinated dibenzo-*p*-dioxin that had physical properties quite similar to the isolated material from which Cantrell, Webb, and Mabis obtained their crystalline material. Moreover, the synthetic compound produced hydropericardium in chickens. Other unpublished information from our laboratory indicates another of the hydropericardium-producing factors to be 1,2,3,6,7,8-hexachlorodibenzo-*p*-dioxin. Since there are a number of nonnatural sources of chlorophenols that could occur as contaminants of agricultural products, the hydropericardium-producing factors may result from subjecting fats containing such phenols to very high temperatures. This possibility is supported by the observation of Higginbotham et al.[134] that the pyrolysis of chlorinated phenols yields chlorinated dibenzo-*p*-dioxins.

ACKNOWLEDGMENTS

I wish to thank A. M. M. Abdellatif, N. R. Artman, J. L. Beare-Rogers, J. A. Campbell, S. Dayton, F. Ederer, M. Gurr, D. C. Herting, M. K. Horwitt, J. F. Mead, M. W. O'Connor, M. L. Pearce, G. Rocquelin, D. Steinberg, and R. O. Vles for supplying me with prepublication copies of their papers and their helpful comments.

REFERENCES

1. E. W. Eckey, Rhoeadales, Chapter 14. In Vegetable fats and oils. Reinhold Publishing Corporation, New York (1954).
2. R. W. Miller, F. R. Earle, and I. A. Wolff, Search for new industrial oils. XIII. Oils from 102 species of Cruciferae. J. Am. Oil Chem. Soc. *42*:817 (1965).

3. B. R. Stefansson, F. W. Hougen, and R. K. Downey, Note on the isolation of rape plants with seed oil free from erucic acid. Can. J. Plant Sci. *41*:218 (1961).

4. J. Krzymanski and R. K. Downey, Inheritance of fatty acid composition in winter forms of rapeseed, *Brassica napus.* Can. J. Plant Sci. *49*:313 (1969).

5. P. Roine, E. Uksila, H. Teir, and J. Rapola, Histopathological changes in rats and pigs fed rapeseed oil. Z. Ernährungswiss. *1*:118 (1960).

6. G. Rocquelin and R. Cluzan, Comparative feeding values and physiological effects of rapeseed oil with a high content of erucic acid and rapeseed oil free from erucic acid. I. Effects on growth rate, feeding efficiency and physiology of various organs in the rat. Ann. Biol. Anim. Biochim. Biophys. *8*:395 (1968).

7. J. L. Beare-Rogers, E. A. Nera, and H. A. Heggtviet, Cardiac lipid changes in rats fed oils containing long-chain fatty acids. Can. Inst. Food Tech. J. *4*:120 (1971).

8. H. J. Thomasson, J. J. Gottenbos, P. L. Van Pijpen, and R. O. Vles, Nutritive value of rapeseed oil. International Symposium for the Chemistry and Technology of Rapeseed Oil and Other Cruciferae Oils, Gdansk (1967).

9. A. M. M. Abdellatif and R. O. Vles, Pathological effects of dietary rapeseed oil in rats. Nutr. Metabol. *12*:285 (1970).

10. A. M. M. Abdellatif and R. O. Vles, Physiopathological effects of rapeseed oil and Canbra oil in rats, p. 423. Proceedings of the International Conference on the Science, Technology and Marketing of Rapeseed and Rapeseed Products. Rapeseed Association of Canada, Winnipeg, Manitoba (1970).

11. G. Rocquelin, J. P. Sergiel, B. Martin, and J. Leclerc, The nutritive value of rapeseed oils: A review. Int. Soc. Fat Res., Chicago (September, 1970).

12. U. M. T. Houtsmuller, C. B. Struijk, and A. Van Der Beek, Decrease in rate of ATP synthesis of isolated rat heart mitochondria induced by dietary erucic acid. Biochim. Biophys. Acta *218*:564 (1970).

13. J. L. Beare-Rogers, Nutritional aspect of long-chain fatty acids, p. 450. Proceedings of the International Conference on the Science, Technology and Marketing of Rapeseed and Rapeseed Products. Rapeseed Association of Canada, Winnipeg, Manitoba (1970).

14. A. M. M. Abdellatif and R. O. Vles, Pathological effects of dietary rapeseed oil in ducklings. Nutr. Metabol. *12*:296 (1970).

15. R. O. Vles and A. M. M. Abdellatif, Effects of hardened palm oil on rapeseed oil-induced changes in ducklings and guinea pigs, p. 435. Proceedings of the International Conference on the Science, Technology and Marketing of Rapeseed and Rapeseed Products. Rapeseed Association of Canada, Winnipeg, Manitoba (1970).

16. G. Rocquelin, B. Martin, and R. Cluzan, Comparative physiological effects of rapeseed and Canbra oils in the rat: Influence of the ratio of saturated to monounsaturated fatty acids, p. 405. Proceedings of the International Conference on the Science, Technology and Marketing of Rapeseed and Rapeseed Products. Rapeseed Association of Canada, Winnipeg, Manitoba (1970).

17. J. Boer, B. C. P. Jansen, and A. Kentie, On the growth-promoting factor for rats present in summer butter. J. Nutr. *33*:339 (1947).

18. H. J. Deuel, Jr., S. M. Greenberg, E. E. Straub, D. Jue, C. M. Gooding, and C. F. Brown, Studies on the comparative nutritive value of fats. X. On the

reputed growth-promoting activity of vaccenic acid. J. Nutr. *35*:301 (1948).

19. H. J. Thomasson, The biological value of oils and fats. I. Growth and food intake on feeding with natural oils and fats. J. Nutr. *56*:455 (1955).

20. J. L. Beare, T. K. Murray, and J. A. Campbell, Effects of varying proportions of dietary rapeseed oil on the rat. Can. J. Biochem. Physiol. *35*:1225 (1957).

21. J. L. Beare, T. K. Murray, H. C. Grice, and J. A. Campbell, A comparison of the utilization of rapeseed oil and corn oil by the rat. J. Biochem. Physiol. *37*:613 (1959).

22. R. Jacquot, J. Raulin, and A. Thoron, Physiopathological effects of unusual fat components. Rapeseed oil. Rev. Fr. Corps Gras *14*:441 (1967).

23. A. Thoron, Interpretation of the particular nutritional character of rapeseed oil. Tests on the pig and the rat. Ann. Nutr. Aliment. *23*:103 (1969).

24. R. E. Salmon, The relative value of rapeseed and soybean oils in chick starter diets. Poult. Sci. *48*:1045 (1969).

25. R. E. Salmon, Soybean versus rapeseed oil in turkey starter diets. Poult. Sci. *48*:87 (1969).

26. H. J. Thomasson and J. Boldingh, The biological value of oils and fats. II. The growth-retarding substances in rapeseed oil. J. Nutr. *56*:469 (1955).

27. J. L. Beare, E. R. W. Gregory, and J. A. Campbell, The effects of different varieties of rapeseed oil on weight gain, and of golden rapeseed oil on reproduction of the rat. Can. J. Biochem. Physiol. *37*:1191 (1959).

28. B. M. Craig and J. L. Beare, Nutritional properties of Canadian Canbra oil. J. Inst. Can. Technol. Aliment. *1*:64 (1968).

29. J. C. Alexander and F. H. Mattson, A nutritional comparison of rapeseed oil and soybean oil. Can. J. Biochem. *44*:35 (1966).

30. J. L. Beare, J. A. Campbell, C. G. Youngs, and B. M. Craig, Effects of saturated fat in rats fed rapeseed oil. Can. J. Biochem. Physiol. *41*:605 (1963).

31. B. M. Craig, C. G. Youngs, J. L. Beare, and J. A. Campbell, Influence of selective and non-selective hydrogenation of rapeseed oil on carcass fat of rats. Can. J. Biochem. Physiol. *41*:51 (1963).

32. H. J. Thomasson, The biological value of oils and fats. III. The longevity of rats fed rapeseed oil- or butterfat-containing diets. J. Nutr. *57*:17 (1955).

33. R. O. Vles and A. M. M. Abdellatif, Long term effects of rapeseed oil in rats and rabbits. Int. Soc. Fat Res., Chicago (September, 1970).

34. J. L. Beare, E. R. W. Gregory, D. M. Smith, and J. A. Campbell, The effect of rapeseed oil on reproduction and on the composition of rat milk fat. Can. J. Biochem. Physiol. *39*:195 (1961).

35. J. P. Carreau, A. Thoron, D. Lapous, and J. Raulin, Erucic acid metabolism. I. Conversion to oleic acid. Bull. Soc. Chem. Biol. *50*:1973 (1968).

36. J. P. Carreau, A. Thoron, and J. Raulin, Erucic acid metabolism and its conversion into oleic acid in the rat. C. R. Acad. Sci. Paris *266*:417 (1968).

37. K. K. Carroll, Metabolism of ^{14}C-labeled oleic acid, erucic acid and nervonic acid in rats. Lipids *1*:171 (1966).

38. A. Bach, P. Metais, J. Raulin, and R. Jacquot, The metabolism of erucic acid. II. The rate of oxidation. Bull. Soc. Chem. Biol. *51*:167 (1969).

39. H. Wagner, E. Sellig, and K. Bernhard, The distribution and biological half-life of erucic acid in rats after dosages of rapeseed oil. Z. Physiol. Chem. *312*:104 (1958).

40. J. L. Sell and G. C. Hodgson, Comparative value of dietary rapeseed oil,

sunflower seed oil, soybean oil and animal tallow for chickens. J. Nutr. *76*: 113 (1962).

41. J. Chudy and J. Batura, Nutrition studies on rapeseed oil. I. Storage of erucic acid in the depot fats in chickens fed rapeseed oil. Zesz. Nauk. Wyzsz. Szk. Roln. Olsytynie *21*:37 (1966).

42. G. B. Stoken and D. M. Walker, The nutritive value of fat in the diet of the milk fed lambs. II. The effect of different dietary fats on the composition of the body fats. Br. J. Nutr. *24*:435 (1970).

43. B. Leclercq, Utilization of colza oil by laying hens; Its influence on genesis and composition of egg lipids. C. R. Acad. Sci. Paris *267*:2235 (1968).

44. J. Chudy, H. Jaworska, J. Jaworski, and A. Rutkowski, Influence of fat contained in feed mixtures on fatty acid composition in hen eggs. Rocz. Technol. Chem. Zywne. *16*:61 (1969).

45. S. Refsum, Heredopathia atactica polyneuritiformis. Acta Psychiatr. Scand., Suppl. *38*:9 (1946).

46. D. Steinberg, Phytanic acid storage disease (Refsum's disease). In Metabolic basis of inherited disease, J. B. Stanbury, J. B. Wyngaarden, and D. S. Fredrickson (eds.). 3rd ed. McGraw-Hill, New York (1971).

47. E. Klenk and W. Kahlke, Über das Vorkommen der 3,7,11,15-Tetramethylhexadecansäure (Phytansäure) in den Cholesterinestern und anderen Lipoidfraktionen der Organe bei einem Krankheitsfall unbekannter Genese Verdacht auf Heredopathia atactica polyneuritiformis (Refsum's syndrome). Hoppe-Seyler's Z. Physiol. Chem. *333*:133 (1963).

48. J. Avigan, The presence of phytanic acid in normal human and animal plasma. Biochim. Biophys. Acta *116*:391 (1966).

49. G. J. Kremer, Über das Vorkommen der 3,7,11,15-Tetramethylhexadecansäure in den Lipoiden von Normalseren. Klin. Wochenschr. *43*:517 (1965).

50. D. Steinberg, J. Avigan, C. Mize, and J. Baxter, Phytanic acid formation and accumulation in phytol-fed rats. Biochem. Biophys. Res. Comm. *19*:412 (1965).

51. E. Klenk and G. J. Kremer, Untersuchungen zum Stoffwechsel des Phytols, Dihydrophytols und der Phytansäure. Hoppe-Seyler's Z. Physiol. Chem. *343*: 39 (1965).

52. R. P. Hansen, F. B. Shorland, and I. A. M. Prior, The fate of phytanic acid when administered to rats. Biochim. Biophys. Acta *116*:178 (1966).

53. D. Steinberg, J. Avigan, C. E. Mize, J. H. Baxter, J. Cammermeyer, H. M. Fales, and P. F. Highet, Effects of dietary phytol and phytanic acid in animals. J. Lipid Res. *7*:684 (1966).

54. C. E. Mize, J. Avigan, D. Steinberg, R. C. Pittman, H. M. Fales, and G. W. A. Milne, A major pathway for the mammalian oxidative degradation of phytanic acid. Biochim. Biophys. Acta *176*:720 (1969).

55. O. Stokke, Alpha-oxidation of fatty acids in various mammals, and a phytanic acid feeding experiment in an animal with a low alpha-oxidation capacity. Scand. J. Clin. Lab. Invest. *20*:305 (1967).

56. J. Avigan, D. Steinberg, A. Gutman, C. E. Mize, and G. W. A. Milne, Alphadecarboxylation, an important pathway for degradation of phytanic acid in animals. Biochem. Biophys. Res. Comm. *24*:838 (1966).

57. C. E. Mize, D. Steinberg, J. Avigan, and H. M. Fales, A pathway for oxidative degradation of phytanic acid in mammals. Biochem. Biophys. Res. Comm. *25*:359 (1966).

58. S.-C. Tsai, J. H. Herndon, Jr., B. W. Uhlendorf, H. M. Fales, and C. E. Mize, The formation of alpha-hydroxyphytanic acid from phytanic acid in mammalian tissues. Biochem. Biophys. Res. Comm. *28*:571 (1967).

59. S.-C. Tsai, J. Avigan, and D. Steinberg, Studies on the alpha-oxidation of phytanic acid by rat liver mitochondria. J. Biol. Chem. *244*:2682 (1969).

60. J. H. Herndon, Jr., D. Steinberg, B. W. Uhlendorf, and H. M. Fales, Refsum's disease: Characterization of the enzyme defect in cell culture. J. Clin. Invest. *48*:1017 (1969).

61. D. Steinberg, J. Avigan, C. Mize, L. Eldjarn, K. Try, and S. Refsum, Conversion of U-C^{14}-phytol to phytanic acid and its oxidation in heredopathia atactica polyneuritiformis. Biochem. Biophys. Res. Comm. *19*:783 (1965).

62. D. Steinberg, C. E. Mize, J. Avigan, H. M. Fales, L. Eldjarn, K. Try, O. Stokke, and S. Refsum, Studies on the metabolic error in Refsum's disease. J. Clin. Invest. *45*:1076 (1966); *46*:313 (1967).

63. D. Steinberg, F. Q. Vroom, W. K. Engel, J. Cammermeyer, C. E. Mize, and J. Avigan, Refsum's disease—A recently characterized lipidosis involving the nervous system. Ann. Int. Med. *66*:365 (1967).

64. C. E. Mize, J. H. Herndon, Jr., J. P. Blass, G. W. A. Milne, C. Follansbee, P. Laudat, and D. Steinberg, Localization of the oxidative defect in phytanic acid degradation in patients with Refsum's disease. J. Clin. Invest. *48*:1033 (1969).

65. D. Steinberg, J. H. Herndon, Jr., B. W. Uhlendorf, C. E. Mize, J. Avigan, and G. W. A. Milne, Refsum's disease: Nature of the enzyme defect. Science *156*: 1740 (1967).

66. D. Steinberg, J. Avigan, C. E. Mize, J. H. Herndon, Jr., H. M. Fales, and G. W. A. Milne, The nature of the metabolic defect in Refsum's disease. Path. Eur. *3*:450 (1968).

67. W. Kahlke and R. Richterich, Refsum's disease (heredopathia atactica polyneuritiformis), an inborn error of lipid metabolism with storage of 3,7,11,15-tetramethyl hexadecanoic acid. II. Isolation and identification of the storage product. Am. J. Med. *39*:237 (1965).

68. N. C. Nevin, J. N. Cumings, and F. McKeown, Refsum's syndrome, heredopathia atactica polyneuritiformis. Brain *90*:419 (1967).

69. J. H. Herndon, D. Steinberg, and B. W. Uhlendorf, Refsum's disease: Defective oxidation of phytanic acid in tissue cultures derived from homozygotes and heterozygotes. N. Engl. J. Med. *281*:1034 (1969).

70. C. E. Mize, J. Avigan, J. H. Baxter, H. M. Fales, and D. Steinberg, Metabolism of phytol-U-^{14}C and phytanic acid-U-^{14}C in the rat. J. Lipid Res. *7*:692 (1966).

71. W. Stoffel and W. Kahlke, The transformation of phytol into 3,7,11,15-tetramethylhexadecanoic (phytanic) acid in heredopathia atactica polyneuritiformis (Refsum's syndrome). Biochem. Biophys. Res. Comm. *19*:33 (1965).

72. J. H. Baxter, Absorption of chlorophyll phytol in normal man and in patients with Refsum's disease. J. Lipid Res. *9*:636 (1968).

73. R. P. Hansen, 3,7,11,15-tetramethylhexadecanoic acid: Its occurrence in sheep fat. N. Z. J. Sci. *8*:158 (1965).

74. R. P. Hansen, Occurrence of 3,7,11,15-tetramethylhexadecanoic acid in ox perinephric fat. Chem. Ind. *303* (1965).

75. S. Patton and A. A. Benson, Phytol metabolism in the bovine. Biochim. Biophys. Acta *125*:22 (1966).

76. R. G. Ackman and J. C. Sipos, Isolation of the saturated fatty acids and branched-chain fatty acids. Comp. Biochem. Physiol. *15*:445 (1965).
77. H. Peters and Th. Wieske, Detection of traces of polybranched fatty acids. Fette, Seifen, Anstrichm. *68*:947 (1966).
78. A. K. Sen Gupta and H. Peters, Isolation and structure determination of poly-branched-chain fatty acids from fish oil. Fette, Seifer, Anstrichm. *68*:349 (1966).
79. L. Eldjarn, K. Try, O. Stokke, A. W. Munthe-Kaas, S. Refsum, D. Steinberg, J. Avigan, and C. Mize, Dietary effects on serum-phytanic-acid levels and on clinical manifestations in heredopathia atactica polyneuritiformis. Lancet *i*:691 (1966).
80. D. Steinberg, C. E. Mize, J. H. Herndon, Jr., H. M. Fales, W. K. Engel, and F. Q. Vroom, Phytanic acid in patients with Refsum's syndrome and response to dietary treatment. Arch. Int. Med. *125*:75 (1970).
81. S. Refsum and L. Eldjarn, Heredopathia atactica polyneuritiformis—An inborn defect in the metabolism of branched-chain fatty acids, p. 36. In Future of neurology, H. G. Bammer (ed.). Georg Thieme Verlag, Stuttgart (1967).
82. R. A. Phelps, F. S. Shenstone, A. R. Kemmerer, and R. J. Evans, A review of cyclopropenoid compounds: Biological effects of some derivatives. Poult. Sci. *44*:358 (1965).
83. American Oil Chemists' Society, Official and tentative methods of the American Oil Chemists' Soc. 3rd ed., revised to 1970. Chicago, Method CB1-25 (1959).
84. F. S. Shenstone and J. R. Vickery, A biologically active fatty acid in Malvaceae. Nature *177*:94 (1956).
85. R. S. Levi, H. G. Reilich, H. J. O'Neill, A. F. Cucullu, and E. L. Skan, Quantitative determination of cyclopropenoid fatty acids in cottonseed meal. J. Am. Oil Chem. Soc. *44*:249 (1967).
86. T. L. Wilson, C. R. Smith, Jr., and K. L. Mikolajczak, Characterization of cyclopropenoid acids in selection seed oils. J. Am. Oil Chem. Soc. *38*:696 (1961).
87. T. W. Hammonds and G. G. Shone, Analysis of fats containing cyclopropenoid fatty acids. Analyst *91*:455 (1966).
88. E. W. Eckey, Malvales, Chapter 18. In Vegetable fats and oils, Reinhold Publishing, New York (1954).
89. T. P. Hilditch and P. N. Williams, The chemical constitution of natural fats. 4th ed. Spottiswoode, Ballantyne, London (1964).
90. A. V. Bailey, J. A. Harris, E. L. Skau, and T. Kerr, Cyclopropenoid fatty acid content and fatty acid composition and crude oils from twenty-five varieties of cottonseed. J. Am. Oil Chem. Soc. *43*:107 (1966).
91. J. A. Harris, F. C. Magne, and E. L. Skau, Methods for the determination of cyclopropenoid fatty acids. IV. Application of the stepwise HBr titration method to the analysis of refined and crude cottonseed oils. J. Am. Oil Chem. Soc. *41*:309 (1964).
92. J. C. Masson, M. G. Vavich, B. W. Heywang, and A. R. Kemmerer, Pink discoloration in eggs caused by sterculic acid. Science *126*:751 (1957).
93. F. S. Shenstone and J. R. Vickery, Substances in plants of the order Malvale causing pink whites in stored eggs. Poult. Sci. *38*:1055 (1959).
94. D. L. Schneider, A. A. Kurnick, M. G. Vavich, and A. R. Kemmerer, Delay of sexual maturity in chickens by *Sterculia foetida* oil. J. Nutr. *77*:403 (1962).

95. H. J. Thomasson, The biological value of oils and fats. I. Growth and food intake on feeding with natural oils and fats. J. Nutr. *56*:455 (1955).

96. D. L. Schneider, E. T. Sheehan, M. G. Vavich, and A. R. Kemmerer, Effect of *Sterculia foetida* oil on weanling rat growth and survival. J. Agric. Food Chem. *16*:1022 (1968).

97. A. M. Rascop, E. T. Sheehan, and M. G. Vavich, Histomorphological changes in reproductive organs of rats fed cyclopropenoid fatty acids. Proc. Soc. Exp. Biol. Med. *122*:142 (1966).

98. F. H. Kratzer, P. N. Davis, and B. J. Marshall, Cottonseed meal in rations for starting poults, growing turkeys and turkey breeder hens. Poult. Sci. *34*:462 (1955).

99. F. W. Lorenz and H. J. Almquist, Effects of malvaceous seeds on stored egg quality. Ind. Eng. Chem. *26*:1311 (1934).

100. H. J. Deuel, Jr., Lipids, 2. Interscience, New York (1955).

101. R. J. Evans, S. L. Bandemer, M. Anderson, J. A. Davidson, Fatty acid distribution in tissues from hens fed cottonseed oil or *Sterculia foetida* seeds. J. Nutr. *76*:314 (1962).

102. E. Allen, A. R. Johnson, A. C. Fogerty, J. A. Pearson, and F. S. Shenstone, Inhibition by cyclopropene fatty acids of the desaturation of stearic acid in hen liver. Lipids *2*:419 (1967).

103. A. R. Johnson, J. A. Pearson, F. S. Shenstone, and A. C. Fogerty, Inhibition of the desaturation of stearic to oleic acid by cyclopropene fatty acids. Nature *214*:1244 (1967).

104. R. J. Evans, J. A. Davidson, J. N. LaRue, and S. L. Bademer, Interference in fatty acid metabolism of laying hens caused by cottonseed oil feeding. Poult. Sci. *42*:875 (1963).

105. P. K. Raju and R. Reiser, Alternate route for the biosynthesis of oleic acid in the rat. Biochim. Biophys. Acta *176*:48 (1969).

106. A. T. James, P. Harris, and J. Bezard, The inhibition of unsaturated fatty acid biosynthesis in plants by sterculic acid. Eur. J. Biochem. *3*:318 (1968).

107. M. I. Gurr, Biosynthesis of polyunsaturated fatty acids in plants. Int. Soc. Fat. Res. Chicago (September, 1970).

108. S. V. Pande and J. F. Mead, Inhibition of the stearyl coenzyme A desaturase system by sterculate. J. Biol. Chem. *245*:1856 (1970).

109. D. C. Herting, Perspective on vitamin E. Am. J. Clin. Nutr. *19*:210 (1966).

110. M. K. Horwitt, Vitamin E and lipid metabolism in man. Am. J. Clin. Nutr. *8*:451 (1960).

111. M. K. Horwitt, Vitamin E in human nutrition—An interpretative review Borden's Rev. Nutr. Res. *22*:1 (1961).

112. M. K. Horwitt, Interrelations between vitamin E and polyunsaturated fatty acids in adult man. Vitam. Horm. *20*:541 (1962).

113. M. K. Horwitt, Tocopherol and polyunsaturated lipid relationships, International Symposium on Vitamin E, Hakone, Japan (September 1970).

114. P. L. Harris and N. D. Embree, Quantitative consideration of the effect of polyunsaturated fatty acid content of the diet on the requirements for vitamin E. Am. J. Clin. Nutr. *13*:385 (1963).

115. F. C. Jager, High linoleic acid intake and vitamin E requirement in rats. Nutr. Diet. *11*:279 (1969).

116. S. Dayton, S. D. Hashimoto, W. J. Dixon, and W. Tomiyasu, A controlled

clinical trial of a diet high in unsaturated fat in preventing complications of atherosclerosis. Circulation, Suppl. II. *40*:1 (1969).

117. S. Dayton, S. Hashimoto, D. Rosenblum, and M. L. Pearce, Vitamin E. Status of humans during feeding of unsaturated fats. J. Lab. Clin. Med. *65*:739 (1965).

118. P. L. Harris, Practical nutritional aspect of vitamin E. Ann. N.Y. Acad. Sci. *52*:240 (1949).

119. L. A. Witting and M. K. Horwitt, Effect of degree of fatty acid unsaturation in tocopherol deficiency-induced creatinuria. J. Nutr. *82*:19 (1964).

120. National Research Council, Food and Nutrition Board, Recommended dietary allowances. 7th ed., National Academy of Sciences, Washington, D.C. (1968).

121. E. L. Hove and P. L. Harris, Note on the linoleic acid–tocopherol relationship in fats and oils. J. Am. Oil Chem. Soc. *28*:405 (1951).

122. M. L. Pearce and S. Dayton, Incidence of cancer in men on a diet high in poly-unsaturated fat. Lancet *i*:464 (1971).

123. F. Ederer, P. Leren, O. Turpeinen, and I. D. Frantz, Cancer among men on cholesterol-lowering diets. Experience from five clinical trials. Lancet *ii*:203 (1971).

124. A. Keys (ed.), Coronary heart disease in seven countries. Circulation, Suppl. I. *61*: (1970).

125. Intersociety Commission for Heart Disease Resources, Primary prevention of the atherosclerotic diseases. Circulation *62*:A55 (1970).

126. N. R. Artman, The chemical and biological properties of heated and oxidized fats, p. 245. In Advances in Lipid Research, 7, R. Poaletti and D. Kritchevsky (eds.). Academic Press, New York (1969).

127. J. S. Andrews, W. H. Griffith, J. F. Mead, and R. A. Stein, Toxicity of air-oxidized soybean oil. J. Nutr. *70*:199 (1960).

128. E. W. Crampton, R. H. Common, F. A. Farmer, A. F. Wells, and D. Crawford, Studies to determine the nature of the damage to the nutritive value of some vegetable oils from heated polymerization. III. The segregation of toxic and non-toxic material from esters of heat-polymerized linseed oil by distillation and by urea. J. Nutr. *49*:333 (1953).

129. E. G. Perkins, S. M. Vachha, and F. A. Kummerow, Absorption by the rat of non-volatile oxidation products of labeled, randomized corn oil. J. Nutr. *100*: 725 (1970).

130. K. Lang and E. H. VonJan, Effect of frying on the nutritional properties of fats for fish frying. Fette, Seifen, Anstrichm. *71*:1032 (1969).

131. C. E. Poling, E. Eagle, E. E. Rice, A. M. Durand, and M. Fisher, Long-term responses of rats to heat-treated dietary fats. IV. Weight gains, food and energy efficiencies, longevity, and histopathology. Lipids *5*:128 (1970).

132. P. Ramel, M. T. Lanteaume, A. M. LeClerc, and J. Rannaud, Influence of heat-ing on physiological effects of some dietary fats. Rev. Fr. Corps Gras *14*:505 (1969).

133. J. S. Cantrell, N. C. Webb, and A. J. Mabis, The identification and crystal structure of a hydropericardium-producing factor: 1,2,3,7,8,9-Hexachlorodi-benzo-*p*-dioxin. Acta Crystall. *B25*:159 (1969).

134. G. R. Higginbotham, A. Huang, D. Firestone, and J. Verrett, Chemical toxi-cological evaluations of isolated and synthetic chloro derivatives of dibenzo-*p*-dioxin. Nature *220*:702 (1968).

10
C. H. VanEtten and
I. A. Wolff

NATURAL
SULFUR
COMPOUNDS*

This review includes work on the isolation, characterization, and biological testing of sulfur-containing compounds from plants that may be deleterious if consumed in large amounts. Little information indicates that these compounds are so distributed or are concentrated as to be harmful to man when the plants containing them are used in a conventional manner. Possible exceptions arise from circumstantial evidence that certain cruciferous plants such as cabbage, turnips, and rutabagas contribute directly or indirectly to a small fraction of the total incidence of goiter in the world population. Biological effects of the goitrogens responsible for this circumstantial evidence and of other substances discussed herein will be described, quantitatively when possible, to indicate the amount of the natural product required to cause acute or chronic harm. Hopefully, this approach may help to anticipate problems that can arise in new food technology concerned with these natural products.

The goitrogens from certain cruciferous plants are derived from a characteristic group of compounds, referred to in the older literature as thioglucosides. The more definitive name *glucosinolates* is now preferred by most authors to refer specifically to the type of starting material in Reaction 1, since it provides a convenient method of chemically naming related compounds as explained in the next section.

* Literature reviewed to February 1972.

Previous reviews include those related to biological effects of ingestion of these plants,[55,57-59,61,129,131] to the chemistry of the glucosinolates,[27,44,77] to problems in the use of rapeseed meals in animal feeds,[12,15,29,108] and to the transfer of deleterious substances into milk from animals fed crucifers.[135,142]

The unique taste and smell of plants of the *Allium* genus, including onions, garlic, and chives, are caused by sulfur-containing compounds that arise from enzyme action on precursors in the plants. Much of the chemistry of these precursors and their transformations has recently been elucidated, and the chemical nature of some of the compounds that can be formed suggests that harm might result if the derived substances were consumed in large amounts. Previous reviews relate to the chemical identity, odor, and lachrymatory properties of these compounds.[23,136]

GLUCOSINOLATES IN THE CRUCIFERAE

Chemistry of the Glucosinolates and Derived Products

The pungent nature of plants in the Cruciferae such as horseradish and mustard has been known from antiquity. Sinigrin was isolated from black mustard seed in 1840[78] and was identified as the precursor of allyl isothiocyanate, the most common of the mustard oils. At the same time a fraction containing an enzyme called "myrosin" was separated from the seed and shown to cause the breakdown of the sinigrin resulting in mustard oil. Prior to World War I, two additional glucosinolates were identified, sinalbin from white mustard and glucocheirolin from wallflower.[44] Up to the present about 65 different glucosinolates have been isolated from plants of the Cruciferae and related families. Of the 1,500 known species of Cruciferae, 300 have been examined and each has been found to contain from one to seven glucosinolates.[78] One or two of the compounds are usually present in relatively large amounts. The glucosinolate structure[45] (Reaction 1) has been confirmed by synthesis.[46] Use of the generic name glucosinolate with an appropriate prefix added to identify the R group provides a nomenclature that clearly defines chemical structures for the large number of glucosinolates that has been found.[43,44]

Reaction 1 shows the products generally formed when glucosinolates are hydrolyzed by thioglucosidase (thioglucoside glucohydrolase, EC 3.2.3.1).[48] Glucose and sulfate ions are always released. The remainder of the glucosinolate molecule, the organic portion of the aglucon, is usually converted to thiocyanate, to nitriles and sulfur, or through a Lossen rearrangement to isothiocyanate. Hydrolysis conditions and prior treatment of the plant material determine which of these products predominate, but a mixture of them is often formed.[129]

Table 1 shows the principal glucosinolates in the crucifers that are grown in quantity for food, condiment, or feed. The glucosinolates in which the *R* group is allyl-, 3-butenyl-, 4-pentenyl-, benzyl-, 2-phenylethyl-, or 4-methylthio-3-butenyl- are the sources of the isothiocyanates that are the steam-volatile mustard oils. Although the mustard oils appear to be the main hydrolysis products from the organic aglucon of the glucosinolates, the nitriles may be formed instead.[27,77,89,97,143] An organic thiocyanate has been reported from benzylglucosinolate in *Lepidium* species such as *L. sativum* (garden cress).[51]

$$R-C\underset{N-O-SO_2O^-}{\overset{S-C_6H_{11}O_5}{\diagup}} \xrightarrow[\text{Thioglucosidase}]{H_2O} \left[R-C\underset{N-}{\overset{S-}{\diagup}} \right] \begin{array}{l} + \text{ Glucose} \\ + \text{ HSO}_4^- \end{array}$$

Glucosinolate

$$R-N{=}C{=}S \qquad R-C{\equiv}N \qquad R-S-C{\equiv}N$$
Isothiocyanate   Nitrile   Thiocyanate
                    + S

Reaction 1

In some instances the isothiocyanates initially formed undergo further transformations. For example, enzymatic hydrolysis of sinalbin (*p*-hydroxybenzylglucosinolate) from white mustard[77] gives *p*-hydroxybenzyl isothiocyanate, which readily degrades into simpler compounds including thiocyanate ion.[72,73] Similarly, 5-vinyloxazolidine-2-thiones are formed by cyclization of the presumed isothiocyanate intermediates indicated in brackets in Reaction 2. This is a specific example of a general cyclization reaction that occurs for all isothiocyanates in which the

$$CH_2{=}CH{-}\overset{*}{C}HOH{-}CH_2{-}C\underset{N-OSO_2O^-}{\overset{S-C_6H_{11}O_5}{\diagup}}$$

Progoitrins

$$CH_2{=}CH{-}\overset{*}{C}HOH{-}CH_2{-}C{\equiv}N + S$$
1-Cyano-2-hydroxy-3-butenes

$$[CH_2{=}CH{-}\overset{*}{C}HOH{-}CH_2{-}N{=}C{=}S]$$

$$\underset{CH_2-CH}{\overset{S}{\diagup\!\!\diagdown}}\overset{*}{C}H{-}\overset{*}{C}HOH{-}CH_2{-}C{\equiv}N$$
1-Cyano-2-hydroxy-3,4-epithiobutanes

$$CH_2{=}CH{-}\overset{*}{C}{-}H \underset{O}{\overset{CH_2-N-H}{\diagup\!\!\!\diagdown}} C{=}S$$
5-Vinyloxazolidine-2-thiones
(Goitrins)

Reaction 2

TABLE 1 Glucosinolates in Familiar Plant Materials from the Cruciferae

Plant	Part	Glucosinolates		Relative Amount	Reference[a]
		Trivial Name	R Group		
FOOD SOURCES					
Brassica oleracea					
Cabbage, kale,	Head,	Sinigrin	Allyl-[b]	Major	31,66,68
brussels sprouts,	leaves,	Glucobrassicin	3-Indolyl-	Major	52,68
cauliflower,	bud		methyl-		
broccoli,		Gluconapin	3-Butenyl-[b]	Minor	66,68
kohlrabi		Progoitrin	(R)-2-Hydroxy-	Minor	1,68,138
			3-butenyl-		
		Neoglucobrassicin	3-(N-Methoxy-	Minor	53,68
			indolyl)methyl-		
B. campestris					
Turnips	Roots	Gluconasturtiin	2-Phenylethyl-[b]	Major	68,88
		Progoitrin	(R)-2-Hydroxy-	Minor	6,68
			3-butenyl-		
			(R)-2-Hydroxy-4-	Minor	123
			pentenyl-		
B. napus					
Rutabaga	Roots	Progoitrin	(R)-2-Hydroxy-3-	Major	6,68
			butenyl-		
		Glucobrassicin	3-Indolylmethyl-	Minor	52,68
		Neoglucobrassicin	3-(N-Methoxy-	Minor	53,68
			indolyl)methyl-		
Lepidium sativum					
Garden cress	Leaves	Glucotropaeolin	Benzyl-[b]	Major	51
Nasturtium officinale					
Watercress	Leaves	Gluconasturtiin	2-Phenylethyl-[b]	Major	111
Raphanus sativus					
Radish	Roots	—	4-Methylthio-3-	Major	49
			butenyl-[b]		
		Glucobrassicin	3-Indolylmethyl-	Minor	52
CONDIMENT SOURCES					
Armoracia lapathifolia,					
A. rusticana					
Horseradish	Roots	Sinigrin	Allyl-[b]	Major	120
		Gluconasturtiin	2-Phenylethyl-[b]	Minor	117
B. carinata					
Ethiopian rapeseed	Seed	Sinigrin	Allyl-[b]	Major	47

TABLE 1 *(Continued)*

Plant	Part	Glucosinolates Trivial Name	R Group	Relative Amount	Reference[a]
B. juncea Indian or brown mustard	Seed	Sinigrin	Allyl-[b]	Major	47,66
B. nigra Black mustard	Seed	Sinigrin	Allyl-[b]	Major	47,66
Sinapis alba White mustard	Seed	Sinalbin	*p*-Hydroxybenzyl-	Major	80
S. arvensis Charlock	Seed	Sinalbin	*p*-Hydroxybenzyl	Major	47
FEED SOURCES					
B. campestris Rape, turnip, turnip rape, Polish rape, rubsen, navette	Seed	Gluconapin	3-Butenyl-[b]	Major	47
		Progoitrin	(*R*)-2-Hydroxy-3-butenyl-	Minor	47
		Glucobrassica-napin	4-Pentenyl-[b]	Minor	47
		Glucoraphanin	4-Methylsulfinyl-butyl-	Minor	47
		Glucoalyssin	5-Methylsulfinyl-pentyl-	Minor	47,113
B. napus Rape, Argentine rape	Seed	Progoitrin	(*R*)-2-Hydroxy-3-butenyl-	Major	6,47,79
		Gluconapin	3-Butenyl-[b]	Major	47,81
		Glucobrassica-napin	4-Pentenyl-[b]	Minor	47,79
		Gluconasturtiin	2-Phenylethyl-[b]	Minor	79
		Glucoiberin	3-Methylsulfinyl-propyl-	Minor	79,112
		Sinalbin	*p*-Hydroxybenzyl-	Minor	79
Crambe abyssinica Crambe, Abyssinian	Seed	*epi*-Progoitrin	(*S*)-2-Hydroxy-3-butenyl-	Major	34,42
		Sinigrin	Allyl-[b]	Minor	39
		Gluconapin	3-Butenyl-[b]	Minor	39
		Gluconasturtiin	2-Phenylethyl-[b]	Minor	39

[a] For the most part, authors who first identified the glucosinolate in the plant material are cited. More details including differences in glucosinolate with variety of *Brassica* are given for the vegetative parts[68] and for the seed.[47]

[b] The glucosinolate is the source of a volatile mustard oil. For example, allylglucosinolate gives allyl isothiocyanate, a typical pungent compound.

R group has an appropriately located hydroxyl substituent. These cyclic products are called goitrins because of their potent goitrogenic activity. Progoitrin from rapeseed (*Brassica napus* or *Brassica campestris*) and *epi*-progoitrin from crambe (*Crambe abyssinica*)* seed are the names given to the precursors, which differ only in stereochemistry at the carbon atom marked with an asterisk. By the glucosinolate method of naming, progoitrin is (*R*)-2-hydroxy-3-butenylglucosinolate, and *epi*-progoitrin is the corresponding (*S*)-compound, where (*R*) and (*S*) designate the stereochemistry at the 2-position by the sequence rule.[20] The nature of this rule is such that compounds in the same stereochemical series may have opposite (*R*)- and (*S*)-designations. Thus progoitrin gives rise to (*S*)-goitrin [(*S*)-5-vinyloxazolidine-2-thione], and *epi*-progoitrin forms (*R*)-goitrin [(*R*)-5-vinyloxazolidine-2-thione].

Depending on conditions during the enzymatic reaction and on the prior treatment of the plant material, an unsaturated nitrile (cyano compound) and two diastereomeric epithio nitriles may be formed instead of (*S*)- or (*R*)-goitrin from either progoitrin or *epi*-progoitrin as shown in Reaction 2. The progoitrins and each of the hydrolysis products have been isolated and characterized.[6,21,34-37] Treatment with ferrous iron, which has been proposed as a means of detoxifying rapeseed meal,[146] causes nonenzymatic degradation of the progoitrins to the unsaturated nitriles and 3-hydroxypent-4-enethionamides.[7,8] Besides the goitrins, other 4- or 5-substituted oxazolidine-2-thiones formed in cruciferous plant material have been isolated and characterized, and their parent glucosinolates have been identified.[44]

Glucobrassicin,[52] 3-indolylmethylglucosinolate, starting material in Reaction 3 (*X* = H), and neoglucobrassicin,[53] 3-(*N*-methoxyindolyl)-methylglucosinolate, starting material in Reaction 3 (*X* = OCH_3), were isolated from cabbage leaves and from rutabaga root. These two glucosinolates form the corresponding nitriles at pH 3 to 4 and presumably the unstable isothiocyanates at pH 3 to 7. The isothiocyanates are believed to be the intermediates that further degrade to thiocyanate ion and 3-hydroxymethylindoles. The indoles may react with ascorbic acid to form a compound called ascorbigen, which is reported to have vitamin C activity.[76,90]

Glucosinolates in Foods, Condiments, and Feeds

Identified glucosinolates from domesticated crucifers are listed in Table 1. Each glucosinolate in a given plant is found in all of the plant parts

---

*Crambe is a potential new oilseed crop in the United States. It is referred to frequently in this chapter because some of the most definitive chemical studies on sulfur-containing glucosides of Cruciferae have been carried out on this species.

Reaction 3

that have been examined except glucobrassicin and neoglucobrassicin, which have not been found in the seed. In general, the glucosinolate concentration is higher in the seed than in other parts of the plant. Because of this fact and the economic importance of some species as oilseeds, the glucosinolate content of *Brassica* seed in particular has been determined more accurately than has that of edible parts of the same plants. Estimates on nondefatted turnip seed from 19 varieties ranged from 0.7 to 2.0 % 3-butenylglucosinolate and 0.0 to 0.1% (R)-2-hydroxy-3-butenylglucosinolate (progoitrin). Nondefatted white cabbage seed from 19 varieties ranged from 0.1 to 2.6% allylglucosinolate (sinigrin) and 0.0 to 0.7% (R)-2-hydroxy-3-butenylglucosinolate.[47] In comparison, fresh edible cabbage contains about 350 ppm allylglucosinolate,[87] traces of three additional mustard oil-forming glucosinolates,[31] at least 0.5 ppm progoitrin,[1] and from 60 to 800 ppm 3-indolylmethylglucosinolate (glucobrassicin).[94] These data show that the edible part of cabbage, used as a food for centuries with no apparent harm, is quite low in glucosinolate content.

A recently developed method for p-hydroxybenzylglucosinolate[69] showed defatted white mustard seed meal to contain from 8.5 to 10.1% of the compound. This range of values was obtained from five varieties of the condiment mustard grown in different localities over several years.[70]

The glucosinolates as sources of toxic compounds from rape and crambe seeds have been examined in some detail because the by-product meals from these oilseed crops will have more value in animal feeds if the harmful compounds can be removed or inactivated. Amino acid contents indicate a high nutritional quality for the protein in meals from cruciferous oilseeds,[99] and feeding studies have confirmed this for crambe.[134] Preliminary work has been done on the preparation and testing of protein isolates from rapeseed for use. in foods.[3,19,41]

Since protein concentrates and isolates from rapeseed and seeds of related plants may in the future find their way into the food chain, the nature of glucosinolate breakdown products, as revealed by animal studies, merits discussion. Earlier indications that more than one toxic substance can be produced[15,64,74,124] have been substantiated by studies on crambe seed meal.[131,133,134] Experimental conditions were developed for causing glucosinolate hydrolysis to occur in order to give either nitriles or goitrin (Reaction 2). The nitrile mixture has eight times the acute toxicity of goitrin toward mice[131] and causes pathological liver and kidney lesions but not thyroid effects in rats.[134] Goitrin caused mild hyperplastic goiter, with slight reduction in weight gain and mild liver enlargement without pathology in rats. The mode of glucosinolate degradation was in part dependent on whether endogenous enzymes present were destroyed before feeding. The experiments cited show results obtained in extreme cases designed to reveal toxic effects. The experimental materials contained high (8–10%) concentrations of glucosinolate and were fed as major (10%) constituents of the rat diet for 90 days. *No analogous results have been reported or are implied for crucifers eaten as human food under usually encountered circumstances.*

Variables that favor formation of goitrin by thioglucosidase hydrolysis in the seed or seed meal include: dry-heat treatment or long storage of the seed under ambient conditions before enzyme hydrolysis; hydrolysis at high pH; high temperature; and low concentration of the seed meal in the aqueous hydrolysis medium. Nitrile formation is favored by autolysis of the seed meal from untreated, recently harvested seed, wetted to a paste at ambient temperature. More detailed studies on thioglucosidase hydrolysis in crambe meal are given in a recent report.[125] Variables affect the nature of the hydrolysis products from the progoitrins in crambe and in rape leaves in a similar manner.[130]

The total glucosinolate content of a natural product that has not been subjected to thioglucosidase hydrolysis may be estimated by measurement of the glucose or the sulfate ion released after adding a source of thioglucosidase. Such methods have been utilized.[93,110,132] However, they do not measure the products released from the organic aglucon of the glucosinolate by the hydrolysis. These products from the aglucon are deleterious and may vary depending on the specific glucosinolate, the prior treatment of the material, and the conditions of hydrolysis. Consequently, analyses for each specific product are often required. On the other hand, attempts to quantitatively determine glucosinolates through measurement of products from the organic aglucon moieties can also give misleading results. In early methods of analyses for progoitrin by conversion to goitrin and measurement of the latter by its ultraviolet absorption, the hydrolysis of the glucosinolate was carried out without control of the pH or at pH 4. Under these conditions analytical results were often low because the progoitrin was not exclusively and quantitatively hydrolyzed to goitrin. By dry heating the seed or seed meal before analysis and by carrying out the thioglucosidase hydrolysis at pH 7, more accurate and higher values have been obtained.[2,129,132] Defatted seed meal from commercial varieties of winter-type rapeseed (*B. napus*) contained 0.8–2.0% (average 1.7%) of glucosinolates that give volatile mustard oils and 2.6–5.5% (average 4.5%) progoitrin. The same method applied to *B. campestris* (winter-type rapeseed) gave 2.8–3.2% (average 3.0%) mustard oil-forming glucosinolates and 0.14–0.65% (average 0.35%) progoitrin.[2] The variability among species and varieties suggests that glucosinolate content may be lowered or removed by the plant geneticist.[40] A summer-type variety of *B. napus* called Bronowski has been found that contains less than 1% total glucosinolate in the defatted seed meal.[71]

Recent gas–liquid chromatographic methods include those for the analyses of the individual mustard oils[147] and for goitrin and each of the organic nitriles from progoitrins.[38] These methods permit complete analysis for all the volatile mustard oils and for all the known thioglucosidase hydrolysis products from the progoitrin aglucon.

Goitrogenic Properties of the Cruciferae

Of the widespread prevalence of human goiter, only about 4% may be due to causes other than that of iodine deficiency.[59] In a detailed study of the etiology of endemic goiter, Roche and Lissitzky[107] state that the cause may often be interactions of factors that vary from case to case. In some areas of the world, cruciferous plants as a part of the diet could be one of the contributing factors. Goiter has been attributed to the consumption of large amounts of cabbage[75] or of kale that was shown to be high in thiocyanate, isothiocyanate, and goitrin.[96]

Experimental goiter due to cruciferous plants was first produced in 1928 by feeding rabbits a ration of high cabbage content,[28] but the experiment could not always be repeated in other laboratories. Later, enlarged thyroids were more consistently obtained in experimental animals when the seed of cabbage or other *Brassica* species was fed.[63] However, with the feeding of the seed, variable poor growth and pathology in body organs other than the thyroid were also observed. From this experimental work it seems plausible that consumption of large amounts of cabbage or related vegetables might cause goiter. In particular, consumption of these vegetables might contribute to the relatively high incidence of the disease in areas of the world where the iodine content of the diet is low.

A brief review of the testing methods for antithyroid activity is necessary in order to more critically evaluate recent pertinent experimental work. Goitrogenic activity was first detected by visual inspection and weight of the thyroid after feeding the test material to experimental animals. Histological examination of the glands gave additional information as to the nature of the agents or the conditions that cause enlargement. Other criteria are growth rate of the test animal, basal metabolism tests, and assays for iodine content of the thyroid and blood. A test developed more recently consists of measuring the reduced radioactive iodine uptake of the thyroid following the feeding of the material under investigation.[118] This procedure has been used with rats,[5] chicks,[126] and humans.[118] Since antithyroid response varies with the species, the test should be used with humans for a more accurate evaluation of a substance for use in food. Advantages of the test are speed and sensitivity. A disadvantage is that the test gives no information on the antithyroid effect of feeding natural products containing goitrogens at low levels over long periods of time. This aspect of the problem requires extended feeding of the test material (usually in a ration of known iodine content) and then examination of the thyroids.[103]

Thiocyanate ion, a product from the enzymatic hydrolysis of the indolylglucosinolates (Reaction 3) and of *p*-hydroxybenzylglucosinolate, causes enlarged thyroids. This fact was first discovered in patients fed the thiocyanate ion to reduce hypertension.[11] Goitrogenic action was attributed to inhibition by the thiocyanate ion of iodine uptake by the thyroid.[127] For this reason the antithyroid effect is most likely to occur when the iodine content of the diet is low.[4] However, based on recent *in vitro* and *in vivo* experiments, higher levels of the thiocyanate ion also inhibit formation of thyroxine and related compounds, even when the iodine supply is not marginal.[62] Analysis of the edible part of fresh cabbage showed thiocyanate ion concentrations ranging from 0.7 to 10.2

mg/100 g.[94] Concentrations were highest in the spring; they varied little with the region where grown, but varied from plant to plant within a field.[95] Ingestion of cabbage by animals or by man caused a rise in thiocyanate ion concentration in the blood and its appearance in the urine.[85] Single feedings of the cabbage to guinea pigs and to rats on a low-iodine ration caused reduced iodine uptake by the thyroid to a greater extent than expected due to the known amount of thiocyanate ion in the plant material.[82,86] A mixture of thiocyanate ion, allyl isothiocyanate, and goitrin was fed to rats on a low-iodine ration at levels equivalent to those in cabbage fed *ad libitum*. Increase in weight and depression of iodine uptake by the thyroid and less synthesis of iodoamino acids occurred about as would be expected to result from the cabbage ration.[84]

It appears that allyl isothiocyanate acts as a goitrogen, because the compound is metabolized to give the thiocyanate ion as one of the products. Doses of 2–4 mg of allyl isothiocyanate mixed with water and fed by stomach tube to rats caused a marked increase in thiocyanate ion in the blood plasma and a decrease in radioactive iodine uptake by the thyroid.[83] This dosage is equivalent to the amount of the compound each rat would get in eating 40 g of cabbage per day. Treating the rats in this manner for 60 days gave histological changes in the thyroid indicative of goiter.[87] The mustard oil cheiroline (3-methylsulfonylpropyl isothiocyanate) when injected into rats also inhibits radioactive iodine uptake by the thyroid.[9] This compound is found in a pasture weed, *Rapistrum rugosum*, that grows in Australia. Since mustard oils are irritating and act as vesicants, they are not likely to be eaten per se, even as a condiment, in large enough amounts to cause malfunction of the thyroid. However, if they were consumed as the glucosinolate over long periods of time and slowly released by the accompanying thioglucosidase or a similar enzyme in the intestinal tract, it is conceivable that they might act as goitrogens through conversion to the thiocyanate ion.

There are reports that daily doses of organic nitriles fed to rabbits caused enlargement of the thyroids that was prevented by increasing the iodine content of the ration.[55] It was observed that most of the nitriles ingested were converted to thiocyanate ion during metabolism by the experimental animals. However, the goitrogenic effect of feeding nitriles could not consistently be repeated by other investigators.[55,134]

A polysulfide fraction and "trithiones" (1,2-dithiocyclopent-4-en-3-thiones) isolated from cabbage juice brought about histological changes in the thyroid of rats similar to those caused by feeding excessive amounts of cabbage.[67] Gas chromatographic and mass spectrometric analyses of volatiles from raw cabbage showed, in addition to thiocyanates, small amounts of tentatively identified mono-, di-, and trisulfides of low molecular weight.[10] The methyl mono-, di-, and trisulfides were the major volatile components from cooked cabbage.[89] Large amounts of methyl-, *n*-propyl-, and allyl disulfides have been reported to have antithyroid activity.[33]

The workers who isolated goitrin (*S*-5-vinyloxazolidine-2-thione) from rapeseed demonstrated that the compound had thyroid-inhibiting activity.[6] The (*R*) isomer of goitrin, which is derived from the major crambe glucosinolate, has equal antithyroid activity.[59] When fed to rats, the goitrins cause slightly less hyperplasia of the thyroid than thiourea (a well-known thyroid-inhibiting drug).[22] The goitrins have 2% and 133% of the goitrogenic activity of the antithyroid drug propylthiouracil as measured by the radioactive iodine method with rats and with man, respectively.[59] After goitrin from crambe was fed to rats as 0.23% of the ration for 90 days, body weights of the animals were 85% of those of the controls, and the thyroids were enlarged with lesions typical of mild hyperplastic goiter.[134] When racemic goitrin was fed to chicks as 0.15% of the ration, growth depression and hyperplasia and hypertrophy of the thyroid gland were observed. During the initial feeding, radioiodine uptake of the thyroid was decreased, and the release of iodine by the gland into the bloodstream was increased.[30] After the goitrin was fed over 3 or 4 weeks, these two measurements returned to normal levels, possibly because the thyroid after enlargement could function normally.

Of the antithyroid agents found in the Cruciferae, the goitrins are the most active. They act presumably by inhibiting the incorporation of iodine into organic compounds to form thyroxin and related compounds; they are not counteracted by larger amounts of iodine in the diet as is the case with thiocyanate ion.[61] Of the many foods from plants and animals that were tested by the radioactive iodine uptake method, turnip and rutabaga consistently gave positive results, with rutabaga about twice as active as turnip.[59] A maximum of 0.13 ppm goitrin can be formed from the 0.5 ppm of progoitrin estimated to be in cabbage.[1] This amount of goitrin is probably negligible in practical nutrition. In contrast, some defatted crucifer seed meals contain progoitrin equivalent to 2.7% goitrin.

Feeding Intact Glucosinolates in the Absence of Thioglucosidase

It was first thought that if foods from the Cruciferae were cooked in such a manner that the thioglucosidase enzyme was inactivated without hydrolysis of the glucosinolates, the goitrogenic properties would be lost.[57] After isolation of pure progoitrin[56] the compound was tested for goitrogenic activity without the accompanying enzyme. By feeding the compound to rats and to man and testing for radioiodine uptake of the thyroid, the progoitrin was found to be active.[60] Goitrin appeared in the blood serum and in the urine. Incubation of progoitrin with rat or human feces gave goitrin as a hydrolysis product. Goitrin formation was prevented by boiling, ultrasonic treatment, or Seitz filtration of the feces. Antibiotics fed with the progoitrin caused a marked decrease in the formation of goitrin. A number of isolated bacteria, including *Paracolobactrum*, commonly found in the mammalian intestinal tract produce thioglucosidase[102] as does the fungus *Aspergillus sydowii* QM 31c.[106] Hydrolysis by the microflora of the intestine as tested was much slower than by the plant thioglucosidase.

Glucosinolate-Derived Substances in Milk

Following the introduction of marrow-stem kale (a crucifer plant) as pasture and hay for dairy cattle in Tasmania, it was reported[32] from a statistical survey that children from the area who consumed the milk developed enlarged thyroids. The suspected milk also caused inhibited thyroid uptake of radioactive iodine following ingestion of test samples. The investigators did not isolate the goitrogens from the milk. They made the hypothesis that antithyroid compounds were being transmitted into the milk in large enough quantity to cause harm. There are reports that animals may develop enlarged thyroids when fed large amounts of cruciferous plants or when grazed on pastures contaminated with cruciferous weeds.[9,104,145] However, surveys made in England[54] and in Holland[128] in areas where crucifer forages are used for dairy cattle gave no indications that the cow's milk was goitrogenic.

As a result of the observations made in Tasmania, experimental work was carried out in Finland to ascertain if goitrogens accumulated in milk when the dairy cow was fed known amounts of crucifer forage or goitrogens known to be in the forage. After a single feeding of progoitrin, goitrin, or rapeseed containing progoitrin equal to that found in a daily full feed of kale or rape forage, only about 0.05% of the ingested goitrin was found in the milk at a maximum concentration of 100 μg/liter.[137]

A positive radioactive iodine test for thyroid inhibition in man requires 20 mg of goitrin. The milk from cows fed 30 kg of marrow-stem kale per day contained 5–8 mg thiocyanate ion per liter compared with milk from cows fed no crucifer plants, which contained 2 mg per liter. By feeding thiocyanate ion equal to that in the 30 kg of marrow-stem kale, a level of 18 mg of thiocyanate ion per liter of milk was achieved.[105] A dose of 200–1,000 mg of thiocyanate ion is required to give a positive radioactive iodine test. These experimental results argue that the goitrogens cannot be transferred to the milk in large enough amounts to cause harm. However, later another Finnish investigator reported that feeding of 0.0, 0.1, 0.5, 1.0, and 2.0 µg of goitrin per day to rats for long periods of time caused larger thyroids as the dose of goitrin was increased. The feeding of milk that contained 50–100 µg goitrin per liter to the rats over long periods of time also caused enlarged thyroids.[103] Thus, while the answer to the question "Can endemic goiter in humans be caused by the ingestion of milk from cows eating cruciferous plants?" appears to be negative for practical purposes, it is not unequivocally so.

In the course of some of this work[105] it was observed that with large amounts of thiocyanate ion in the ration, the iodine content of the cow's milk was lowered markedly but increased to normal levels when thiocyanate feeding was stopped. This observation has been made by other investigators.[50, 98] Possibly, ingestion of thiocyanate ion by a lactating mammal could cause goiter in her young or in those consuming her milk because of its low iodine content.

Although not considered toxic as consumed by the dairy cow, land cress (*Coronopus didymus*) contains benzylglucosinolate, which is the source of off-flavors in milk that increased during pasteurization. This problem is the subject of a recent review.[142]

Safety of Edible Products from Glucosinolate-Containing Plants

Little information is available on the effect of simple processing of the vegetable *Brassicas*, such as the shredding of cabbage to make slaw, or fermenting to make kraut. Similarly, the maximum amount of condiment seed (i.e., white mustard, table mustard, or horseradish) that may be consumed without harm is not known. In view of the diversity of products from glucosinolates and the chemically active nature of many of these products, it is difficult to evaluate specifically harm that might occur from consumption of these plants under all conceivable circumstances. However, their use as vegetables and condiments as currently practiced causes no known harm and adds nutritional value and variety to the diet.

COMPOUNDS FROM ONION, GARLIC, AND CHIVE

Volatile Oils from Allium Species

Throughout the history of man, species from the *Allium* genus of the Liliaceae have been used as vegetables, spices, and folk medicines for the cure of various diseases. Of the greatest practical interest are onions (*A.*

cepa L.), garlic (*A. sativum* L.), and chive (*A. schoenoprasum* L.). The volatile compounds from these plants, most of which contain sulfur, appear to be the sources of the flavor, odor, lachrymatory, and antibiotic properties attributed to them. These compounds are the products of enzyme action on precursor substrates stored in the intact plant.

The precursors are *S*-substituted cysteine sulfoxides or peptides containing them,[114] of which (+)-*S*-allyl-L-cysteine sulfoxide (alliin)[119] is the major one in garlic, present at about 2.4 mg/g.[121] Products formed from alliin are given in Reaction 4. Allicin (allylthiosulfinate) is a labile compound that has the odor of fresh garlic; it also has antibiotic activity.[26] Compounds have been isolated from onions that are analogous to alliin but have the allyl group (*R* in the starting material in Reaction 4) replaced, respectively, with methyl, propyl, and *trans*-1-propenyl radicals.[24,25,116,140] The (+)-*S*-methyl-L-cysteine sulfoxide has been isolated from other plants, including turnip root, cabbage, kohlrabi, together with mustard leaves, cauliflower flowers, and broccoli stems of the crucifer family.[101,122] All three substituted cysteine sulfoxides form the labile thiosulfinates by action of alliinase.[92] The thiosulfinates slowly decompose by disproportionation to give thiosulfonates and disulfides. The disulfides are volatile and are responsible for part of the characteristic odor of the crushed plants that contain them. The thiosulfinates have antibiotic activity.[115] A series of mono-, di-, and trisulfides with methyl, propyl, isopropyl, 1-propenyl, and allyl groups, combinations of two of these, dimethylthiophenes, hydrogen sulfide, and methyl-, propyl-, and allyl-thiols has been found in fresh onion, dehydrated onion, distilled onion oil,[13,14,16,17] and garlic.[65] It seems likely that these sulfides are derived from substituted cysteine sulfoxides.

$$
\begin{array}{c}
\underset{\text{Alliin}}{\underset{\displaystyle \text{COOH}}{\underset{\displaystyle |}{\underset{\displaystyle \text{CHNH}_2}{\underset{\displaystyle |}{2\ \underset{\displaystyle |}{\text{CH}_2}+\text{H}_2\text{O}}}}}}
\quad\xrightarrow{\text{Alliinase}}\quad
\underset{\substack{\text{2-Propenyl-2-}\\\text{propenethiolsulfinate}\\\text{(Allicin)}}}{\underset{\displaystyle R}{\underset{\displaystyle |}{\underset{\displaystyle S}{\underset{\displaystyle |}{S\to O}}}}}
\ +\ 2\ \text{CH}_3\overset{\displaystyle O}{\overset{\displaystyle ||}{\text{C}}}\text{COOH}\ +\ 2\,\text{NH}_3
$$

$$\downarrow$$

$$\text{R—S—S—R} + \text{R—[SO}_2\text{]—S—R}$$

Allyl Disulfide   Allyl Thiosulfonate

$$R = CH_2{=}CH{-}CH_2{-}$$

Reaction 4

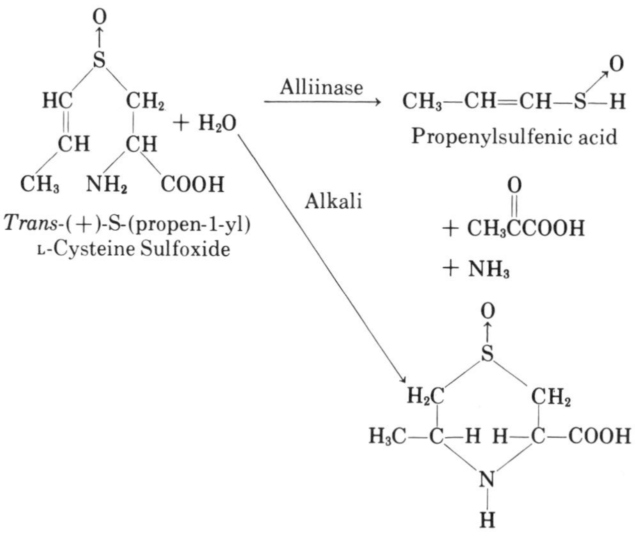

Reaction 5   Cycloalliin

The major cysteine sulfoxide in onion is *trans*-(+)-*S*-(propen-1-yl)-L-cysteine sulfoxide[24,116] (Reaction 5), present at about 2 mg/g fresh weight.[91] Alliinase hydrolysis gives the very labile propenylsulfenic acid with the structure shown, which is based on mass spectrometry of the compound within 1 min after it was formed.[100] This compound or a closely related substance appears to be the major lachrymator from onion.* The decomposition products from the lachrymator have not been clearly established. When the precursor cysteine sulfoxide is treated with alkali, the compound cycloalliin is obtained.[139] Cycloalliin is inert to enzymes in the onion and apparently makes no contribution to onion flavor. From gas-chromatographic and mass-spectrometric studies, volatiles from chives contain methyl propyl disulfide, propyl disulfide, and propenyl propyl disulfide (*cis* and *trans*), but there is no evidence for propenyl or allyl disulfide.[141]

Evidence for Goitrogenic Properties of Allium *Species*

There is little evidence that the sulfur-containing compounds in the *Allium* species are harmful as consumed in edible products. It has been suggested, however, that the known high occurrence of endemic goiter

---

*After this manuscript was completed, the labile lachrymatory factor from onion was shown to be thiopropanal *S*-oxide, the structure of which ($CH_3CH_2CH=S=O$) was confirmed by synthesis.[18]

in the valleys of mountainous areas of Lebanon may be due in part to the large amount of onions in the diet.[109] By the radioactive iodine method, with rats as the test animal, methyl-, *n*-propyl-, and allyl disulfides; allyl sulfide; and allyl alcohol were assayed for antithyroid activity. The disulfides depressed radioiodine uptake by the thyroid when the rats were fed a high level (30–60 μl) of the compounds. The allyl sulfide had little effect. The allyl alcohol was toxic at levels above 25 μl per rat.[33] These results do not imply that any of the vegetables and spices that contain these compounds at relatively low levels are harmful when used in a conventional manner; indeed, there are no direct observations in support of harm occurring in the use of these vegetables and spices. However, it is believed that due consideration should be given to the chemistry and biological effect of these compounds when new ways of processing food materials containing them are developed, especially if the processing could conceivably involve fractionation and concentration of the natural sulfur compounds or deleterious products derived from them.

COMPOUNDS FROM SOURCES OTHER THAN THE CRUCIFERAE AND *ALLIUM*

The antithyroid action of cyanide from cyanogenic glycosides due to cyanide detoxification by conversion to the thiocyanate ion is covered in Chapter 14, p. 303. The sulfur-containing peptides from mushrooms that are toxic are described in Chapter 5, p. 120, the toxic amino acid djenkolic acid in Chapter 21, p. 466.

By a careful restudy, reported in 1949, of the antithyroid activity claimed for ergothionine, it was shown that there is no significant antithyroid activity of the compound in the rat, monkey, or man.[144] No later reports were found in the literature that disagree with this conclusion.

NOTE

According to a report that appeared after completion of this chapter [C.-S. Tang, *Phytochemistry 12*:769 (1973)], the dried latex from the green, immature fruit of papaya (*Carica papaya,* Caricaceae) contains 73 to 116 mg potassium benzylglucosinolate per gram of dried material. The ground dried latex from the unripe papaya is the source of papain, a proteolytic enzyme with important food and medicinal uses. However, no reports have been found that the crude enzyme preparations from this source are harmful.

REFERENCES

1. M. R. Altamura, L. Long, Jr., and T. Hasselstrom, Goitrin from fresh cabbage. J. Biol. Chem. *234*:1847 (1959).
2. L. A. Appelqvist and E. Josefsson, Method for quantitative determination of *iso*thiocyanates and oxazolidinethiones in digests of seed meals of rape and turnip rape. J. Sci. Food Agric. *18*:510 (1967).
3. M. M. Aref, Development of protein concentrates and isolates from rapeseed. International Conference on the Science, Technology and Marketings of Rapeseed and Rapeseed Products. Session 6. Agriculture Fisheries and Food Products Branch, Department of Industry, Trade, and Commerce, Ottawa, Canada (1970). (Abstr.)
4. E. B. Astwood, The chemical nature of compounds which inhibit the function of the thyroid gland. J. Pharmacol. Exp. Ther. *78*:79 (1943).
5. F. B. Astwood, A. Bissell, and A. M. Hughes, Further studies on the nature of compounds which inhibit the function of the thyroid gland. Endocrinology *37*:456 (1945).
6. E. B. Astwood, M. A. Greer, and M. G. Ettlinger, L-5-Vinyl-2-thiooxazolidone, an antithyroid compound from yellow turnip and from *Brassica* seeds. J. Biol. Chem. *181*:121 (1949).
7. F. L. Austin, C. A. Gent, and I. A. Wolff, Degradation of natural thioglucosides with ferrous salts. J. Agric. Food Chem. *16*:752 (1968).
8. F. L. Austin, C. A. Gent, and I. A. Wolff, Enantiomeric 3-hydroxypent-4-enethionamides from thioglucosides of crambe and brassica seeds by action of ferrous salts. Can. J. Chem. *46*:1507 (1968).
9. H. S. Bachelard, M. T. McQuillan, and V. M. Trikojus, Studies on endemic goiter. III. An investigation of the antithyroid activities of isothiocyanates and derivatives with observations on fractions of milk from goitrous areas. Aust. J. Biol. Sci. *16*:177 (1963).
10. S. D. Bailey, M. L. Bazinet, J. L. Driscoll, and A. I. McCarthy, The volatile sulfur components of cabbage. J. Food Sci. *26*:163 (1961).
11. M. H. Barker, The blood cyanates in the treatment of hypertension. J. Am. Med. Assoc. *106*:762 (1936).
12. J. M. Bell, The nutritional value of rapeseed oil meal, a review. Can. J. Agric. Sci. *35*:242 (1955).
13. R. A. Bernhard, Comparative distribution of volatile disulfides derived from fresh and dehydrated onions. J. Food Sci. *33*:298 (1968).
14. M. Boelens, P. J. de Valois, H. J. Wobben, and A. van der Gen, Volatile flavor compounds from onion. J. Agric. Food Chem. *19*:984 (1971).
15. J. P. Bowland, D. R. Clandinin, and L. R. Wetter (eds.), Rapeseed meal for livestock and poultry—A review. Publ. 1257. The Canada Department of Agriculture, Ottawa (1965).
16. M. H. Brodnitz and C. L. Pollock, Gas chromatographic analysis of distilled onion oil. Food Technol. *24*:78 (1970).
17. M. H. Brodnitz, C. L. Pollock, and P. P. Vallon, Flavor components of onion oil. J. Agric. Food Chem. *17*:760 (1969).
18. M. H. Brodnitz and J. V. Pascale, Thiopropanol *S*-oxide: A lachrymatory factor in onions. J. Agric. Food Chem. *19*:269 (1971).

19. J. M. Butt, O. Yunus, and F. H. Shah, Preparation of bland protein meal from mustard seed cake. Pak. J. Sci. Ind. Res. 9:130 (1966).

20. R. S. Cahn, An introduction to the sequence rule, a system for the specification of absolute configuration. J. Chem. Educ. 41:116 (1964).

21. K. D. Carlson, D. Weisleder, and M. E. Daxenbichler, Intramolecular hydrogen bonding, an infrared and nuclear magnetic resonance study of diasteriomeric episulfides. J. Am. Chem. Soc. 92:6232 (1970).

22. K. K. Carroll, Isolation of an anti-thyroid compound from rapeseed (Brassica napus). Proc. Soc. Exp. Biol. Med. 71:622 (1949).

23. J. F. Carson, Onion flavor, p. 390. In Chemistry and physiology of flavors, H. W. Schultz, E. A. Day, and L. M. Libbey (eds.). Avi, Westport, Conn. (1967).

24. J. F. Carson, R. E. Lundin, and T. M. Lukes, The configuration of (+)-S-(1 propenyl)-L-cysteine S-oxide from Allium cepa. J. Org. Chem. 31:1634 (1966).

25. J. F. Carson and F. F. Wong, Isolation of (+)-S-methyl-L-cysteine sulfoxide and of (+)-S-n-propyl-L-cysteine sulfoxide from onions as their N-2,4-dinitrophenyl derivatives. J. Org. Chem. 26:4997 (1961).

26. C. J. Cavallito and J. H. Bailey, Allicin—The antibacterial principal of Allium sativum. I. Isolation, physical properties and antibacterial action. J. Am. Chem. Soc. 66:1950 (1944).

27. F. Challenger, The natural mustard oil glucosides and the related isothiocyanates and nitriles, p. 115. In Aspects of the organic chemistry of sulfur, Butterworth's Scientific Publications, London (1959).

28. A. M. Chesney, T. A. Clawson, and B. Webster, Endemic goitre in rabbits. I. Incidence and characteristics. Bull. Johns Hopkins Hosp. 43:261 (1928).

29. B. C. Christian, Rapeseed, mustard-seed, and poppy-seed meals, p. 577. In Processed plant protein foodstuffs, A. M. Altschul (ed.). Academic Press, New York (1958).

30. D. R. Clandinin, L. Bayly, and A. Caballero, Rapeseed meal studies. 5. Effects of (+)-5-vinyl-2-oxazolidinethione, a goitrogen in rapeseed meal, on the rate of growth and thyroid function of chicks. Poult. Sci. 45:833 (1966).

31. R. C. Clapp, L. Long, G. P. Dateo, F. H. Bissett, and T. Hasselstrom, The volatile isothiocyanates in fresh cabbage. J. Am. Chem. Soc. 81:6278 (1959).

32. F. W. Clements and J. W. Wishart, A thyroid-blocking agent in the etiology of endemic goiter. Metabol. Clin. Exp. 5:623 (1956).

33. J. W. Cowan, A. R. Saghir, and J. P. Salji, Antithyroid activity of onion volatiles. Aust. J. Biol. Sci. 20:683 (1967).

34. M. E. Daxenbichler, C. H. VanEtten, and I. A. Wolff, A new thioglucoside, (R)-2-hydroxy-3-butenylglucosinolate from Crambe abyssinica seed. Biochemistry 4:318 (1965).

35. M. E. Daxenbichler, C. H. VanEtten, and I. A. Wolff, (S)- and (R)-1-Cyano-2-hydroxy-3-butene from myrosinase hydrolysis of epi-progoitrin and progoitrin. Biochemistry 5:692 (1966).

36. M. E. Daxenbichler, C. H. VanEtten, W. H. Tallent, and I. A. Wolff, Rapeseed meal autolysis. Formation of diastereomeric (2R)-1-cyano-2-hydroxy-3,4-epithiobutanes from progoitrin. Can. J. Chem. 45:1971 (1967).

37. M. E. Daxenbichler, C. H. VanEtten, and I. A. Wolff, Diastereomeric episulfides from epi-progoitrin upon autolysis of crambe seed meal. Phytochemistry 7:989 (1968).

38. M. E. Daxenbichler, G. F. Spencer, R. Kleiman, C. H. VanEtten, and I. A. Wolff, Gas-liquid chromatographic determination of products from the progoitrins in crambe and rapeseed meals. Anal. Biochem. *38*:373 (1970).

39. M. E. Daxenbichler, C. H. VanEtten, F. S. Brown, and Q. Jones, Oxazolidinethiones and volatile isothiocyanates in enzyme-treated seed meals from 65 species of Cruciferae. J. Agric. Food Chem. *12*:127 (1964).

40. R. K. Downey, B. M. Craig, and C. G. Youngs, Breeding rapeseed for oil and meal quality. J. Am. Oil Chem. Soc. *46*:121 (1969).

41. K. E. Eapen, N. W. Tape, and R. P. A. Sims, New process for the production of better-quality rapeseed oil and meal. II. Detoxification and dehulling of rapeseeds—Feasibility study. J. Am. Oil Chem. Soc. *46*:252 (1969).

42. F. R. Earle, J. E. Peters, I. A. Wolff, and G. A. White, Compositional differences among crambe samples and between seed components. J. Am. Oil Chem. Soc. *43*:330 (1966).

43. M. G. Ettlinger and J. P. Dateo, Jr., Studies of mustard oil glucosides. Contract No. DA 19-129 QM-1059, Project No. 7-84-06-032, Simplified food logistics, final report, p. 1–96. Department of Chemistry, Rice Institute, Houston, Texas (1961).

44. M. G. Ettlinger and A. Kjaer, Sulfur compounds in plants, p. 59. In *Recent Advances in Phytochemistry*, Vol. 1, T. J. Mabry (ed.). Appleton-Century-Crofts, New York (1968).

45. M. G. Ettlinger and A. J. Lundeen, The structures of sinigrin and sinalbin: An enzymatic rearrangement. J. Am. Chem. Soc. *78*:4172 (1956).

46. M. G. Ettlinger and A. J. Lundeen, First synthesis of a mustard oil glucoside: The enzymatic Lossen rearrangement. J. Am. Chem. Soc. *79*:1764 (1957).

47. M. G. Ettlinger and C. P. Thompson, Studies of mustard oil glucosides (II). Contract No. DA 19-129-QM-1689, Project No. 7-99-01-001, Simplified food logistics, final report, p. 1–106. Department of Chemistry, Rice Institute, Houston, Texas (1962).

48. M. Florkin and E. H. Stotz, p. 142. In Comprehensive biochemistry, Vol. 13, M. Florkin and E. H. Stotz (eds.). Elsevier, New York (1965).

49. P. Friis and A. Kjaer, 4-Methylthio-3-butenyl isothiocyanate, the pungent principle of radish root. Acta Chem. Scand. *20*:698 (1966).

50. R. J. Garner, B. F. Sanson, and H. G. Jones, Fission products and the dairy cow. III. Transfer of I^{131} to milk following single and daily dosing. J. Agric. Sci. *55*:283 (1960).

51. R. Gmelin and A. I. Virtanen, A new type of enzymatic cleavage of mustard oil glucosides. Formation of allylthiocyanate in *Thlaspi arvense* L. and benzylthiocyanate in *Lepidium ruderale* L. and *Lepidium sativum* L. Acta Chem. Scand. *13*:1474 (1959).

52. R. Gmelin and A. I. Virtanen, Glucobrassicin the precursor of the thiocyanate ion, 3-indolylacetonitrile, and ascorbigen in *Brassica oleracea* (and related) species. Ann. Acad. Sci. Fenn. Ser. *A2*:1071 (1961).

53. R. Gmelin and A. I. Virtanen, Neoglucobrassicin a second thiocyanate ion precursor from an indolyl in *Brassica* species. Acta Chem. Scand. *16*:1378 (1962).

54. H. F. Greene and R. F. Glascock, Goitrogens in milk. J. Endocrinol. *17*:272 (1958).

55. M. A. Greer, Nutrition and goiter. Physiol. Rev. *30*:513 (1950).

56. M. A. Greer, Isolation from rutabaga seed of progoitrin, the precursor of the naturally occurring antithyroid compound, goitrin (L-5-vinyl-2-thiooxazolidone). J. Am. Chem. Soc. 78:1260 (1956).
57. M. A. Greer, Goitrogenic substances in food. Am. J. Clin. Nutr. 5:440 (1957).
58. M. A. Greer, The significance of naturally occurring antithyroid compounds in the production of goiter in man. Borden's Rev. Nutr. Res. 21:61 (1960).
59. M. A. Greer, The natural occurrence of goitrogenic agents. Recent Prog. Horm. Res. 18:187 (1962).
60. M. A. Greer and J. M. Deeney, Antithyroid activity elicited by the ingestion of pure progoitrin, a naturally occurring thioglucoside of the turnip family. J. Clin. Invest. 38:1465 (1959).
61. M. A. Greer, J. W. Kendall, and M. Smith, Antithyroid compounds, p. 357. In The thyroid gland, R. Pitt-Rivers and W. R. Trotter (eds.). Butterworths, Washington, D.C. (1964).
62. M. A. Greer, A. K. Stott, and K. A. Milne, Effect of thiocyanate, perchlorate and other anions on thyroidal iodine metabolism. Endocrinology 79:237 (1966).
63. C. E. Hercus and H. B. Purves, Studies on endemic goiter. J. Hyg. 36:182 (1936).
64. W. B. Holmes and R. Roberts, A perotic syndrome in chicks fed extracted rapeseed meal. Poult. Sci. 42:803 (1963).
65. J. V. Jacobsen, R. A. Bernhard, L. K. Mann, and L. K. Saghir, Infrared spectra of some asymmetric disulfides produced by Allium. Arch. Biochem. Biophys. 104:473 (1964).
66. K. A. Jensen, J. Conti, and A. Kjaer, isoThiocyanates II. Volatile isothiocyanates in seeds and roots of various Brassicae. Acta Chem. Scand. 7:1267 (1953).
67. L. Jirousek and L. Starka, Concerning the occurrence of trithiones (1,2-dithiocyclopenta-4-ene-3-thione) in Brassica plants. Naturwissenschaften 45:386 (1958).
68. E. Josefsson, Distribution of thioglucosides in different parts of Brassica plants. Phytochemistry 6:1617 (1967).
69. E. Josefsson, Method for quantitative determination of p-hydroxybenzyl isothiocyanate in digests of seed meal of Sinapis alba L. J. Sci. Food Agric. 19:192 (1968).
70. E. Josefsson, Content of p-hydroxybenzylglucosinolate in seed meals of Sinapis alba as affected by heredity, environment and seed part. J. Sci. Food Agric. 21:94 (1970).
71. E. Josefsson and L. A. Appelqvist, Glucosinolates in seed of rape and turnip rape as affected by variety and environment. J. Sci. Food Agric. 19:564 (1968).
72. S. Kawakishi and K. Muramatsu, Studies on the decomposition of sinalbin. Part I. The decomposition products of sinalbin. Agric. Biol. Chem. 30:688 (1966).
73. S. Kawakishi, M. Namiki, H. Watanabe, and K. Muramatsu, Studies on the decomposition of sinalbin. Part II. The decomposition products of sinalbin and their degradation pathways. Agric. Biol. Chem. 31:823 (1967).
74. T. H. Kennedy and H. D. Purves, Studies on experimental goitre. I. The effect of brassica seed diets on rats. Br. J. Exp. Pathol. 22:241 (1941).
75. F. C. Kelly and W. W. Snedden, Prevalence and geographical distribution of

endemic goitre, p. 91. In Endemic goitre, World Health Organ. Monog. Ser. No. 44. World Health Organization, Geneva (1960).

76. M. Kiesvaara and A. I. Virtanen, Synthetic ascorbigen as a source of vitamin C for guinea pigs II. Acta Chem. Scand. *17*:849 (1963).

77. A. Kjaer, Naturally derived *iso*thiocyanates (mustard oils) and their parent glucosides, p. 122. In The chemistry of organic natural products, L. Zechmeister (ed.). Springer-Verlag, Vienna (1960).

78. A. Kjaer, *iso*Thiocyanates of natural origin. Pure Appl. Chem. *7*:229 (1963).

79. A. Kjaer and R. Boe Jensen, *iso*Thiocyanates XX. 4-Pentenyl *iso*thiocyanate, a new mustard oil occurring as a glucoside (glucobrassicanapin) in nature. Acta Chem. Scand. *10*:1365 (1956).

80. A. Kjaer and K. Rubinstein, *iso*Thiocyanates VIII. Synthesis of *p*-hydroxybenzyl *iso*thiocyanate and demonstration of its presence in the glucoside of white mustard (*Sinapis alba* L.). Acta Chem. Scand. *8*:598 (1954).

81. A. Kjaer, J. Conti, and K. A. Jensen, *iso*Thiocyanates III. The volatile *iso*thiocyanates in seeds of rape (*Brassica napus* L.). Acta Chem. Scand. *7*:1271 (1953).

82. P. Langer, Studies concerning the relation between thiocyanate formation and goitrogenic effects of foods. IV. Concerning the relation between the thiocyanate content of different plant foods and their inhibiting influence on radioactive iodine uptake in the guinea pig thyroid. Hoppe-Seyler's Z. Physiol. Chem. *323*:194 (1961).

83. P. Langer, Relations between thiocyanate formation, and goitrogenic effect of foods. VI. Thiocyanogenic activity of allylisothiocyanate, one of the most frequently occurring mustard oils in plants. Hoppe-Seyler's Z. Physiol. Chem. *339*:33 (1964).

84. P. Langer, Antithyroid action in rats of small doses of some naturally occurring compounds. Endocrinology *79*:1117 (1966).

85. P. Langer and N. Michajlovskij, The relation between thiocyanate formation and the goitrogenic effect of foods. II. The thiocyanate content of foods, the chief cause of thiocyanate excretion in urine of man and animals. Hoppe-Seyler's Z. Physiol. Chem. *312*:31 (1958).

86. P. Langer and V. Stolc, Relationship between thiocyanate formation and goitrogenic effect of foods. V. Comparison of the effect of white cabbage and thiocyanate on the rat thyroid gland. Hoppe-Seyler's Z. Physiol. Chem. *335*:216 (1964).

87. P. Langer and V. Stolc, Goitrogenic activity of allylisothiocyanate—A widespread natural mustard oil. Endocrinology *76*:151 (1965).

88. E. P. Lichtenstein, F. M. Strong, and D. G. Morgan, Naturally occurring insecticides, identification of 2-phenylethylisothiocyanate as an insecticide occurring naturally in the edible part of turnips. J. Agric. Food Chem. *10*:30 (1962).

89. A. J. Macleod and G. Macleod, Volatiles of cooked cabbage. J. Sci. Food Agric. *19*:273 (1968).

90. K. Matano and N. Kato, Studies on synthetic ascorbigen as a source of vitamin C for guinea pigs. Acta Chem. Scand. *21*:2886 (1967).

91. E. J. Matikkala and A. I. Virtanen, On the quantitative determination of the amino acids and γ-glutamylpeptides of onion. Acta Chem. Scand. *21*:2891 (1967).

92. M. Mazelis, Demonstration and characterization of cysteine sulfoxide lyase in the Cruciferae. Phytochemistry 2:15 (1963).

93. J. E. McGhee, L. D. Kirk, and G. C. Mustakas, Methods for determining thioglucosides in *Crambe abyssinica*. J. Am. Oil Chem. Soc. 42:889 (1965).

94. N. Michajlovskij and P. Langer, The relation between thiocyanate formation and the goitrogenic effects of foods. I. The preformed thiocyanate content of some foods. Hoppe-Seyler's Z. Physiol. Chem. 312:26 (1958).

95. N. Michajlovskij and P. Langer, The relation between thiocyanate formation and the goitrogenic effect of foods. III. The occurrence of preformed thiocyanate in some vegetables with regard to seasonal and regional differences. Hoppe-Seyler's Z. Physiol. Chem. 317:30 (1959).

96. N. Michajlovskij, J. Sedlak, M. Jusic, and R. Buzina, Goitrogenic substances of kale and their possible relations to the endemic goiter on the Island of Krk (Yugoslavia). Endocrinol. Exp. 3(2):65 (1969).

97. H. E. Miller, The aglucone of sinigrin. Thesis, Rice University, Houston, Texas. (1965).

98. J. K. Miller, E. W. Swanson, and R. G. Cragle, Effect of feeding thiocyanate to dairy cows on absorption and clearance of intramammary iodine. J. Dairy Sci. 48:1118 (1965).

99. R. W. Miller, C. H. VanEtten, C. McGrew, I. A. Wolff, and Q. Jones, Amino acid composition of seed meals from forty-one species of Cruciferae. J. Agric. Food Chem. 10:426 (1962).

100. T. Moisio, C. G. Spåre, and A. I. Virtanen, Mass spectral studies of the chemical nature of the lachrymatory factor formed enzymically from S-(1-propenyl)-cysteine sulfoxide isolated from onion (*Allium cepa*). Suom. Kemistilehti B 35:29 (1962).

101. C. J. Morris and J. F. Thompson, The identification of (+)-S-methyl-L-cysteine sulfoxide in plants. J. Am. Chem. Soc. 78:1605 (1956).

102. E. L. Oginsky, A. E. Stein, and M. A. Greer, Myrosinase activity in bacteria as demonstrated by the conversion of progoitrin to goitrin. Proc. Soc. Exp. Biol. Med. 119:360 (1965).

103. P. Peltola, The role of L-5-vinyl-2-thiooxazolidone in the genesis of endemic goiter in Finland, p. 872. In Current topics in thyroid research, C. Cassano and M. Andreoli (eds.). (1965).

104. P. Peltola and A. Vartiainen, Effect of the prophylactic use of iodine on the thyroid of cattle in the endemic goitre district of Finland. Ann. Med. Intern. Fenn. 43:209 (1954).

105. E. Piironen and A. I. Virtanen, The effect of thiocyanate in nutrition on the iodine content of cow's milk. Z. Ernaehrungswiss. 3:140 (1963).

106. E. T. Reese, R. C. Clapp, and M. Mandels, A thioglucosidase in fungi. Arch. Biochem. Biophys. 75:228 (1958).

107. J. Roche and S. Lissitzky, Etiology of endemic goitre, p. 351. In Endemic goitre, World Health Organ. Monog. Ser. No. 44. World Health Organization, Geneva (1960).

108. A. Rutkowski, The feed value of rapeseed meal. J. Am. Oil Chem. Soc. 48:863 (1971).

109. A. R. Saghir, J. W. Cowan, and J. P. Salji, Goitrogenic activity of onion volatiles. Nature (London) 211:87 (1966).

110. M. Sandberg and O. M. Holly, Myrosin. J. Biol. Chem. 96:443 (1932).

111. O. E. Schultz and R. Gmelin, Paper chromatography of mustard oil drugs. Z. Naturforsch. B 7:500 (1952).

112. O. E. Schultz and R. Gmelin, Das Senfölglukosid "Glucoiberin" und der Bitterstoff "Ibamarin" von *Iberis amora* L. (Schleifenblume). Arch. Pharm. *287*:404 (1954).

113. O. E. Schultz and W. Wagner, Glucoalyssin, ein neus Senfölglukosid aus *Alyssum*-Arten. Z. Naturforsch. B *11*:417 (1956).

114. S. Schwimmer, Enzymatic conversion of γ-L-glutamyl cysteine peptides to pyruvic acid, a coupled reaction for enhancement of onion flavor. J. Agric. Food Chem. *19*:980 (1971).

115. L. D. Small, J. H. Bailey, and C. J. Cavallito, Alkyl thiosulfinates. J. Am. Chem. Soc. *69*:1710 (1947).

116. C. G. Spåre and A. I. Virtanen, On the lachrymatory factor in onion (*Allium cepa*) vapors and its precursor. Acta Chem. Scand. *17*:641 (1963).

117. M. A. Stahmann, K. P. Link, and J. C. Walker, Mustard oils in crucifers and their relation to resistance to clubroot. J. Agric. Res. *67*:49 (1943).

118. M. M. Stanley and E. B. Astwood, Determination of the relative activities of antithyroid compounds in man using radioactive iodine. Endocrinology *41*: 66 (1947).

119. A. Stoll and E. Seebeck, *Allium* compounds. I. Alliin, the true mother compound of garlic oil. Helv. Chim. Acta *31*:189 (1948).

120. A. Stoll and E. Seebeck, The isolation of sinigrin as the true, crystallized mother substance of horse-radish oil. Helv. Chim. Acta *31*:1432 (1948).

121. A. Stoll and E. Seebeck, Chemical investigations on alliin, the specific principle of garlic. Adv. Enzymol. *11*:377 (1951).

122. R. L. M. Synge and J. C. Wood, (+)-(S-Methyl-L-cysteine S-oxide) in cabbage. Biochem. J. *64*:252 (1956).

123. B. A. Tapper and D. B. MacGibbon, Isolation of (L-5-allyl-2-thiooxazolidone) from *Brassica napus* L. Phytochemistry *6*:749 (1967).

124. H. L. Tookey, C. H. VanEtten, J. E. Peters, and I. A. Wolff, Evaluation of enzyme-modified, solvent-extracted crambe seed meal by chemical analyses and rat feeding. Cereal Chem. *42*:507 (1965).

125. H. L. Tookey and I. A. Wolff, Effect of organic reducing agents and ferrous ion on thioglucosidase activity of *Crambe abyssinica* seed. Can. J. Biochem. *48*:1024 (1970).

126. W. P. VanderLaan and A. Bissell, The influence of selected goitrogenic compounds on the thyroid gland of the chick. Endocrinology *38*:308 (1946).

127. J. E. VanderLaan and W. P. VanderLaan, The iodide-concentrating mechanism of the rat thyroid and its inhibition by thiocyanate. Endocrinology *40*:403 (1947).

128. H. E. VanderVeen and P. C. Hart, The occurrence in milk of compounds which cause struma. Voeding *16*:12 (1955).

129. C. H. VanEtten, Goitrogens, p. 103. In Toxic constituents in plant foodstuffs, I. E. Liener (ed.), Academic Press, New York (1969).

130. C. H. VanEtten and M. E. Daxenbichler, Formation of organic nitriles from progoitrins in leaves of *Crambe abyssinica* and *Brassica napus*. J. Agric. Food Chem. *19*:194 (1971).

131. C. H. VanEtten, M. E. Daxenbichler, and I. A. Wolff, Natural glucosinolates (thioglucosides) in foods and feeds. J. Agric. Food Chem. *17*:483 (1969).

132. C. H. VanEtten, M. E. Daxenbichler, J. E. Peters, I. A. Wolff, and A. N. Booth, Seed meal from *Crambe abyssinica*. J. Agric. Food Chem. *13*:24 (1965).

133. C. H. VanEtten, M. E. Daxenbichler, J. E. Peters, and H. L. Tookey, Variation in enzymatic degradation products from the major thioglucosides in *Crambe abyssinica* and *Brassica napus* seed meals. J. Agric. Food Chem. *14*: 426 (1966).

134. C. H. VanEtten, W. E. Gagne, D. J. Robbins, A. N. Booth, M. E. Daxenbichler, and I. A. Wolff, Biological evaluation of crambe seed meals and derived products by rat feeding. Cereal Chem. *46*:145 (1969).

135. A. I. Virtanen, On the chemistry of the *Brassica* factor: Its effect on the function of the thyroid gland and its transfer to milk. Experientia *17*:241 (1961).

136. A. I. Virtanen, Studies on organic sulfur compounds and other labile substances in plants. Phytochemistry *4*:207 (1965).

137. A. I. Virtanen, M. Kreula, and M. Kiesvaara, The transfer of L-5-vinyl-2-thio-oxazolidone (oxazolidine-thione) to milk. Acta Chem. Scand. *12*:580 (1958).

138. A. I. Virtanen, M. Kreula, and M. Kiesvaara, Investigations on the alleged goitrogenic properties of cow's milk. Z. Ernaehrungswiss. Suppl. *3*:23 (1963).

139. A. I. Virtanen and E. J. Matikkala, The structure and synthesis of cycloalliin isolated from *Allium cepa*. Acta Chem. Scand. *13*:623 (1959).

140. A. I. Virtanen and E. J. Matikkala, The isolation of S-methylcysteine sulfoxide and S-n-propylcysteine-sulfoxide from onion (*Allium cepa*) and the antibiotic activity of crushed onions. Acta Chem. Scand. *13*:1898 (1959).

141. Ö. Wahlroos and A. I. Virtanen, Volatiles from chives (*Allium schoenoprasum*). Acta Chem. Scand. *19*:1327 (1965).

142. N. J. Walker and I. K. Gray, The glucosinolate of land cress (*Coronopus didymus*) and its enzymic degradation products as precursors of off-flavor in milk— A review. J. Agric. Food Chem. *18*:346 (1970).

143. F. E. Weber II, Physical and chemical characteristics of bottled fresh and dehydrated horseradish. Diss. Abstr. *25*:1142 (1964).

144. M. L. Wilson and D. A. McGinty, Antithyroid activity of ergothioneine. Am. J. Physiol. *156*:377 (1949).

145. E. Wright and D. P. Sinclair, The concentration of radioiodine by the fetal thyroid gland and its relationship to congenital goitre in sheep. N. Zealand J. Agric. Res. *2*:933 (1959).

146. C. G. Youngs and A. S. Perlin, Fe(II)-catalyzed decomposition of sinigrin and related thioglycosides. Can. J. Chem. *45*:1801 (1967).

147. C. G. Youngs and L. R. Wetter, Microdetermination of the major individual isothiocyanates and oxazolidinethiones in rapeseed. J. Am. Oil Chem. Soc. *44*:551 (1967).

11 K. C. Hayes and
D. Mark Hegsted

TOXICITY
OF THE
VITAMINS*

This chapter reviews the toxicity of vitamins, with special emphasis upon the effects in man. Data obtained with various animal species have been included where these are considered to be especially relevant. Much of the material has been previously reviewed by Molitor and Emerson,[1] Robinson,[2] Sebrell and Harris,[3] Spies et al.,[4] and in the previous edition of this monograph.[5]

The toxicity of excessive levels of essential nutrients, such as the vitamins, may be of particular interest in view of the recent public concern about toxicants of all kinds. The distinction between enough and too much is not easily made by the average consumer or, indeed, in some cases by physicians or nutritionists. There is also a movement in this country toward the fortification of increasing numbers and kinds of foods, a trend that has potential risks. The need for rational solutions based upon substantial evidence must be emphasized. It may be especially pertinent to note that a few cases of clear toxicity are likely to provoke much more public outcry than greater numbers of deficiency diseases.

Even though some of the vitamins and essential minerals may be considered relatively toxic materials, it is obvious that prohibiting their inclusion in foodstuffs would be ridiculous. The fact that vitamins do

* Literature reviewed to April 1971.

235

qualify as toxic emphasizes the need for rational decisions regarding the amounts of toxicants that may be allowed in the food supply. At the same time it should be recognized that relatively concentrated vitamin preparations are available in the marketplace and are promoted for their health benefits.

FAT-SOLUBLE VITAMINS

Vitamin A

Vitamin A active substances are consumed by man in two forms from either plant or animal sources. Plants contain the ultimate source in the form of the carotenoid pigments, particularly β-carotene, which can be cleaved in the intestinal mucosa to form two molecules of vitamin A (retinol).[6] Cleavage and conversion by man are poor, however, amounting to 20–30% efficiency. Vitamin A is stored in the liver and fat of animals as the palmitate ester; this ester provides a sizable component of man's vitamin A when meat, milk, and eggs are dietary staples. Vitamin A is also synthesized commercially and is supplied as the palmitate or acetate ester in vitamin supplements.

Although the literature contains approximately 200 reports of vitamin A toxicity in man, toxicity rarely results from ingestion of natural foodstuffs. Those exceptions result from the consumption of polar-bear liver by Arctic explorers, or from ingestion of fish livers from those large fishes (shark, halibut, cod) capable of storing high concentrations.[7] The usual cause of toxicity is the prolonged consumption of large vitamin supplements, often initiated for dermatologic reasons. There is no evidence that carotenoids are toxic, as massive oral loading does not result in elevated serum vitamin A[8] and may even depress circulating levels.[9] Children may develop a yellow pigmentation of the skin (xanthosis) when consuming pureed baby foods rich in carotenoids. Pigmentation slowly disappears when the dietary source of pigment is removed.[10]

Acute toxicity in the adult requires a dose in the range of 2–5 million IU or above[11,12] and ingestion of as much as 30 million IU has been reported.[7] Such cases occur after ingestion of polar-bear or fish livers, the latter of which contain up to 100,000 IU/g.[7,11] Ingestion of a comparable amount in vitamin capsules would be unlikely. In the infant, doses as low as 75,000 to 300,000 IU can precipitate acute toxic signs generally following an accidental overdose or unwitting supplementation by an overzealous mother.[11,13,14]

Chronic toxicity developing in a few months is most commonly encountered in infants and children,[15-18] whereas chronic toxicity in adults may take several months or even years (up to 8) to develop.[19-22] Although the chronic dose necessary to induce toxicity varies with the individual for reasons yet to be defined, reported cases of toxicity would indicate that chronic intakes in excess of 1,000 μg (approximately 3,000 IU)/kg body weight/day are likely to produce toxicity in man. Reports range from 18,000 to 60,000 IU/day for infants less than 1 yr old, and from 80,000 to 500,000 IU/day for the 1-5-yr-old age group.[15,22,23] Consumption of 100,000 IU or more per day has generally been associated with toxicity in man, whereas one half this intake apparently did not induce toxicity during 17 yr in an adult male.[24]

Signs of acute toxicity in adults have developed in 6-8 h following ingestion of vitamin A; these include severe headache centered in the forehead and eyes, dizziness, drowsiness, and nausea with vomiting followed in 12-20 h by redness and erythematous swelling of the skin, which eventually begins to peel. These changes may become most severe where the epidermis is thickest, in the palms of the hands and soles of the feet, and may persist for several weeks before returning to normal.[7] In infants, bulging fontanelles, anorexia, hyperirritability, and vomiting generally occur in 12 h, followed in a few days by a fine cutaneous desquamation.[11,13]

Chronic toxicity in man results in anorexia, headache, blurred vision, muscle soreness after exercise, hair loss, maculoerythematous eruptions on the shoulders and back, and general drying and flaking of the skin with pruritis, cracking and bleeding of lips, reddened gingiva, and nosebleeds. The liver and spleen may be palpably enlarged, and anemia may be present.[19,20] Often painful subcutaneous swelling and cortical hyperostoses are present in the regions of muscle attachments on long bones.[14] An increased angle of metaphyseal flare (pagoda effect) has been described in growing bones of children.[18,25] Increased cerebrospinal fluid pressure or pseudotumor cerebri with papilledema[26,27] seem to be symptomatic of chronic intake in somewhat less than half the cases reported in adults, whereas this syndrome in infants is generally diagnosed on the basis of bulging fontanelles.

Interestingly, there are no recorded deaths unequivocally ascribed to vitamin A excess, perhaps the most serious implied sequelae to toxicity being irreparable damage to the liver, resulting in cell death, fibrosis, and cirrhosis[19,20] or permanent stunting of bone growth due to cell death in the growing endochondral plate.[23,25] In essentially all cases, complete withdrawal of vitamin A results in regression of signs and symptoms in a matter of days, with no apparent changes remaining in a few weeks.

Diagnosis is best established by estimating the vitamin A concentration in plasma or serum from a fasting blood sample utilizing a colorimetric procedure, or more accurately by microfluorometry utilizing the natural fluorescence of the vitamin. Values in excess of 100 μg/100 ml (normal 20–60) can be considered suspect with values appreciably greater than that indicative of toxicity.

Vitamin A intoxication has been extensively studied in animals but almost exclusively in the young. Ability to induce toxicity varies widely with species, the calf[28] and pig[29] being in a range of susceptibility comparable to man (approximately 1,000–3,000 μg/kg body weight/day), whereas the rat[30] and carnivores such as the dog,[29,31] cat,[32] and probably the polar bear and seal can tolerate extremely large (20,000–60,000 μg/kg) daily doses before being clinically affected. Systemic toxicity probably reflects liver saturation and overflow into the general circulation, which would indicate that herbivores and, to a lesser extent, omnivores are less well equipped for handling the large doses of preformed retinol and retinyl esters that carnivorous species consume. In adult monkeys the rise in plasma vitamin A associated with toxic intake was not accompanied by an equal rise in the carrier, retinol-binding protein (RBP),[33] suggesting that "unbound" retinol or excessive retinyl esters may be the damaging agent in toxicity.

Toxicity in animals results in anorexia, weight loss, and cessation of growth, including bone, which becomes thin and brittle with a tendency to fracture.[30,34,35] Skin changes include hair loss, erythema, eczema of the axillary region and groin, with drying and desquamation of skin in the more exposed areas.[29,30,33,34] Bleeding from small hemorrhages subcutaneously and in the viscera may result in death.[30] Massive parenteral doses of a water-miscible form of vitamin A have produced calcification of arteries in rats.[36] Teratogenic changes, including cleft palate, spina bifida, deformities of the brain, and anomalies of other organ systems, can be induced when toxic doses are administered to the pregnant animal during critical periods of fetal development.[37] The developing mesenchymal cell seems particularly prone to toxicity.[38] Interestingly, in contrast to human beings, chronic toxicity has not resulted in elevated cerebrospinal fluid pressure in those animals studied experimentally,[39] with the possible exception of fetal rats affected *in utero*.[40]

The mechanism of *in vivo* toxicity is undefined, although it would appear to be related to the membrane-labilizing potential of retinol demonstrated to damage cell organelles and cause excessive release of hydrolytic enzymes.[41,42] Such changes are disruptive to the point of cell death, especially in mesenchymal cells normally containing hydrolytic enzymes. The likelihood that this is a pharmacologic effect related to the physical characteristics of the vitamin is emphasized by the fact that α-retinol, an isomer of retinol, produces bone changes characteristic of toxicity in rats but has almost no physiological potential for promoting growth.[43]

An important aspect of the toxicity of fat-soluble vitamins, which has not been considered in most studies or case reports, is the interrelationship demonstrated to exist between them. Vitamins A and D diminish the toxic effects of each other,[44,45,46] which may explain why toxicity imposed by cod-liver oil can require a long induction period and why the observed toxicity may not be due clearly to either vitamin A or D as the relative concentrations of each may vary. Vitamin E also spares the toxic effect of vitamin A[47]; conversely, muscle weakness and degeneration described in vitamin A or D toxicity may reflect a relative vitamin E deficiency.[28,48] Similarly, nosebleeds, hemorrhagic diatheses, and prolongation of prothrombin time associated with vitamin A toxicity respond to vitamin K.[49,50] These may reflect competitive absorption and bulk displacement by the excessive vitamin, although this is not firmly established.

α-Retinol

Vitamin D

Unlike other vitamins, vitamin D can be made in the body where it is formed in the skin by the conversion of biologically synthesized 7-dehydrocholesterol to cholecalciferol (D_3). Ultraviolet irradiation from sunlight provides energy for this conversion, making this sterol-vitamin a sunlight-dependent hormone. Garments of civilized man, a cloistered life, or existence in northern latitudes, especially in cities, have necessitated an exogenous source of this vitamin supplied commercially by the irradiation of yeast ergosterol to form ergocalciferol (D_2). Vitamin D_3 can also be formed by irradiation of food. Vitamin D is also found in fish-liver oil, which was the original source of the antirachitic vitamin and still is incriminated as a source of toxicity. There are no recorded cases of vitamin D toxicity from overexposure to sunlight. Extensive exposure has evolved a means of protection by increasing the skin pigmentation, thereby filtering large amounts of ultraviolet irradiation.[51] By this means negroid populations seem to have established higher requirements and greater tolerance for vitamin D, as they appear more prone to rickets when inhabiting northern climes and appear less susceptible to toxicity.[52]

Vitamin D is considered to be safe when consumed in the 400 IU/day dose as recommended,[53] although there is a growing awareness that it may be an etiologic factor in idiopathic hypercalcemia of infancy (see below) at doses approximating the recommended daily allowance. The source of vitamin D affects its potency. Ergocalciferol (D_2) was reported to be more toxic than that from tuna-fish oil for cardiovascular and renal toxicity in the rat,[54] whereas D_3 was more toxic than D_2 in the pig.[55] In the New World monkey, which requires the vitamin as D_3, this form, but not D_2, was capable of inducing toxicity.[56] The relative toxicity of the two forms has apparently not been reported in man. The vehicle for administration is important, too. Vitamin D was found to be 3–10 times more potent when supplied in milk than in corn oil.[57] The toxicity of vitamin D induced by cod-liver oil may be quite variable, probably due to the fact that its vitamin A content can ameliorate the vitamin D toxicity, and vice versa.

Symptoms of acute toxicity take several days (2–8) to develop and include anorexia, nausea, vomiting, diarrhea, headache, polyuria, and polydipsia. In chronic cases weight loss, pallor, constipation, and fever are other clinical findings.[58–62]

The dose range reported to induce toxicity in children varies from 10,000 IU/day for 4 months to 200,000 IU/day for 2 weeks, with most cases ranging from 25,000 to 60,000 IU/day for 1 to 4 months.[60,61,63,64] An exceptional case where 0.5 million IU/day was consumed for 2 yr is also reported.[65] Although these figures represent clinical cases, lower doses may produce subclinical damage that goes undiagnosed. Data from a small sample of children indicate that an intake of 1,800 IU/day of ergocalciferol may impair linear skeletal growth,[66] but this is not supported by data from infants supplemented with up to 2,170 IU/day.[67] Nonetheless, as much as 2,000 IU/day have been and probably are consumed by many infants regularly without effect.[52,53] The Committee on Nutrition of the American Academy of Pediatrics has set a dose of 1,000 to 3,000 IU/kg body weight/day as dangerous.[53]

Those symptoms associated with vitamin D toxicity are rather nonspecific, suggesting a systemic metabolic derangement or toxicity. The metastatic calcification produced may result from physiological exaggeration of the vitamin's normal functions of calcium absorption from the intestine and mobilization of calcium from bone.[68] The resulting hypercalcemia is compounded by the damaging pharmacologic effects this fat-soluble vitamin has on membranes,[69] the combination resulting in calciphylaxis and deposition of mineral in soft tissues, including the basement membrane of renal tubules, myocardium, arterial walls, stomach wall, and alveolar septa of the lung.[70] Subsequent damage may result in hypertension and cardiac insufficiency with abnormal electrocardiograms[71]; and in renal failure, azotemia, and hypochromic anemia.[72] In contrast to the case with vitamin A, tissue damage and metastatic calcification from vitamin D can result in death.[63, 70, 73] However, most people recover when vitamin D and calcium are restricted and cortisone therapy is instituted.[74, 75] A case of decompensated hypertension during pregnancy has been recorded 12 yr following the clinical manifestation of vitamin D toxicity.[76] Bones may have increased periosteal thickening and intense calcification of the provisional zone in the epiphysis as serum calcium rises, accompanied by rarefaction of the diaphysis due to stimulation of bone resorption.[77]

During the past two decades numerous cases of an idiopathic hypercalcemia of infants have been reported. These children, generally consuming a formula diet, have developed clinical symptoms of anorexia, vomiting, irritability, constipation, weight loss, or failure to grow during the first few weeks or months of life. Renal and cardiac damage develop and are followed by severe mental retardation and peculiar "elfin" facies. Incidence of the syndrome peaked in Britain during the 1950's when milk was fortified at approximately 1,600 IU/quart; this problem subsided after fortification returned to 400 IU/quart in 1957. Excessive calcium absorption (with hypercalcemia) and abnormal metabolism of derivatives of vitamin D have been noted in this syndrome and have caused many to speculate that it represents genetic variation and hyperreactivity to vitamin D or a defect in the metabolism of the vitamin.[52] Concern has been expressed that the infant syndrome may be dependent on maternal ingestion of high doses of vitamin D during pregnancy,[78] but a retrospective survey of the involved mothers did not support the hypothesis.[52]

In light of the fact that a supplement of 400 IU/day of vitamin D is entirely adequate for the prevention of rickets (particularly when milk is the supplemented vehicle) and that a hypersensitivity phenomenon exists, it seems unjustified to allow supplementation of foods other than milk or milk replacers. Such an allowance would unnecessarily approach toxic levels without producing significant changes in the amount of corresponding deficiency disease.

Massive doses of vitamin D in the range of 0.2–10.0 mg/day in mice, rats, guinea pigs, rabbits, cats, and dogs resulted in pathologic changes and death in 6 days to 3 months. Calcification of arteries, kidney, heart, and other soft tissues was the predominant alteration, with kidney calcification being the earliest and most severe.[79] Although mineralization is most conspicuous, cellular injury is not dependent upon calcium deposition. This is indicated by deterioration of oxidative phosphorylation with large doses of vitamin D,[80] changes in lipid and protein metabolism,[58] seromucoid accumulations in arterial lesions prior to calcification,[81] and data from man[58] and New World monkeys[56] indicating that kidney malfunction and death (in monkeys) can result from vitamin D intoxication without the usual observable pathologic changes such as nephrocalcinosis.

Muscle atony and degenerative changes in skeletal muscle are common[82]; the inner portions of the myocardium degenerate and are replaced by calcium deposits,[83] possibly indicating concomitant vitamin E deficiency, as vitamin E has been found to prevent or mitigate aortic and kidney calcification from vitamin D_3 and D_2 intoxication, respectively.[69, 84] Bone resorption increases, and bones become brittle with prolonged toxicity. Vitamin D toxicity in the rabbit is enhanced by pre-existing hepatocellular damage and cirrhosis, or by nicotine administration,[85] leading to the suggestion that toxicity may affect calcium ions for the release and activation of the biogenic amines.

In a study on fertility and pregnancy in rats, an oral dose of 20,000 IU of vitamin D_2/day, given prior to or during pregnancy, produced infertility in the first instance and fetal resorption when administered before the seventh day of gestation in the latter. Dosage after day 7 resulted in normal pups.[86]

Vitamin D toxicity is most commonly assessed by measurement of serum calcium and can be suspected with concentrations greater than 12 mg/100 ml. Elevations in blood citrate and cholesterol and decreased alkaline phosphatase are also clinical findings. Analytical methods for measuring circulating concentrations of vitamin D have been developed but are not in general use clinically.

Vitamin E

Vitamin E, or tocopherol, is a substituted hydroquinone formed in plants. Alpha-tocopherol has the highest biological activity of the seven known tocopherols and is normally ingested in its hydroxyl form. It occurs in the lipid fraction of plants. It is susceptible to oxidation when exposed to heat, light, and air. The acetate and succinate esters, commonly available commercial preparations, are relatively stable forms of the vitamin.

Vitamin E is relatively innocuous and has been given to patients for months both orally and parenterally at a dosage level of 300 mg/day without effect.[87] However, in another study 6 of 13 patients on a similar dose complained of headache, nausea, fatigue, giddiness, and blurred vision.[88] Consumption of 40 g/day for as long as 1 month by 6 men produced no side effects.[89] On the other hand, an intake of 4–12 g for prolonged periods has been suspected of disrupting gonadal function,[87] and consumption of 2–4 g/day for 3 months produced slight creatinuria and chapping, cheilosis, angular stomatitis, gastrointestinal disturbances, and muscle weakness in an isolated case; symptoms ceased within 2 weeks when vitamin E was discontinued.[90] Hypoglycemia and depressed prothrombin levels have also been reported,[91] the latter suggesting a relative vitamin K deficiency.

Several nonspecific degenerative changes have been reported in many tissues of experimental animals dosed with toxic levels of vitamin E.[5] In most reports the vitamin was administered by injection, with gonadal degeneration being the most common alteration recorded.[92]

Vitamin K

Vitamin K is available as several compounds consisting of naphthoquinone rings with various aliphatic side chains. The original form isolated from alfalfa concentrates is designated Vitamin K_1 (phylloquinone); it is fat soluble and is the safest form to use. The water-soluble analogs and derivatives of menadione (synthetic vitamin K_3) are widely employed but may produce toxic side effects in the newborn when administered parenterally.

Hypoprothrombinemia and hemorrhagic disease of the newborn are not uncommon obstetrical complications thought to be indicative of

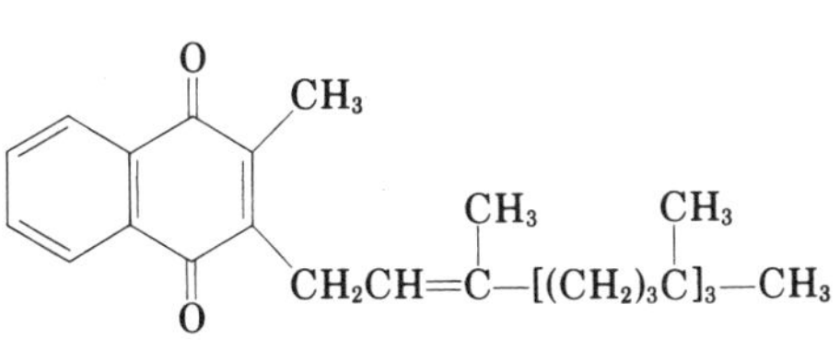

Phylloquinone (Vitamin K_1)

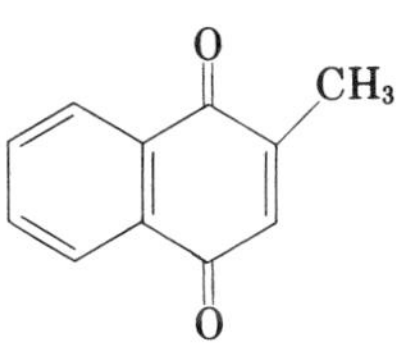

Menadione (Vitamin K_3)

vitamin K deficiency. Doses up to 10–25 mg of vitamin K have been administered to pregnant women prior to and during delivery or to the newborn infant to prevent this circumstance. Hemolytic anemia, hyperbilirubinemia, and kernicterus have been observed in infants following parenteral administration (vomiting may follow oral administration) of large doses of the water-soluble analogs, especially in premature infants. Hemolytic anemia occurred with 5–10 mg daily of menadiol sodium diphosphate (Synkayvite). Kernicterus and death occurred in six premature infants given 10 mg three times a day for 3 days. On the other hand, vitamin K_1 apparently is not harmful when given in doses of 10–25 mg.[93]

The mechanism of toxicity involves red-cell hemolysis and subsequent overloading of an immature liver with bilirubin, which cannot be sufficiently conjugated and which, in turn, proves toxic to the neonatal brain (kernicterus). Vitamin K may increase the susceptibility of the red blood cell to hemolysis by lowering the blood glutathione essential to red-cell stabilization or by acting as an oxidizing hemolysin,[94] a process enhanced by a concomitant vitamin E deficiency that is often present in premature infants.[95] The possibility that the vitamin K impaired the conjugation of bilirubin glucuronide was not supported by *in vitro* and *in vivo* studies of glucuronyl transferase, the enzyme mediating this reaction.[96]

Prolonged prothrombin time resulting from primary liver damage and an inability to synthesize prothrombin will not be remedied by vitamin K, and the vitamin may prove detrimental if administered in large doses. The water-soluble analogs are ineffective and contraindicated in cases of drug-induced (dicumarol) hypoprothrombinemia, in which cases the fat-soluble natural form (K_1) is required.[97]

WATER-SOLUBLE VITAMINS

Vitamin C

Toxicity due to ascorbic acid has not been reported, but the current fad endorsing its consumption in doses of 10–15 g/day to prevent the common cold[98] is not without danger. There is evidence that increasing the daily intake from 4 to 9 g can more than double the oxalic acid excreted in the urine of man,[99] and intravenous injection of 0.5 g on two successive days reportedly elevated the uric acid concentration in blood and urine.[100] Urinary calcium slightly increased, while sodium was reduced to one half its normal excretion by an oral dose of 1 g every 4 h administered to acidify the urine.[101] These factors may enhance formation of oxalate or urate crystals to produce kidney or bladder stones.[102, 103] On the other hand, ascorbic acid has been reported to reduce cystine excretion in cystinuria.[104] Abortion in guinea pigs[105] and rats[106] was apparently achieved by doses in the range of 1 g/kg body weight, and an attempt at therapeutic abortion in women has induced menstrual bleeding following 6 g/day for 3 days.[105] The possibility that 400 mg/day of vitamin C taken by women during pregnancy may have increased the requirement for ascorbic acid in the newborn was suggested by two cases of scurvy in infants receiving supposedly adequate intakes of ascorbic acid.[107] Similar experimental observations were reported in guinea pigs delivered of females given extraordinary doses (1 g or more by injection) during pregnancy.[108] The significance of these observations has not been determined.

Ascorbic acid is readily oxidized to dehydroascorbic acid, which is reduced by glutathione in blood. Although repeated intravenous injection of 80 mg dehydroascorbic acid was reported to be diabetogenic in rats,[109] oral consumption of 1.5 g/day of ascorbic acid for 6 weeks had no effect on glucose tolerance or glycosuria in 12 normal men and produced no change in blood glucose concentration in 80 diabetics after 5 days. The same report noted that a 100-mg intravenous dose of dehydroascorbic acid given daily for prolonged periods produced no signs of diabetes.[110]

Although the mechanism of action is not clear, ascorbic acid has been found to block the anticoagulant effect of heparin or dicumarol in experimental animals and has similarly interfered with the prophylactic use of dicumarol in a woman in whom a doubled prothrombin time was reduced to normal.[111]

Niacin

High doses of niacin (nicotinic acid), but not niacinamide (nicotinamide), cause vasodilation in the skin and increased intracranial blood flow. One hundred to 300 mg of niacin orally, or 20 mg intravenously, induced flushing and caused headache, cramps, and nausea.[4] Although used primarily to treat pellagra, large doses (2–6 g/day) of nicotinic acid have lowered serum cholesterol by 10–15%. Transient side effects, including pruritis, desquamation, and pigmented dermatosis, were reported, although no changes were found in liver biopsies after 1 yr of treatment.[112] Nicotinamide produces no side effects, nor does it affect serum cholesterol, but it has inhibited growth and produced fatty livers in rats when fed as 1% of a diet high in fat and low in choline.[113]

Blood glucose values were elevated by injections of 100 mg/day into rabbits without observable clinical effects.[114] In similar experiments phosphorylated pyridoxine derivatives decreased, while unphosphorylated pyridoxal increased, in urine,[115] and serum glutamic oxaloacetic transaminase declined, all of which resulted in the suggestion that a vitamin B_6 deficiency was induced.[116]

Pantothenic Acid

Pantothenic acid has a wide margin of safety. Neither oral administration of 50–200 mg/kg of body weight in monkeys, dogs, and rats for 6 months,[117] nor 100 mg/kg in man,[4] have produced any toxic manifestations. Depending on the route of administration, death by respiratory failure has been induced with doses of 0.8–10 g/kg in mice and rats.[117]

Pyridoxine

In natural sources pyridoxine is also found as pyridoxamine and pyridoxal, the latter of which is two to five times as toxic as the other two,[118] although none is considered toxic by normal standards. An intravenous dose of 200 mg was nontoxic in man,[119] and daily oral doses of 100–300 mg have been administered for the alleviation of drug-induced neuritis without side effects.[4]

Choline

Choline and its derivative, acetylcholine, behave pharmacologically as vasodilators and blood pressure depressants and are marked stimulants of secretory activity. However, 50 mg/day for a week produced no toxic symptoms in man.[4]

Folic Acid

The common therapeutic dose of folic acid in man is 5 mg/day. Based on experimental data in animals, a maximum daily injection of 20 mg should not be exceeded in infants.[120] In adults no effect has been noted after 400 mg/day for 5 months, or 10 mg/day for 5 yr.[4] In doses greater than 1 mg/day, folic acid may correct the pernicious anemia of vitamin B_{12} deficiency but will not counter the progressive degeneration of nerves in the posterolateral columns of the spinal cord found in that deficiency. Thus, folic acid in excess of the 25–250 µg needed to correct the anemia of folic-acid deficiency can mask megaloblastic anemia (generally relied upon in the diagnosis of vitamin B_{12} deficiency) and therefore can result in severe neurologic damage. For these reasons, excessive intake of folic acid is to be avoided.[121,122] Intravenous injection of 500 mg/kg body weight of folic acid in rats decreased renal filtration, increased kidney size, and produced epithelial degeneration in the proximal convoluted tubules.[123]

Thiamine

No toxic effects of thiamine have been reported following oral dosing; this is probably due to the fact that 5 mg is the maximum quantity that can be absorbed from a given dose.[124] Parenteral administration is indicated only when deficiency is evident, because repeated injections at levels of 10–100 mg may produce anaphylactic shock with vasodilation, nausea, tachycardia, and dyspnea.[125]

REFERENCES

1. H. Molitor and G. Emerson, Vitamins as pharmacologic agents. Vitam. Horm. *6*:69 (1948).
2. F. A. Robinson, The vitamin B complex. Wiley, New York (1951). P. 62.
3. W. Sebrell and R. Harris (eds.), The vitamins, chemistry, physiology, pathology. Academic Press, New York (1954).
4. T. Spies, R. Hillman, S. Cohlan, B. Kramer, and A. Kanof, Vitamins and avitaminoses. In Diseases of metabolism, G. Duncan (ed.). Saunders, Philadelphia (1959).
5. R. Ostwald and G. M. Briggs, Toxicity of the vitamins. In Toxicants occurring naturally in foods, National Research Council. National Academy of Sciences, Washington, D.C. (1966).
6. D. S. Goodman and H. S. Huang, Biosynthesis of vitamin A with rat intestinal enzymes. Science *149*:879 (1965).
7. J. P. Nater and H. M. G. Doeglas, Halibut liver poisoning in 11 fishermen. Acta Derm. *50*:109 (1970).
8. R. Greenberg, T. Cornbleet, and A. I. Jeffay, Accumulation and excretion of vitamin A-like fluorescent material by sebaceous glands after oral feeding of various carotenoids. J. Invest. Dermatol. *32*:599 (1959).
9. M. Dagadu and J. Gillman, Hypercarotenaemia in Ghanaians. Lancet *ii*:531 (1963).
10. H. W. Josephs, Hypervitaminosis A and carotenemia. Am. J. Dis. Child. *67*:33 (1944).
11. A. G. Knudson and P. E. Rothman, Hypervitaminosis A. A review with a discussion of vitamin A. Am. J. Dis. Child. *85*:316 (1953).
12. A. Gerber, A. Raab, and A. Sobel, Vitamin A poisoning in adults: Description of a case. Am. J. Med. *16*:729 (1954).

13. J. Marie and G. See, Acute hypervitaminosis of the infant. Am. J. Dis. Child. *87*:731 (1954).

14. W. K. Woodard, L. J. Miller, and O. Legant, Acute and chronic hypervitaminosis A in a 4-month old infant. J. Pediatr. *59*:260 (1961).

15. B. Persson, R. Tunell, and K. Ekengren, Chronic vitamin A intoxication during the first half year of life. Description of 5 cases. Acta Paediatr. Scand. *54*:49 (1965).

16. R. C. Breslau, Hypervitaminosis A. Arch Pediatr. *74*:139 (1957).

17. T. K. Oliver, Jr., Chronic vitamin A intoxication: Report of a case in an older child and review of the literature. Am. J. Dis. Child. *95*:57 (1958).

18. G. Bartolozzi, G. Bernini, L. Marianelli, and E. Corvaglia, Chronic vitamin A excess in infants and children. Description of 2 cases and a critical review of the literature. Riv. Clin. Pediatr. *80*:231 (1967).

19. M. D. Muenter, H. O. Perry, and J. Ludwig, Chronic vitamin A intoxication in adults. Am. J. Med. *50*:129 (1971).

20. E. Rubin, A. L. Florman, T. Degnan, and J. Diaz, Hepatic injury in chronic hypervitaminosis A. Am. J. Dis. Child. *119*:132 (1970).

21. J. W. Smit and D. P. Hofstede, Vitamin A poisoning in adults. Ned. Tijdschr. Geneeskd. *110*:10 (1966).

22. R. J. DiBenedetto, Chronic hypervitaminosis A in an adult. J. Am. Med. Assoc. *201*:700 (1967).

23. P. Ammann, K. Herwig, and T. Baumann, Vitamin A excess. Helv. Paediatr. Acta *23*:137 (1968).

24. R. F. Krause, Liver lipids in a case of hypervitaminosis A. Am. J. Clin. Nutr. *16*:455 (1965).

25. C. N. Pease, Focal retardation and arrestment of growth of bones due to vitamin A intoxication. J. Am. Med. Assoc. *182*:980 (1962).

26. A. D. Lascari and W. E. Bell, Pseudotumor cerebri due to hypervitaminosis A. Clin. Pediatr. *9*:627 (1970).

27. M. H. Feldman and N. S. Schlezinger, Benign intracranial hypertension associated with hypervitaminosis A. Arch. Neurol. *22*:1 (1970).

28. D. G. Hazzard, C. G. Woelfel, M. C. Calhoun, J. E. Rousseau, Jr., H. D. Eaton, S. W. Nielsen, R. M. Grey, and J. J. Lucas, Chronic hypervitaminosis A in Holstein male calves. J. Dairy Sci. *47*:391 (1964).

29. H. D. Hurt, R. C. Hall, Jr., M. C. Calhoun, J. E. Rousseau, Jr., H. D. Eaton, R. E. Wolke, and J. J. Lucas, Chronic hypervitaminosis A in weanling pigs. Univ. Conn. Agric. Exp. Stn. Bull. 400 (1966).

30. K. Rodahl, Hypervitaminosis A in the rat. J. Nutr. *41*:399 (1950).

31. C. L. Maddock, S. B. Wolbach, and S. Maddock, Hypervitaminosis A in the dog. J. Nutr. *39*:117 (1949).

32. A. A. Seawright, P. B. English, and R. J. W. Gartner, Hypervitaminosis A and deforming cervical spondylosis of the cat. J. Comp. Pathol. *77*:29 (1967).

33. K. C. Hayes and D. S. Goodman, Unpublished data.

34. R. E. Wolke, S. W. Nielsen, and J. E. Rousseau, Jr., Bone lesions of hypervitaminosis A in the pig. Am. J. Vet. Res. *29*:1009 (1968).

35. A. Khogali, Bone strength and calcium retention of rats in hypervitaminosis-A. Q. J. Exp. Physiol. *51*:120 (1966).

36. R. F. Strebel, R. J. Girerd, and B. M. Wagner, Cardiovascular calcification in rats with hypervitaminosis A. Arch. Pathol. *87*:290 (1969).

37. J. Langman and G. W. Welch, Effect of vitamin A on development of the central nervous system. J. Comp. Neurol. *128.*
38. M. Marin-Padilla, Mesodermal alterations induced by hypervitaminosis A. J. Embryol. Exp. Morphol. *15*:261 (1960).
39. H. D. Eaton, Chronic bovine hypo- and hypervitaminosis A and cerebrospinal fluid pressure. Am. J. Clin. Nutr. *22*:1070 (1969).
40. M. H. Bass, The relation of vitamin A intake to cerebrospinal fluid pressure: A review. J. Mount Sinai Hosp., N.Y. *24*:713 (1957).
41. J. T. Dingle and J. A. Lucy, Vitamin A, carotenoids, and cell function. Biol. Rev. *40*:422 (1965).
42. S. Bazin and A. Delaunay, Influence of vitamin A excess on the constitution of the connective tissue and on the collagenolytic activity of normal or inflamed tissues. Ann. Inst. Pasteur *110*:487 (1966).
43. G. A. J. Pitt, Comments. In International symposium on the metabolic function of vitamin A, G. Wolf (ed.). Am. J. Clin. Nutr. *22*:1045 (1969).
44. T. G. Taylor, K. M. L. Morris, and J. Kirkley, Effects of dietary excesses of vitamins A and D on some constituents of the blood of chicks. Br. J. Nutr. *22*:713 (1968).
45. I. Clark and C. A. L. Bassett, The amelioration of hypervitaminosis D in rats with vitamin A. J. Exp. Med. *115*:147 (1962).
46. A. Billitteri and Y. Raoul, Antagonism between vitamins A and D in mitochondria and lysosomes. C. R. Soc. Biol. *159*:1919 (1965).
47. L. W. McCuaig and I. Motzok, Excessive dietary vitamin E: Its alleviation of hypervitaminosis A and lack of toxicity. Poult. Sci. *49*:1050 (1970).
48. L. V. Krjukova, I. I. Ulasevic, and V. S. Medvedskaja, Interrelation of vitamins A and E in the live animal. Bjull. Eksp. Biol. Med. *6*:59 (1969); Nutr. Abstr. Rev. *40*:448 (1970).
49. J. T. Matschiner and E. A. Doisy, Jr., Role of vitamin A in induction of vitamin K deficiency in the rat. Proc. Soc. Exp. Biol. Med. *109*:139 (1962).
50. P. Griminger, Vitamin K activity in chickens: Phylloquinone and menadione in the presence of stress agents. J. Nutr. *87*:337 (1965).
51. W. F. Loomis, Skin-pigment regulation of vitamin D biosynthesis in man. Science *157*:501 (1967).
52. M. S. Seelig, Vitamin D and cardiovascular, renal, and brain damage in infancy and childhood. Ann. N.Y. Acad. Sci. *147*:537 (1969).
53. Committee on Nutrition, The prophylactic requirement and the toxicity of vitamin D. Pediatrics *31*:512 (1963).
54. R. S. Harris, B. D. Ross, and J. W. M. Bunker, Histological study of hypervitaminosis D. The relative toxicity of the vitamin D of irradiated ergosterol and tuna liver oil. Am. J. Dig. Dis. *6*:81 (1939).
55. H. Burgisser, C. Jacquier, and M. Leuenberger, Vitamin D poisoning in the pig. Schweiz. Arch. Tierheilkd. *106*:714 (1964).
56. R. D. Hunt, F. G. Garcia, and D. M. Hegsted, Hypervitaminosis D in new world monkeys. Am. J. Clin. Nutr. *22*:358 (1969).
57. J. J. Lewis, Clinical experience with crystalline vitamin D: The influence of the menstruum on the effectiveness of antirachitic factor. J. Pediatr. *6*:326 (1935).
58. M. I. Sevljagina, N. I. Gulinova, R. I. Gordon, I. M. Raskin, and A. S. Pipko, Vitamin D excess in adults. Klin. Med. Moscow *46*:31 (1968); Nutr. Abstr. Rev. *39*:562 (1969).

59. D. Rosenberg, J. A. Roux, A. Frederich, N. Philippe, J. Peytel, and P. Monnet, Facial paralysis as a result of vitamin D poisoning. Pediatrie *23*:565 (1968).
60. A. Berio and P. Moscatelli, Hypervitaminosis D. Minerva Pediatr. *19*:972 (1967).
61. C. Calandi, C. Calzolari, M. DiMaria, and U. Pierro, Vitamin D poisoning in infancy (12 clinical cases). Riv. Clin. Pediatr. *77*:3 (1966).
62. G. De Luca and M. Cozzi, Syndrome of vitamin D excess. Minerva Pediatr. *16*:210 (1964).
63. S. G. Ross and W. E. Williams, Vitamin D intoxication in infancy. Am. J. Dis. Child. *58*:1142 (1939).
64. J. M. Pereda, P. Arnal, J. M. Cavanilles, F. Miranda Gonzales, and J. L. Facal, Vitamin D poisoning with radiologically visible nephrocalcinosis. Rev. Clin. Esp. *110*:61 (1968); Nutr. Abstr. Rev. *39*:1276 (1969).
65. P. Davies, Vitamin D poisoning: A report of two cases. Ann. Intern. Med. *53*: 1250 (1960).
66. P. C. Jeans and G. Stearns, The effect of vitamin D on linear growth in infancy. J. Pediatr. *13*:730 (1938).
67. S. J. Foman, M. K. Younoszai, and L. N. Thomas, Influence of vitamin D on linear growth of normal full-term infants. J. Nutr. *88*:345 (1966).
68. H. G. De Luca, Recent advances in the metabolism and function of vitamin D. Fed. Proc. *28*:1678 (1969).
69. W. B. Spirichev and N. V. Blazheievich, Mechanism of toxicity of vitamin D. Int. Z. Vitaminforsch. *39*:30 (1969).
70. K. Kimura, Y. Nozawa, S. Kitamura, H. Takahashi, M. Ota, H. Norimatsu, and H. Wada, An autopsy case of hypervitaminosis D. Acta Pathol. Jap. *17*: 377 (1967).
71. L. M. O. Pljaskova, Damage to the cardiovascular system by excess vitamin D_2 in infants. Pediatrija, No. 7, 39 (1966); Nutr. Abstr. Rev. *37*:192 (1967).
72. L. M. O. Pljaskova, Anaemia of vitamin D excess in young children. Pediatrija, No. 12, 49 (1968); Nutr. Abstr. Rev. *39*:1276 (1969).
73. H. P. Kaserer, H. J. Gibitz, and O. Witontky, Fatal vitamin D poisoning in an adult. Wien. Klin. Wochenschr. *78*:463 (1966).
74. J. Winberg and R. Zetterström, Cortisone treatment of vitamin D intoxication. Acta Paediatr. *45*:96 (1956).
75. J. Marie, A. Hennequet, H. Marandian, and A. Momenzadeh, Vitamin D_2 excess due to daily ingestion of an excessive dose of a water-alcohol solution containing 400 IU per drop. Recovery on a diet free of Ca and with corticosteroid. Sem. Hop. Ann. Pediatr. *45*:24 (1969); Nutr. Abstr. Rev. *39*:1275 (1969).
76. F. Pfaffenschlager, Late effects of vitamin D_2 poisoning. Wien. Klin. Wochenschr. *76*:935 (1964).
77. H. Hungerland, Metabolism of calcium and phosphorus, p. 884. In Thaunhauser's textbook of metabolism and metabolic disorders, N. Zollner (ed.). 2nd ed. Grune & Stratton, New York (1964).
78. W. F. Friedman, Vitamin D as a cause of the supravalvular aortic stenosis syndrome. Am. Heart J. *73*:718 (1967).
79. H. Krietmair and T. Moll, Hypervitaminose durch grosse Dosen Vitamin D, Munch. Med. Wochenschr. *37*:637 (1928).
80. L. P. Scipicyna, Effect of toxic doses of vitamin D_2 on the dissociation of oxidative phosphorylation. Bjull. Eksp. Biol. Med. No. 9, 60 (1966); Nutr. Abstr. Rev. *37*:405 (1967).

81. R. Eisenstein and W. A. Groff, Experimental hypervitaminosis D: Hypercalcemia hypermucoproteinemia and metastatic calcification. Proc. Soc. Exp. Biol. Med. *94*:441 (1957).
82. J. Gillman and C. Gilbert, Calcium, phosphorus and vitamin D as factors regulating the integrity of the cardiovascular system. Exp. Med. Surg. *14*:136 (1956).
83. E. N. Coleman, Electrocardiographic changes in idiopathic hypercalcemia of infancy. Lancet *2*:467 (1959).
84. M. Cantin, J. M. Dieudonne, and H. Selye, Effects of vitamin E on cardiomuscular calciphylactic lesions. Exp. Med. Surg. *20*:318 (1962).
85. G. M. Hass, D. E. Henson, R. A. Scott, E. C. McClain, and A. Hemmens, Influence of cirrhosis on production of atheroarteriosclerosis and thromboarteritis with vitamin D and dietary cholesterol. Am. J. Pathol. *57*:405 (1969).
86. L. Nebel and A. Ornstein, Effect of hypervitaminosis D_2 on fertility and pregnancy in rats. Isr. J. Med. Sci. *2*:14 (1966).
87. R. Beckman, Vitamin E physiology, pathological physiology and clinical significance. Z. Vitam. Horm. Fermentforsch. *7*:153, 281 (1955).
88. R. A. King, Vitamin E therapy in Dupuytren's contracture. J. Bone Joint Surg. *31B*:443 (1949).
89. I. J. Greenblatt, Use of massive doses of vitamin E in humans and rabbits to reduce blood lipids. Circulation *16*:508 (1957).
90. R. Hillman, Tocopherol excess in man: Creatinuria associated with prolonged ingestion. Am. J. Clin. Nutr. *5*:597 (1957).
91. A. B. Vogelsang, E. V. Shute, and W. E. Shute, Vitamin E in heart disease. Med. Record *160*:279 (1947).
92. L. Piedrabuena, Experiments on the production of hypervitaminosis E in birds by giving DL-a-tocopheryl acetate. An. Inst. Invest. Vet. (Madrid) *18–19*:153 (1968–69); Nutr. Abstr. Rev. *40*:48 (1970).
93. Committee on Nutrition, Vitamin K compounds and the water-soluble analogues. Pediatrics *28*:501 (1961).
94. R. Wynn, Relationship of menadiol tetrasodium diphosphate (Synkayvite) to bilirubinemia and hemolysis in the adult and newborn rat. Am. J. Obstet. Gynecol. *86*:495 (1963).
95. A. C. Allison, Danger of vitamin K to newborn (letter to the editor). Lancet *1*:669 (1963).
96. B. Jones, Negative effects of vitamin K preparations on glucuromyl transferase activity, Pediatrics *40*:993 (1967).
97. J. A. Udall, Don't use the wrong vitamin K. Cal. Med. *112*:65 (1970).
98. L. Pauling, Vitamin C and the common cold. W. H. Freeman and Co., San Francisco (1970).
99. M. P. Lamden and G. A. Chrystowski, Urinary oxalate excretion by man following ascorbic acid ingestion. Proc. Soc. Exp. Biol. Med. *85*:190 (1954).
100. A. Pena, J. L. del Arbol, J. A. Garcia Torres, and J. Mora Lara, Effect of vitamin C on excretion of uric acid. Rev. Clin. Esp. *89*:101 (1963); Nutr. Abstr. Rev. *34*:195 (1964).
101. F. J. Murphy and S. Zelman, Ascorbic acid as a urinary acidifying agent. 1. Comparison with the ketogenic effect of fasting. J. Urol. *94*:297 (1965).
102. S. N. Gershoff, The formation of urinary stones. Metabolism *13*:875 (1964).
103. M. P. Lamden, Dangers of massive vitamin C intake. N. Engl. J. Med. *284*:336 (1970).

104. M. Sarnecka-Keller, J. Noworytko, T. Ciba, and S. Kos, Effect of some amino acids and ascorbic acid on the level of metabolites of N and S in urine in a patient with cystinuria. Pol. Tyg. Lek. *19*:1881 (1964); Nutr. Abstr. Rev. *35*: 793 (1965).

105. E. P. Samborskaja and T. D. Ferdman, Mechanism of interruption of pregnancy by ascorbic acid. Bjull. Eksp. Biol. Med. *62*:96 (1966); Nutr. Abstr. Rev. *37*:73 (1967).

106. E. P. Samborskaja, Effect of large doses of ascorbic acid on course of pregnancy and progeny in the guinea pig. Bjull. Eksp. Biol. Med. *60*:105 (1964); Nutr. Abstr. Rev. *34*:988 (1964).

107. W. A. Cochrane, Overnutrition in prenatal and neonatal life: A problem? Canad. Med. Assoc. J. *93*:893 (1965).

108. T. Gordonoff, Should one administer excessive doses of water-soluble vitamins? Experiments with vitamin C. Schweiz. Med. Wochenschr. *90*:726 (1960).

109. J. W. Patterson, The diabetogenic effect of dehydroascorbic and dehydroisoascorbic acids. J. Biol. Chem. *183*:81 (1950).

110. H. Mehnert, H. Forster, and V. Funke, The effects of ascorbic acid on carbohydrate metabolism. Ger. Med. Mon. *11*:360 (1966).

111. G. Rosenthal, Interaction of ascorbic acid and warfarin. J. Am. Med. Assoc. *215*:1671 (1971).

112. W. Parsons and J. Flinn, Reduction in elevated blood cholesterol levels by large doses of nicotinic acid. J. Am. Med. Assoc. *165*:234 (1957).

113. P. Handler and W. Dann, Inhibition of rat growth by nicotinamide. J. Biol. Chem. *146*:357 (1942).

114. T. L. Frateschi, Glucose in blood of rabbits given large doses of nicotinamide by muscle. Ann. Fac. Med. Vet. Pisa 1968 *21*:243 (1969); Nutr. Abstr. Rev. *40*:466 (1970).

115. D. Spisni and A. P. Mariani, Pyridoxine in urine of rabbits given large parenteral doses of nicotinamide. Ann. Fac. Med. Vet. Pisa 1968 *21*:238 (1969); Nutr. Abstr. Rev. *40*:466 (1970).

116. A. P. Mariani, Glutamic oxaloacetic transaminase (GOT) in blood serum of rabbits given large parenteral doses of nicotinamide. Ann. Fac. Med. Vet. Pisa 1968 *21*:254 (1969); Nutr. Abstr. Rev. *40*:467 (1970).

117. K. Unna and J. Greslin, Toxicity of pantothenic acid. Proc. Soc. Exp. Biol. Med. *45*:311 (1940).

118. P. Holtz and D. Palm, Pharmacological aspects of vitamin B_6. Pharmacol. Rev. *16*:113 (1964).

119. C. Weigand, C. Eckler, and K. K. Chen, Action and toxicity of vitamin B_6 hydrochloride. Proc. Soc. Exp. Biol. Med. *44*:147 (1940).

120. W. J. Darby, The rational use of vitamins in medical practice. Med. Clin. N. Am. *48*:1203 (1964).

121. W. Crosby, The danger of folic acid in multivitamin preparations. Mil. Med. *125*:233 (1960).

122. T. Sheehy, How much folic acid is safe in pernicious anemia. Am. J. Clin. Nutr. *9*:708 (1961).

123. W. Brade, H. Herken, and H. J. Merker, Disturbance of function and stimulation of growth of the kidneys by large doses of folic acid. Klin. Wochenschr. *46*:1232 (1968).

124. T. Friedemann, T. Kmieciak, P. Keegan, and B. Sheft, The absorption, destruction and excretion of orally administered thiamine by human subjects. Gastroenterology *11*:100 (1948).

125. A. Tetreault and I. Beck, Anaphylactic shock following intramuscular thiamine chloride. Ann. Intern. Med. *45*:134 (1956).

12 J. C. Somogyi

ANTIVITAMINS*

INTRODUCTION

The exact meaning of the term *antivitamin* is controversial. According to the classical definition of Woolley[1] and Shaw,[2] an active agent should be considered an antivitamin only when the following conditions are fulfilled:

1. Similarity of the chemical structure
2. Similarity of the symptoms produced by the antivitamin and by the lack of the vitamin
3. Competitive in its effect with the respective vitamin

However, a number of compounds that are antivitamins do not fulfill one or more of these criteria. It seemed necessary to extend the definition of antivitamin. Without the extension of the concept, a great number of substances—nearly all naturally occurring vitamin antagonists—could not be considered antivitamins, e.g., avidin, the antithiamine factors of fern and carp, and certain antagonists of pyridoxine and vitamin D.

*Literature reviewed through June 1970.

254

Some of these were the very first active agents that were observed to show biological antagonism.

Some years ago, therefore, it was proposed by Somogyi[3] to divide the antimetabolites and antivitamins into two groups: structurally similar compounds, i.e., antivitamins as a specific type of antimetabolite; and structure-modifying antivitamins, i.e., substances, mainly of biological origin, that destroy or decrease the effect of a vitamin as by modifying the molecule itself or forming complexes with the vitamin. This classification parallels that used for the inhibitors in enzymology. The structurally similar antivitamins correspond to the competitive inhibitors, and the structure-modifying antivitamins to the noncompetitive inhibitors.

Accordingly, an antivitamin may be defined as a compound that diminishes or abolishes the effect of a vitamin in a specific way. It is difficult, if not altogether impossible, to offer a more precise definition, since the mechanism of action of many vitamin antagonists is still unknown.

Mellanby,[4] in 1926, was the first to report an antivitamin action. He observed that certain cereals were antagonistic to vitamin D. Only many years later, in 1939, after Bruce and Callow[5] had described the inhibition of calcium absorption by phytic acid, was it possible for Harrison and Mellanby[6] to demonstrate that the antivitamin D substance in cereals is actually phytic acid itself.

Similarly, the antagonistic action of avidin against biotin was based on observations that had been known for a long time. These studies are also noteworthy because the inhibitor was discovered first and the vitamin later. In 1916 Bateman[7] reported that raw egg white is toxic. Boas[8] observed that certain foods contain an organic material that counteracted the toxic effect of the egg white. Many years later Eakin and co-workers[9,10] showed that the toxicity of egg white is due to a protein (named avidin) that forms an insoluble complex with biotin. Today, feeding of raw egg white is generally used for the production of a biotin deficiency state.[11]

Green[12] first described the so-called Chastek paralysis as a vitamin B_1 deficiency that appeared in silver foxes fed raw fish. It is now known that the viscera of these fish contain a thiamine antagonist.

In the period between 1940 and 1950, the investigations of antivitamins, stimulated by the above observations as well as the clarification by Woods[13] of the mechanism of action of the sulfonamides as antagonists of p-aminobenzoic acid, were greatly expanded; in addition to the naturally occurring antagonists, a very large number of compounds resembling almost all of the vitamins were synthesized.

ANTAGONISTS OF THIAMINE

Thiamine antagonists can be divided into two groups according to the above definition of antivitamin, i.e., *structurally similar* or *structure-modifying* antithiamine compounds.

In this article we shall deal with the naturally occurring antivitamins of thiamine, which all belong to the group of structure-modifying vitamin antagonists. The earlier work on structure-altering antithiamine factors (prior to 1955) has been thoroughly reviewed by Somogyi,[14] Lee,[15] Yudkin,[16] Bär,[17] Fujita,[18] and Jancarik.[19]

History

In 1932 a new illness in silver foxes was observed on the farm of J. S. Chastek (a U.S. fox breeder). Green[12,20] described this illness and reported that it occurred only in those foxes that had been fed raw fish (carp). He called the disease "Chastek paralysis."

Foxes that ate raw carp for a few weeks gradually lost their appetite so that finally they were not eating. About 2 weeks after the onset of anorexia, a stiff gait appeared that generally progressed into spastic paralysis, and the animals could no longer stand. A further characteristic symptom was a great sensitivity to pain in the extremities; the foxes generally died within 12 h after the appearance of the paralysis. The basal diet of the affected animals before addition of carp contained approximately the same level of vitamin B_1 as the diets of healthy animals.[21]

On the basis of the symptoms, Green suspected that the disease was a B_1-avitaminosis. The illness did not appear if the diet contained less than 10% carp or if the carp was not fed with the rest of the ration.[22] Viscera, skin, and heads of carp produced the above described symptoms, but fillets produced no illness.[23]

Green, Carlson, and Evans[24] succeeded in preventing Chastek paralysis by adding 20 mg of thiamine daily to the feed. However, why the feeding of raw carp produced a B_1-avitaminosis was still not known at this time. Similar observations concerning a disease of silver foxes in Sweden were reported by Carlström and Jonsson[25] and in Norway by Ender and Helgebostad.[26] That antithiamine compounds were also present in plants was first recognized a few years later by Bhagvat and Devi[27] and by Rutishauser.[28] The work of Japanese authors (beginning in 1949) also showed that certain bacteria likewise contain antithiamine compounds. (See p. 261.)

Antagonists from Cold-Blooded Animals

Sources Although antithiamine factors occur predominantly in the viscera of carp (*Cyprinidiae*), they are also found in other freshwater and marine fishes. Thus, antithiamine compounds were recognized by Deutsch and Hasler[29] in 15 of 21 species of freshwater fish (including 4 species of the carp family); by Neilands[30] in fish of the waters of Nova Scotia; and by Jacobsohn and Azevedo[31] in fish from the waters of Portugal. Ågren and co-workers,[32,33] who investigated 30 fish species of Swedish lakes and the Baltic Sea, found antithiamine factors in 9 species of carp. Somogyi[14,34] found a significant antithiamine activity in the viscera of carp and various species of trout. Among marine fishes, antithiamine factors are contained in the viscera of herring (*Clupea harengus, Cl. pallasus*),[35] in swordfish (*Belone acus*),[32] and in many other species.

Antithiamine compounds were also found by Jacobsohn and Azevedo[31] in a species of crab (*Penacus caramote*) and in mussels (*Tellina*), by Lee[15] in seastars (*Asterias sorbesi*), by Ceh et al.[154] in *Mallotus villosus* (an Arctic fish of the salmon family), and by Hilker and Peter[155] in 21 Hawaiian fish species. Oser et al.[36] were among the first to point out that mussels of the Atlantic coast (*Venus mercenaria, Mya arenaria*), which are frequently consumed by man, can cause complete destruction of thiamine.

Distribution in Various Organs Sealock et al.[37] showed by *in vitro* experiments that the extracts of the spleen, liver, and intestines of carp possess the highest antithiamine activity. Somogyi[38] partly confirmed these results and reported that the extract from heart muscle was very high in antithiamine activity, that from brain and mesentery was moderate, and that from striated muscle had no activity.

Mechanism of Action Krampitz and Woolley[39] clarified the manner in which thiamine is inactivated by an extract of carp viscera (ECV). Their *in vitro* experiments showed that the thiamine molecule is split by ECV at the methylene bridge. They isolated from the reaction mixture about 82% of the thiazole moiety of the vitamin (2-methyl-5-hydroxyethyl-thiazole), but only 41% of the pyrimidine portion (2-methyl-4-amino-5-hydroxymethylpyrimidine) was isolated. Barnhurst and Hennessy[40,41] later isolated a conjugate of the pyrimidine portion and called it ichthi-amine. Further work by Kupstas and Hennessy[42,43] established the exact chemical structure of ichthiamine as 4-amino-5-(2-aminoethane-

sulfonyl)-methyl-2-methylpyrimidine. This finding was confirmed by
Somogyi and von Brasch.[156]

Purification and Isolation   Japanese investigators, in particular Fujita
and co-workers,[18] as well as Murata and co-workers, have worked on the
isolation of antithiamine compounds from cold-blooded animals, ferns,
and bacteria. This work was reviewed by Murata.[44] These investigators
claim that these organisms should contain two different thiamine-
destroying enzymes: "thiaminase I" in fish, shellfish, ferns, *Bacillus
thiaminolyticus,* and *Clostridium thiaminolyticum*; and "thiaminase II"
in bacteria (particularly *Bacillus aneurolyticus*), yeast, and fungi.

Somogyi and co-workers have concentrated on the isolation of the
antithiamine compound from carp viscera. Lüscher *et al.*[157] and
Somogyi[158] succeeded in purifying an antithiamine factor by repeated
precipitation with ammonium sulfate at the isoelectric point (pH 5.0).
A purification method was developed later, thus permitting isolation of
the active compound as a dark brown crystalline substance[159] having an
activity about 200 times that of the crude extract. The product was
soluble in water at pH 7 and above, in Na_2CO_3, in 10 N formic acid, in
pyridine, and in ethanolamine; it was insoluble in ethyl alcohol and in
acetone, and it decomposed at 260–270 °C. It was nondialyzable and was
not inactivated by heating at 100 °C for 1 h. The substance had a molecular weight in the range of 75,000–100,000. One milligram dry weight of
this compound destroyed 1.8–2.2 mg of thiamine in *in vitro* tests in which
the remaining intact thiamine was determined by both the thiochrome
and microbiological methods.

Further studies by these authors[45] on the purified active compound
revealed that it was partly proteinaceous in nature and that a portion of
the antithiamine activity could be recovered after enzymatic or acid hydrolysis of the protein. The active factor, designated substance K, was
recovered from the hydrolysis mixture by column chromatography on
Sephadex 50 and Sephadex 25 and was shown by a variety of analytical
and spectral methods to resemble hemin very closely.[46]

Hemin or a very similar compound is, accordingly, the thermostable
antithiamine factor contained in carp viscera. Whether additional antithiamine compounds are also present is an open question. The thiamine
degradation produced by substance K proceeds equally well under both
aerobic and anaerobic conditions.

Iron plays a role in the inactivation of thiamine only when it is a component of substance K or hemin.[46] Inorganic iron compounds are ineffective. To produce an antithiamine activity corresponding to that of
substance K, the iron content of test solutions—depending on the indi-

vidual compound used—must be 3,000–10,000-fold higher than that of substance K.

Hematoporphyrin, the iron-free parent compound of the hemin molecule, shows only a very slight antithiamine activity. Thus, the thiamine-degrading action of heme-containing compounds seems to be a property of the intact heme molecule. Other heme-containing substances (crystalline antithiamine compounds, hemoglobin, catalase, etc.) show antithiamine activity corresponding to their heme content.

Antagonists from Warm-Blooded Animals

Although Sure and Ford[47] detected the decomposition of thiamine by animal tissues as early as 1943, for many years there was a general feeling that no antithiamine compounds were present in the organs of warm-blooded animals. According to Bojo,[48] negative results were obtained from testing the tissues of pigeons, guinea pigs, and cattle. Somogyi[49] was able to recognize antithiamine activity in organs of rabbits and hens, particularly in spleen and heart-muscle extracts. In contrast to carp, the intestinal extracts of warm-blooded animals inactivated thiamine only to a very slight degree. Striated muscles from these animals also showed no antithiamine activity.

Antagonists in Higher Plants

Sources and Distribution Bhagvat and Devi[27] detected thiamine antagonists in ragi (*Eleusine cora*), a kind of bean (*Phaseolus radiatus*), mustardseed, cottonseed, and flax seed. The activity was confirmed by experiments[50] with mosquito larvae, rats, and guinea pigs. The antithiamine factor of these plants was thermostable and largely dialyzable.

Weswig and co-workers[51] produced experimental "fern poisoning" by feeding bracken fern (*Pteridium equilinum*) to rats, just as it occurs in cattle and sheep. High thiamine doses cured the sick animals. Watanabe[52] and Parsons[53] separately demonstrated reduced thiamine excretion in human subjects given 15–20 g bracken fern/day. Haag *et al.*[54] showed that the antithiamine factor of bracken fern was very stable to heat; it was water soluble but was not soluble in ether, petroleum ether, acetone, or ethanol. Inactivation of thiamine by bracken-fern extract (FE) proceeded rapidly.[55] Further studies by various investigators showed that FE inactivates thiamine *in vitro*,[56] that bracken fern has higher activity than other ferns,[57–59] and that the thiamine antagonist of ferns is a small, thermostable molecule that, in electric fields, migrates exclusively toward the anode.[60]

A thiamine-inactivating effect was detected in blackberries, blue-berries, black currants, red cicerone, red beets, brussel sprouts, and red cabbage; somewhat smaller amounts were found in watercress, green cicerone, kefen, spinach, crisped cabbage, raspberries, and black cherries.[61] Rice bran also contains a thiamine antagonist.[27,62,63] Purified preparations from red cabbage and from blueberries[64] were similar to and possibly identical with the antithiamine compound in ferns.

Purification and Isolation   According to the earlier investigations of Somogyi and co-workers,[65,66] fern extracts contain two thermostable antithiamine factors: so-called hydrolysates I and II. The exact chemical nature of these phenol-like compounds was at that time still unknown. The significant antithiamine action of hydrolysates I and II was confirmed not only by microbiological tests but also through electrophysiological experiments.[160]

Later Berüter and Somogyi[67] prepared an antithiamine factor from bracken fern in a pure crystalline form. The purified factor was an acidic, thermostable organic compound and also seemed to be a phenol. It was identified as 3,4-dihydroxy cinnamic acid (caffeic acid) on the basis of its UV, IR, and NMR spectra; by its behavior on thin-layer chromatograms; and by other characteristic properties (melting point, molecular weight microanalyses, etc.).[68] Complete (95–99%) inactivation, as measured by both the thiochrome and microbiological assay methods, occurred when an aqueous (pH 7.8) solution of thiamine and caffeic acid (molar ratio 1:3) was held at 37 °C for 16 h.[69] Similar inactivation was brought about by various o-dihydric phenols. A close connection between chemical constitution and antithiamine activity was observed.[69]

Compounds that possess the aliphatic side-chain of caffeic acid, but that have no or only one OH-group, show no antithiamine activity. According to experiments,[69] the number and the position of the OH-groups are of primary importance for the antithiamine effect. Molecules with *ortho*-hydroxy groups show a marked antithiamine effect and those with OH-groups in the *para*-position a medium one; phenols with OH-groups in the *meta*-position are inactive.

Heavy metals such as iron and copper do not affect the inactivation of thiamine by caffeic acid. The main part of the inactivation reaction of thiamine by caffeic acid or catechol is blocked under anaerobic conditions.

In further experiments, Davis and Somogyi[70] investigated the mechanism of thiamine inactivation by o-dihydric phenols (caffeic acid, catechol). The reaction consists of two phases, which are distinguished by their marked difference in reaction rate and reversibility and by their dependency on temperature, oxygen, and pH. The initial phase (readily reversed by the addition of a reducing agent) has a high reaction-rate constant, and over a wide range it is independent of pH and temperature. The second phase is characterized by its irreversibility under these conditions; by a much lower rate of reaction; and by its dependence on oxygen, pH, and temperature. Although thiamine is rendered chemically and biologically inactive by caffeic acid, there is as yet no evidence for an addition product. The observation that one mole of *o*-dihydric phenols can inactivate several moles of thiamine, together with the results of chromatographic experiments, would indicate, rather, that each reactant is mutually altered in an oxidation–reduction reaction.

Antagonists from Bacteria

The presence of thiamine antagonists in bacteria was recognized by Japanese investigators. Three bacterial species are known to destroy thiamine. Matsukawa and Misawa[71,72] isolated one such organism from human feces and named it *Bacillus thiaminolyticus*; this was supposed to contain a "thiaminase I." Another type of thiamine-degrading bacterium is *Bacillus aneurolyticus,* which was isolated by Kimura and Aoyama[73] from hay and soil. This bacillus produces "thiaminase II." Later Kimura and Liao[74] discovered another agent in feces that produces "thiaminase I": *Clostridium thiaminolyticum.* Aoki[75] found a strain of *Trichosporum* that destroys thiamine and named it *Trichosporum aneurinolyticum.* Other yeast-like fungi, such as *Torulaspora, Torulopsis,* and *Thodotorula,* also contain "thiaminase II" according to Ozawa.[76] Recently, Kawasaki and Ono[161] reported that not only "thiaminase I" but also a thermostable thiamine antagonist is contained in the fungus *Lentinus edodes.*

Inoue[77] succeeded in culturing thiamine-splitting bacilli from the feces of beriberi patients. A method of determining "thiaminase I" (actually a determination of antithiamine activity) in feces was reported by Fujimiya[78] as well as by Kimura and co-workers.[79] Through the use of these methods the antithiamine activity in the feces of a great number of people in Japan was determined. About 3% of the people studied by Hamada[80] showed antithiamine activity in the feces, whereas Kimura and Aoyama[81] found activity in about 7–10% of the subjects in their investigation.

The "thiaminase I" of *Bacillus thiaminolyticus,* according to Douthit and Airth,[82] is predominantly extracellular. The formation of "thiaminase I" (i.e., the increase of antithiamine activity) was inhibited by the addition of thiamine.[83] Further purification and characterization of these thiaminases have recently been undertaken by Wittlife and Airth.[84] Both enzymes have been purified extensively and appear to be homogenous.[85] "Thiaminase I" catalyzes a base-exchange reaction, whereby the thiazole moiety of thiamine is replaced by another base (e.g., an amine) and the vitamin activity is lost. "Thiminase II" catalyzes breakdown of thiamine by simple hydrolysis. Both enzymes are destroyed by heating at 60 °C or above and would, therefore, not survive normal cooking of food.[85]

The significance of "thiaminase I and/or II" in human nutrition and health is regarded by Murata[44] as very slight, although habitual intake of large amounts of raw shellfish and raw ferns should probably be avoided.

ANTAGONISTS OF RIBOFLAVIN

Until a few years ago no riboflavin (vitamin B_2) antagonist was known whose activity could not be directly or indirectly accounted for by its structural similarity to riboflavin. In 1960 Fox and Miller[86] reported that the so-called "vomiting sickness" in Jamaica, which is caused by a toxin of the ackee plum (*Blighia sapida*) and not infrequently has a fatal outcome, may be the result of a riboflavin deficiency. (See Chapter 21, p. 472.) Administration of ribofalvin prevented the loss of body weight and death of rats that usually result from the feeding of this fruit. In further experiments, Fox and Miller[86] showed that the toxicity of 60 mg/kg subcutaneous hypoglycin A (the ackee toxin) was significantly diminished by simultaneous subcutaneous administration of 120 mg/kg riboflavin. It therefore appeared to them possible that hypoglycin exerted its action as an antimetabolite of riboflavin.

This assumption is supported by the earlier work of Hill,[87] who reported that severe riboflavin deficiency was established for the overwhelming majority of patients who were ill after consumption of the ackee plum. There is as yet no definitive proof that hypoglycin A is a structure-altering riboflavin antagonist, and, further, there has been no clarification of its mechanism of action.

ANTAGONISTS OF NIACIN

It is known that people and experimental animals whose nourishment consists preponderantly of corn often show symptoms of niacin deficiency. Since corn has a rather good niacin content (1–3 mg/100 g), it has been suspected that the vitamin exists in corn in a bound form unavailable to man and animals. Christianson and co-workers[88] reported briefly on the isolation, from the gluten fraction of corn, of such a complex consisting of 35% carbohydrates, 2% peptides, 0.6% nicotinic acid, and 62% aromatic or heterocyclic nitrogenous compounds. A complex of similar chemical composition (designated as niacytin) had already been prepared by Kodicek and Wilson[89] from wheat bran. Treatment with alkaline solutions freed the bound niacin and rendered it utilizable, as could be demonstrated by animal experiments.[90,91]

On the other hand, Gontzea and Sutzescu[92] claim that alkali treatment of corn failed to improve the symptoms caused by a high-corn diet but made them even worse, possibly by destruction of other vitamins. These authors felt that the dystrophic action of corn was caused less by the unavailability of the bound nicotinamide than by the presence of toxic substances having antinicotinamide properties. Thus Borrow *et al.*[93] found that corn bran retarded the growth of rats and that the addition of 5 mg of nicotinamide/100 g diet was necessary to overcome this inhibition. Cooperman *et al.*[94] were able to prevent the retardation of growth caused by borrelidin, an antibiotic also occurring in corn, by the addition of niacin or tryptophan.

Gopalan[95] suspected still another mechanism of action based on the observation that pellagra occurs in certain regions of India where millet constitutes the chief component of an otherwise protein-poor diet. Millet contains a sufficient content of free nicotinic acid, but—like corn—it also has a high leucine content. It was suggested that leucine interferes with niacin metabolism in amino acid imbalanced diets in such a way that the NAD and NADP content is increased and the NMN (nicotinamide mononucleotide) content diminished in the erythrocytes. (See Chapter 6, p. 144.) However, only when it is exactly known which factor or factors from corn and wheat produce the symptoms of nicotinamide deficiency will it be possible to decide whether specific antivitamin actions contribute to the appearance of these symptoms.

ANTAGONISTS OF BIOTIN

Feeding of large quantities of raw egg white can produce symptoms of biotin avitaminosis in man and animals. Raw egg white contains a protein, avidin, which in the intestinal tract forms a stable complex with biotin and renders it biologically inactive. Likewise, biotin-containing enzymes (e.g., pyruvate carboxylase,[96,97] oxalacetate-decarboxylase,[98] carbamyl-phosphate synthetase[99]) can be inactivated *in vitro* by avidin. (See Chapter 5, p. 107, and Chapter 13, p. 279.)

Avidin is present in the white of bird eggs, in the jelly of amphibian eggs,[100] and in the ovarian tissues of birds during the laying period.[101] Because of the localized occurrence of these proteins, Hertz and co-workers[102] investigated the influence of sex hormones on avidin synthesis. They were able to show that the synthesis of avidin was induced in ovarian tissue by injection of stilbestrol and progesterone, not only in immature hens but also in those that were no longer laying. The two hormones were inactive individually. These discoveries have been confirmed,[103-107] and the mechanism of action of these hormones in avidin synthesis has been clarified.

Avidin was isolated in 1940 by Eakin and co-workers[9] and somewhat later by Woolley and Longworth.[108] The compound is a basic protein (molecular weight 60,000) containing 10% carbohydrate (hexoses and hexosamines) and 6% tryptophan.[109] The tryptophan residues play an important role in the formation of the biotin–avidin complex. Destruction of only two of the tryptophan residues of the avidin molecule reduces the binding capacity about 10%; one molecule of avidin binds four of biotin.[110] In ion-free aqueous solution no binding occurs.[111,112] The biotin–avidin complex is very stable against alteration by pH, heating, or the action of proteolytic enzymes.

Gilgen and Leuthardt[113] isolated from chicken liver a protein fraction that binds added biotin quickly and irreversibly. In contrast to avidin, however, the quantity of biotin bound by a definite quantity of this protein fraction depends on the biotin concentration supplied. As a possible clarification of this behavior, the authors suggest that the binding of the biotin and the protein perhaps becomes irreversible only when the protein is denatured. This assumption is supported by Vallotton and Leuthardt,[114] who observed that denaturation of the protein with urea more than doubles the quantity of biotin bound. A further protein fraction with similar properties was isolated from human serum by Vallotton et al.[115]

Even though the property of combining with biotin is certainly not a general property of proteins, it nevertheless seems that proteins that do have this capacity are much more widely distributed than had previously been assumed, and this raises the question of their importance or significance.

ANTAGONISTS OF PYRIDOXINE

In 1946 Kratzer reported that the growth of chickens was retarded by the feeding of flax seed,[116,117] and according to Kratzer and Williams[118]

this growth retardation was diminished by pyridoxine (vitamin B_6).
From these and later experiments[119] they conclude that flax seed contains antivitamin B_6 factors that are water soluble and heat stable and are counteracted by pyridoxine, pyridoxal, and/or pyridoxamine.

Further exhaustive studies by Klosterman *et al.*[120-123] led to the isolation, characterization, and synthesis of the active substance. They suggested for the antagonist the name linatine (derived from the botanical designation of flax, *Linum usitatissimum*). Linatine is the only naturally occurring structure-altering vitamin B_6 antagonist known to date.

The tests used during the isolation were the inhibition of the growth of chickens and *Azotobacter vinelandii*. It turned out that the active factor is the γ-glutamyl derivative of 1-amino-D-proline. It is easily hydrolyzed into glutamic acid and 1-amino-D-proline, the last-named product being the antivitamin.

γ-Glutamyl-1-amino-D-proline 1-Amino-D-proline Glutamic Acid
(Linatine)

Synthetic linatine shows the same physical, chemical, and biological properties as does the naturally occurring compound from flax.[123] Its antagonistic action against vitamin B_6 can be understood in that the hydrolytically cleaved 1-amino-D-proline forms a stable complex with pyridoxalphosphate, as does avidin with biotin.[123] The growth inhibition by extracts of flax seed was also confirmed on various bacterial strains by Tjostem.[124]

ANTAGONIST OF VITAMIN B_{12}

Apparently no natural vitamin B_{12} antagonist is known to occur in plants or animals used as human food.

ANTAGONISTS OF PANTOTHENIC ACID

Smashevskii[125-127] recently reported the isolation of a pantothenic acid antagonist from pea seedlings. This compound—not yet identified chemically—inhibits the growth of *Saccharomyces cerevisiae*. The effect is enhanced by asparagine and lessened by pantothenic acid as well as by β-alanine. Also, the activity of the antivitamin can be counteracted by methionine.

ANTAGONISTS OF VITAMIN A

As is well known, vitamin A and carotenoids, because of their unsaturated character, are easily destroyed by oxidizing agents. Vitamin E appears to be a natural antioxidant for vitamin A, and not a few publications have reported reciprocal action between these two vitamins.[128-131] Thus, even small doses of vitamin E improved the utilization of β-carotene and vitamin A. However, with large vitamin E doses an antagonistic effect, instead of a vitamin A sparing action, appears. From the experiments of Hickman and co-workers,[132,133] it can be concluded that the vitamin A sparing action cannot be exclusively an antioxidative protection. These authors found that alpha, beta, gamma and delta-tocopherol show the same protection *in vivo,* although these substances *in vitro* have very different antioxidative properties. Even the oxidized product, tocopherylquinone, exerted as great a protective action as did the tocopherols themselves. From the reciprocal effects between vitamins A and E, Brubacher and co-workers[129] developed the hypothesis that there are two superimposed effects: (a) an antioxidative effect, and (b) a genuine antagonistic effect, which results from the displacement of vitamin A by high vitamin E doses, or vice versa.

ANTAGONISTS OF VITAMIN D

There are a number of naturally occurring substances that antagonize the action of vitamin D; the mechanisms of their effects are still unknown. In 1944 Fitch and Ewer[134] described the appearance of rickets and growth disturbances in New Zealand lambs that had been fed green oats and other green feeds during the winter months. These observations were later confirmed by Ewer and Bartrum,[135] as well as by Ewer,[136] in experiments with lambs and guinea pigs. Administration of vitamin D cured the sick animals. Grant[137,138] fed a chloroform extract from green oats to rats and was able to show that this diminished the activity of particular levels of vitamin D on the mineral content of the bones and that these effects were not caused by interference with vitamin absorption. He concluded that the β-carotene present in the green oats was probably responsible for this antagonistic effect. These assumptions were supported by the investigations of Weits.[139-141] Weits found that, after feeding hay to rachitic rats, the degree of healing observed was less than that expected from the amount of vitamin D present in the hay. Chromatographic separation of the nonsaponifiable portion of the hay lipids yielded a fraction that lessened the action of vitamin D in the rat test. The active substance was identified as β-carotene.

Another compound with antivitamin D character was isolated by Raoul and co-workers[142] from the stems and leaves of fresh vegetables. About 0.2 μg of this product per day decreased by about 50% the activity of a curative dose of vitamin D_3 in hens. The chemical reactions of this compound indicated a steroid structure; it was, therefore, possible that the compound was a structure-related antagonist. A decision on this point, however, is not possible on the basis of currently available data.

Substances with antivitamin D properties also occur in pig liver, according to Coates and Harrison.[143] These are partly soluble in organic solvents, but partly soluble also in water. Twenty grams of pig liver contain enough activity to nullify the action of 3 IU of vitamin D in hens.

ANTAGONISTS OF VITAMIN E

Several components of foods are known that diminish or prevent the biological action of vitamin E *in vivo*. To be considered in this connection are: (1) the reciprocal action between vitamin A and E, (2) a relation between polyenic acids and vitamin E, and (3) the antivitamin E action of unknown materials in beans.

It is known from many publications that an elevated intake of polyenic acids by animals causes an increased need for vitamin E. This antagonism could have at least two causes. The vitamin E might be acting as a natural antioxidant to protect from degradation the easily oxidizable polyenic acids in the diet and in the GI tract. On the other hand, the vitamin E might function as an antioxidant in the tissues of the organism[144]; or it may be necessary for the metabolism of long-chained fatty acids[145] so that, with a large intake of polyenic acids and insufficient vitamin E, the former could not be decomposed and therefore might exert a damaging effect.[146] (See Chapter 9.)

The behavior of the antivitamin E factors in beans (*Phaseolus vulgaris*), described by Hintz and Hogue,[147] is similarly unclear. These factors—one heat stable and ether soluble, the other heat labile and ether insoluble—prevent the protection offered by vitamin E against development of nutritional muscular dystrophy in hens. The heat-stable compound is said to be linoleic acid.

ANTAGONISTS OF VITAMIN K

The best known antagonists of vitamin K are dicumarol (3,3′-methylene-bis-4-hydroxy coumarin), isolated by Stahmman et al.[148] from spoiled sweet clover hay (Melilotus alba), and related synthetic products, particularly the rodenticide and anticoagulant warfarin. However, none of these substances has been found in any human food.

Another vitamin K antagonist is vitamin A. Light and co-workers[149] reported that high doses of vitamin A in rats produce hypoprothrombinemia and hemorrhaging, which can be relieved by administration of vitamin K. Quick and Stefanini[150] assumed that these difficulties arose from an influence on the intestinal synthesis of vitamin K, but this opinion was contradicted by the work of Wostmann and Knight[151] with germ-free rats. The observed effects may result from a specific antagonism.[152] Matschiner et al.[153] believe the antagonistic effect depends on interference with the absorption of the K vitamins, since only orally administered retinoic acid lowers the prothrombin content, while intracardially or intraperitoneally injected retinoic acid shows no influence at all.

REFERENCES

1. D. W. Woolley, A study of antimetabolites. Wiley, New York (1952).
2. E. Shaw, Antimetabolites—A review. Metabolism 2:103 (1953).
3. J. C. Somogyi, Metaboliten und Antimetaboliten, p. 141. In Ergebnisse der medizinischen Grundlagenforschung, K. F. Bauer (ed.). Thieme, Stuttgart (1956).
4. E. Mellanby, The presence in foodstuffs of substances having specific harmful effects under certain conditions. J. Physiol. 61:24 (1926).
5. H. M. Bruce and R. K. Callow, Cereals and rickets. The role of inositolhexaphosphoric acid. Biochem. J. 28:517 (1934).
6. D. C. Harrison and E. Mellanby, Phytic acid and the rickets-producing action of cereals. Biochem. J. 33:1660 (1939).
7. W. G. Bateman, The digestibility and utilization of egg proteins. J. Biol. Chem. 26:263 (1916).
8. M. A. Boas, The effect of desiccation upon the nutritive properties of egg-white. Biochem. J. 21:712 (1927).
9. R. E. Eakin, E. E. Snell, and R. J. Williams, A constituent of raw egg-white capable of inactivating biotin in vitro. J. Biol. Chem. 136:801 (1940).
10. R. E. Eakin, E. E. Snell, and R. J. Williams, The concentration and assay of avidin, the injury-producing protein in raw egg-white. J. Biol. Chem. 140:535 (1941).
11. A. Hertz, Biotin and the avidin-biotin complex. Physiol. Rev. 26:479 (1946).
12. R. G. Green, Chastek paralysis. Minn. Wildl. Dis. Inv. 3:83 (1937).

13. D. D. Woods, The relation of *p*-aminobenzoic acid to the mechanism of the action of sulphanilamide. Br. J. Exp. Pathol. *21*:74 (1940).

14. J. C. Somogyi, Die Antineurin-Faktoren. Hans Huber Verlag, Bern (1952).

15. C. F. Lee, Thiaminase in fishery products: A review. Comm. Fish. Rev. *10*:7 (1948).

16. W. H. Yudkin, Thiaminase, the Chastek-paralysis factor. Physiol. Rev. *29*: 389 (1949).

17. F. Bär, Vitamin B_1-inaktivierende Stoffe aus Tieren und Pflanzen. Antithiaminfaktoren, Thiaminasen. Arzneimittelforsch. *2*:365, 427, 486 (1952).

18. A. Fujita, Thiaminase. Adv. Enzymol. *15*:389 (1954).

19. A. Jancarik, Die Antithiamine und ihre Bedeutung für Nutztiere. Vitam. Horm. *7*:430 (1957).

20. R. G. Green, Chastek paralysis—A new disease of foxes. Minn. Wildl. Dis. Inv. *2*:106 (1936).

21. G. Lunde, Is "Chastek paralysis" caused by feeding too much fresh fish? Am. Nat. Fur Mark. J. *18*:5 (1939).

22. R. G. Green, W. E. Carlson, and C. A. Evans, The inactivation of Vitamin B_1 in diets containing whole fish. J. Nutr. *23*:165 (1942).

23. R. G. Green, C. A. Evans, W. E. Carlson, and F. S. Swale, Chastek paralysis in foxes. J. Am. Vet. Med. Assoc. *100*:394 (1942).

24. R. G. Green, W. E. Carlson, and C. A. Evans, A deficiency disease of foxes produced by feeding fish. J. Nutr. *21*:243 (1941).

25. B. Carlström and G. Jonsson, Ataxi, konvulsioner och acetonemi i samband med B_1-avitaminos. Scand. Vet. Tidskr. *28*:144 (1938).

26. F. Ender and A. Helgebostad, Eksperimentell beriberi hos sölvrev. Scand. Vet. Tidskr. *29*:1232 (1939).

27. K. Bhagvat and P. Devi, Inactivation of thiamine by certain foodstuffs and oilseeds. Indian J. Med. Res. *32*:131 (1944).

28. F. Rutishauser, Lähmungen und Krämpfe bei Silberfüchsen. Schweiz. Pelz-Gewerbe 649 (1944).

29. H. F. Deutsch and A. D. Hasler, Distribution of a vitamin B_1 destructive enzyme in fish. Proc. Soc. Exp. Biol. Med. *53*:63 (1943).

30. J. B. Neilands, Thiaminase in aquatic animals of Nova Scotia. J. Fish. Res. Board Can. *7*:94 (1947).

31. K. P. Jacobsohn and M. D. Azevedo, On the enzymatic destruction of thiamine. Arch. Biochem. *14*:83 (1947).

32. H. Lieck and G. Ågren, Thiamine inactivating factor in some species of Swedish fish. Acta. Physiol. Scand. *8*:205 (1944).

33. T. Wiken and G. Ågren, Studies on the occurrence of the thiamin inactivating factor in tissues of cattle, pigeon, toad and bream by means of the phycomyces assay method. Ark. Kem. Miner. Geol. *24*A:436 (1947).

34. J. C. Somogyi, Inaktivierung von Aneurin durch Karpfendarmextrakt. Helv. Physiol. Acta *7*:C24 (1949).

35. P. M. Sautier, Thiamine assays of fishery products. Comm. Fish. Rev. No. *126*:17 (1946).

36. D. Melnick, M. Hochberg, and B. L. Oser, Physiological availability of the vitamins. II. The effect of dietary thiaminase in fish products. J. Nutr. *30*:81 (1945).

37. R. R. Sealock, A. H. Livermore, and C. A. Evans, Thiamine inactivation by the freshfish or Chastek-paralysis factor. J. Am. Chem. Soc. *65*:935 (1943).

38. J. C. Somogyi, Inactivation of aneurin by extracts of animal and plant tissues. Int. Z. Vitaminforsch. 21:341 (1949).
39. L. O. Krampitz, and D. W. Woolley, The manner of inactivation of thiamine by fish tissue. J. Biol. Chem. 152:9 (1944).
40. J. D. Barnhurst and D. J. Hennessy, The action of fish tissue on thiamine. I. The isolation of icthiamin. J. Am. Chem. Soc. 74:353 (1952).
41. J. D. Barnhurst and D. J. Hennessy, The action of fish tissue on thiamine. II. Identification of the pyrimidine moiety of icthiamin. J. Am. Chem. Soc. 74: 356 (1952).
42. E. E. Kupstas and D. J. Hennessy, The action of fish tissue on thiamin. III. The further elucidation of the structure of icthiamin. J. Am. Chem. Soc. 79:5217 (1957).
43. E. E. Kupstas and D. J. Hennessy, The action of fish tissue on thiamin. IV. The synthesis of icthiamin. J. Am. Chem. Soc. 79:5220 (1957).
44. K. Murata, Thiaminase. Review of Japanese literature on beriberi and thiamine. Vitam. B Res. Comm. Jap. Tokyo 220 (1965).
45. H. Kündig and J. C. Somogyi, Isolation of the active moiety of the antithiamine compound from carp viscera. Int. Z. Vitaminforsch. 37:476 (1967).
46. J. C. Somogyi and H. Kündig, Inaktivierung des Thiamins durch Substanz K und andere Hämverbindungen sowie durch verschiedene Eisensalze. Int. Z. Vitaminforsch. 38:503 (1968).
47. B. Sure and Z. W. Ford, Influence of incubation at 37 °C on the stability of thiamine and riboflavine in cow's milk. Proc. Soc. Exp. Biol. (N.Y.) 54:83 (1943).
48. H. Bojo, Hukuoka Acta Med. 33:130 (1940).
49. J. C. Somogyi, Inaktivierung von Aneurin durch Organextrakte von Warmblütern. Helv. Physiol. Acta 8:C75 (1950).
50. K. Bhagvat and P. Devi, Inactivation of thiamine by certain foodstuffs and oil seeds. Part II. Indian J. Med. Res. 32:123 (1944).
51. P. H. Weswig, A. M. Freed, and J. R. Haag, Antithiamine activity of plant materials. J. Biol. Chem. 165:737 (1946).
52. H. Watanabe, Studies on the nutritional value of fern (3) thiamine content of the fern and its assay. Kokumin Eisei 21:134 (1953). Cited by Murata.
53. H. T. Parsons and S. Samruatruamphol, An antithiamine effect produced in human subjects by bracken ferns. J. Am. Diet. Assoc. 31:790 (1955).
54. J. R. Haag, P. H. Weswig, and A. M. Freed, Antithiamine activity of bracken fern. Fed. Proc. 6:408 (1947).
55. J. R. Haag and P. H. Weswig, Further observations concerning antithiamine activity in plants. Fed. Proc. 7:157 (1948).
56. K. P. Jacobson, Sur une thiaminase végétable. Arch. Port. Sci. Biol. 10:52 (1948).
57. G. Fabriani, A. Fratoni, and M. A. Spadoni, Azione biologica della tiamina nella modificazione in essa provocata da un fattore contenuto nelle folie di felce di macchia (Pteris aquilina). Q. Nutr. 10:295 (1948).
58. B. Thomas and H. F. Walker, The inactivation of thiamin by bracken (Pteris aquilina). J. Soc. Chem. Ind. 68:6 (1949).
59. J. C. Somogyi and A. von Muralt, Inaktivierung von Aneurin durch Farnkrautextrakte. Helv. Physiol. Acta 7:C56 (1949).
60. J. C. Somogyi, Die elektrische Wanderung von Antianeurin-Wirkstoffen verschiedenen Ursprungs. Helv. Physiol. Acta 9:C79 (1951).

61. H. Kündig and J. C. Somogyi, Antithiaminwirkstoffe in pflanzlichen Nahrungsmitteln. Int. Z. Vitaminforsch. *34*:135 (1964).

62. D. K. Chaudhuri, Antithiamine factor of rice-bran. Sci. Cult. *28*:384 (1962).

63. D. K. Chaudhuri, Purification of antithiamine factor from rice-bran. Sci. Cult. *30*:97 (1964).

64. D. Hilker, Antithiamine factors in blueberries. Int. Z. Vitaminforsch. *38*:387 (1968).

65. J. C. Somogyi and A. Koller, Ueber die chemische Natur eines Antianeurinwirkstoffes im Farnkraut. Int. Z. Vitaminforsch. *29*:234 (1959).

66. A. Koller and J. C. Somogyi, Weitere Versuche zur Isolierung eines thermostabilen Antianeurinwirkstoffes aus Adlerfarnkraut. Int. Z. Vitaminforsch. *31*:230 (1961).

67. J. Berüter and J. C. Somogyi, Isolation of a crystalline antithiamine factor from fern. Proc. Int. Congr. Nutr. *5*:543 (1966).

68. J. Berüter and J. C. Somogyi, 3,4-Dihydroxycinnamic acid an antithiamine factor of fern. Experientia *23*:996 (1967).

69. J. C. Somogyi and R. Bönicke, Connection between chemical structure and antithiamine activity of various phenol derivatives. Int. Z. Vitaminforsch. *39*: 65 (1969).

70. J. S. Davis and J. C. Somogyi, Reaction mechanism of the inactivation of thiamine by 3,4-dihydroxycinnamic acid. Int. J. Vitam. Res. *39*:401 (1969).

71. T. Matsukawa and H. Misawa, Proc. Comm. Vitam. Res. *31*:16 (1949).

72. T. Matsukawa and H. Misawa, Studies on fecal thiaminase. 17. Isolation of thiamine-decomposing bacterium. Vitamins *2*:137 (1950).

73. R. Kimura and S. Aoyama, On a new thiamine-decomposing bacterium. Vitamins *4*:366 (1951).

74. R. Kimura and T. H. Liao, A new thiamine decomposing anaerobic bacterium, *Clostridium thiaminolyticum*. Proc. Jap. Acad. *29*:132 (1953).

75. F. Aoki, Studies on the yeast-like enmyces which has thiaminase action. I. Biochemical characters of the thiaminase. Vitamins *9*:48 (1955).

76. K. Ozawa, Studies on the destruction of thiamine by microorganisms. I. Thiamine destruction by certain fungi. Vitamins *13*:9 (1957).

77. N. Inoue, Properties of thiaminase of a bacillus isolated from the faeces of a beriberi patient. J. Ferm. Technol. *29*:422 (1951).

78. M. Fujimiya, Studies in fecal aneurinase (3), Percentages of thiaminase disease among Japanese people. Vitamins *3*:270 (1951).

79. R. Kimura, R. Hayashi, and H. Nakayama, The method of separation of aneurinase bacterium. Vitamins *3*:290 (1951).

80. K. Hamada, Studies on dispositions of carriers of *B. thiaminolyticus* in the intestinal canal. I. On so-called thiaminosis-patients and carriers of *B. thiaminolyticus*. Vitamins *6*:951 (1953).

81. R. Kimura and S. Aoyama, Distribution of aneurinase bacteria in Kyoto City and thiamine value in the blood of people who had thiaminase bacteria in their feces. Vitamins *4*:205 (1951).

82. H. A. Douthit and R. L. Airth, Thiaminase I of *Bacillus thiaminolyticus*. Arch. Biochem. Biophys. *113*:331 (1966).

83. L. Wang and R. L. Airth, Repression of thiaminase I in *Bacillus thiaminolyticus*. Biochem. Biophys. Res. Commun. *27*:325 (1967).

84. J. L. Wittlife and R. L. Airth, The extracellular thiaminase I of *Bacillus thi-*

aminolyticus. I. Purification and physicochemical properties. Biochemistry 7:736 (1968).

85. J. L. Wittlife and R. L. Airth, Thiaminase I. E.C. 2.5.1.2., Method. Enzymol. *18A*:229 (1970); Thiaminase II, E.C. 3.5.99.2, Method. Enzymol. *18A*:234 (1970).

86. H. C. Fox and D. S. Miller, Ackee toxin: A riboflavin antimetabolite? Nature *186*:561 (1960).

87. K. R. Hill, The vomiting sickness of Jamaica. W. Indian Med. J. *1*:243 (1952).

88. D. D. Christianson, J. S. Wall, R. J. Dimler, and A. N. Booth, Nutritionally unavailable niacin in corn. Isolation and biological activity. J. Agric. Food Chem. *16*:100 (1968).

89. E. Kodicek and P. W. Wilson, The isolation of niacytin, the bound form of nicotinic acid. Biochem. J. *76*:27P (1960).

90. R. O. Cravioto, G. H. Massieu, O. Y. Cravioto, and F. Figuera, Effect of untreated corn and Mexican tortilla upon the growth of rats on a niacin-tryptophan deficient diet. J. Nutr. *48*:453 (1952).

91. E. Kodicek, The effect of treating maize and other materials with sodium hydroxide. Br. J. Nutr. *14*:13 (1960).

92. I. Gontzea and P. Sutzescu, Natural antinutritive substances in foodstuffs and forages. Karger, Basel (1968).

93. A. Borrow, L. Fowdon, M. M. Stedman, J. C. Waterlow, and R. A. Webb, A growth-retarding factor in maize bran. Lancet *1*:752 (1948).

94. J. M. Cooperman, S. H. Rubin, and B. Tabenkin, Effect of niacin and tryptophan in counteracting toxicity of crystalline Borrelidin for rat. Proc. Soc. Exp. Biol. (N.Y.) *76*:18 (1951).

95. C. Gopalan, Leucine and pellagra. Nutr. Rev. *26*:323 (1968).

96. J. J. Cazzulo and A. O. M. Stoppani, Purification and properties of pyruvate carboxylase from baker's yeast. Arch. Biochem. *121*:596 (1967).

97. M. C. Scrutton and A. S. Mildvan, Pyruvate carboxylase. XI. Nuclear magnetic resonance studies of the properties of the bound manganese after interaction of the biotin residues with avidin. Biochemistry *7*:1490 (1968).

98. J. R. Stern, Oxalacetate decarboxylase of *Aerobacter aerogenes.* I. Inhibition by avidin and requirement for sodium ion. Biochemistry *6*:3545 (1967).

99. V. P. Wellner, J. I. Santos, and A. Meister, Carbamyl phosphate synthetase. A biotin enzyme. Biochemistry *7*:2848 (1968).

100. P. D. Jones and M. H. Briggs, The distribution of avidin. Life Sci. *1*:621 (1962).

101. R. Hertz and W. H. Sebrell, Occurrence of avidin in the oviduct and secretions of the genital tract of several species. Science *96*:257 (1942).

102. R. Hertz, R. M. Fraps, and W. H. Sebrell, Induction of avidin formation in the avian oviduct by stilbestrol plus progesterone. Proc. Soc. Exp. Biol. (N.Y.) *52*:142 (1943).

103. B. W. O'Malley, In vitro hormonal induction of a specific protein (avidin) in chick oviduct. Biochemistry *6*:2546 (1967).

104. B. W. O'Malley and S. G. Korenman, Studies on the mechanism of hormone induction of a specific protein. Immunological identity and kinetic studies of avidin synthesized in vitro by the chick oviduct. Life Sci. *6*:1953 (1967).

105. B. W. O'Malley, W. L. McGuire, and S. G. Korenman, Estrogen stimulation of synthesis of specific proteins and RNA polymerase activity in the immature chick oviduct. Biochim. Biophys. Acta *145*:204 (1967).

106. B. W. O'Malley and W. L. McGuire, Studies on the mechanism of action of progesterone in regulation of the synthesis of specific protein. J. Clin. Invest. *47*:654 (1968).

107. P. O. Kohler, P. M. Grimley, and B. W. O'Malley, Protein synthesis: Differential stimulation of cell-specific proteins in epithelial cells of chick oviduct. Science *160*:86 (1968).

108. D. W. Woolley and L. G. Longworth, Isolation of an antibiotin factor from egg-white. J. Biol. Chem. *142*:285 (1942).

109. M. D. Melamed and N. M. Green, Avidin. II. Purification and composition. Biochem. J. *89*:591 (1963).

110. N. M. Green, Avidin. III. The nature of the biotin-binding site. Biochem. J. *89*:599 (1963).

111. R. D. Wei and L. D. Wright, Heat stability of avidin and avidin-biotin complex and influence of ionic strength on affinity of avidin for biotin. Proc. Soc. Exp. Biol. (N.Y.) *117*:341 (1964).

112. C. H. Pai and H. C. Lichstein, The use of avidin in bacteriological media. Proc. Soc. Exp. Biol. (N.Y.) *116*:197 (1964).

113. A. Gilgen and F. Leuthardt, Die Fixierung von ^{14}C-Biotin an die Leberproteine des Hühnchens. Helv. Chim. Acta *45*:1833 (1962).

114. M. Vallotton and F. Leuthardt, Étude de la fixation spontanée de la biotine (C^{14}) à diverses protéines. Helv. Physiol. Pharmacol. Acta *21*:C67 (1963).

115. M. Vallotton, U. Hess-Sander, and F. Leuthardt, Fixation spontanée de la biotine à une protéine dans la sérum humaine. Helv. Chim. Acta *48*:126 (1965).

116. F. H. Kratzer, The treatment of linseed meal to improve its feeding value for chicks. Poult. Sci. *25*:541 (1946).

117. F. H. Kratzer, Effect of duration of water treatment on the nutritive value of linseed meal. Poult. Sci. *26*:90 (1947).

118. F. H. Kratzer and D. E. Williams, The relation of pyridoxine to the growth of chicks fed rations containing linseed oil meal. J. Nutr. *36*:297 (1948).

119. F. H. Kratzer, D. E. Williams, B. Marshall, and P. N. Davis, Some properties of the chick growth inhibitor in linseed oil meal. J. Nutr. *52*:555 (1954).

120. H. J. Klosterman, R. B. Olsgaard, W. C. Lockhart, and J. W. Magill, Proc. N. Dak. Acad. Sci. *14*:87 (1960).

121. H. J. Klosterman, T. M. Farley, J. L. Parsons, and G. L. Lamoureux, The antipyridoxine factor in flaxseed. Abstr. Div. Agric. Food Chem. American Chemical Society, New York , September 9–13 (1963).

122. H. J. Klosterman, G. L. Lamoureux, J. L. Parsons, and A. Diner, Isolation and characterization of an antipyridoxine factor from flaxseed. Abstracts, Great Lakes Regional Meeting of the American Chemical Society, Chicago, Ill., June 17 (1966).

123. H. J. Klosterman, G. L. Lamoureux, and J. L. Parsons, Isolation, characterization, and synthesis of linatine. A vitamin B_6 antagonist from flaxseed (*Linum usitatissimum*). Biochemistry *6*:170 (1967).

124. J. L. Tjostem, Microbiological studies on the vitamin B_6 antagonist found in flaxseed. Proc. Iowa Acad. Sci. *72*:51 (1965).

125. N. D. Smashevskii, Isolation of an antivitamin from young pea sprouts. Uch. Zap., Khabarovsk. Gos. Ped. Inst., Biol. Khim. Nauk. *11*:79 (1964); Chem. Abstr. *63*:3315e (1965).

126. N. D. Smashevskii, A natural antivitamin of pantothenic acid. Nauchn. Dokl. Vysshei Shk. Biol. Nauk. *182* (1966); Chem. Abstr. *65*:2677e (1966).

127. N. D. Smashevskii, Amino acid inactivation of a natural pantothenic acid anti-vitamin, pizamine, and possible mechanism of its action. Biol. Nauk. *80* (1968); Chem. Abstr. *70*:1157p (1969).

128. J. Green, Interrelationship between vitamin E and other vitamins and the ubiquinones. Vitam. Horm. *20*:485 (1962).

129. G. Brubacher, K. Schärer, A. Studer, and O. Wiss, Ueber die gegenseitige Beeinflussung von Vitamin E, Vitamin A und Carotinoiden. Z Ernährungswiss. *5*:190 (1965).

130. Anonymous, Interrelationships between vitamins A and E. Nutr. Rev. *23*:82 (1965).

131. F. Weber and O. Wiss, Wechselwirkung zwischen Vitamin E und anderen Nahrungsbestandteilen. Bibl. Nutr. Diet. *8*:54 (1966).

132. K. C. D. Hickman, M. Woodside Kaley, and P. L. Harris, The sparing action of natural tocopherol concentrates on vitamin A. J. Biol. Chem. *152*:303 (1944).

133. K. C. D. Hickman, M. Woodside Kaley, and P. L. Harris, The sparing equivalence of the tocopherols and mode of action. J. Biol. Chem. *152*:321 (1944).

134. L. W. N. Fitch and T. K. Ewer, Aust. Vet. J. *20*:220 (1944); T. K. Ewer, Nature *166*:732 (1950).

135. T. K. Ewer and P. Bartrum, Aust. Vet. J. *24*:73 (1948).

136. T. K. Ewer, Rachitogenicity of green oats. Nature *166*:732 (1950).

137. A. B. Grant, Antivitamin D factor. Nature *168*:789 (1951).

138. A. B. Grant, Carotene, a rachitogenic factor in green-feeds. Nature *172*:627 (1953).

139. J. Weits, A factor in hay inhibiting the action of vitamin D. Nature *170*:891 (1952).

140. J. Weits, The influence of carotene and vitamin A on the anti-rachitic action of vitamin D. Int. Z. Vitaminforsch. *30*:399 (1960).

141. J. Weits, On an antagonist of vitamin D. Bibl. Nutr. Diet. *8*:44 (1966).

142. Y. Raoul, C. Marnay, N. le Boulch, M. Prelot, A. Guerillot-Vinet, R. Bazier, and C. Baron, Isolement d'une antivitamine D des parties aériennes des végétaux. C. R. Acad. Sci. (Paris) *244*:954 (1957).

143. M. E. Coates and G. E. Harrison, A rachitogenic factor in pig's liver. Proc. Nutr. Soc. *16*:21 (1957).

144. F. Weber and O. Wiss, Wechselwirkungen zwischen Vitamin E und anderen Nahrungsbestandteilen. Bibl. Nutr. Diet. *8*:54 (1966).

145. J. Green, A. T. Diplock, J. Bunyan, D. McHale, and I. R. Muthy, Vitamin E and stress. I. Dietary unsaturated fatty acid stress and the metabolism of alpha-tocopherol in the rat. Br. J. Nutr. *21*:69 (1967).

146. A. L. Tappel, Vitamin E as the biological lipid antioxidant. Vitam. Horm. *20*:493 (1962).

147. H. F. Hintz and D. E. Hogue, Kidney beans (*Phaseolus vulgaris*) and the effectiveness of vitamin E for prevention of nutritional muscular dystrophy in the chick. J. Nutr. *84*:283 (1964).

148. M. A. Stahmann, C. F. Huebner, and K. P. Link, Studies on the hemorrhagic sweet clover disease. V. Identification and synthesis of the hemorrhagic agent. J. Biol. Chem. *138*:513 (1941).

149. R. F. Light, R. Alscher, and C. Frey, Vitamin A toxicity and hypothrombinemia. Science *100*:225 (1944).

150. A. J. Quick and M. Stefanini, Experimentally induced changes in the prothrombin level of the blood. IV. The relation of vitamin K deficiency to the

intensity of dicumarol action and to the effect of excess vitamin A intake. J. Biol. Chem. *175*:945 (1948).

151. B. S. Wostmann and P. L. Knight, Antagonism between vitamins A and K in the germfree rat. J. Nutr. *87*:155 (1965).

152. Anonymous, The antagonistic effect of vitamin A on vitamin K in the germfree rat. Nutr. Rev. *24*:125 (1966).

153. J. T. Matschiner, J. M. Amelotti, and E. A. Doisy, Mechanism of the effect of retinoic acid and squalene on vitamin K deficiency in the rat. J. Nutr. *91*:303 (1967).

154. L. Ceh, A. Helgebostad, and F. Ender, Thiaminase in capelin (*Mallotus villosus,* an arctic fish of the Salmonidae family). Int. Z. Vitaminforsch. *34*:189 (1964).

155. D. M. Hilker and O. F. Peter, Antithiamine activity in Hawaii fish. J. Nutr. *89*:419 (1966).

156. J. C. Somogyi and A. von Brasch, In J. C. Somogyi, Inactivation of aneurin by extracts of animal and plant tissues. Int. Z. Vitaminforsch. *21*:341 (1949).

157. E. Lüscher, G. Bührer, and J. C. Somogyi, In J. C. Somogyi, Metaboliten und Antimetaboliten, p. 141. In Ergebnisse der medizinischen Grundlagenforschung, K. F. Bauer (ed.). Thieme, Stuttgart (1956).

158. J. C. Somogyi, On the antimetabolites of thiamin. Bibl. Nutr. Diet. *1*:77 (1960).

159. J. C. Somogyi and H. Kündig, Die Isolierung eines kristallinen Antithiaminwirkstoffes aus Karpfeneingeweide. Acta Chem. Scand. *17*:302 (1963).

160. S. F. Petropulos, The action of an antimetabolite of thiamine on single myelinated nerve fibres. J. Cell. Comp. Physiol. *56*:7 (1960).

161. M. Kawasaki and T. Ono, Thiaminase of fungi. I. Thiaminase of *Lentinus edodes.* Vitamin *37*:44 (1968); Chem. Abstr. *68*:46 513 (1968).

13 J. R. Whitaker and R. E. Feeney

ENZYME
INHIBITORS
IN FOODS*

An inhibitor may be defined broadly as any substance that reduces enzyme activity. Excluded from this broad definition is loss in activity due to denaturation caused by extremes of pH, temperature, and organic solvents. *In vivo,* a substance can decrease the activity of an enzyme as a result of:

1. Affecting binding and transformation of the substrate to products
2. Rendering the substrate unavailable
3. Interfering with biosynthesis of the enzyme
4. Increasing the rate of turnover of enzyme
5. Affecting a hormone, which in turn affects the level of enzyme activity

The first type of inhibitor has been most frequently reported in foods.

Substances that affect the binding and transformation of the substrate to products include: (a) substrate analogs, such as many of the naturally occurring cholinesterase inhibitors; (b) cofactor analogs of riboflavin,[1] pyridoxine,[2] niacin,[3] and vitamin K[4]; (c) allosteric effectors, which cause changes in conformation and active concentra-

*Literature reviewed to February 1971. Researches providing the background for the chapter were supported by NIH grants AM-13165 and AM-13686.

tions of enzymes, (d) compounds such as cyanide and thiocyanate, which form covalent or strong coordination bonds with essential groups of the enzyme; (e) specific proteins, which form strong inactive complexes with enzymes such as proteolytic enzyme inhibitors, amylase inhibitors, and antibodies; and (f) nonspecific macro-ions such as nucleic acids, protamines, and tannins.

An example of a substance in food that renders a substrate unavailable to enzymatic degradation has been reported in navy beans. Navy beans contain two types of compounds that decrease pancreatic amylase activity.[5,6] One is a protein (see below), the other an ether-extractable oil. It appears that the fat-soluble fraction specifically combines with starch in such a manner as to prevent its hydrolysis by pancreatic α-amylase.

The amount of an enzyme synthesized *in vivo* is the net result of genetic factors, environmental influence on the transcription and translation processes, and nutritional state. Aflatoxins are thought to exert their effect by interfering with the genetic code and thus transcription in the pathway of biosynthesis of enzymes. Lactose toxicity and favism are due to inborn errors of metabolism in which the respective enzymes β-galactosidase[7] and glucose-6-phosphate dehydrogenase[8] are not synthesized. (See Chapter 22, p. 477.) Many other examples of enzyme deficiency nutritional diseases can be cited.[9] Any substance that affects the availability of essential amino acids or energy for biosynthesis will act as an enzyme inhibitor *in vivo.*

In the normal individual, there is a delicate balance between the rate of biosynthesis and the rate of degradation of an enzyme. Any substance that upsets this balance in favor of rate of turnover will appear as an enzyme inhibitor. Conditions leading to increased proteolytic enzyme activity (such as those occurring in nutritional and genetic muscular dystrophy, infections, and bruises) give temporary or permanent imbalance between synthesis and degradation.

Modulation of enzyme activity may be the result of the action of a substance on a hormone. It is well known that various hormones affect the activity of certain enzymes *in vivo*; for example, epinephrine affects adenyl cyclase activity, which in turn controls the level of the very important cyclic 3',5'-adenosine monophosphate.[10] Any substance that decreases the level of a hormone having either a primary or secondary effect on an enzyme will be an *in vivo* inhibitor of that enzyme.

Enzyme inhibitors occur naturally in the human body. Examples of naturally occurring inhibitors of enzymes in humans include the pancreatic proteolytic enzyme inhibitors, blood-clotting enzyme inhibitors, tissue kallikrein inhibitor, one or more protein inhibitors (which interfere with glycogenolysis by affecting activity of protein kinase[10]), liver nicotinamide deamidase inhibitor,[11] and hyaluronidase inhibitor.[12] In the case of the hyaluronidase inhibitor, for example, the inhibitor concentration remains within a well-defined "normal" range and is thought to perform a physiological function in controlling the metabolic turnover of intercellular ground substance. The amount of inhibitor is significantly increased in human beings suffering from various viral and bacterial infections, malignancies, and rheumatic diseases.[13]

Because of different levels of enzymes, all humans are not equally susceptible to constituents of foods. Lactose is toxic to many non-Caucasians because of a deficiency of β-galactosidase[9] (see Chapter 22, p. 477); phenylalanine is toxic to many people, particularly infants, because of deficiency of phenylalanine hydroxylase[9] (see Chapter 6, p. 146); and favism is a result of stress induced by eating broad bean because of deficiency of glucose-6-phosphate dehydrogenase.[8] (See Chapter 22, p. 489.) The sympathomimetic amine, tyramine (see Chapter 8, p. 147) is present in cheese in considerable amounts (up to 200 mg/100 g) and is normally detoxified by monoamine oxidase present in the intestine and liver. Some patients treated with drugs that inhibit monoamine oxidase (e.g., tranylcypromine) have shown hypertensive attacks as the result of eating cheese.[14] Alcohol is occasionally fatal when consumed in conjunction with certain drugs.

It must be emphasized that the more thoroughly studied enzyme inhibitors occurring naturally in foods are those that interfere with the binding and transformation of substrate to products; these are treated in detail in this chapter. Detailed treatment of this one category of enzyme inhibitors, however, must not be permitted to overshadow and thus delay a determination of the importance of inhibitors of the other categories. Our lack of knowledge on these subjects points up the need for good basic research in these largely unexplored areas.

There are many deficiencies in our knowledge of the inhibitors that interfere with the binding and transformation of substrate to products. Much of the work on proteolytic enzyme inhibitors has been performed using bovine enzymes; thus, the work can not necessarily be translated to their effects on human enzymes.[15] Little is known about the effect of these inhibitors on the bacterial systems (and their enzymes) of the gastrointestinal tract. Yet these bacterial systems play an extremely important function in human nutrition and health. Because of our lack of knowledge in these areas, we have included enzyme inhibitors (e.g., subtilisin, ficin, and papain inhibitors) that have not yet been studied extensively with enzymes derived from humans.

It must not be overlooked that a number of the enzyme inhibitors discussed below are proteins and that their activity may be lost on cooking. For example, eggs and legumes contain large amounts of substances that have been shown to inhibit human proteolytic enzymes. These inhibitors, although relatively heat stable, are destroyed during proper cooking.

PROTEIN INHIBITORS OF PROTEOLYTIC ENZYMES

A great variety of protein inhibitors, particularly against the pancreatic proteolytic enzymes of vertebrates, occurs in plant and animal tissues.[16,17] The principal studies of inhibitors from plants have been with those from soybeans, lima beans, peas, and potatoes. The principal studies of inhibitors from animal sources have been with those from the pancreas, colostrum, blood plasma, and avian egg white of different species. These, however, are only a few of the many inhibitors studied. For example, inhibitors have also been found in seminal fluid, lung tissue, submandibular gland, urine, and certain intestinal parasites.

Not only do inhibitors occur in diverse biological systems, they also exist in many different structural forms and inhibit many different proteolytic enzymes (Table 1). Their specificities for inhibiting different proteinases vary widely, and it is frequently difficult to predict the specificity of any particular inhibitor.

The logical function of the inhibitors of proteolytic enzymes in biological systems might be to control the activities of proteolytic enzymes. Possible examples are the inhibitors of pancreatic enzymes found together with the zymogens of proteolytic enzymes in the pancreas and the inhibitors in blood plasma where proteolytic enzymes related to the clotting of blood and the dissolving of blood clots exist. Recent reports also indicate the importance of control of proteolytic enzymes involved in sperm penetration of the ovum. However, no functions have been found for the inhibitors present in many other places such as in avian egg whites and in many different plant tissues.

Trypsin Inhibitors

Trypsin inhibitors are probably the most widely distributed among the inhibitors of proteolytic enzymes. Part of this wide distribution may be more apparent than real, since most studies have been done against bovine trypsin and only in the past decade or so have their effects against other proteolytic enzymes been measured. Nevertheless, the wide distribution of inhibitors of trypsin is in agreement with the dis-

TABLE 1 Some Naturally Occurring Inhibitors of Proteolytic Enzymes

Source	Type	pI	Molecular Weight (g/mole)	Enzymes Inhibited	Remarks	References
Egg white						
Chicken	Ovomucoid	3.8–4.4	28,000	Tryp.[a]	Contains approx. 20% carbohydrate	18–20
	Ovoinhibitor	—	46,500	Tryp., chym., subtilisin, A. oryzae proteinase	Tryp. and chym. inhibited simultaneously; chym. and subtilisin compete	21
	Papain inhibitor	—	12,700	Papain, ficin	Papain and ficin compete	22
Tinamou	Ovomucoid	4–5	28,000	Chym., subtilisin	—	24
Turkey	Ovomucoid	4–5	28,000	Tryp., chym., subtilisin	Tryp. and chym. inhibited simultaneously	23
Penguin	Ovomucoid	4–5	28,000	Tryp., chym., subtilisin	Subtilisin strongly inhibited	25
Quail (Japan)	Ovomucoid	4–5	28,000	Tryp.	Human trypsin inhibited[a]	15
Pancreas						
Bovine	Tissue (basic)	10.1	6,513	Tryp., chym.	Human trypsin strongly inhibited	26,27
	Juice (Kazal)	—	6,155	Tryp.	—	16,28,29
Porcine	Juice (Kazal)	—	6,024	Tryp.	—	16,30
Blood						
Human	α_1	4.0	45,000	Tryp., chym.	Greater affinity for chym.	31,32
	1	2.8	16,400	Tryp., chym.	Weak inhib. of chym.	33
Bovine	—	3.8	39,000–71,000[b]	Tryp., chym.	Weak inhib. of chym.	34
Ovine	—	4.3	40,600	Tryp., chym., plasmin, proteinase A	—	35

Source						
Bovine	–	4.2	10,500	Tryp.	Human trypsin strongly inhibited[c]	15,36,37
Porcine	–	–	–	Tryp.	Resistant to pepsin	38
Ascaris lumbricoides var. *suis*	–	–	8,000	Tryp.	Chym. inhibitors also present	39
Soybean	Crystalline (Kunitz)	4.5	21,000	Tryp.	Has tryptophan	16,40
	"Acetone insol."	4.2	24,000	Tryp., chym.	No tryptophan	41
	STI A$_1$	4.5	14,300	Tryp.	–	42
	STI A$_2$[c]		21,600	Tryp.	–	42
	1.9 S inhibitor	4.0	16,400	Tryp., chym.	High cystine, no glycine	43
	F$_1$	–	–	Tryp., chym.	Has tryptophan	44
	F$_2$	–	–	Tryp., chym.	Has tryptophan	44
	F$_3$	–	–	Tryp.	Has tryptophan, no tyrosine	44
Lima bean	–	3.6	10,000	Tryp., chym.	Resolved into 4 comp; strongly inhibits human trypsin[a]	15,45–47
Navy bean	–	–	23,000	Tryp.	No data for chym.	48
Pea (black-eyed)	–	–	17,000	Tryp., chym.	–	49
Potato	1	–	38,000	Tryp., chym., *B. subtilis* proteinase, *S. griseus* proteinase, carboxypeptidase B	Tryp. only inhibited with casein as substrate	50–52

[a] Tryp. and chym. refer to bovine trypsin and bovine chymotrypsin, respectively. Chicken ovomucoid and nine other ovomucoids tested do not inhibit human trypsin. Japanese quail ovomucoid, lima bean inhibitor, bovine colostrum inhibitor, and bovine Kunitz pancreatic inhibitor are good inhibitors of human trypsin[15] (adapted from Feeney and Allison[16]).

[b] The molecular weight obtained from trypsin inhibition studies is 39,000 g/mole, and 71,000 g/mole is the molecular weight obtained by sedimentation–diffusion studies. It has been suggested that the inhibitor may exist in solution as a dimer.

[c] The acetone-soluble inhibitor and the A$_2$ (STI$_2$) inhibitor of Rackis *et al.*[42] are both believed to be similar to Kunitz's soybean inhibitor.

281

tribution of trypsin-like enzymes, although the presence of the inhibitor of the enzyme in the same material does not necessarily follow. One of the characteristics evident from the data of Table 1 is that the structures and properties of inhibitors of trypsin vary widely. In addition to the property of inhibiting trypsin, they also share a resistance to proteolysis and frequently are relatively resistant to other environmental factors such as heat. The total structure of the bovine Kunitz pancreatic inhibitor (one of the smallest of the inhibitors) has recently been reported.[53] With the information available on both the primary sequence and the x-ray crystallographic structure, investigators are now in a position to plan more precise studies on the structural interactions between this inhibitor and trypsin.

Studies during the past decade have clearly demonstrated the importance of determining the activities of trypsin inhibitors (as well as inhibitors of other enzymes) against homologous trypsins from different species. In a preliminary report[54] it was shown that whereas soybean trypsin inhibitor inhibited bovine, porcine, ovine, and human trypsin, chicken ovomucoid inhibited only the trypsin of the first three species and did not inhibit human trypsin. Feeney and co-workers[15] studied this in more detail and reported that human trypsin was strongly inhibited by three apparently unrelated inhibitors—lima-bean trypsin inhibitor, bovine colostrum inhibitor, and bovine Kunitz pancreatic inhibitor—and inhibited to lesser degrees by Kunitz soybean inhibitor, soybean inhibitor AA, kidney-bean inhibitor, blackeyed-bean inhibitor, navy-bean inhibitor, and quail (*Coturnix coturnix*) ovomucoid. However, human trypsin was essentially uninhibited by bovine Kazal pancreatic inhibitor, porcine Kazal pancreatic inhibitor, potato inhibitor, chicken ovoinhibitor, and 10 avian ovomucoids, including chicken ovomucoid. Many of these latter inhibitors strongly inhibited bovine trypsin. Thus, it was clearly demonstrated that the inhibition of bovine trypsin by naturally occurring inhibitors is no index of activity against human trypsin.

Chymotrypsin Inhibitors

For some strange reason the testing of inhibitors of proteolytic enzymes against the readily available bovine α-chymotrypsin was not done for many years. Two earlier studies showed that some inhibitors are strongly inhibitory for bovine α-chymotrypsin. One inhibitor was from the parasitic worm *Ascaris lumbricoides* var. *suis*,[39] and the other from avian egg whites (e.g., golden pheasant ovomucoid[23]). Many inhibitors were then shown to have activity against α-chymotrypsin as well as trypsin. Some of the inhibitors are "double-headed" and inhibit trypsin and chymotrypsin simultaneously. In many instances, the inhibitory sites appear to be independent and nonoverlapping, that is, the inhibitors inhibit trypsin and α-chymotrypsin independently or simultaneously, but the inhibition of one enzyme does not affect the simultaneous inhibition of the other enzyme.[16] In some cases, multiple binding sites for chymotrypsin have been observed. One such example is the potato inhibitor, which apparently can bind and inhibit up to four molecules of chymotrypsin per molecule of inhibitor.[50,51] Only very recently have studies been made of the inhibition of human chymotrypsin by protein inhibitors.[55] Lima-bean trypsin inhibitor completely inhibited the proteolytic activity of both human trypsin and human chymotrypsin. These human enzymes were, however, only partially inhibited even at very high concentrations of soybean trypsin inhibitor, Kunitz pancreatic trypsin inhibitor, and by chicken ovomucoid.

Subtilisin Inhibitors

A report on inhibition of subtilisin, a proteolytic enzyme of *Bacillus subtilis*, by chicken ovoinhibitor[56] was the first well-documented example of protein inhibitors of this enzyme. The great similarity between subtilisin and bovine α-chymotrypsin is shown by their competition for the same interacting sites on all the inhibitors so far studied.[16,57]

Different inhibitors vary a great deal in their relative inhibitory activities against bovine α-chymotrypsin and subtilisin. In some cases, as with turkey ovomucoid, the activity against α-chymotrypsin is greater than against subtilisin, while in others (such as penguin ovomucoid) the activity against subtilisin is much greater than against chymotrypsin.

Elastase Inhibitors

A small protein of molecular weight about 10,000 that is stable at 90 °C at pH 2 and to pepsin treatment has been isolated from kidney beans.[58] It forms a 1:1 enzyme–inhibitor complex with bovine trypsin, with pancreatic elastase, and at low concentration with human plasmin and bovine chymotrypsin. The inhibitor has separate binding sites for trypsin and chymotrypsin. The protein has no effect on pepsin, on papain, or on carboxypeptidase A; however, it decreases the activity of carboxypeptidase B and thrombin slightly. Soybean trypsin inhibitor and bovine lung kallikrein were reported to strongly inhibit the proteolytic activity of elastase on casein, hemoglobin, and fibrin, but they were without effect on its elastolytic properties.[59] The inhibition of porcine elastase by soybean trypsin inhibitor has been confirmed; however, it was found that some tyrosinate-splitting enzymes associated with purified elastase are inhibited more strongly.[60] In view of the marked homology between trypsin and elastase, it is not surprising that both enzymes should be inhibited by the same protein.

Plasmin Inhibitors

Plasmin is inhibited by proteins from blood serum,[61] kidney bean,[15,58] lima bean,[15,62] and soybean[15,61] and by tissue kallikrein inhibitor[63] and pancreatic inhibitor.[15,61] It is significant that all of these inhibitors also inhibit trypsin. The fraction of human serum designated as C'1 esterase inhibitor has also been found to inhibit plasmin.[64] C'1 esterase inhibitor is antigenically identical with α_2-neuraminoglycoprotein.[65]

Kallikrein Inhibitors

Tissue kallikrein inhibitor, particularly from bovine lung (Trasylol), is well known.[63] The inhibitor from bovine lung has a strong action on hog pancreatic kallikrein, human plasmin, and bovine trypsin and a slight activity on human plasma kallikrein. C'1 esterase inhibitor of human serum also decreases kallikrein activity.[64] Two types of kallikrein inhibitors from potatoes have been isolated[66]; both have molecular weights of about 25,000. They are readily soluble in neutral salt and are unstable on heating. The inhibitors differ in having isoelectric points of 5.6 and 6.4. The purified compounds inhibited human plasma kallikrein strongly; hog pancreatic kallikrein and human plasmin only slightly; and bovine trypsin and chymotrypsin very slightly. They did not inhibit *Seratia* protease, pronase-P, pepsin, and papain. The inhibitors were present in 16 kinds of Japanese potatoes and 22 other kinds in amounts from 60 to 190 kallikrein inhibitor units per g potato. They were shown to be different from potato chymotrypsin inhibitor I.[51]

Papain Inhibitors

Proteins that inhibit papain have been reported in soybeans,[67,68] haricot beans,[68] garden peas,[68] broad beans,[68] wheat flours,[69] egg white,[22] and various blood sera.[61,63] The inhibitor in soybeans is water soluble, and heat labile and is concentrated almost totally in the germ. The protein of wheat flour inhibits activity of papain and ficin; it is water soluble and nondialyzable. It is found in all grades of flours and in higher concentration in wheat bran. The egg-white papain inhibitor also inhibits ficin. It is a protein of molecular weight 12,000 and is different from ovomucoid and ovoinhibitor (see above). Blood sera have very weak inhibitory activity on papain and ficin,[70] which are not found in man; however, enzymes with similar properties may be present in organisms of the intestinal flora.

NUTRITIONAL AND TOXICOLOGICAL EFFECTS OF PROTEOLYTIC ENZYME INHIBITORS

It has been recognized for many years that a ration containing raw soybeans inhibits growth in rats, chicks, and some other monogastric animals. The obvious implication is that the soybean inhibitors of proteolytic enzymes are responsible for this effect. Unfortunately, much of the data in the older literature must now be reassessed because no consideration was given to the effects on α-chymotrypsin as well as on trypsin. In addition, the many studies on the effect of chicken egg white in humans must be reconsidered in the light of the observation that the principal inhibitor in egg white, ovomucoid, does not inhibit human trypsin.[15] Nevertheless, the nutritional studies with laboratory and farm animals indicate relationships between the presence of the soybean inhibitor and growth-retardation effects.

Soybean trypsin inhibitor enhances the formation or the release of a humoral pancreozymic-like substance that markedly stimulates external secretion of the rat pancreas.[71] When the plasma from rats that were fed soybean trypsin inhibitor was perfused through an isolated rat pancreas, amylase secretion was increased two to three times that of a pancreas perfused with plasma from rats fed the same diet without the trypsin inhibitor. Hyperplasia of some of the pancreatic cells occurs as a result of feeding trypsin inhibitors. In studies of the adaptive effects of exocrine pancreatic enzymes of rats fed soybean flour, it was found that the pancreases of rats that were fed diets containing unheated soybean flour contained less amylase and similar amounts of lipase and esterase but more trypsinogen and chymotrypsinogen than the pancreases of rats fed heated soybean flour.[72] Pancreatic enlargement has also been observed when the low-molecular-weight trypsin inhibitor p-aminobenzamidine is fed.[73] However, there apparently is not always a correlation between the hypertrophy of the pancreas and the inhibition of growth. Some investigators believe that, at least insofar as growth retardation is concerned, the effect is primarily a nutritional one and is caused by unavailability of amino acids. It has been suggested that in the case of navy beans there is a disproportionately high amount of cystine in the trypsin inhibitor and that the poor digestibility of the inhibitor leads to a deficiency in cystine.[74]

Unfortunately, in spite of the extensive research activity and the apparent excellence of some of the investigations, the answer to this important problem is still not clear.

MECHANISM OF INHIBITION OF PROTEOLYTIC ENZYMES

There currently appears to be general agreement among investigators that:

1. Inhibitors of proteolytic enzymes form strong complexes with the enzymes they inhibit.
2. The enzyme and inhibitor undergo some type of enzyme–substrate interaction.
3. The inhibitors are resistant to proteolysis, although some peptide-bond splitting may occur in the interaction.

Small but important differences in interpretations as to the relative importance of various of the events exist, however.

One of the earlier insights into the specificity and mechanism of action of inhibitors was gained through the work of Fraenkel-Conrat and co-workers,[45] who showed that the amino groups of the lima-bean trypsin inhibitor were important for inhibitory action against bovine trypsin. This was the forerunner of the many later observations on the essentiality of either the ϵ-amino group of lysine or the guanidino group of arginine for inhibition of trypsin by all trypsin inhibitors studied.[16,57] Workers in Nord's laboratory[75] suggested the possibility of an enzyme–substrate interaction between chicken ovomucoid and bovine trypsin. These workers stated that "a substrate which is acted upon only very slowly but forms a stable enzyme–substrate complex will, therefore, act as an inhibitor." Ozawa and Laskowski have shown that peptide-bond splitting may occur at specific sites in the inhibitor, which they named "reactive sites."[76] These same workers suggested that proteolytic action of the enzyme is essential for inhibition to occur, and many laboratories have confirmed the hydrolysis of specific bonds in the complex.[77] However, workers in other laboratories have shown that competitive complexes may be formed between the inhibitor and inactive derivatives of trypsin, of chymotrypsin, and subtilisin,[78,79] and of papain.[22] From these and other studies, it can be concluded that the enzyme and inhibitors definitely interact in a manner suggestive of an enzyme–substrate complex, but the interaction stops at some stage, leaving the enzyme still bound to the inhibitor. Model building allows for seven hydrogen bonds and about 200 Van der Waals contacts in the complex of bovine pancreatic trypsin inhibitor and bovine trypsin or α-chymotrypsin.[80] Such numerous noncovalent forces should be sufficient to form a strongly associated complex, but the formation of the inhibitor enzyme covalent bond is still possible. The resolution of this problem most likely will be best done by further model building and x-ray studies.

PROTEIN INHIBITORS OF OTHER ENZYMES

Amylase Inhibitors

Protein inhibitors of various amylases have been reported in wheat,[81,82] beans (*Phaseolus vulgaris*),[83-85] taro root (*Colocasia esculenta*),[86] unripe mangoes,[87] unripe bananas,[87] and leaves of rice plants infected with *Helminthosporium oryzae*.[88] The inhibitor from wheat was found in similar amounts in all 13 varieties examined but was not found in barley (5 varieties), maize (5 varieties), oats, millet, rice, and 6 varieties of sorghum. Two samples of rye gave about 60% the reduction in amylase activity found for an equivalent amount of wheat protein. The protein from wheat, purified some 750-fold, was precipitated by protein precipitants, and was nondialyzable; it was inactivated by nitrous acid or by digestion with ficin and pepsin and was readily denatured at 95 °C in 10–15 min at alkaline pH. However, it was more stable at acid pH.[82] It had maximal inhibitory action on salivary α-amylase and less on pancreatic α-amylase and certain bacterial amylases, but it did not inhibit all bacterial amylases nor β-amylase. It is stable during the baking of bread.

Pancreatic amylase inhibitor from beans was destroyed by heating at 100 °C for 15 min; it was nondialyzable and was not retarded on Sephadex G-75.[85] The feeding of white-bean or tapiramo-bean diets to rats gave copious light-colored feces containing undigested starch. On autopsy the rats had bloated, white intestines.[84] It is not clear that the abnormal conditions were caused by the α-amylase inhibitor. The inhibitor from taro roots was nondialyzable and stable at boiling temperatures; it was precipitated by the usual protein precipitants. It strongly inhibited salivary α-amylase but had no activity on pancreatic amylase, soybean β-amylase, taka diastase, and bacterial α-amylase.[86] The inhibitors from unripe mangoes and bananas were heat-labile nondialyzable proteins.[87]

Invertase Inhibitors

A protein of molecular weight 17,000, purified 1,000-fold from potatoes, inhibited potato invertase and a great variety of other plant invertases but not yeast, *Neurospora*, weeping birch, tulip, and sunflower invertases.[89] Action of the inhibitor on human invertase has not been studied. The inhibitor was rapidly inactivated by foaming, by heating above 50 °C and by storage overnight at pH 7 and 3 °C. It was quite stable at pH 4.5 and 3 °C.[90] The *in vivo* function of the inhibitor appears to be a regulation of invertase activity. It increases severalfold in concentration in potatoes stored at room temperature and decreases at cooler temperatures.[91,92] Combination of inhibitor with invertase is pH dependent with maximum binding occurring at the pH optimum of invertase. This results in a double pH optimum for invertase in the presence of inhibitor.[90,93] Because of the heat lability of the inhibitor it is unlikely that it is nutritionally important in cooked potatoes. A protein inhibitor of invertase has also been reported in artichoke tubers and carrot roots.[94]

Peroxidase and Catalase Inhibitors

Most of the reported inhibitors have activity against hydrolases, but two oxidative enzyme inhibitors have been reported. A peroxidase inhibitor was purified approximately 300-fold from green mangoes and was shown to be a heat-labile, nondialyzable protein.[87] It was stable at 0 °C but lost most of its activity at 30 °C in 12 h. It formed a reversible complex with peroxidase with a K_i of 1.1×10^{-7} M. A similar inhibitor was reported in green bananas.[87] A catalase inhibitor was also reported in green mangoes and green bananas.[87]

NONPROTEIN INHIBITORS

Cholinesterase Inhibitors

The most intensively studied naturally occurring nonprotein enzyme inhibitors are those with activity against acetylcholinesterase. Orgell has studied the effect of aqueous extracts of 256 plant species on human plasma cholinesterase.[95] Among the list were 17 edible vegetables and fruits. The most potent cholinesterase inhibitors, as measured *in vitro*, are found in the potato family (*Solanaceae*), although some activity has been found in the fruits of the apple and eggplant, in the roots and leaves of tomatoes, and in the roots of sugar beets. Many other nonfood plants contain cholinesterase inhibitors, including petunia, boxwood, periwinkle, and poppy. The most potent inhibitor of all is physostigmine from the West African calabar bean. The carbamate insecticides are modeled after this compound.

Several cases of poisoning, and even death, on eating potatoes (*Solanum tuberosum*) have been reported.[96,97] There are several glycoalkaloids in potatoes that may, in combination, lead to the toxicity of certain batches of potatoes. Most workers have analyzed toxicity on the basis of the alkaloid solanine (present in the greatest amount), although there is a poor correlation between the anticholinesterase activity of potatoes and the solanine content.[98] Nishie *et al.* found that, despite *in vivo* anticholinesterase activity, little cholinergic effect was found on injection of solanine into rabbits.[99] The normal range of solanine in potatoes is 2–13 mg/100 g fresh weight,[100] although the bulk of market potatoes contain 3–6 mg/100 g fresh weight. In certain isolated cases the solanine concentration may increase to as high as 80–100 mg/ 100 g fresh weight as in "greening" in smaller tubers (since solanine is concentrated in the skin) or in certain experimental varieties. For example, the experimental variety Lenape was found to have excellent solids content and chipping properties[101] but was unacceptable because of an unusually high total glycoalkaloid content.[102] Because of this recent varietal problem, all existing and newly developed varieties of potatoes are now monitored for alkaloid content. It is generally accepted that 20 mg/ 100 g fresh weight of solanine is the upper limit of safety for food.[103-105] Solanine, being water insoluble and stable, is not lost or destroyed when potatoes are cooked.

The clinical symptoms described for the isolated cases of potato poisoning in man and farm animals generally involve gastrointestinal disturbances and certain neurological disorders.[96,105-107] A semicomatose state has been observed to precede death caused by solanine poisoning.[96] Solanine also has saponin-like properties that cause hemolytic and hemorrhagic damage to the gastrointestinal tract.[108]

Sensitivity to solanine varies considerably among animals. In humans an oral dose of 200 mg (approximately 2.8 mg/kg body weight) caused drowsiness, hyperesthesia, and dyspnea, while higher doses caused vomiting and diarrhea.[109] Oral doses of 225 mg/kg of solanine given to sheep had no lethal effects but did produce blood dyscrasias.[108] In rats the oral LD_{50} was reported to be 590 mg/kg of solanine[108]; in mice 1,000 mg/kg of solanine given orally had no effect.[99]

The method of administering solanine has a pronounced effect on its toxicity. It is relatively nontoxic when given orally because of (1) its poor absorption from the gastrointestinal tract as shown by low blood levels, (2) the rapid (within 12 h) fecal and urinary excretion of most of the ingested solanine, and (3) hydrolysis of solanine in the gastrointestinal tract to the less toxic and very poorly absorbed solanidine.[99] As a result of rapid excretion, solanine does not accumulate in the body. In contrast to low oral toxicity, the Intraperitoneal (IP) LD_{50} was reported to be 75 mg/kg of solanine in rats[110] and 42 mg/kg in mice.[99] The aglycone, solanidine, was nontoxic to mice when given IP at a dose level of 500 mg/kg.[99] An IP dose of 20 mg/kg of solanine caused death in a rabbit overnight, while 30 mg/kg caused death in 6¼ h. When given intravenously, 10 mg/kg of solanine caused death in a rabbit in 2 min.[99] The LD_{50} value of solanine in chick embryos was reported to be 18.8 mg/kg.[99]

Solanine has some effect on the nervous system of animals, although, in general, its effect is of low level[99] compared with other anticholinesterase compounds. In mice, at a level of 10 mg/kg of solanine given IP, there was approximately a twofold reduction in spontaneous motor activity, and at 20 mg/kg IP there was approximately a 50% increase in the pentobarbital sleeping time. Dose levels of 50 and 100 µg/ml of solanine were comparable to 0.005 and 0.01 µg/ml of acetylcholine in causing contraction in guinea pig ileum strips. This is considerably less anticholinesterase activity than reported for *in vitro* studies on solanine.[95] In unanesthetized rabbits solanine, at levels of 15–30 mg/kg given intraperitoneally, produced tachycardia, initial tachypnea, and terminal bradypnea.[99] There was an initial slight activation of the EEG followed by delta waves associated with bradypnea and cyanosis.[99]

The toxic lipid-like fractions from several fish species[111] have a low anticholinesterase activity *in vitro.* Presently it is thought that the effect of these fractions on cholinesterase activity *in vivo* is not important.

Amylase Inhibitors

A substance extracted from Leoti sorghum grain has been reported to inhibit many amylases, including β-amylase.[112] Cereal amylases are most sensitive to the inhibitor, while fungal amylases are least sensitive. The compound, which disappears when sorghum is germinated, is precipitated from basic but not acidic solution by acetone, ethanol, isopropyl alcohol, or calcium chloride. It is stable in 1 M HCl and 1 M NaOH and to autoclaving at pH 2.9 or 10.5 for 30 min at 15 lb/in^2. It appears to be a high molecular weight organic acid that differs from the amylase inhibitor from Kafir bran, kafiroic acid.[112,113] This inhibitor, effective against salivary and pancreatic amylases, is inactivated by water extracts of cereals, presumably because of its combination with starch, and may not be of dietary significance.

An ether-soluble fraction extracted from navy beans inhibits starch digestion by pancreatic amylase,[5] presumably by rendering the substrate inaccessible to the enzyme.

Liver Nicotinamide Deamidase Inhibitor

The endogenous inhibitor of liver nicotinamide deamidase has been isolated and shown to be a mixture of free fatty acids, predominately oleic, linoleic, and arachidonic.[11] The fatty acids are effective at about 2 μM. It is postulated that the regulation of NAD synthesis from nicotinamide is regulated by hormonal control of levels of free fatty acids, which in turn affect activity of the enzyme nicotinamide deamidase.

Phosphoglucomutase Inhibitor

A dialyzable potato phosphoglucomutase inhibitor, soluble in water, benzene, chloroform, and diethyl ether, has been reported in onion bulbs.[114] The inhibitor had no effect on potato starch phosphorylase. The dietary significance, if any, of this inhibitor has not been determined.

Oxidative Phosphorylation Inhibitor

Consumption of the thistle (*Atractylis gumnifera*) of North Africa and the Mediterranean area each year causes several cases of serious toxicity and sometimes death in man and animals. The active compound is atractyloside, a sulfated glucoside usually isolated as the dipotassium salt,

Potassium Atractylate

potassium atractylate.[115,116] The compound interferes with oxidative phosphorylation[117,118] by inhibiting the ADP–ATP carrier responsible for transporting these nucleotides across the mitochondrial membrane.[119] Bongkrek acid (see Chapter 20) acts similarly. It is probable that atractyloside is an artifact of isolation and the active substance in the plant is gumniferin,[116] a carboxy atractyloside.[120]

Soybean Saponins

Soybean and alfalfa saponins inhibit α-chymotrypsin, proteases from the midgut of *Tribolium* larvae, and cholinesterase.[121,122] The inhibition is nonspecific and appears to be a general protein–saponin interaction. The most recent studies do not substantiate the original toxicity ascribed to these compounds.

Phenolic Compounds

The majority of plant phenolic compounds either have no inhibitory properties on enzymes or have only a low level of inhibition. Tannins and other plant phenolics (see Chapter 15) form precipitates with proteins, and there is some evidence that this retards proteolysis in the small intestine.

At a concentration of 0.1 mM, phloretin (see Chapter 15) was found to produce 63% inhibition of ATPase activity in isolated mitochondrial membranes from rat kidney cortex.[123]

REFERENCES

1. H. C. Fox and D. S. Miller, Ackee toxin: A riboflavin antimetabolite. Nature *186*:561 (1960).
2. H. J. Klosterman, G. L. Lamoureux, and J. L. Parsons, Isolation, characterization and synthesis of linatine. A. Vitamin B_6 antagonist from flaxseed (*Linum usitatissimum*). Biochemistry *6*:170 (1967).
3. B. Belavady and C. Gopalan, Production of black tongue in dogs by feeding diets containing jowar (*Sorghum vulgare*). Lancet *2*:1220 (1965).
4. G. C. Collentine and A. J. Quick, The interrelationship of vitamin K and dicoumarin. Am. J. Med. Sci. *222*:7 (1951).
5. D. E. Bowman, The ether soluble fraction of navy beans and the digestion of starch. Science *98*:308 (1943).
6. D. E. Bowman, Amylase inhibitor of navy beans. Science *102*:358 (1945).
7. V. Schwartz, L. Goldberg, G. M. Kommower, and A. Holzel, Some disturbances of erythocyte metabolism. Biochem. J. *62*:34 (1956).
8. J. Mager, A. Razin, and A. Hershko, Favism, p. 293. In Toxic constituents of plant foodstuffs, I. E. Liener (ed.). Academic Press, New York (1969).

9. W. E. C. Wacker and T. L. Coombs, Clinical biochemistry: Enzymatic methods: Automation and atomic absorption spectroscopy. Ann. Rev. Biochem. *38*:539 (1969).

10. M. A. Brostrom, E. M. Reimann, D. A. Walsh, and E. G. Krebs, A cyclic 3',5'-AMP-stimulated protein kinase from cardiac muscle, p. 191. In Advances in enzyme regulation, Vol. 8, G. Weber (ed.). Pergamon Press, New York (1970).

11. P. Greengard, B. Petrack, and H. J. Kalinsky, Identification of hormonally controlled endogenous inhibitor of liver nicotinamide deamidase. Biochim. Biophys. Acta *184*:148 (1969).

12. J. K. Newman, G. S. Berenson, M. B. Mathews, E. Goldwasser, and A. Dorfman, The isolation of the non-specific hyaluronidase inhibitor of human blood. J. Biol. Chem. *217*:31 (1955).

13. M. B. Mathews and A. Dorfman, Inhibition of hyaluronidase. Physiol. Rev. *35*:396 (1955).

14. B. Blackwell and E. Marley, Interactions of cheese and its constituents with monoamine oxidase inhibitors. Br. J. Pharmacol. Chemother. *26*:120 (1966).

15. R. E. Feeney, G. E. Means, and J. C. Bigler, Inhibition of human trypsin, plasmin, and thrombin by naturally occurring inhibitors of proteolytic enzymes. J. Biol. Chem. *244*:1957 (1969).

16. R. E. Feeney and R. G. Allison, Evolutionary biochemistry of proteins. Homologous and analogous proteins from avian egg whites, blood sera, milk, and other substances, Wiley–Interscience, New York (1969).

17. H. Fritz and H. Tschesche (ed.), Proceedings of the First International Research Conference on Proteinase Inhibitors. Institut für Klinische Chemie und Klinische Biochemie der Universität München, Munich, Germany. Walter de Gruyter, New York (1971).

18. M. Bier, L. Terminiello, J. A. Duke, R. J. Gibbs, and F. F. Nord, Investigations on proteins and polymers. X. Composition and fractionation of ovomucoid. Arch. Biochem. Biophys. *47*:465 (1953).

19. E. Fredericq and H. F. Deutsch, Studies on ovomucoid. J. Biol. Chem. *181*:499 (1949).

20. H. F. Deutsch and J. I. Morton, Physical–chemical studies of some modified ovomucoids. Arch. Biochem. Biophys. *93*:654 (1961).

21. Y. Tomimatsu, J. J. Clary, and J. J. Bartulovich, Physical characterization of ovoinhibitor, a trypsin and chymotrypsin inhibitor from chicken egg white. Arch. Biochem. Biophys. *115*:536 (1966).

22. K. Fossum and J. R. Whitaker, Ficin and papain inhibitor from chicken egg white. Arch. Biochem. Biophys. *125*:536 (1968).

23. M. B. Rhodes, N. Bennett, and R. E. Feeney, The trypsin and chymotrypsin inhibitors from avian egg whites. J. Biol. Chem. *235*:1686 (1960).

24. D. T. Osuga and R. E. Feeney, Biochemistry of the egg-white protein of the ratite group. Arch. Biochem. Biophys. *124*:560 (1968).

25. J. C. Bigler and R. E. Feeney, Properties of penguin ovomucoid. (Manuscript in preparation).

26. B. Kassell, M. Radicevic, S. Berlow, R. J. Peanasky, and M. Laskowski, Sr., The basic trypsin inhibitor of bovine pancreas. I. An improved method of preparation and amino acid composition. J. Biol. Chem. *238*:3274 (1963).

27. B. Kassell and R. B. Chow, Modification of the basic trypsin inhibitor of bovine pancreas. The ϵ-amino groups of lysine and the amino-terminal sequence. Biochemistry *5*:3449 (1966).

28. L. J. Greene, M. Rigbi, and D. S. Fackre, Trypsin inhibitor from bovine pancreatic juice. J. Biol. Chem. *241*:5610 (1966).
29. L. J. Greene, J. J. DiCarlo, A. J. Sussman, and D. C. Bartelt, Two trypsin inhibitors from porcine pancreatic juice. J. Biol. Chem. *243*:1804 (1968).
30. E. W. Cerwinsky, P. J. Burck, and E. L. Grinnan, Acidic bovine pancreatic trypsin inhibitor. I. Purification and physical characterization. Biochemistry *6*:3175 (1967).
31. F. C. Moll, S. F. Sunden, and J. R. Brown, Partial purification of the serum trypsin inhibitor. J. Biol. Chem. *233*:121 (1958).
32. H. F. Bundy and J. W. Mehl, Trypsin inhibitors of human serum. II. Isolation of the α_1-inhibitor and its partial characterization. J. Biol. Chem. *234*:1124 (1959).
33. N. R. Shulman, A proteolytic inhibitor with anticoagulant activity separated from human urine and plasma. J. Biol. Chem. *213*:655 (1955).
34. F. C. Wu and M. Laskowski, Crystalline acid labile trypsin inhibitor from bovine blood plasma. J. Biol. Chem. *235*:1680 (1960).
35. C. J. Martin, Inhibition of trypsin, chymotrypsin, and plasmin by an inhibitor isolated from sheep serum. J. Biol. Chem. *237*:2099 (1962).
36. R. Haynes, D. T. Osuga, and R. E. Feeney, Modification of amino groups in inhibitors of proteolytic enzymes. Biochemistry *6*:541 (1967).
37. M. Laskowski, Jr., P. H. Mars, and M. Laskowski, Comparison of trypsin inhibitor from colostrum with other crystalline trypsin inhibitors. J. Biol. Chem. *198*:745 (1952).
38. M. Laskowski, B. Kassell, and G. Hagerty, A crystalline trypsin inhibitor from swine colostrum. Biochim. Biophys. Acta *24*:300 (1957).
39. J. Pudles, F. H. Rola, and A. K. Matida, Studies on the proteolytic inhibitors from *Ascaris lumbricoides* var. *suis*. II. Purification, properties, and chemical modification of the trypsin inhibitor. Arch. Biochem. Biophys. *120*:594 (1967).
40. Y. V. Wu and H. A. Scheraga, Studies on soybean trypsin inhibitor. I. Physicochemical properties. Biochemistry *1*:698 (1962).
41. Y. Birk, A. Gertler, and S. Khalef, A pure trypsin inhibitor from soya beans. Biochem. J. *87*:281 (1963).
42. J. J. Rackis, H. A. Sasame, R. K. Mann, R. L. Anderson, and A. K. Smith, Soybean trypsin inhibitors: Isolation, purification, and physical properties. Arch. Biochem. Biophys. *98*:471 (1962).
43. M. Yamamoto and T. Ikenaka, Studies on soybean trypsin inhibitors. I. Purification and characterization of two soybean trypsin inhibitors. J. Biochem. *62*:141 (1967).
44. V. Frattali and R. F. Steiner, Soybean inhibitors. I. Separation and some properties of three inhibitors from commercial crude soybean trypsin inhibitor. Biochemistry *7*:521 (1968).
45. H. Fraenkel-Conrat, R. C. Bean, E. D. Ducay, and H. S. Olcott, Isolation and characterization of a trypsin inhibitor from lima beans. Arch. Biochem. Biophys. *37*:393 (1952).
46. G. Jones, S. Moore, and W. H. Stein. Properties of chromatographically purified trypsin inhibitors from lima beans. Biochemistry *2*:66 (1963).
47. R. Haynes and R. E. Feeney, Fractionation and properties of trypsin and chymotrypsin inhibitors from lima beans. J. Biol. Chem. *242*:5378 (1967).
48. L. P. Wagner and J. P. Riehm, Purification and partial characterization of a

trypsin inhibitor isolated from the navy bean. Arch. Biochem. Biophys. *121*: 672 (1967).

49. M. M. Ventura and J. X. Filho, A trypsin and chymotrypsin inhibitor from black-eyed pea. I. Purification and partial characterization. Acad. Bras. Cienc. Anais *38*:553 (1966).
50. A. K. Balls and C. A. Ryan, Concerning a crystalline chymotryptic inhibitor from potatoes, and its binding capacity for the enzyme. J. Biol. Chem. *238*: 2976 (1963).
51. C. A. Ryan, Chymotrypsin inhibitor I from potatoes: Reactivity with mammalian, plant, bacterial, and fungal proteinases. Biochemistry *5*:1592 (1966).
52. C. A. Ryan, Personal communication (1968).
53. R. Huber, D. Kukla, A. Ruhlmann, O. Epp, and H. Formanek, The basic trypsin inhibitor of bovine pancreas. I. Structure analysis and conformation of the polypeptide chain. Naturwissenschaften *57*:389 (1970).
54. F. F. Buck, M. Bier, and F. F. Nord, Some properties of human trypsin. Arch. Biochem. Biophys. *98*:528 (1962).
55. M. H. Coan and J. Travis, Interaction of human pancreatic proteinases with naturally occurring proteinase inhibitors, p. 294. In Proceedings of the International Research Conference on Proteinase Inhibitors, H. Fritz and H. Tschesche (eds.). Institut für Klinische Chemie und Klinische Biochemie der Universität München. Walter de Gruyter, New York (1971).
56. K. Matsushima, An undescribed trypsin inhibitor in egg white. Science *127*: 1178 (1958).
57. W. H. Liu, G. E. Means, and R. E. Feeney, The inhibitory properties of avian ovoinhibitors against proteolytic enzymes. Biochim. Biophys. Acta *229*:176 (1971).
58. A. Pusztai, General properties of a protein inhibitor from the seeds of kidney bean. Eur. J. Biochem. *5*:252 (1968).
59. R. L. Walford and B. Kickhöfen, Selective inhibition of elastolytic and proteolytic properties of elastase. Arch. Biochem. Biophys. *98*:191 (1962).
60. T. H. Marshall, J. R. Whitaker, and M. L. Bender, Porcine elastase. II. Properties of the tyrosinate-splitting enzyme and the specificity of elastase. Biochemistry *8*:4671 (1969).
61. D. Grob, Proteolytic enzymes. III. Further studies on protein, polypeptide and other inhibitors of serum proteinase, leucoproteinase, trypsin and papain. J. Gen. Physiol. *33*:103 (1949).
62. J. H. Lewis and J. H. Ferguson, The inhibition of fibrinolysin by lima bean inhibitor. J. Biol. Chem. *204*:503 (1953).
63. N. Back and R. Steger, Effect of inhibitors on kinin-releasing activity of proteases. Fed. Proc. *27*:96 (1968).
64. O. D. Ratnoff, J. Pensky, D. Ogston, and G. B. NAff, Inhibition of plasmin, plasma kallikrein, plasma permeability factor and the $C'1r$ subcomponent of the first component of complement by serum $C'1$ esterase inhibitor. J. Exp. Med. *129*:315 (1969).
65. J. Pensky, H. Schwick, and H. Gerhard, Human serum inhibitor of $C'1$ esterase: Identity with α_2-neuraminoglycoprotein. Science *163*:698 (1969).
66. H. Moriya, Y. Hojima, C. Moriwaki, and T. Tajima, Specificity of potato kallikrein inhibitors for kalibreins. Experientia *26*:720 (1970).
67. E. M. Learmonth, The influence of soya flour on bread doughs. I. A papain-inhibiting fraction in soya beans. J. Sci. Food Agric. *2*:447 (1951).

68. E. M. Learmonth, The influence of soya flour on bread doughs. III. The distribution of the papain-inhibiting factor in soya beans. J. Sci. Food Agric. *9*: 269 (1958).
69. B. D. Hites, R. M. Sandstedt, and L. Schaumburg, Study of proteolytic activity in wheat flour doughs and suspensions. II. A papain inhibitor in flour. Cereal Chem. *28*:1 (1951).
70. K. Fossum, personal communication.
71. H. Khayambashi and R. L. Lyman, Secretion of rat pancreas perfused with plasma from rats fed soybean trypsin inhibitor. Am. J. Physiol. *217*:646 (1969).
72. A. M. Konijn, Y. Birk, and K. Guggenheim, Pancreatic enzyme pattern in rats as affected by dietary soybean flour. J. Nutr. *100*:361 (1970).
73. J. D. Geratz and J. P. Hurt, Regulation of pancreatic enzyme levels by trypsin inhibitors. Am. J. Physiol. *219*:705 (1970).
74. M. L. Kakade, R. L. Arnold, I. E. Liener, and P. E. Waibel, Unavailability of cystine from trypsin inhibitors as a factor contributing to the poor nutritive value of navy beans. J. Nutr. *99*:34 (1969).
75. J. Sri Ram, L. Terminiello, M. Bier, and F. F. Nord, On the mechanism of enzyme action. LVII. Interaction between trypsin and ovomucoid. Arch. Biochem. Biophys. *52*:451 (1954).
76. K. Ozawa and M. Laskowski, Jr., The reactive site of trypsin inhibitors. J. Biol. Chem. *241*:3995 (1966).
77. M. Laskowski, Jr., R. W. Duran, W. R. Finkenstadt, S. Herbert, H. F. Hixson, Jr., D. Kowalski, J. A. Luthy, J. A. Mattis, R. E. McKee, and C. W. Niekamp, Kinetics and thermodynamics of interaction between soybean trypsin inhibitor (Kunitz) and bovine β trypsin, p. 117. In Proceedings of the International Research Conference on Proteinase Inhibitors, H. Fritz and H. Tschesche (eds.). Institut für Klinische Chemie und Klinische Biochemie der Universität München. Walter de Gruyter, New York (1971).
78. G. Feinstein and R. E. Feeney, Interaction of inactive derivatives of chymotrypsin and trypsin with protein inhibitors. J. Biol. Chem. *241*:5183 (1966).
79. R. J. Foster and C. A. Ryan, Reactions of potato inhibitor with modified chymotrypsin. Fed. Proc. *24*:473, Abstr. #999 (1968).
80. D. M. Blow, C. S. Wright, D. Kubla, A. Ruhlmann, W. Steigemann, R. Huber, A model for the association of bovine pancreatic trypsin inhibitor with chymotrypsin and trypsin. J. Mol. Biol. *69*:137 (1972).
81. E. Kneen and R. M. Sandstedt, Distribution and general properties of an amylase inhibitor in cereals. Arch. Biochem. *9*:235 (1946).
82. W. Militzer, C. Ikeda, and E. Kneen, The preparation and properties of an amylase inhibitor of wheat. Arch. Biochem. *9*:309 (1946).
83. D. E. Bowman, Amylase inhibitor in navy beans. Science *102*:358 (1945).
84. W. G. Jaffé and C. L. V. Lette, Heat-labile growth-inhibitory factors in beans. J. Nutr. *94*:203 (1968).
85. A. Hernandez and W. G. Jaffé, Inhibitor of pancreatic amylase from beans (*Phaseolus vulgaris*). Acta Cient. Venez. *19*:183 (1968).
86. M. Narayana Rao, K. S. Shurpalekar and O. E. Sundaravalli, An amylase inhibitor in *Colocasia esculenta*. Indian J. Biochem. *4*:185 (1967).
87. A. K. Mattoo and V. V. Modi, Partial purification and properties of enzyme inhibitors from unripe mangoes. Enzymologia *39*:237 (1970).
88. J. Shishiyama, T. Oguchi, and S. Akai, Biochemical properties of the protein

fractions in diseased leaves of rice plants in the early stages of *Helmintho-sporium oryzae* infection. Nippon Shokubutsu Byori Gakkaiko *34*:23 (1968); Chem. Abstr. *69*:57506y (1968).

89. R. Pressey, Invertase inhibitor from potatoes: Purification, characterization, and reactivity with plant invertases. Plant Physiol. *42*:1780 (1967).

90. R. Pressey, Separation and properties of plant invertase and invertase inhibitor. Arch. Biochem. Biophys. *113*:667 (1966).

91. S. Schwimmer, R. U. Makower, and E. S. Rorem, Invertase and invertase inhibitor in potato. Plant Physiol. *36*:313 (1961).

92. R. Pressey and R. Shaw, Effect of temperature on invertase, invertase inhibitor and sugars in potato tubers. Plant Physiol. *41*:1657 (1966).

93. E. S. Rorem and S. Schwimmer, Double pH optimum of potato invertase. Experientia *19*:150 (1963).

94. M. J. Bradshaw, J. M. Chapman, and J. Edelman, Enzyme formation in higher plant tissues. Protein inhibitor of invertase synthesis secreted by tissue slices of plant storage organs. Planta *90*:323 (1970).

95. W. H. Orgell, Inhibition of human plasma cholinesterase *in vitro* by alkaloids, glycosides, and other natural substances. Lloydia *26*:36 (1963).

96. S. G. Willimot, An investigation of solanine poisoning. Analyst *58*:431 (1933).

97. A. A. Hanson, Two fatal cases of potato poisoning. Science *61*:340 (1925).

98. D. C. Abbott, K. Field, and E. I. Johnson, Observations on the correlation of anticholinesterase effect with solanine content of potatoes. Analyst *85*:375 (1960).

99. K. Nishie, M. R. Gumbmann, and A. C. Keyl, Pharmacology of solanine Toxicol. Appl. Pharmacol. *19*:81 (1971).

100. M. J. Wolf and B. M. Duggar, Estimation and physiological role of solanine in the potato. J. Agric. Res. *73*:1 (1946).

101. R. V. Akeley, W. R. Mills, C. E. Cunningham, and J. Watts, Lenape: A new potato variety high in solids and chipping quality. Am. Potato J. *45*:142 (1968).

102. A. Zitnak and G. R. Johnson, Glycoalkaloid Content of B5141-6 Potatoes, Amer. Potato J. *47*:256 (1970).

103. A. Bömer and H. Mattis, The solanine content of potatoes. Z. Nahr. Genussm. *47*:97 (1924).

104. H. J. Oslage, Über das Solanin in der Kartoffel und seine Wirkung auf das Tier. Kartoffelbau *7*:204 (1956).

105. N. Sapeika, Food pharmacology, p. 67. Charles C Thomas, Springfield, Ill. (1969).

106. W. F. van Oettinger, Poisoning, p. 462. P. B. Hoeber–Harper and Brothers, New York (1952).

107. T. A. Gonzalez, M. Vance, and C. J. Umberger, Legal medicine pathology and toxicology, p. 868. Appleton Century Crofts, New York (1954).

108. H. König and A. Staffe, Beiträge zur Wirkung des Solanins auf Blutbild und Katalase beim Schaf. Dtsch. Tieraerztl. Wochenschr. *60*:150 (1953).

109. R. Rühl, Beitrag zur Pathologie und Toxikologie des Solanins. Arch. Pharm. *284*:67 (1951).

110. D. D. Gull, Chlorophyll and solanine changes in tubers of *Solanum tuberosum* induced by fluorescent light, and a study of solanine toxicology by bioassay technique, Diss. Abstr. *21*:2242 (1960).

111. A. H. Banner, P. Helfrick, P. J. Scheuer, and T. Yoshida, Research on Cigua-

tera in the tropical Pacific. Proc. Gulf Caribb. Fish Inst., 16th Ann. Sess., p. 84 (1963).

112. B. S. Miller and E. Kneen, The amylase inhibitor of Leoti sorghum. Arch. Biochem. Biophys. *15*:251 (1947).

113. L. L. Woods and C. W. Colver, The isolation of karifoic acid from Kafir bran. J. Am. Chem. Soc. *67*:653 (1945).

114. I. S. Bhatia and S. Singh, Effect of an inhibitor isolated from onion (*Allium cepa* Linn) bulbs on the activity of some enzymes involved in starch biosynthesis. Experientia *26*:1078 (1970).

115. F. Piozzi, A. Quilico, R. Mondelli, T. Ajello, Y. Spiro, and A. Melera. Stereochemistry of atractyligenin. Chem. Ind. (Milan) *48*:371 (1966).

116. P. V. Vignais, P. M. Vignais, and G. Defaye, Gumniferin, an inhibitor of the adenine nucleotide translocation. Its binding properties to mitchondria. Fed. Eur. Biochem. Soc. Lett., *17*:281 (1971).

117. P. V. Vignais, P. M. Vignais, and E. Stanilas, Action of potassium atractylate on oxidative phosphorylation in mitochondria and in submitochondrial particles. Biochim. Biophys. Acta *60*:284 (1962).

118. D. W. Allman, R. A. Harris, and D. E. Green, Site of action of atractyloside in mitochondria. II. Inhibitor of oxidative phosphorylation. Arch. Biochem. Biophys. *122*:766 (1967).

119. E. D. Duée and P. V. Vignais. Kinetics of phosphorylation of intramitochondrial and extramitochondrial adenine nucleotides as related to nucleotide translocation. J. Biol. Chem. *244*:3932 (1969).

120. G. Defaye, P. M. Vignais, and P. V. Vignais, Experimental evidence for the identity of gumniferin with carboxy atractyloside. C. R. Acad. Sci. Ser. D *273*:2671 (1971).

121. I. Ishaaga and Y. Birk, Soybean saponins. IV. The effect of proteins on the inhibitory activity of soybean saponins on certain enzymes. J. Food Sci. *30*: 118 (1965).

122. Y. Birk, Saponins, p. 169. In Toxic constituents of plant foodstuffs, I. E. Liener, (ed.). Academic Press, New York (1969).

123. M. T. Tellez de Inon, Inhibition of mitochondrial ATPase by phlorizin. Acta Physiol. Latinoam. *18*:268 (1968).

14 Eric E. Conn

CYANOGENETIC GLYCOSIDES*

The cyanogenetic glycosides are compounds that yield hydrogen cyanide (HCN) upon treatment with acid or appropriate hydrolytic enzymes. These compounds have a wide distribution among the higher plants, but they are also found in ferns, moths, and insects. More than 1,000 species of plants are reported to be cyanophoric; that is, HCN is released when tissues of the plant are crushed or otherwise disrupted. Although the production of HCN is usually attributed to the presence in the plant of one or more of the 20 known glycosides of α-hydroxynitriles (cyanohydrins), the parent glycoside has been positively identified in fewer than 50 species. The cyanogenetic glycosides have been the subject of recent reviews.[1,2]

Table 1 lists several of the more common cyanogenetic glycosides, some plants in which they occur, and the products formed on hydrolysis. The well-known toxicity of these compounds is due to the production of HCN, a potent respiratory inhibitor. The site of inhibition is the enzyme cytochrome oxidase, the terminal respiratory catalyst of aerobic organisms. Also usually produced on decomposition of a cyanogenetic glycoside is an aldehyde or ketone with which the HCN was combined as a cyanohydrin (Figure 1). The glycosides may contain as their sugar

* Literature reviewed to November 1971.

299

TABLE 1   Some Cyanogenetic Glycosides[1,3,4]

Glycoside	Plant Source	Hydrolysis Products		
Amygdalin	Members of the Rosaceae, including almond, apple, apricot, cherry, peach, pear, plum, quince	Gentiobiose	+ HCN	+ benzaldehyde
Prunasin	Members of the Rosaceae, including cherry laurel; *Eucalyptus cladocalyx; Linaria striata* Dc.	D-Glucose	+ HCN	+ benzaldehyde
Sambunigrin	*Sambucus nigra* L. (elderberry), *Acacia* sp. (Australian acacias)	D-Glucose	+ HCN	+ benzaldehyde
Vicianin	*Vicia* sp. (common vetch)	Vicianose	+ HCN	+ benzaldehyde
Dhurrin	*Sorghum* sp. (sorghums, Kaffir corns)	D-Glucose	+ HCN	+ p-hydroxybenzaldehyde
Taxiphyllin	*Taxus* sp.	D-Glucose	+ HCN	+ p-hydroxybenzaldehyde
Linamarin	*Phaseolus lunatus* L. (lima bean, many varieties); *Linum usitatissimum* L. (linen flax); *Manihot* sp. (cassava or manioc); *Trifolium repens* L. (white clover); *Lotus* sp. (trefoils); *Dimorphotheca* sp.	D-Glucose	+ HCN	+ acetone
Lotaustralin	Occurs with linamarin	D-Glucose	+ HCN	+ 2-butanone
Acacipetalin	*Acacia* sp. (South African acacias)	D-Glucose	+ dimethylketene cyanohydrin	
Triglochinin[5]	*Triglochin maritimum* L. (arrow grass)	D-Glucose	+ HCN	+ triglochinic acid

component a monosaccharide (usually glucose) or disaccharides such as vicianose and gentiobiose. The carbon atom to which the glycosyl moiety is attached may be asymmetric and may provide the possibility of two diastereomeric forms yielding the same products on hydrolysis[1] (e.g., prunasin and sambunigrin, dhurrin and taxiphyllin).

Table 1 also shows that there is no obvious pattern in the distribution of cyanogenetic glycosides in nature. There is a fairly common occurrence in the rose family of two of the five cyanogens that produce benzaldehyde on hydrolysis. A third, sambunigrin, was first reported in *Sambucus nigra* L. (family Caprifoliaceae); it also occurs together with vicianin in some legumes. While linamarin and lotaustralin are also found in several legumes, they are not restricted to that family. It is unwise to

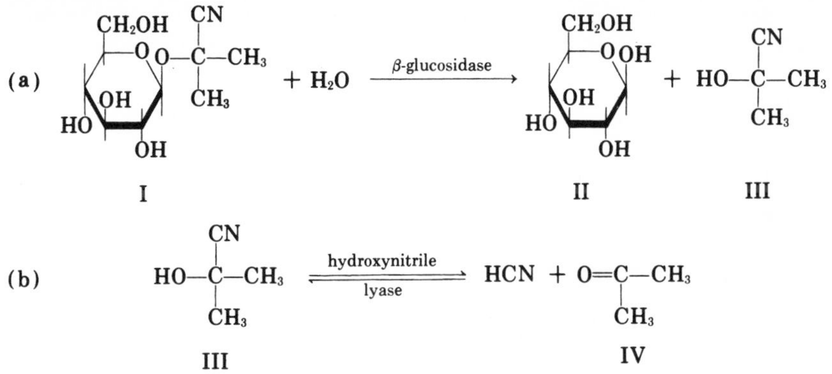

FIGURE 1 The decomposition of linamarin by plant enzymes. In reaction (a), linamarin [2-(β-D-glucopyranosyloxy)isobutyronitrile] (I) is hydrolyzed by the β-glucosidase linamarase to form β-D-glucopyranose (II) and 2-hydroxyisobutyronitrile or acetone cyanohydrin (III). In reaction (b), the dissociation of the cyanohydrin to HCN and acetone (IV) is catalyzed by a hydroxynitrile lyase.

generalize regarding which parts of a cyanophoric plant contain the cyanogenetic glycosides; they have been found in roots, tubers, stems, leaves, flowers, and seeds. Seeds of a cyanophoric species may not necessarily contain the glycoside, however. For example, sorghum seed with its high starch content can be safely consumed as food because it is lacking or very low in cyanogen. On germination, however, the dark-grown sorghum seedling may reach a concentration of 0.3–0.5% HCN (dry weight) within a period of 3 or 4 days, and young, green leaves are a rich source of dhurrin.[2]

Knowledge of the manner in which cyanogenetic glycosides give rise to HCN permits one to better understand some of the information that is available on poisoning by these substances. The action of two enzymes usually found in plants that contain cyanogenetic glycosides is illustrated in Figure 1 for linamarin, a cyanogen occurring in cassava (*Manihot* sp.), linen flax (*Linum usitatissimum* L.), and lima beans (*Phaseolus lunatus* L.). The initial reaction involves the hydrolysis by a β-glycosidase of the β-glycosidic bond between the sugar and the aglycone (in this case, 2-hydroxyisobutyronitrile or acetone cyanohydrin) of the glycoside. β-Glycosidases catalyzing the reaction have been partially purified from linen flax and white clover.[1,6] Similar enzymes acting on amygdalin and dhurrin have been obtained from almonds and sorghum.[1] These enzymes are highly specific for the β-glycosidic linkage that is characteristic of the cyanogenetic glycosides. The plant enzymes therefore differ from the α-glycosidases (amylases) of the mammalian digestive tract that hydrolyze only α-glycosidic bonds.

Although the α-hydroxynitriles (cyanohydrins) produced by the action of plant glycosidases will dissociate nonenzymatically, hydroxynitrile lyases that catalyze the dissociation of these compounds are present in cyanophoric plants.[1] In the presence of the lyase, the cyanohydrin dissociates to produce HCN and the product ketone (or aldehyde). While an enzyme catalyzing the dissociation of acetone cyanohydrin (Figure 1) has not been studied in a higher plant, such an enzyme has been reported in a fungus.[7] The hydroxynitrile lyases of almonds and sorghum have been extensively examined.[1]

The literature on cyanogenesis occasionally refers to the "HCN content" of a plant or plant tissue. It should be emphasized, however, that the HCN is produced, according to Figure 1, only after disruption of the plant cell has occurred. Presumably in the intact plant the degradative enzymes are spatially separated from the cyanogenetic glycoside. Moreover, little, if any, free HCN would be expected to accumulate in the cell since, being volatile, it would escape to the atmosphere. HCN is also actively metabolized by many plants, the nitrile group being converted to the amide group of asparagine.[2]

From the above it is clear why the ingestion of fresh, cyanophoric plant material by livestock can result in the death of the animal. Maceration by the animal of the fresh plant tissue as it is ingested initiates the enzymatic breakdown of the glycoside by the plant enzymes described above. Therefore, the animal merely needs to eat enough of a plant that is sufficiently rich in cyanogen and enzymes to be poisoned. Members of the rose family (apples, mountain mahogany, choke cherries) have been cited for loss of much livestock in the United States[8]; leaves of the eastern wild cherries may produce 200 mg HCN/100 g. According to Kingsbury, ¼ lb of those leaves could kill a 100-lb animal. Cyanophoric species of acacia have been blamed for the death of sheep and cattle in Australia,[9] South Africa,[10] and the United States.[8] In general, it was the leafy foliage of these plants that was consumed. It is common knowledge among farmers in the United States that their cattle must not be permitted to graze on young sorghum plants until "the cane is belly-high on the cow." The young sorghum leaves are particularly rich in dhurrin, and only in the older plants does the concentration become low enough to permit grazing. When the sorghum plant is taken for ensilage, the cellular breakdown and fermentation that occur in the silo release the HCN, which then escapes.

Several methods are available for determining both the presence and the amount of cyanogenetic glycosides in plants.[8,11-15] These are based on maceration and extraction of the tissue with a buffer or H_2O, followed by hydrolysis by the enzymes that are usually present in the plant. If these enzymes are absent or low in activity, preparations of β-glucosidase (emulsin from almonds; linamarase from flax) can be added to accomplish the hydrolysis. The HCN released can be detected qualitatively with filter paper that contains picric acid.[8,11] For quantitative estimates, the HCN released can be determined in the hydrolysate by direct potentiometric measurement,[12] or it can be removed by distillation,[13] aeration,[14] or diffusion[15] and then determined.

There is an extensive literature[8] on the cyanide content of forage crops such as sorghums (*Sorghum* sp.), white clover (*Trifolium repens* L.), and bird's-foot trefoil (*Lotus corniculatus* L.), some as it is influenced by different environmental conditions. In clover[11] and trefoil,[16] two genes determining the cyanophoric nature of these species have been recognized. One gene is dominant for the production of the glycoside, while another controls the production of a β-glycosidase that hydrolyzes the glycoside. The four phenotypes exist in nature and of course can be obtained by selective breeding. Those strains with little or no glycoside can be safely used for forage.

Although the cyanide-producing capacity of a plant is important in determining its toxicity, other factors must also be considered: the size and kind of subject; the speed of ingestion; the type of food ingested simultaneously with the cyanogen; the presence of active degradative enzymes both in the plant and in the subject's digestive tract; and the subject's ability to detoxify the HCN. The minimum lethal dose for humans of HCN taken orally has been estimated at between 0.5 mg and 3.5 mg per kg of body weight.[17] The poison is rapidly absorbed from the gastrointestinal tract and produces recognizable symptoms at both fatal and nonfatal levels. With fatal doses, death results from the general anoxic condition caused by the inhibition of cytochrome oxidase. With nonfatal doses, the inhibition of cellular respiration can be reversed, due to the removal of HCN by respiratory exchange or by a metabolic detoxification process. In the latter instance, HCN is metabolized by reaction with thiosulfate to form thiocyanate and sulfite:

$$CN^- + S_2O_3^= \longrightarrow CNS^- + SO_3^=$$

Rhodanase, the enzyme that catalyzes this reaction, is widely distributed in animal tissues.[17] The thiocyanate produced is excreted in the urine. While the conversion of cyanide to thiocyanate represents a detoxification of the HCN, it should be noted that thiocyanate in turn is a goitrogenic agent. (See Chapter 10, p. 219.)

The accidental poisoning of humans who ate bitter almonds or the pits of peaches or apricots is recorded.[8] There is one case of poisoning of children who had eaten large amounts of western choke cherries without removing the stones.[18] These instances of human poisoning are similar to those involving livestock in that the fresh plant material provides both the cyanogenetic glycoside and the enzymes responsible for the production of the lethal HCN. If the enzyme had been totally lacking in these plants, one might think that modest amounts of the intact glycoside could be safely ingested, for mammals do not appear to contain digestive enzymes that hydrolyze β-glycosidic bonds. There are, however, conflicting reports regarding the toxicity of purified glycosides administered orally to experimental animals.[8,19-21]

The occurrence of cyanogenetic glycosides in plants (Table 1) that are commonly taken by man as food can result in acute cyanide poisoning. In some instances the poisoning occurred with cooked plant material, suggesting that care was not taken to remove HCN released during soaking and prior to cooking of the plant. In a review on the medical significance of cyanogenetic glycosides in plants, Montgomery[21] has cited numerous references to the poisoning of humans by cassava and lima beans. The sweet potato or yam, maize, bamboo, chick pea, and sorghum are also mentioned as food plants capable of producing HCN. Viehoever[22] has documented numerous cases of poisonings by lima beans, a species that is widely distributed in the world and one of the important edible legumes.

The HCN-producing capacity of lima beans is known to vary, with native American strains containing less than those originating in the East.[21,22] While a white American variety produced only 10 mg HCN/100 g of seed, a white Burma variety yielded 200 mg, and a black Puerto Rican variety produced 300 mg HCN/100 g of seed. Since the lethal dose of HCN for the adult human is in the range of 50-250 mg, 100 g of seed of the wrong variety could easily prove fatal. In some areas where legumes are a staple of the diet, the daily intake may reach 200-300 g of beans.[21] Today, the importation of lima beans is restricted by several countries, including the United States, to varieties yielding less than 20 mg HCN/100 g of seed. Selective breeding of low-cyanide varieties has also been encouraged.

The toxicity of cassava has long been recognized.[21,23] However, it remains an important food plant because the peoples employing it have developed means of preparation that serve to remove or hydrolyze the linamarin and lotaustralin and to destroy the β-glucosidase that is present. Thus, the cassava, which is rich in starch, is scraped or grated, then soaked in water, and allowed to "ferment" for several days. Under these conditions, the cyanogen is extensively hydrolyzed, and both it and its hydrolysis products leached out. The soaked plant tissue is then dried, pounded into a flour, and, depending on the local traditions, made into cassava bread or boiled into a paste. Obviously such procedures can greatly reduce the cyanogen content of this important food, but Osuntokun[24] cites the following figures as evidence that certain preparations of cassava common in Nigeria can still remain a source of cyanide and result in chronic cyanide poisoning. Osuntokun states that the amount of HCN released from fresh cassava root (38 mg/100 g) is reduced to 1.1 mg HCN/100 g in a cassava preparation known as "gari." Another preparation known as "purupuru," which is not as extensively washed, can yield 4–6 mg HCN/100 g of cassava. Some Nigerians may consume 750 g of cassava per day; this corresponds to 8 mg of HCN if the food is taken as "gari." This amount, however, would increase to 32–48 mg HCN if "purupuru" is eaten. These values, which approach the lower limits of the lethal dose of HCN (35 mg) cited earlier, represent HCN that can be released by further enzymatic hydrolysis, distillation, and determination. Whether all of the "available" HCN in this preparation would be released in the consumer is doubtful, unless, as frequently suggested, the bacteria of the lower digestive tract can degrade the cyanogenetic glycoside.

In a series of reports, Osuntokun and co-workers have described recent evidence linking the degenerative disease known as tropical ataxic neuropathy to chronic cyanide intoxication of dietary origin.[24-27] These papers implicate the high consumption of cassava in the disease in a group of Nigerians. The subjects exhibited an increased level of thiocyanate in the plasma and an increased excretion of this compound in the urine. Since thiocyanate is the compound formed when cyanide is detoxified in the animal body,[17] an increased cyanide intake was indicated in these patients. Moreover, these individuals exhibited higher levels of plasma cyanide (free and bound) than controls.[28]

Montgomery, in reviewing the question of chronic cyanide poisoning, points out[21] that tropical amblyopia (blindness) is common in West Africa. He cites others who proposed that cyanide in cassava was the cause. Related neuropathies have been described in Jamaica and Malaya, where cassava is consumed. A diet of millet (sorghum) consumed by Senegalese may be responsible for a syndrome similar to ataxic neuropathy.[24] Some prisoners of war subsisting on a diet composed mainly of rice, cassava, sweet potato, and mung beans developed amblyopia.[21] While chronic cyanide toxicity may be a major factor in each of these conditions, attention must be paid to the possibility of dietary imbalance, which may increase an individual's susceptibility to trace amounts of cyanide. It should also be emphasized that ataxic neuropathy is different from lathyrism, the disease produced by consumption of certain lathyrus peas (see Chapter 7, p. 155). While the toxic compounds in those legumes are nitriles (i.e., they contain the $-C\equiv N$ functional group), they do not give rise in metabolism to HCN and therefore are not cyanogenetic.

As attention focuses on the possibility of chronic cyanide toxicity from dietary sources of HCN, notice should be paid to other sources of HCN as well as to possible therapeutic measures. The blindness occurring in some heavy smokers (tobacco amblyopia) may be due to poisoning by the HCN that is a component of cigarette smoke.[21,29] This condition in man, and other neurological conditions induced in animals receiving dietary cyanide, has been treated therapeutically with the hydroxocobalamin form of Vitamin B_{12}, which has a high affinity for cyanide.[30] Earlier mention has been made of the fact that thiocyanate formed by detoxification of HCN is itself a goitrogenic agent (p. 303). It is not surprising, therefore, that a widespread incidence of goiter has been reported in eastern Nigeria[31] where a dry, unfermented form of cassava is a major item of the diet.

In view of the problems associated with the consumption of cyanophoric plants by man and other animals, it is interesting to note the biosynthetic origin of the cyanogenetic glycosides.[1,2] Most of the glycosides listed in Table 1 are formed from four naturally occurring amino acids: valine, isoleucine, phenylalanine, and tyrosine. A biosynthetic pathway leading from these amino acids to the aglycones of the glycosides has been proposed, and supporting evidence has been cited.[1] In recent work, enzymes catalyzing certain of the reactions in the pathway have been partially purified from linen flax and sorghum and their properties examined. Of considerable biochemical interest are two facts: the $-CN$ or nitrile moiety of the aglycones is derived from the α-carbon and nitrogen atoms of the parent amino acid; and the intermediates involved are compounds not previously encountered in the metabolism of amino acids in animals and microorganisms.

REFERENCES

1. E. E. Conn, Cyanogenic glycosides. Agric. Food Chem. *17*:519 (1969).
2. E. E. Conn and G. W. Butler, The biosynthesis of cyanogenic glycosides and other simple nitrogen compounds, p. 47. In Perspectives in phytochemistry, J. B. Harborne and T. Swain (eds.). Academic Press, London (1969).
3. G. Dilleman, Composés cyanogénétiques, p. 1050. In Handbuch der Pflanzenphysiologie, Vol. VIII, W. Ruhland (ed.). Springer, Berlin (1958).
4. R. Eyjolfsson, Recent advances in the chemistry of cyanogenic glycosides. Fortsch. Chem. Organ. Naturst. *28*:74 (1970).

5. R. Eyjolfsson, Isolation and structure determination of triglochinin, a new cyanogenic glucoside from *Triglochin maritimum*. Phytochemistry *9*:845 (1970).

6. M. A. Hughes, Studies on the β-glucosidase system of *Trifolium repens* L. J. Exp. Bot. *19*:427 (1968).

7. D. L. Stevens and G. A. Strobel, Origin of cyanide in cultures of a psychrophilic basidiomycete. J. Bacteriol. *95*:1094 (1968).

8. J. M. Kingsbury, Poisonous plants of the United States and Canada. Prentice-Hall, Englewood Cliffs, N.J. (1964).

9. E. Hurst, The poison plants of New South Wales. Snelling Printing Works, Sydney (1942).

10. D. G. Steyn and C. Rimington, The occurrence of cyanogenetic glucosides in South African species of Acacia. I. Onderstepoort J. Vet. Sci. An. Ind. *4*:51 (1935).

11. L. Corkill, Cyanogenesis in white clover (*Trifolium repens*) V. The inheritance of cyanogenesis. N. Zealand J. Sci. Technol. *B 23*:178 (1942).

12. W. J. Blaedel, D. B. Easty, L. Anderson, and T. R. Farrell, Potentiometric determination of cyanide with an ion selective electrode. Anal. Chem. *43*:890 (1971).

13. W. O. Winkler, Report on hydrocyanic glucosides. J. Assoc. Off. Agric. Chem. *34*:541 (1951).

14. T. Akazawa, P. Miljanich, and E. E. Conn, Studies on the cyanogenic glycoside of *Sorghum vulgare*. Plant Physiol. *35*:535 (1960).

15. K. Hahlbrock and E. E. Conn, The biosynthesis of cyanogenic glycosides in higher plants. I. J. Biol. Chem. *245*:917 (1970).

16. D. A. Jones, On the polymorphism of cyanogenesis in *Lotus corniculatus* L. Selection by animals. Can. J. Genet. Cytol. *8*:556 (1966).

17. R. D. Montgomery, Cyanogens. In Toxic constituents of plant foodstuffs, I. E. Liener (ed.). Academic Press, New York (1969).

18. M. Pijoan, Cyanide poisoning from choke cherry seed. Am. J. Med. Sci. *204*: 550 (1942).

19. H. R. Seddon and R. O. C. King, The fatal dose for sheep of cyanogenetic plants containing sambunigrin or prunasin. J. Counc. Sci. Ind. Res. Aust. *3*:14 (1930).

20. I. E. Coop and R. L. Blakley, The metabolism and toxicity of cyanides and cyanogenetic glucosides in sheep. N. Zealand J. Sci. Technol. *31A* (5):44 (1950).

21. R. D. Montgomery, The medical significance of cyanogen in plant foodstuffs. Am. J. Clin. Nutr. *17*, 103 (1965).

22. A. Viehoever, Edible and poisonous beans of the lima type (*Phaseolus lunatus* L.). Thai Sci. Bull. *2*:1 (1940).

23. A. Clark, Report on the effects of certain poisons contained in food-plants of West Africa upon the health of the native races. J. Trop. Med Hyg. *39*:269 (1936).

24. B. O. Osuntokun, An ataxic neuropathy in Nigeria. Brain *91*:215 (1968).

25. B. O. Osuntokun, G. L. Monekosso, and J. Wilson, Relationship of a degenerative tropical neuropathy to diet. Br. Med. J. *1*:547 (1969).

26. B. O. Osuntokun, S. P. Singh, and F. D. Martinson, Deafness in tropical nutritional ataxic neuropathy. Trop. Geogr. Med. *22*:281 (1970).

27. B. O. Osuntokun, Cassava diet and cyanide metabolism in Wistar rats. Br. J. Nutr. *24*:797 (1970).

28. B. O. Osuntokun, A. Aladetoyinbo, and A. O. G. Adenja, Free-cyanide levels in tropical ataxic neuropathy. Lancet *ii*:372 (1970).

29. Anonymous, Chronic cyanide neurotoxicity. Lancet *ii*:942 (1969).

30. J. Wilson, J. C. Linnell, and D. M. Matthews, Plasma-cobalamins in neuro-ophthalmological diseases. Lancet *i*:259 (1971).

31. O. L. Ekpechi, A. Dimitriadou, and R. Fraser, Goitrogenic activity of cassava (a staple Nigerian food). Nature *210*:1137 (1966).

15 V. L. Singleton and
F. H. Kratzer

PLANT PHENOLICS*

INTRODUCTION

The phenols and biochemically related substances of natural origin in
plants can be divided roughly into two groups: the botanically widespread and structurally common ones, and those with exotic structures
and limited specific occurrence. The first group consists of 25 or so
substances such as *p*-coumaric, caffeic, ferulic, sinapic, and gallic acids
or their derivatives. Included are the flavonoids with the common and
analogous variations in the 5,7,3',4',5'-hydroxyl or 3',5'-methoxyl substituents in the anthocyanidin, catechin, flavone, flavonol, and leucoanthocyanidin series. Lignin, hydrolyzable and condensed tannins (p.
328), ellagic acid, and derivatives such as depsides and glycosides substantially complete the first group. Some of these substances almost invariably are contained in plant-derived foods, at least in traces and
sometimes in fairly large amounts.

The second group is heterogeneous and includes most of the few
dozen phenolic derivatives known to have high toxicity or potent physiological activity in animals.[1] These substances may also be present in
very significant amounts in the particular plant tissues that contain
them. A third group perhaps worthy of consideration would be the

* Literature reviewed to January 1971.

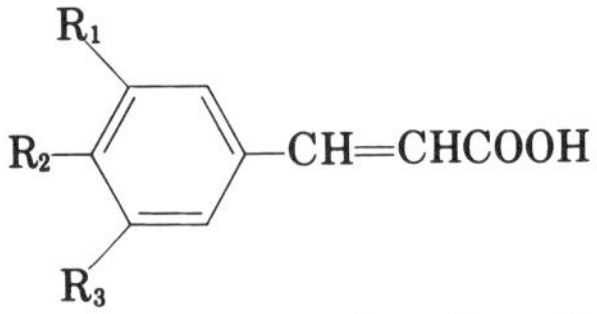

	R₁	R₂	R₃
p-Coumaric Acid	H	OH	H
Caffeic Acid	OH	OH	H
Ferulic Acid	OCH₃	OH	H
Sinapic Acid	OCH₃	OH	OCH₃

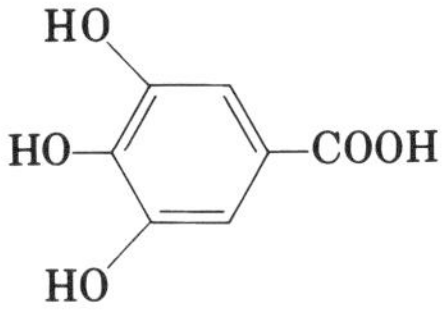

Gallic Acid

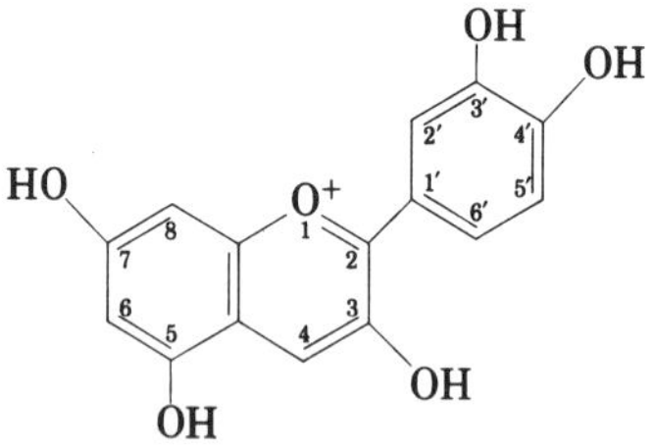

Cyanidin (an anthocyanidin)

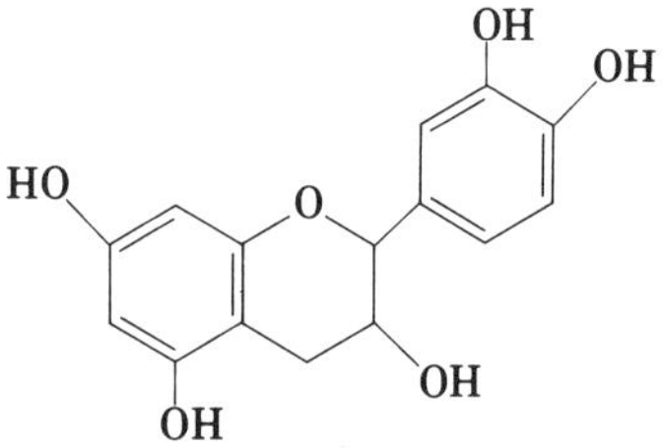

Catechin (a flavanol)

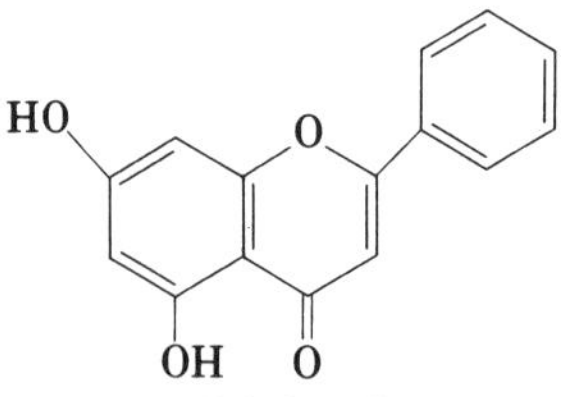

5,7-Dihydroxyflavone

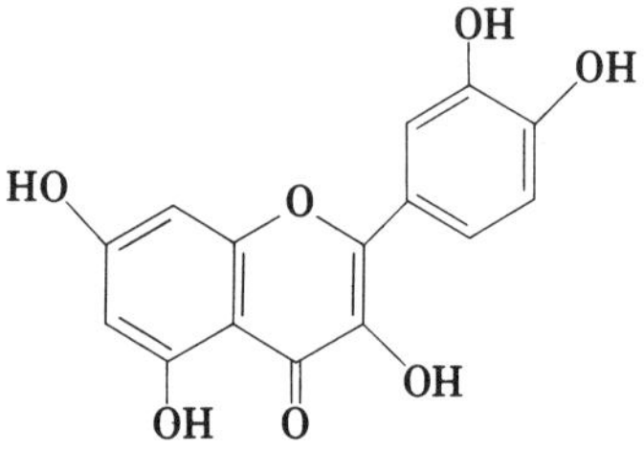

Quercetin (a flavonol)

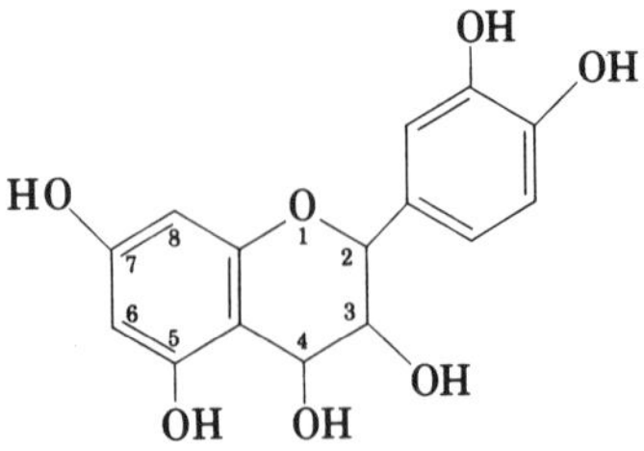

Leucoanthocyanidin (a flavan-3,4-diol)

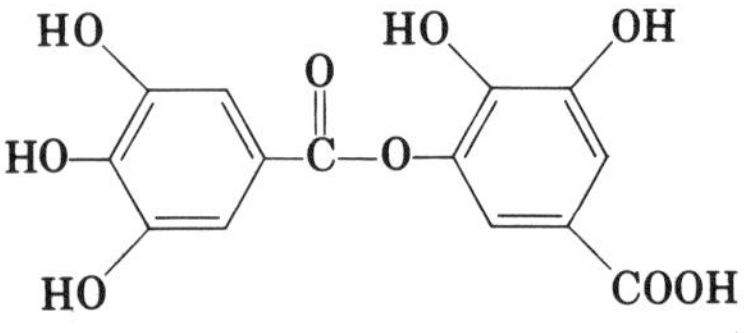

m-Digallic Acid (a depside)

smaller phenols produced by reactions such as pyrolysis. They could appear in foods as a result of smoking or other processing.

Owing, presumably, to long evolutionary adaptation, the common plant phenolics as usually consumed are readily detoxified. It appears[1] that carnivores tend to be more susceptible than herbivores to the acute toxicity of phenols, such as those from plants. Omnivores, for example, man and rats, appear to be intermediate. This relative sensitivity seems to be true parenterally as well as orally, so that it does not appear to be exclusively an effect of digestive-tract microflora. Considering that the diet of a herbivore may contain nearly 20% of its dry weight as lignin and other plant phenols, and that the diet of a carnivore has nearly none, an evolved difference in phenol tolerance seems reasonable. A case can be made for the concept that all phenols have some properties in common that render them potentially toxic to animals[1]; the fact that most plant phenols are harmless as usually encountered in the diet is largely the result of the animal's effective detoxification or nonabsorption of them. This leads to the corollary that if the animal's detoxification mechanisms can be overloaded by massive amounts of phenolic derivatives in the diet or circumvented by unusual structures of the phenols or unusual circumstances of ingestion, toxicity is likely to become manifest.

With a few exceptions,[1,2] it has been the fashion to consider effects of plant phenols according to botanical origin (mycotoxins, toxic plants, etc.), type of effect (antibiotics, antioxidants, carcinogens, estrogens, flavors, photosensitizers, etc.), or structures (cinnamates, coumarins, flavonoids, isoflavones, quinones, tannins, etc.). This practice tends to prevent recognition of general relationships in phenol toxicity, although to a degree it is continued in the present volume.

The reader is also referred to additional chapters in this volume in which other potential phenolic relationships are discussed: nitrogenous phenols such as tyrosine (Chapter 6) and mescaline (Chapter 8); phenolic vitamin E and quinoidal vitamin K (Chapter 11); phenolic enzyme inhibitors (Chapter 13); mycotoxins such as aflatoxin (Chapter 18); flavoring components such as myristicin and coumarin (Chapter 20); safrole (Chapter 23); dihydromethysticin and other kava components (Chapter 21); tremetol and related substances from white snakeroot in milk (Introduction); isoflavones and other phenols as estrogens (Chapter 24); and hypericin and psoralen relatives such as photosensitizers (Chapter 25).

Here some apparently general correlations of toxicity of nitrogen-free phenols from higher plants will be discussed, as well as a few exotic toxic phenols not covered in other chapters, notably gossypol. Some

Tremetone

consideration will be given to the more widespread plant phenols, flavonoids, and tannins as related to food toxicity.

PLANT PHENOLS AS ACUTE TOXICANTS

The primary concern in this report is the significance of plant phenols as present or potential toxicants in human foods, but some useful perspective appears possible from brief consideraton of their participation in poisoning of animals or in "medicine cabinet" and "novices afield" accidents. Of about 300,000 species of plants, an estimated 700 have caused death or serious illness in this hemisphere, and doubtless many have yet to be recognized as poisonous.[3] Many instances go unreported, but thousands of persons receive medical treatment and hundreds of thousands of animals die annually from consuming poisonous plants.[3] Intoxications from plant ingestion are responsible for about 4% of all accidental poisonings in this country, and in most cases small children are involved.[4]

Implicated in 1,051 plant ingestions reported to poison control centers in the 50 states, Puerto Rico, and the Canal Zone during 1959–1960, plus several hundred reports from other years, were at least 175 plants in addition to mushrooms.[5] Of these, 11 plants, involving at least 123 patients and 5 fatalities, were those whose intoxicating properties are attributed at least in part to phenols. Other summaries[3-8] of plants with reported acute effects on humans attributable to phenols give a combined list including aloe, *Cassia, Rhamnus,* rhubarb, St. John's wort, and buckwheat containing anthraquinone derivatives; cashew, mango, poison ivy, and *Ginkgo biloba* containing vesicant phenols with long hydrocarbon side chains; and *Areca catechu,* aspidium, buckeye (*Aesculus*), daphne, *Derris,* hawthorn, marihuana, mayapple, nutmeg, and sassafras containing several different active phenolics. Examining these reports quickly leads to the conclusion that, although acute poisoning of people by plants with toxic phenols is real enough and some of the vectors are readily available, such poisoning is more often either a nonfatal nuisance (as with poison ivy) or a relatively rare event in modern times.

Some of the listed plants may be toxic primarily because of compounds other than phenols. The anthraquinones of rhubarb are mainly in the root, and the cathartic drug is prepared from less edible varieties. Human poisonings occur mainly from eating rhubarb leaves (see Chapter 16), and the petioles, of course, are good food. The leaf poison is commonly thought to be oxalate, but other factors, possibly the quinones, may more likely be involved (see Chapter 16).[7] Daphne and *Aesculus* poisonings have been attributed to their content of the coumarin glycosides daphnin and esculin. There is not general agreement on this, however, and it appears that much of their acute toxicity should be attributed to an acid anhydride in daphne[4] and a saponin in buckeye or horse chestnut.[4,9,10] On the other hand, the toxicants in many plants have not been identified, and many toxicants are doubtless waiting in the wings to make an appearance. For example, 27 soldiers suddenly and permanently lost their sight after consuming the Australian finger cherry, *Rhodomyrtus macrocarpa.* The rhodomyrtoxin apparently is or contains completely substituted dibenzofurans derived from phloroglucinol.[11] The pure dibenzofuran was present in immature fruit at levels of at least 3,500 mg/kg fruit and was toxic to mice at oral doses of 30 mg/kg body weight.[11] Similar compounds had been found previously in lichens but not in higher plants.

A few of the plants listed as producing human toxicity are also of considerable practical importance in losses of farm animals, notably St. John's wort and white snakeroot. However, most of the economically significant phenolic plant poisons, such as dicumarol (the sweet clover anticoagulant), cocklebur, oak tannins, plant estrogens, and cottonseed gossypol, have evidently not directly caused human accidents. This is apparently because the plant materials are not likely to be consumed by humans and because, except for cocklebur, their most serious effects require repeated dosage. The apparent unlikelihood of human consumption is not always valid, however. Daphne, buckeye, and buckwheat toxins (possibly phenolics) are reportedly present in honey (see Chapter 22, p. 495) drawn from these plants.[5,8] Cashew oil, although removed and detoxified in preparing the nuts for sale, has been used as a coating for vanilla beans and thereby has caused irritation.

In terms of human lives lost from phenols originating in plants, the salicylate aspirin is probably the most dangerous. Aspirin is now obtained synthetically, but salicyl derivatives were first known from willow (*Salix*). Accidental and suicidal consumption of salicylates produces deaths of the order of four per million population per year.[12] Other

medicinal preparations such as aspidium and podophyllin, particularly
in former times, offered considerable danger not only in the home but
also to the gatherers and processors.

Only a few plant phenols are so highly toxic or so physiologically
active that potentially lethal effects would result from a single dose that
readily occurs in a natural product. Aspidium,[13] the anthelminthic drug
(for elimination of tapeworms) prepared from male fern (*Dryopteris
filix-mas*), contains at least 6.5% oleoresin, 24% or more of which is a
mixture of substituted and oligomeric phloroglucinols. The oleoresin at
a 1–5 g oral dose for humans produces headache, dizziness, nausea, and
visual disturbances. At least one human fatality is known. An isolated
constituent, desaspidin, had an acute oral LD$_{50}$ of 595 mg/kg to mice,
but its toxicity rose to 195–280 mg/kg when mixed with the nontoxic
oils, etc., present in an ether extract of fern.[14] Filicin, another constituent, had an acute oral LD$_{50}$ to rats of 1,076 mg/kg, but 90 mg/kg daily
produced a number of toxic symptoms, including a gradual loss of the
ability to generate sperm.[15] Cotoin[13,16] (2,6-dihydroxy-4-methoxy-
benzophenone) from coto bark, formerly an antidiarrheal, is lethal at
8 mg/kg subcutaneously to frogs.

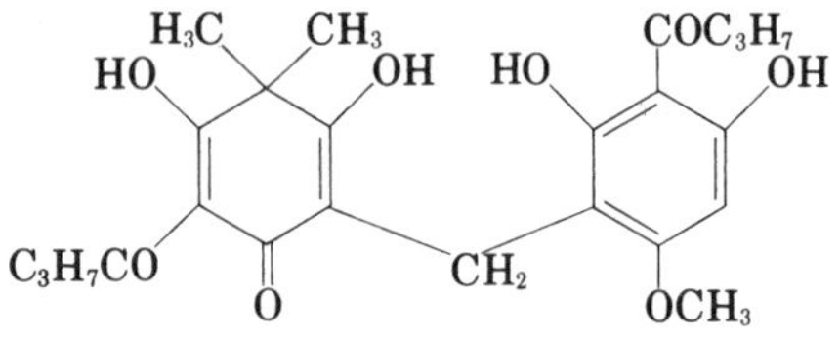

Desaspidin

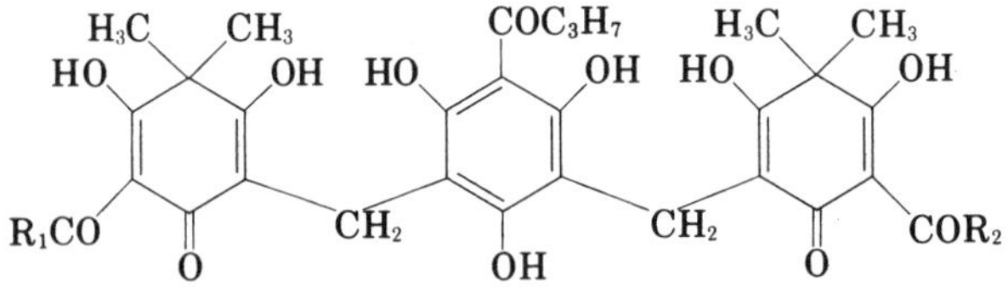

Filicin (a mixture of similar substances)
BBB, R$_1$ = R$_2$ = C$_3$H$_7$; PBB, R$_1$ = C$_2$H$_5$, R$_2$ = C$_3$H$_7$; PBP, R$_1$ = R$_2$ = C$_2$H$_5$

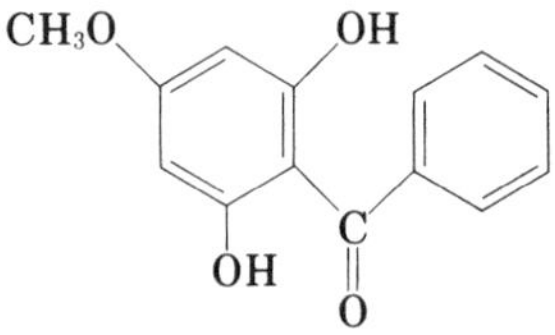

Cotoin

The mayapple, *Podophyllum peltatum,* contains in the dry roots about 8% of the resin podophyllin, of which about 20% consists of podophyllotoxin (a lignan) plus other related substances. The resin has irritant, cytotoxic, and cathartic effects, and a 130-mg medical dose has caused death.[16] The ripe fruits are often eaten with no effect or a mild catharsis, but green fruits are dangerous.[17] Podophyllotoxin has an oral LD_{50} to mice of 90 mg/kg.[13,16] Derris root powder has an oral LD_{100} to rats of about 400 mg/kg,[16] and the rotenone it contains has an LD_{50} of 133 mg/kg orally and 5 mg/kg intraperitoneally.[1,13] Of value as a natural fish poison and insecticide, rotenone (an isoflavone derivative) is ordinarily handled carefully but is considered relatively low in toxicity and in residual persistence compared to other insecticides. The lethal oral dose for humans has been estimated to be as low as 200 mg,[13] although this has been disputed.[18] The compound has cumulative toxicity on long exposure and is more toxic when inhaled.[13,18]

Most other phenols are less acutely toxic. Hydroquinone is the most toxic of the simple phenols at oral LD_{50} 320 mg/kg for the rat.[1,16] It is the toxicant in cocklebur seeds and sprouts that has caused much loss when animals consume the cotyledon stage of seedlings.[1,6] The seeds (not including the burrs) are toxic at about 3 g/kg of body weight, and apparently the hydroquinone is not present as a glycoside, in contrast to

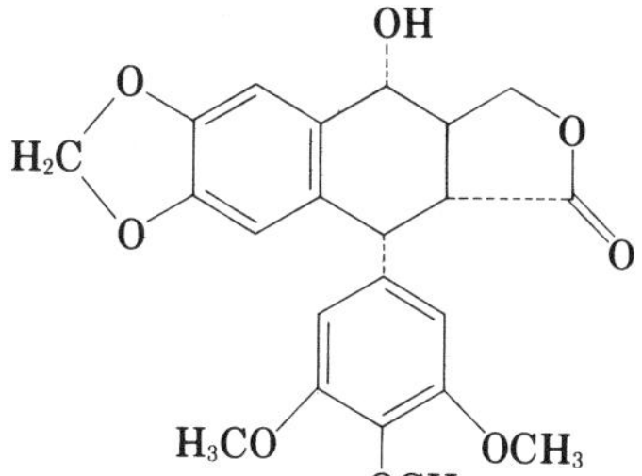

Podophyllotoxin

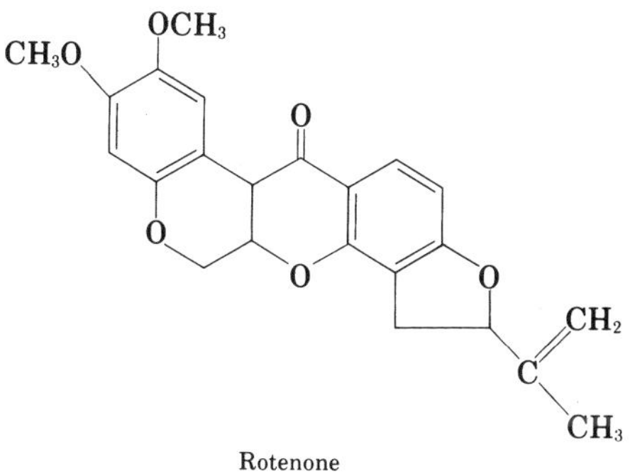

Rotenone

the usual situation.[6] The acute toxicities of the other phenols of the plant type are nearly all in the range considered only slight in oral toxicity, i.e., LD_{50} 500–5,000 mg/kg, or even less toxic. Some representative acute oral toxicity values, not necessarily determined in a strictly comparable way,[1,13,16] are: vanillin 1,580, methyl salicylate 887, coumarin 680, thymol 980, safrole 1,950, menadione (a synthetic vitamin K) 1,000, dicumarol 542, and tannic acid 6,000 mg/kg.

Few values have been found for the lethal dose of common flavonoids or cinnamates, because they are essentially nontoxic in a single dose; however, they might be toxic if administered at high levels for a long time. Coumarin and safrole are no longer permitted additions to food, since, among other tests, long-term (nearly 1 yr to 6 yr) oral dosage of dogs at as little as 25 and 5 mg/kg, respectively, produced deleterious liver changes.[5] Higher levels, of course, gave more serious effects.

In general, flavonoids of the botanically usual types have negligible toxicity and show no harmful effects at oral doses of at least 500 mg/ kg.[19] Rutin required 19.5 g/kg intraperitoneally to produce an LD_{95} in rats, and similar levels given orally to guinea pigs were only marginally toxic.[20] Rutin is the 3-rhamnoglucoside of quercetin (see Chapter 25, p. 565). Daily feedings of 850 mg/kg for 3 months gave insignificant *gains* in growth rate of rats. In the same trials the sodium salt of the ethereal sulfate of 4-methylesculetin gave similar results (LD_{95} intraperitoneally rat of 8.22 g/kg) and normal growth with 555 mg/kg daily for 3 months. A number of studies on naringin, hesperidin, rutin, quercetin, quercitrin (quercetin-3-rhamnoside), and dihydroquercetin have shown no acute toxicity, nor was toxicity noted when fed to rats at 1%

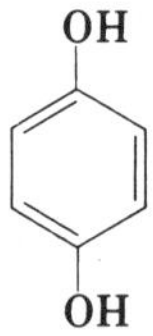

Hydroquinone

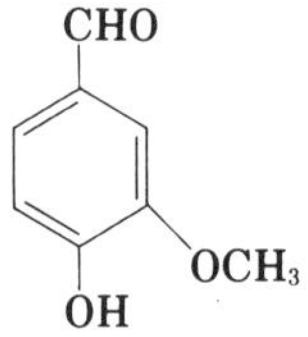

Vanillin

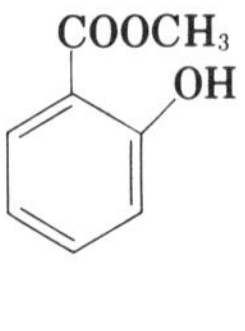

Methyl Salicylate

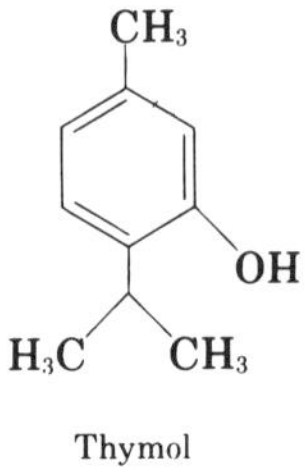

Thymol

of the diet for 200 days or longer.[21] The lethal dose of chlorogenic acid (3-caffeoylquinic acid) to mice intraperitoneally was 3.5 g/kg, but 4–5 g/kg orally or subcutaneously gave no toxicity.[22] Oral dosage of humans for 60 days with 1.5 g/day of 1,4-dicaffeoylquinic acid gave only favorable effects.[23] Parenteral toxicity of some of these substances is sometimes high, however, particularly that of the substances with high protein affinity of the tannin type. The IP LD$_{50}$ of a leucocyanidin to rats was about 100 mg/kg[24] (although oral LD$_{50}$ to mouse was 3 g/kg), and the tannic acid intravenous LD$_{100}$ to mice was 80 mg/kg.[16]

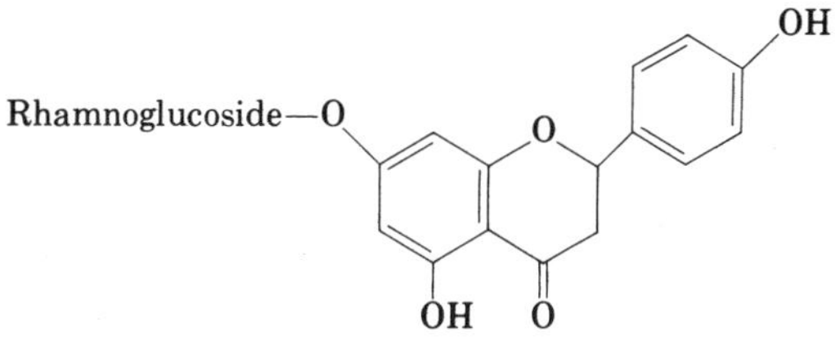

Naringin

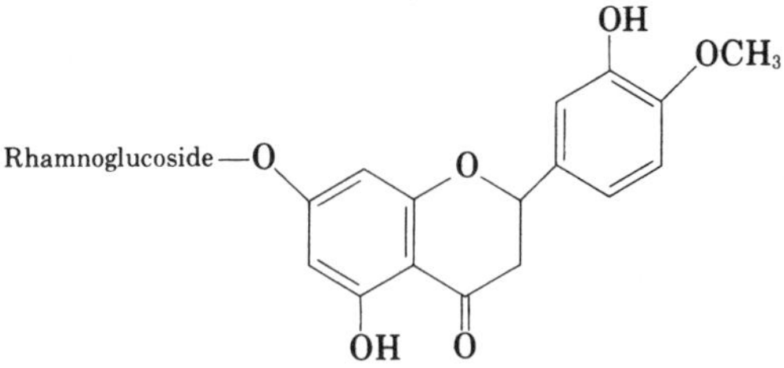

Hesperidin

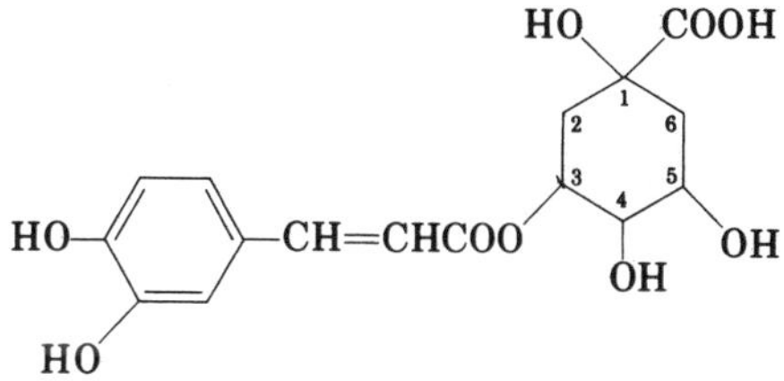

Chlorogenic Acid

SPECIFIC PLANT PHENOLIC TOXICANTS

It has been mentioned that several of the most important phenolic toxicants are being covered in other chapters. Several more have been discussed in the preceding sections, but, owing to their minimal significance in human foods, they need little elaboration here. A few others,
however, deserve more consideration not only because of real or potential hazard to humans but also to illustrate some aspects of phenolic
toxicity with, perhaps, general applicability.

Gossypol

A yellow phenol characteristic of the genus of cotton, *Gossypium*,
gossypol would have probably remained insignificant as a natural hazard, but it has assumed importance because of the use of seed meal recovered from cotton production as a protein supplement for animal, and
now human, diets. With major production in Brazil, Egypt, India, Mexico, and Pakistan, cottonseed is the protein-rich oilseed most widely
available for supplementation of inadequate diets in tropical and subtropical countries.[25,26] For each 500-lb bale of cotton fiber, about 840
lb of seed is produced.[27] Total world production of cottonseed is as
much as 25 million tons/yr, and about 3–6 million tons have been produced in the United States,[26] depending on fiber demand. Each ton of
seed produces about 335 lb of oil and 945 lb of feed-grade meal.[27] If
refined 60% protein cottonseed flour is prepared for human use, 300–
400 lb/ton is produced; the remainder of the meal can be diverted to
animal feed.[28] It is estimated that only one fourth of the cottonseed
flour potentially available could satisfy the present serious deficiencies
in protein in diet-deficient nations, and the protein is of high nutritional
quality.[29]

There are no known instances of toxic effects of gossypol ingestion
in humans, and there have been several reports on the absence of deleterious effects when cottonseed meal with low gossypol content has been
consumed in moderate amounts, such as 60 g daily for 4.5 months of
heated cottonseed cake originally containing 0.11–0.20% free gossypol.[30] A number of agencies have studied the use of cottonseed flour in
foods, notably the Instituto de Nutricion de Centro America y Panama
(INCAP), which developed Incaparina, a food containing 38% cottonseed flour.[31] Maximum gossypol in cottonseed preparations for human
use has been set at 0.045% (450 mg/kg) free gossypol in the United
States. Less than 0.06% free and 1.2% total is recommended by international groups.[25] Use of Incaparina by small children under close clini-

cal supervision for over 2 yr failed to cause any toxicity, and there was much improved protein status over an unsupplemented diet.[25] The product is already a commercial and nutritional success in some countries, notably Guatemala, and some families have used it for more than 4 yr without any indication of difficulty.[25,29,31]

Nevertheless, gossypol is a potential toxicant, and the fact that it is now possible to use processed cottonseed flour safely in the human diet depends on information developed in animal studies.

Gossypol is 1,1',6,6',7,7'-hexahydroxy-5,5'-diisopropyl-3,3'-dimethyl-[2,2'-binaphthalene]-8,8'-dicarboxaldehyde:

Gossypol

It occurs in the three equilibrium forms: the aldehyde, its enolic quinoid tautomer, and as the hemiacetal with the *peri*-hydroxyl.[1,25,32] It is strongly acidic for a phenol, is readily oxidizable, and acts as an antioxidant. It is soluble in most solvents of intermediate polarity but is not readily soluble in hexane or water. Along with it in cottonseed are found at least 15 related pigments in smaller amounts, including purple, orange, blue, and green substances. As far as they have been studied, they are derivatives of gossypol, or gossypol can be generated from them by treatments with acid, etc.[25] Biosynthesis is via the isoprenoid pathway, apparently by a specific cyclization of *cis-cis*-farnesyl pyrophosphate.[33] Gossypol pigments are confined in the cotton plant to "glands" (ovospheroidal bodies about 100–400 μm long) present in all but the woody tissues. Cotton without glands in the seed kernels (and therefore free of gossypol in the meal) has been bred and is beginning to be planted commercially. It remains to be seen if differing pest and disease resistance, fiber yield, quality, etc. will enable cotton with glandless seed to displace the glanded forms.[25,28,29,31]

The pigment glands represent about 2.4–4.8% of the kernel in varieties grown in the United States, and gossypol is about 20.6–39.0% of the weight of the glands; the other pigments contain about 2%.[25] In present commercial processes a small portion of the gossypol appears in the unrefined cottonseed oil, but it imparts color and is removed to a low level by refining and bleaching processes.[25,27] Heating in the presence of moisture disrupts the glands and causes the conversion of much of the free gossypol to bound forms. The lack of toxicity of cottonseed, even with intact glands, to ruminants is attributed to prolonged mastication, water contact, and increased time in the rumen, which result in binding of gossypol to protein.[34] Gossypol can be determined by spectrophotometry of the aniline derivative at 440 nm.[25] Total gossypol is that recovered after hydrolysis with oxalic acid in methyl ethyl ketone or after heating with 3-amino-1-propanol in N,N-dimethylformamide. Free gossypol is that extracted at room temperature with aqueous acetone or similar solvents; bound, of course, is total minus free.

Present commercial processes for cottonseed meal production all involve the use of heat and other processes to remove, destroy, or bind as much as possible (80–99%) of the gossypol.[25,28,31,35] The four types of processes for oil removal are screw pressing, pressing then solvent extraction, direct solvent extraction, and hydraulic pressing. The residual-oil and free-gossypol contents of typical commercial meal products prepared in these four ways would be about 2.5–5% and 0.02–0.05%, 0.4–1% and 0.02–0.07%, 1% and 0.1–0.5%, and 4.5–7.5% and 0.04–0.10%, respectively. The residual total gossypol is about the same for all and is in the range of 0.5–1.2%. Hydraulic pressing has nearly disappeared. The trend is toward solvent extraction, particularly prepress solvent extracting, at the expense of screw pressing, although the latter still accounts for about half of the production in the United States.

Bound gossypol is considered essentially nontoxic to animals. The toxicity of cottonseed meal to nonruminants is usually attributed to free gossypol, although there are complications. A simple analysis of the free and total gossypol content does not truly measure the biological activity under all circumstances. The activity is affected by the pH and composition of the diet, the source and method of incorporation of the gossypol, the test animal, etc.[25,36,37,38] It has been suggested that there are several forms of both free and bound gossypol, each with different activities,[37] or that toxicants in addition to gossypol are present in cottonseed.[38] Cyclopropenoid fatty acids (p. 196) do occur in the residual lipids of the meals, but, with a few exceptions such as pinking of egg white from hens fed cottonseed meal, it has been difficult to attribute the extra toxicity to them.[25,29]

Pigment glands can be isolated intact. They are quite variable in action but may be as much as four times as toxic as pure gossypol in equivalent amounts. The acute oral toxicity of gossypol is not high for most animals. On a single-dose basis the oral LD_{50} to rats is about 2,400–3,340 mg/kg (averaging 2,630 mg/kg) when administered in water; it is about 10% more toxic when administered in oil.[38] The water-soluble equimolar glycine adduct did not reach LD_{50} values at 6,000 mg/kg. Intact glands have given acute oral LD_{50} values with rats of 925–2,170 mg/kg in water and were slightly less toxic in oil.[38] The three most toxic samples had the highest gossypol content (36.9–40.0%) and the least toxic the lowest (28.6%), but intermediate correlations were not proportionate. It appears that potentiation of absorption by oil and possibly by unidentified gland components, together with lesser inactivation in the gut or en route to a sensitive site (and possible synergism among the various forms of gossypol pigments) could account for the extra toxicity of glands and variable results with other preparations. So far at least, no different natural toxicant species has been identified, and gossypol pigments appear to be the significant toxicant of cottonseed meal.

In experimental animals, sensitivity to gossypol toxicity appears to decrease in the order guinea pig, rabbit, mouse, and rat.[38] Dogs appear quite sensitive; repeated oral dosage at 10–200 mg/kg/day is usually fatal in less than a month. Chickens are about as sensitive as rats, but pigs are more sensitive. Fed toxic levels of gossypol, pigs may appear normal for a few weeks to a year, then abruptly begin to gasp for breath (thump) and die in a few days with severe anemia and other complications.[1,6,32] Commercial meal with 0.04% or less free gossypol is believed to be safe as a supplement in balanced diets for chicks and pigs,[27] but 0.02% gossypol in the diet is the approximate borderline between toxic and nontoxic levels in the pig[39]; for safety, 0.01% or less free gossypol (or not over 9 percent cottonseed meal) in the diet is recommended.[40]

Common symptoms[6,25] with cumulative gossypol or cottonseed meal toxicity are loss of appetite; weight loss; hypoprothrombinemia[41]; diarrhea; hair discoloration; lowering of hemoglobin, red cell count, and serum protein; edematous fluid in body cavities, lungs, and heart; degenerative changes in liver and spleen; hemorrhages of liver, small intestine, and stomach; and yolk discoloration and decreased hatchability of eggs. Gossypol is more rapid but less effective than dicumarol in suppressing prothrombin formation, and the effect is antagonized by some forms of vitamin K; however, this effect is evidently contributory rather than primary in hemorrhage induction and the toxicity of gossypol.[41]

Gossypol forms stable, equimolar chelates of low water solubility with many metallic cations, apparently by linking through the carbonyl and *ortho*-hydroxyl groups.[42,43] The Schiff's base adducts formed between gossypol and amines (such as aniline) still chelate metals, though slightly less strongly. It appears that gossypol produces anemia by its binding of iron. Addition of iron salts to diets with free gossypol decreases their toxicity, increases the proportion of the gossypol found in the feces, and at high levels can hasten the elimination of gossypol from the body and produce normal hematology.[44,45,46] Iron alone, however, does not prevent all toxic effects of gossypol, but the addition of 1% calcium hydroxide to the diet with iron did fully prevent gossypol toxicity at the levels involved.[44] This appears to be partly from rendering the iron complexes less soluble,[47] but could also be due to the fact that gossypol is unstable to alkali,[25] probably owing to catalysis of oxidation. Iron also appears to catalyze loss of the formyl group, and, although a major part of this action takes place in the digestive tract, it seems to be an important detoxification pathway for gossypol.[45] Little gossypol is eliminated via the urine, bile being the major excretory route.[45]

Combination, apparently of the Schiff's base type, between the carbonyls of gossypol and amino groups of amino acids and proteins is a major factor in the toxicity of gossypol and its cumulative effects. Part of the toxicity of gossypol can result from rendering amino acids unavailable by this reaction, particularly lysine via its terminal amino group, thus lowering the biological value of the diet.[48,50] A high intake of quality protein or supplementation of the diet with excess lysine lowers but does not abolish the toxicity of high gossypol levels.[39,50] The binding with gossypol lowers the digestibility of the protein and increases the proportion of the gossypol in the feces.[49,51,52] Bound gossypol suppresses liberation of some other amino acids by enzymatic digestion more than by the liberation of lysine.[53] Since both carbonyls of gossypol will link with amino groups, cross linking between protein chains could have a profound effect on enzymic hydrolysis.[49] The free carbonyls of gossypol could, of course, similarly link with enzyme protein to bind and inactivate it. Hill and Totsuka[56] showed that the addition of gossypol to a chick diet reduced the metabolizable energy of the diet. Rojas and Scott[57] observed increased metabolizable energy in chick diets in which the cottonseed meal was treated with phytase. Ferrous sulfate addition also improved the metabolizable energy value of diets containing glanded cottonseed meal but not glandless meal.

The development of an olive discoloration in egg yolk from hens fed cottonseed meal is due to the reaction between gossypol and iron in the yolk. Cyclopropenoid fatty acids, also from the cottonseed, enhance the discoloration by accelerating an increase in pH during storage, making the iron more readily available.[35] Removing the fat containing the cyclopropenoid fatty acids and reducing the amount of available gossypol are, therefore, both desirable objectives in processing cottonseed meal. The measurement of a gossypol-cephalin fraction in eggs from hens fed cottonseed meal has been used as an assay for the available gossypol in meals.[58]

Gossypol at superphysiological levels inhibits oxidative enzymes *in vitro*, but enzymes in liver mitochondria from animals showing gossypol toxicity were not inhibited when oxygen uptake was measured.[54] However, respiration involvement certainly seems indicated, and (by analogy to dicumarol and other phenols) uncoupling of oxidative phosphorylation, rather than inhibition of oxygen uptake, would be suspected as a gossypol effect.

The binding between gossypol and proteins no doubt also explains the high residual gossypol and cumulative effect of gossypol in the body. In the body, gossypol is especially high in the epithelial lining of the stomach and in the liver; considerable amounts are also bound in the kidney, spleen, blood, and muscle.[45,51,52] The liver may reach 900 mg of gossypol/kg in poisoned pigs; after cessation of intake, the level in the liver declined from 520 to 100 mg/kg total gossypol in 34 days.[46] The half-life of gossypol in the rat body, including the digestive tract, following a single small oral dose was about 48 h without—and 23 h with—added iron.[45] The ratio of extractable to residual gossypol in the tissues increased with time.[45] This indicates that gossypol was being eliminated by hydrolysis of the proteins to which it was bound and by excretion of the nontoxic[38] but soluble amino acid or peptide adduct. In trout,[55] evidence has been found of a slow buildup of gossypol bound in the tissues over an extended period of gossypol feeding. After a year or more of gossypol intake, shifting to a gossypol-free diet gave a decrease in free gossypol in body tissues, but bound gossypol decreased little—or even increased in certain tissues—over a 10-week period.

Tangeretin

The completely methylated flavonoids tangeretin, nobiletin, and the flavonol analog of nobiletin (3,3',4',5,6,7,8-heptamethoxyflavone) occur in citrus, the first two in tangerine, mandarin, and orange, and the latter in grapefruit.[59] They, of course, cannot occur as glycosides and are evidently confined to the oil receptacles such as those in the fruit peel (but not in the flesh). Juice pressed from orange peel contains about 20 mg/liter of nobiletin and perhaps 3 mg/liter of tangeretin. Along with other flavones and flavanones, tangeretin is nontoxic in various acute tests, including 500 mg/kg intraperitoneally to mice and 1,000 mg/kg orally to dogs (some diarrhea). However, tangeretin was second only to podophyllotoxin as a cytotoxin to zebra-fish embryos. It affected 50% of the embryos at 24 h at 0.2–0.4 mg/liter; nobiletin was less active but was not tested beyond 1 mg/liter.[60] With 10 mg/kg/day of tangeretin subcutaneously to rats during gestation, 83% of the offspring, although appearing normal, were born dead or died within 3 days.[61] The natural

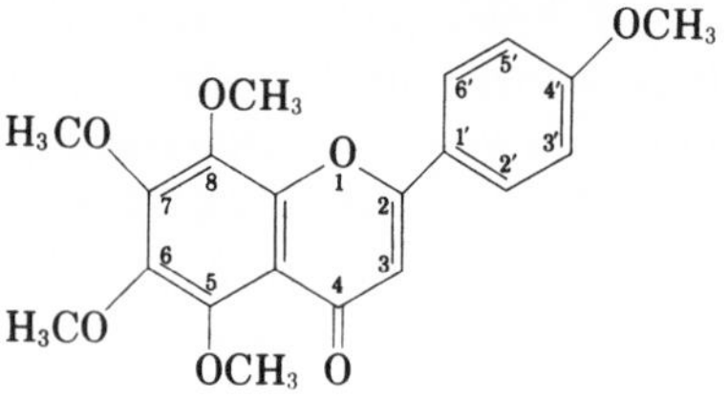

Tangeretin

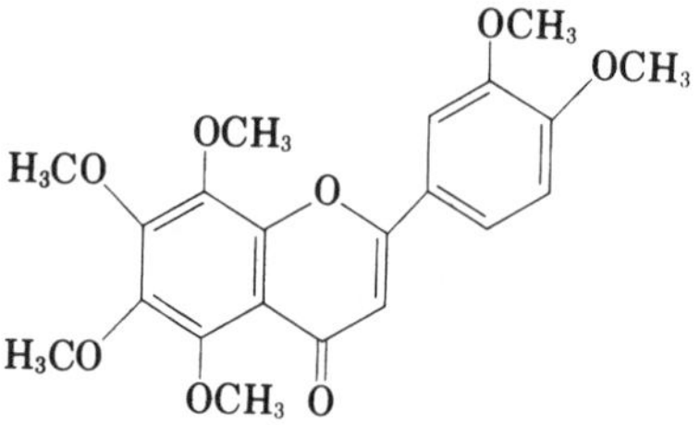

Nobiletin

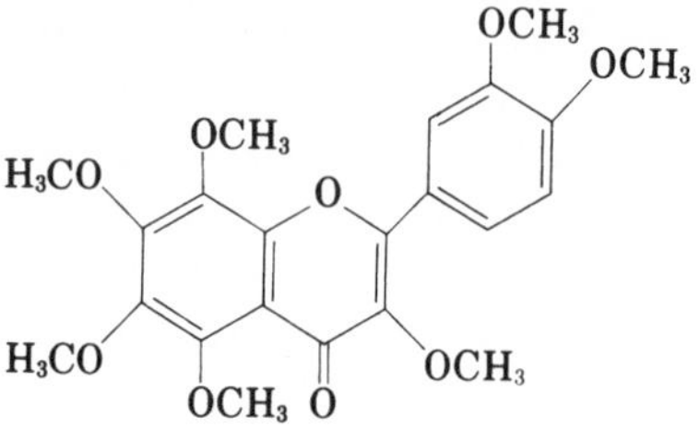

3,3',4',5,6,7,8-Heptamethoxyflavone

hazard of fruit to humans seems very small or absent. Pending further testing, regular consumption in copious amounts of tangerine peeling, and perhaps that of other citrus fruits, should be discouraged and is unlikely in any event. Its lipid solubility and completely substituted phloroglucinol ring would be suspected factors in tangeretin toxicity.

Phlorizin

The dihydrochalcones and their glycosides are of very limited and specific occurrence in plants.[59] Most of them have not been investigated toxicologically, even though some occur in toxic plants. Phloretin, 2',4',6'-trihydroxy-3-(p-hydroxyphenyl)propiophenone, occurs in apple as the 2'-glucoside (phlorizin) at levels of up to 1% in the fresh leaf, over 12% in the root bark (dry-weight basis), and about 300–400 mg/kg in

Phloretin

the fruit core and seeds.[62,63] Phlorizin produces the toxic effect of pronounced glucosuria in man and animals with oral doses of the order of 200–400 mg/kg of body weight.[64,65] The specific physiological effect is to block the active transport of glucose from kidney-tubule urine back into peritubular blood against the concentration and osmotic gradient by affecting the epithelial cells. Absorption of glucose in the small intestine is also inhibited.

The actual concentration of phlorizin at the active site in the kidney is very low, i.e., the substance is very potent. Phloretin is nearly inactive orally, and part of the activity loss en route to the kidney is probably due to hydrolysis of phlorizin.[64,65] Methylated phlorizin is inactive. Treatment of rats with 500 mg/kg subcutaneously of phlorizin for 6 days gave a slight weight loss, drowsiness, and—in spite of glucosuria—an increase in kidney glycogen.[66] This latter effect also occurs in liver and evidently results from inhibition of oxidation of carbohydrate. Phloretin (and to a lesser extent phlorizin) inhibits mitochondrial ATPase noncompetitively.[67] Phlorizin diminishes the efficiency of phosphorylation in mitochondria and causes them to swell. This swelling can be prevented by ATP addition. In plants, phlorizin and phloretin inhibit oxidative phosphorylation and have a distinct uncoupling effect,[68] phloretin being more active. Phloretin inhibits photophosphorylation by chloroplasts (phlorizin is about one third as effective) by affecting both transphosphorylation and electron transport during ATP synthesis.[69] Chloroplast ATPase is also inhibited. Studies with the absorbing cells of hamster intestinal and kidney epithelium have indicated that phlorizin is adsorbed instantaneously and strongly on a readily accessible receptor site.[70] There are a maximum of about 4×10^8 of these sites per absorbing cell membrane, and their binding would appear competitively to affect glucose uptake. However, the actual poison appears to be phloretin, which is liberated by hydrolase activity in the membrane; phlorizin serves only as a carrier of phloretin capable of penetrating some selective barrier in the membrane. Since glucose absorption is energy requiring, the phloretin would presumably act by interfering with

ATP production for this purpose, and the apparent conflict between the relative activity of phloretin and phlorizin in plants and animals would be reconciled.

Anthraquinone Cathartics

Vegetable purgatives of wide use (perhaps weekly by 30% of the elderly[71]) such as senna leaf and related products from *Cassia* spp., cascara and frangula barks from Rhamnaceae, aloe sap preparations, and rhubarb root (*Rheum* spp.) are active because of their content of anthraquinone derivatives. The species of rhubarb used are not the same as the garden food plant but are closely related.[72] Except for—or perhaps because of—the sometimes violent purging action, these compounds appear to be of low oral toxicity. A *Cassia* preparation of unknown content (but probably about 1% total anthraquinone derivatives) produced a single-dose oral LD_{50} to rats of 10 g/kg.[73] The total anthraquinone content of the natural dry drugs is usually 1–3% but may be up to 11% in fresh cascara bark. Typical laxative doses would contain 10–100 mg of anthraquinone derivatives,[13] but gross anthraquinone content is a poor measure of cathartic power.

The mixture of these substances and their chemistry is complex.[2,74,75,76] In the fresh plant the anthrone form is present, and apparently during drying and aging of the drug, dianthrones (usually two similar units but not always) and anthraquinones form or at least increase.[77] This is accompanied by a decrease in the violence and potency of the drug's action.[2] There appears to be a synergistic effect of the components. Both *C*- and *O*-glycosides are present, with the former considerably predominant. The anthraquinones present in these drugs include rhein (1,8-dihydroxyanthraquinone-3-carboxylic acid) and several others with more reduced substituents in position 3 or with additional hydroxyls. The particular group of substances present is, of course, variable by plant source. They may be biosynethsized by the acetate–malonate pathway as would be expected, or alternatively in higher plants such as *Cassia* and *Rheum* by a shikimic acid pathway as are cinnamates and flavonoids.[79]

Rhein

High purgative activity is favored in these compounds by prevention of absorption en route to the site of action, the large intestine.[80] This is favored by high molecular weight and retention of glycosidation. Retention of dianthrone and reduced forms by prevention of oxidation increases activity; the more water-soluble aglycone is usually more active. The specific toxic action seems to be to initiate strong peristalsis in the large intestine; it may be related to 5-hydroxytryptamine metabolism since this substance appears to control peristalsis and it is more than just an "irritant" effect.[1] More serious and permanent effects appear related to destruction of nervous tissue in the intestinal wall, which seems to be a factor in the "cathartic colon" problem, particularly in the elderly after long dosage.[71] Rhein in dilute solution is an inhibitor of electron transport in mitochondrial NAD-linked oxidations. Only slight uncoupling of oxidative phosphorylation was observed and, unlike rotenone (p. 315), its effect was not reversed by synthetic vitamin K.[78,79] Rhein also tends to bind various proteins, but its effect is apparently not through HS-groups.[81,82,83]

Tannins

Any plant polyphenolic substance with a molecular weight greater than about 500 can be considered to be a tannin. The two distinctive groups are the hydrolyzable and the condensed tannins.[84] They have in common protein-binding and leather-forming activities, but they usually differ considerably in botanical distribution, other properties, and breakdown products. Tannic acid is typical of the hydrolyzable tannins. It is readily hydrolyzed enzymatically or hydrolyzes spontaneously to glucose and gallic acid (p. 310) with about 7 or less gallic acid units per glucose. Other tannins of this group may yield as hydrolysis products[84] ellagic acid, which replaced gallic acid, or quinic acid, which replaces glucose.

Tannic Acid

The condensed tannins (flavolans) are polymeric flavonoids composed predominantly of leucoanthocyanidin (p. 310) units linked carbon-to-carbon from the 4-position of one unit to the 6- or 8-position of the next.[84] They do not break down readily under physiological conditions; when treated drastically, they usually produce either less soluble polymeric "phlobaphenes" or flavonoid monomers, particularly catechins and anthocyanidins.[84]

Condensed Tannin (flavolan)

Tannic acid has been the tannin most used in medical treatment; its single-dose oral acute toxicity is low, the LD_{50} to 160-g rats by gastric intubation being $2,260 \pm 83$ mg/kg.[85] One reason for the low oral toxicity is that tannic acid is hydrolyzed in passing through the normal gut, and only gallic acid or metabolic products thereof appear in blood or urine.[86] The absorption of an intact protein-binding, nondialyzable tannin macromolecule, whether hydrolyzable or condensed, seems quite unlikely, and the best evidence seems to be that it does not occur in the normally functioning alimentary tract of an animal.[1]

Liver and kidney toxicity and human fatalities, however, were produced when 3–5% tannic acid solution was used as a treatment on burned tissue. Absorption into the bloodstream must have occurred, since gallic acid does not produce the same effect.[87] Condensed tannins are somewhat less toxic in burn treatment. When injected, all tannins are rather toxic, as might be expected for powerful precipitants of proteins. A purified condensed tannin from hawthorn had LD_{50} values in mice of 300 mg/kg subcutaneously and 130 mg/kg intraperitoneally,[88] while another from spruce bark given intraperitoneally to rats had an LD_{50} of 100 mg/kg.[24] The LD_{100} value of tannic acid administered intravenously to mice was 80 mg/kg.[16]

Carcinogenicity seems to be a definite component in tannin toxicity.[87] The production of liver cancer in rats by repeated subcutaneous application of tannin has been demonstrated.[87,89] Habitual chewers of betel nut (*Areca catechu*) have a high incidence of buccal carcinoma that has been attributed to the 11–26% condensed tannins contained in the nut, although other components may be involved.[90,91] A series of epidemiological, demographic, and dietary correlations[92] present some evidence for human esophageal cancer related to food or beverage tannin. Perhaps the most nearly convincing case is the unusually high incidence of esophageal cancer in certain areas of the Transkei of South Africa when high-tannin sorghum is consumed. The cancer appears to result from chronic irritation of the mucous membranes of the throat caused by high consumption of the grain in Bantu beer and porridge; the incidence is particularly high in drought periods when high-tannin "bird-proof" grain sorghums are utilized to produce sufficient food.

Tannic acid has been used in barium enemas to improve definition of the colon wall in diagnostic x-rays. Severe acute liver damage, sometimes fatal, was produced in a small proportion of the patients.[1,93] The toxicity of tannic acid when administered rectally is about twice that of the substance when given orally.[85] The incidence of serious reactions after tannin enemas was greater when administered to juvenile patients, when the enemas were given repeatedly, when the patients had pre-existing ulcers or inflammation, when the enemas were retained in the bowel for increased periods of time, or when the tannin concentration was increased.[94,95,96] Liver injury from rectal tannic acid appears to result from damage to the intestinal wall that allows absorption of intact tannin. The damage is related to the tannin concentration; 0.25% or less in the enema preparation appears to be safe.[95] Tannic acid inhibits the absorption of glucose and methionine in the mouse intestine; this is believed to be the result of denaturation of the proteins of the protective outer cellular layer of the mucous membrane.[97] Localized destruction of epithelium of the gastrointestinal tract has been found to occur following oral administration of tannic acid and to be more severe in newborn than in older rats.[98]

A small injection of tannic acid gives recognizable cellular and subcellular changes within 1 h in kidney and liver and, if the animals recover, cells of these organs return to normal after about 7 days.[99,100,101] Effects include decreased liver glycogen, proteinuria, altered mitochondria, and fragmentation of polyribosomes with associated strong inhibition of protein and ribonucleic acid synthesis in the liver.

There are instances of significant farm-animal losses owing to high-tannin consumption in natural feed. Periodic losses in England from high consumption of oak acorns were attributed to the approximately 6%

tannin in the acorns, since no other toxic fraction was identified.[102] In the southwestern United States, annual losses of livestock may exceed $10 million from consuming shin oak (*Quercus havardi*) foliage at a time when other forage is lacking.[1,103] The toxicity results from a high level of hydrolyzable tannin, which produces liver necrosis and other effects similar to those described for other tannins. Some substances when added to the diet (e.g., iron salts, calcium salts, high protein levels) oxidize, precipitate, or bind the tannin and thus aid in avoiding this toxicity.[104]

Experimental feeding of diets with known or added tannins to chicks and to rats have shown growth depression with levels of the order of 1% of the diet, but effects are somewhat variable. Chicks are apparently more sensitive than rats. As much as 0.5% of various tannins in the drinking water of mice for 3 months gave no liver carcinoma and minimal other effects.[89] Condensed tannin, a pectinase inhibitor from sericea (*Lespedeza cuneata*) used in pickles, was fed to rats at 2% of the diet for as long as 150 days without effect on growth or other toxic effects.[105] Condensed tannin from grapes also produced no histopathological changes in rats fed 2% in their diet for 700 days.[105] Even intramuscular injection with 0.75 mg/kg of tannic acid in mice every other week for 18 months produced only a weak local reaction and no signs of cancer or other liver damage in one study.[106]

It appears that there are several causes of the growth-depressing and toxic effects of tannins, and the interplay between them and the experimental conditions account for variable observations. High tannin in the diet makes it astringent, and the animals must be starved to force them to eat it. Weight loss during this period is more serious for smaller, younger animals and seems to be at least one reason that larger animals are more tolerant of a high-tannin diet.[107] Paired feeding (i.e., the animal on the normal diet is limited to the intake of the animal on the high-tannin diet) shows that feed intake and presumably palatability are major but not the only factors in growth depression by high-tannin diets.[107,108,109]

The feeding of tannin also leads to lowered energy conversion from food and to the excretion of high levels of nitrogen in the feces.[109,110,111,112] The high nitrogen excretion results largely from the binding of dietary protein by tannin into an indigestible form. Any protein added in excess of the amount required to bind the tannin is utilized by the animal, resulting in greatly improved growth; the residual nitrogen in the feces remains about as it was before the addition.[112] Supplementation with 40% casein and 5% tannic acid gave growth equal to that of pair-fed rats without these supplements.[107] The protein–tannin complex appears to be formed by multiple hydrogen bonding, as in leather tanning, because treatment of feces with urea liberates some of the tannin.[111] Similar nonspecific binding accounts for the highly inhibitory effect of free tannin on digestive enzymes[111] and, since the body responds to high-tannin diets by synthesizing severalfold as much proteolytic enzymes,[112] part of the high nitrogen excretion is endogenous enzyme protein. A net loss of nitrogen would be possible on protein-poor and high-tannin diets, and this would be expected to be most deleterious to young animals during the period of rapid muscular growth.

Depending upon the situation, supplementation with choline, methionine and ornithine, or arginine sometimes partially counteracts dietary tannic acid toxicity.[113,114] Since no arginine or ornithine conjugate was found in the excreta,[114] their effects would presumably reflect mere supplementation of a deficient diet. Free amino acids do not bind strongly with tannin. The methyl donors (choline and methionine), however, are necessary for detoxification of gallic acid to 4-*O*-methylgallic acid, a major excretory product when tannic acid is fed.[113,114] Methylated products are also important in the detoxification of flavonoids.[21] Thus a high absorption of tannin-breakdown products would deplete the supply of the essential amino acid methionine and place further stress on the animal unless methionine or other methyl donors are plentiful in the diet. Fatty livers, a symptom of methyl-donor deficiency, were produced by 5% gallic acid, but not with 5% tannic acid in the diet of rats.[107] Catechin is also growth depressing, although it and gallic acid are less toxic than tannic acid; they do not bind protein, and they appear to affect palatability less.[109,112,115] Additional load and nutrient loss may be occasioned by other similar mechanisms. For example, gallic acid is apparently partly detoxified, at least in the rabbit, by conjugation with glucuronic acid, since the urinary excretion of glucuronic acid is increased 10-fold following gallic-acid feeding, reaching values as high as 250 mg/100 ml of urine.[116] Two metabolic products from tannic acid, pyrogallol and pyrocatechol, are highly toxic to the chicken.[113,114]

It would appear from the data now available that tannins can be seriously toxic, perhaps carcinogenic, if they enter the bloodstream. However, it seems that unless high concentrations of soluble tannins *not*

Pyrogallol

Pyrocatechol

complexed with protein or other binding agent contact mucosa in such a way as to damage it, or unless they contact burns or other unprotected areas, they are not absorbed. Unless absorbed intact, their effects seem related only to either the systemic effects of breakdown products known to be low in toxicity, or to "external" effects (particularly on palatability) and protein digestion. Since they tend to break down more, hydrolyzable tannins would be expected to be more toxic than condensed tannins in the systemic sense. The no-effect level for food-grade tannic acid in rats has been established to be 800 mg/kg body weight/day, and the total acceptable daily intake for a man is 560 mg.[96] This, however, is below the total intake of "tannin" by some persons, which may be of the order of 1,000 mg/day in coffee, tea, cocoa, etc. Mueller[117] has estimated that a child fed his entire milk intake as chocolate milk and eating additional candy might consume 160 mg/kg/day of cocoa tannin.

GENERAL CORRELATIONS AND PERSPECTIVE

Many other examples of reported plant phenol toxicity could be cited in addition to those noted above and elsewhere in this volume. However, it seems more useful to attempt to achieve some overall perspective on their various roles as a class of compounds including toxic members.[1] The phenolic substances that normally occur in foods are generally considered to be nontoxic[1,2,118,119] and certainly long history of apparently safe consumption in food and use in various experimental medical treatments[35,119-121] would bolster this view. In fact, many favorable effects have been claimed, although often later refuted or unsubstantiated, following administration of certain flavonoids and cinnamates.[35,120,121]

Some reports of toxicity of common phenols appear to result from the specific experimental conditions. Commercial rutin from eucalyptus produced cataracts after oral doses of about 25 mg to rats, but pure quercetin or rutin from other sources did not have this effect, which was evidently from contaminants.[122] In mice and rats with implanted tumors, the maximum tolerable (and tumor-inhibiting) oral dose of cyanidin-3,5-diglucoside was 350 mg/kg.[123] Purified mixtures of anthocyanidin glycosides from currants, blueberries, and elderberries produced no deaths in mice or rats with oral doses of 20 g/kg; the intravenous LD_{50} was 240 mg/kg in rats and 40 mg/kg in mice.[124] Oral doses of 6 g/day to rats for 3 months produced no gross or microscopic abnormalities. Anthocyanins and most other natural flavonoids are not very readily absorbed when fed, but rabbits fed 500 mg of grape anthocyanins excreted 1–2% of the pigment in the urine, and dogs injected intravenously with the same pigment excreted portions of it within 20 min in both bile and urine.[125] Oral doses of 750 mg of anthocyanins to humans produced no toxic effects but produced in man and animals accelerated regeneration of visual purple and dark adaptation.[126,127] The flavonoids without glycosidation and with higher lipid solubility seem more toxic; flavone, for example, had an oral LD_{50} to mice of 400 mg/kg.[128] However, in the course of studies of the metabolism of flavonoids by humans, ingestion of 2-g samples of several common flavonoids produced no significant toxic effects.[21]

The common detoxification path of flavonoids in animals involves the destruction of the phloroglucinol "A" ring[129] and the excretion of the "B" ring products in forms like those predicted from cinnamic acid metabolism.[21] Of significance to our discussion, methylation of phenolic hydroxyls and conjugation with glucuronic acid or glycine are common reactions leading to the excreted metabolites. As already discussed with tannins, this metabolic loss of methionine, glycine, and metabolizable carbohydrate would be stress producing and in marginal situations could produce or aggravate toxicity. This would appear to be the toxic mechanism for the simpler and common plant phenols, very high dietary levels of which are ordinarily required to demonstrate toxic effects experimentally. In general, feeding at 1% of the diet to experimental animals for prolonged periods has produced little or no effect on growth or other significant toxicity for naringin, hesperidin, rutin, quercetin, dihydroquercetin, quercitrin, catechin, or gallic acid.[21,115] At 2% and more of the diet, gallic acid and catechin cause increasing growth depression[115] in the rat. Bioflavonoids from citrus at 2.5% in the diet did not depress chicken growth but 5% did.[130]

From these data, it would appear to be very unlikely that the plant phenols usually present in human diets would produce significant toxic effects. In some cases, however, the amounts of phenols consumed may reach high levels and may produce some negative effects, especially when the diet is suboptimal (as may be caused by famine or idiosyncrasy, for example). Unripe persimmons have a total phenol content of the order of 13 g/kg; although only about half this amount can be recovered from the ripe fruit, the remainder probably is present but insoluble.[131] Some bananas are nearly as high in total phenols as persimmon. If grapes are consumed, seeds and all, they could contribute about 5.6 g of total phenols/kg.[132] Nearly all other fruits and vegetables have caffeic and other cinnamic acid derivatives of the order of 100–300 mg/kg fresh weight and many have as much as 500 mg/kg of flavonoids in addition.[133] Coffee and tea may contribute 1 g of total phenols/day[96] in the habitual diet in this country; in other countries consumption of an exhaustive decoction of 100 g tea/day, contributing up to 30 g of polyphenols to the diet, has led to toxic symptoms.[134] There appear to be significant positive (and some negative) correlations between cancer mortality of specific types and national per capita consumption of tea and coffee as well as cigarettes and other potential carcinogens such as solid fuels.[135]

A common observation in natural phenolic toxicity studies has been synergism, as reflected in the fact that the isolated components are not as toxic as they are when present in the natural mixture or added back together. Synergism of this general type is noted[1] with aspidium,[14] gossypol, anthraquinone cathartics, dihydromethysticin and kava components, myristicin and nutmeg components, and others. Perhaps the most striking example is the synergistic augmentation of rotenone's insecticidal activity by nontoxic phenols such as sesamin.[136] One component of such synergism appears to be the placing of extra demands on the animal's adaptive detoxification mechanisms when they are already having difficulty in coping with a toxicant. From this it would appear that normally innocuous plant phenols could increase the effect of toxic phenols. It is not uncommon to find a considerable percentage of usual, nontoxic phenols occurring in the same plant material with the unusual and toxic ones.

Sesamin

The toxicity of tangeretin would appear to be partly related to its lipid solubility and lack of glycosidation, but it also seems to depend on the animal's inability to metabolize its completely substituted phloroglucinol A-ring directly to carbon dioxide as is the case with the common flavonoids.[21,129] It seems highly significant that many of the most toxic or most physiologically potent phenolic derivatives are, or appear to be, derived from mevalonic acid–terpenoid biosynthesis: gossypol, tetrahydrocannabinol (from marihuana), and tremetone (from snakeroot), for example. Other toxic phenols appear to be derived primarily from the acetate pathway but seem to have been further modified so that they cannot be metabolized as simple phloroglucinol derivatives, e.g., anthraquinones, hypericin, aspidium components, and rhodomyr-toxin. The shikimic acid biosynthetic pathway seems to give rise to rela-tively few toxic cinnamate or flavonoid components; when they are toxic they also are substituted in additional, unusual ways (e.g., tanger-etin, isoflavones, rotenone, dicumarol, etc.). A common feature is the methylene dioxy grouping that is found in safrole and myristicin and is necessary in sesamin-type rotenone synergy.[1]

In addition to protecting the phenols from metabolism by usual ani-mal detoxification mechanisms so that they can reach vulnerable sites and cause toxicity, substitutions of the types mentioned—methylation, methylene dioxy groups, polycyclization, alkyl substituents, etc.—would increase lipid solubility, and this tends to enhance toxicity. Administra-tion of many phenolic toxicants in oil aids their absorption and increases the toxic effect; myristicin and gossypol afford two examples.[1] Related but opposite effects were noted with anthraquinone cathartics in that the glycosides (especially nonhydrolyzable *C*-glycosides) enable the medication to reach the lower bowel and act without absorption earlier. Phloretin to be active must reach the kidney as the glucoside phlorizin, even though the liberation of the aglycone in passing through the kidney cell membrane may be required for the actual toxic process.

The combination of lipid- and water-soluble properties of phenols appears important in their toxicity, membrane transfer, and penetra-tion to active sites. Phenol itself is an extraordinary solvent for proteins and is used in the laboratory to extract proteins from nucleic acids, for example. A small amount of phenol spilled on appreciable skin area is rapidly absorbed and may easily be fatal. Penetration through the skin is a feature of some forms of natural phenol toxicity, notably poison ivy urushiol and related cashew and mango dermatitis and photosensiti-zation (see Chapter 25) from topically applied psoralen.[1] Cumarin in ointment rubbed on the skin leads to the same urinary excretory prod-ucts as does parenteral administration.[137] This ready penetration applies to internal tissues as well. Esters of salicylic acid applied to the skin in ointment rapidly penetrate into the muscles directly below but not lateral to the application.[138] Aspirin is rapidly absorbed through the stomach wall; since many phenols have the required properties of rather small molecular size, polarity, and nonionizability at stomach pH, they should be absorbed also.[139]

It appears to us that this solvent action and ready penetration by phenols may explain the observations that phenols can serve as pro-moters of carcinoma. Under certain conditions, repeated application of phenols following a single application of a carcinogen such as benzo-pyrene produced skin cancers (although a single application of a carcino-

gen to animal skin did not produce cancer and phenols alone did not);
similar promoting effects are found in inhalation-induced lung cancer.[140,141] Black tea contains phenol, cresols, and other small phenols.
An initial application to skin of 3,4-benzopyrene followed by frequent
applications of brewed tea produced epithelial carcinoma in 6 of 15
treated mice.[142] Pyrolysis produces smaller phenols such as guaiacol and
4-vinylguaiacol from lignin, ferulic acid, and other larger natural phenols;
however, carcinogenic hydrocarbons and phenols are also among the
products of pyrolysis of cellulose, glucose, fructose, sodium acetate,
proteins, amino acids, etc.[143]

Urushiol

The analyzed content of phenols in the surface layer of smoked meat
is only of the order of 37 mg/kg, although it appears this is about half
the true value.[144] At this dilute level of phenol content, tumor promotion by solubilization of carcinogenic hydrocarbons and by carrying
them along as the cells are penetrated would seem unlikely. Although
the possibility of tumor promotion by phenols seems to be real enough
and it should not be forgotten, as a food hazard it seems small, in view
of the long and apparently safe use of smoked foods without demonstrated adverse effects.[144]

An action of phenols generally, including natural plant phenols, is
the uncoupling of oxidative phosphorylation in the mitochondria so
that respiration energy is not trapped in usable form as ATP but is
wasted. This effect can be predicted from physical and chemical data on
a series of substituted phenols, taking into account hydrophobic (lipophilic) character and tendency to ionize.[145] These data predict about
equally well the relative toxicity and uncoupling activities. Highly ionizable phenols tend to be more active in phosphorylation uncoupling,
and the nitrophenols are much more active than the natural phenols.
However, a major action involved in the toxicity of rotenone and dicumarol is the uncoupling of oxidative phosphorylation. The specific
site of action is apparently different, since they are affected differently
by antagonists such as vitamin K. Concentration of the phenol at or in
specific membranes seems to be involved (thus lipoidal solubility), and
inhibition of energy requiring membrane transport is a frequent effect,
as seems to be the case with phlorizin in glucosuria. The pain-relieving

effect of salicylates is believed to involve inhibition of oxidative phosphorylation at specific pain receptors.[12]

Common features of phenol toxicity are the cumulative effect and the relatively prolonged retention of the substance in the body. This is the case with gossypol, dicumarol, tetrahydrocannabinol, urushiol, hypericin, psoralen, and podophyllin.[1] These effects involve binding of the phenol to body constituents. In some cases, for example, with gossypol and perhaps tremetone, the binding is primarily via nonphenolic functionality. In other instances, it appears to involve hydrogen bonding and other linking dependent upon the phenolic character. Certainly the effect of tannin in tying up dietary protein is a related example. Urushiols from poison ivy are rapidly bound as the skin is penetrated.[1] Tetrahydrocannabinol binds to plasma lipoproteins.[146] Salicylates bind to albumin in blood and are no longer dialyzable.[1] Salicylates and phenylbutazone potentiate the effect of coumarin anticoagulants, such as dicumarol, apparently by displacing them from nonspecific binding sites in the liver and blood-plasma proteins.[147,148] The binding, however, need not be simple, readily displaced complexing. Covalent linking has been demonstrated between the catechol portion of urushiols and proteins.[149] The mechanism involves oxidation of the catechol to *ortho*-quinone and then linking of the protein groups (particularly sulfhydryl) to the activated, unsubstituted positions on the quinone ring. This strong binding mechanism is available to many plant phenols, including gossypol, which contains the common catechol type of substitution.

Another potential toxic effect involves metal chelation, as is evident in anemia related to gossypol and tannin toxicity and some other conditions such as prolonged overdosing with aspirin. Many phenols, including common ones with low toxicity, bind metal ions rather strongly through vicinal functional groups.

Since phenols are commonly detoxified by methylation, competitive inhibition of O-methyltransferase by plant phenols is apparently the reason they often prolong the action of adrenaline.[1,21] Interference with nerve-regulating animal phenols appears to be involved in the central-nervous-system effects reported for the active phenolic constituents of marihuana, nutmeg, sassafras, marking nut, and kava. Similar peripheral effects are indicated by trembling, analgesia, peristalsis, etc., as shown by salicylates, anthraquinone cathartics, tremetone, and hypericin.[1]

A mild goitrogenic action by anthocyanins from various sources, by catechin, quercitrin, and phloroglucinol, appears to result from the binding of iodine with these phenols instead of with tyrosine to form thyroxine.[150,151]

Irradiation of psoralen produces activation, which enables interstrand cross linking with DNA; this effect is related to photosensitizing activity in animals.[152] Light activation, production of free radicals, etc., are common properties of plant phenols, but these specific effects seem limited to substances that have a certain molecular structure. Similarly, the estrogenic activity of isoflavones and coumestrol appears to result from the positioning of two phenolic hydroxyls a certain distance apart in a relatively planar molecule.[1]

CONCLUDING REMARKS

Although some plant phenols are quite toxic, and a few phenols have caused occasional serious human poisonings or serious losses of animals, these are mostly caused by phenolic structures uncommon in human food. The common phenols are of low toxicity under most circumstances. However, this low toxicity appears to result from efficient barriers developed by animals through long contact with common plant phenols. Several toxic mechanisms appear to be potentially available for most plant phenols, but if natural defenses are overloaded (by large amounts) or evaded (by unusual forms of administration or unusual derivatives), toxicity may result. Barring accidental consumption of plant material or medicines not normally considered to be food for humans, the most likely toxicity to humans would appear to be marginal effects from unusually high consumption of a high-phenol beverage or food, coupled with a poor diet. Such effects appear rare and are difficult to demonstrate. They would be more likely in juvenile, senile, or debilitated individuals. Some suggestive relationships (such as those between mouth cancer and the chewing of high-tannin areca nut, or throat cancer and high-tannin grain sorghum consumption) need further investigation to be considered proved, but caution is certainly suggested.

REFERENCES

1. V. L. Singleton and F. H. Kratzer, Toxicity and related physiological activity of phenolic substances of plant origin. J. Agric. Food Chem. *17*:497 (1969).
2. J. W. Fairbairn (ed.), The pharmacology of plant phenolics. Academic Press, New York (1959).
3. J. M. Kingsbury. Deadly harvest, a guide to common poisonous plants. Holt, Rinehart and Winston, New York (1965).
4. K. F. Lampe and R. Fagerström, Plant toxicity and dermatitis, a manual for physicians. Williams & Wilkins, Baltimore (1968).
5. S. B. O'Leary, Poisoning in man from eating poisonous plants. Arch. Environ. Health *9*:216 (1964).

6. J. M. Kingsbury, Poisonous plants of the United States and Canada. Prentice-Hall, Englewood Cliffs, N.J. (1964).
7. J. W. Hardin and J. M. Arena, Human poisoning from native and cultivated plants. Duke University Press, Durham, N.C. (1969).
8. H. G. Scott, Poisonous plants and animals. In Food-borne infections and intoxications, H. Riemann (ed.). Academic Press, New York (1969).
9. F. Corcilius, Die Wirkstoffe der Rosskastanie und ihre Biochemischen Funktionen bei Erkrankungen des Venensystems. Q. J. Crude Drug Res. 7:1005 (1967).
10. G. Vogel, M. L. Marek, and R. Oertner, Untersuchungen zum Mechanismus der therapeutichen und toxischen Wirkung des Rosskastanien-Saponins Aescin. Arzneïmittel-Forsch. 20:699 (1970).
11. N. H. Anderson, W. D. Ollis, J. G. Underwood, and R. M. Scrowston, Constitution of the dibenzofuran *psi*-rhodomyrtoxin, isolated from *Rhodomyrtus macrocarpa* Benth. J. Chem. Soc. C. 2403 (1969).
12. M. J. H. Smith and P. K. Smith, The salicylates: A critical bibliographic review. Wiley, New York (1966).
13. P. G. Stecher (ed.), The Merck index. 8th ed. Merck and Co., Rahway, N.J., p. 107 (1968).
14. M. J. Mattila and S. Takki, The effect of non-phloroglucinol residues of fern extracts on the toxicity and absorption of desaspidin. Ann. Med. Exp. Biol. Fenn. 45:357 (1967).
15. A. Georges, Y. Gerin, and J. Denef, Toxic effects of purified fern extracts. Proc. Eur. Soc. Stud. Drug Toxicity 10:218 (1969).
16. W. S. Spector, Handbook of toxicology, Vol. 1. W. B. Saunders, Philadelphia, (1956).
17. R. Chatterjee, Indian Podophyllum. Econ. Bot. 6:342 (1952).
18. A. Heyndrickx, Toxicology of insecticides, rodenticides, herbicides, and phytopharmaceutical compounds. Prog. Chem. Toxicol. 4:179 (1969).
19. K. Böhm, Die Flavonoide. Arzneimittel-Forsch. 9:539,647,778 (1959); 10: 54,139,188,468,547 (1960).
20. S. Radouco-Thomas, P. Grumback, G. Nosal, and F. Garcin, Etude toxicologique de quelques facteurs P. Therapie 20:879 (1965).
21. F. De Eds, Flavonoid metabolism, In Comprehensive biochemistry, M. Florkin and E. H. Stotz (eds.). 20:127–171. Elsevier, Amsterdam (1968).
22. F. Chassevent, L'Acide chlorogenique ses actions physiologiques et pharmacologiques. Ann. Nutr. Aliment. 23:1 (1969).
23. M. Mancini, P. Oriente, and L. D'Andrea. Hypocholesterolemic effects of quinic acid 1,4-dicaffeate in atheroscloerotic patients, p. 533–537. In S. Garattini and R. Paoletti (eds.) Drugs affecting lipid metabolism. Proceedings of a Symposium on Drugs Affecting Lipid Metabolism. Elsevier, Amsterdam (1961).
24. P. Claveau and M. Masquelier, Le metabolisme du leucocyanidol chez le rat. Can. J. Pharm. Sci. 1:74 (1966).
25. L. C. Berardi and L. A. Goldblatt. Gossypol, p. 211. In Toxic constituents of plant foodstuffs, I. E. Liener (ed.). Academic Press, New York (1969).
26. K. M. Decossas, L. J. Molaison, A. de B. Kleppinger, and V. L. Laporte, Cottonseed oil and meal utilization. J. Am. Oil. Chem. Soc. 45:52A (1968).
27. A. M. Altschul, C. M. Lyman, and F. H. Thurber. Cottonseed meal, p. 469. In Processed plant protein foodstuffs, A. M. Altschul (ed.). Academic Press, New York (1958).

28. U.S. Department of Agriculture, Proceedings of the 1967 Cottonseed Processing Clinic. ARS 72-61 Washington, D.C. (1967).

29. F. E. M. Gillham, Cotton in a hungry world. S. Afr. J. Sci. 65:173 (1969).

30. A. A. Adamova and M. A. Lebedeva, Khlopkovyi zhmykh kak dopolnitelnyi istochnik pitaniya. Gig. Sanit. 12:33 (1947).

31. G. A. Harper and K. J. Smith. Status of cottonseed protein. Econ. Bot. 22:63 (1968).

32. R. Adams, T. A. Geissman, and J. D. Edwards, Gossypol, a pigment of cottonseed. Chem. Rev. 60:555 (1960).

33. P. F. Heinstein, D. L. Herman, S. B. Tove, and F. H. Smith, Biosynthesis of gossypol. Incorporation of mevalonate-2-^{14}C and isoprenyl pyrophosphates. J. Biol. Chem. 245:4658 (1970).

34. R. Reiser and H. C. Fu, The mechanism of gossypol detoxification by ruminant animals. J. Nutr. 76:215 (1962).

35. R. A. Phelps, Cottonseed meal for poultry. World's Poult. Sci. J. 22:86 (1966).

36. R. Bressani, L. G. Elias, and A. Porras, Effect of pH on the free and total gossypol and nutritive value of cottonseed and protein concentrate. Arch. Latinoam. Nutr. 19:367 (1969).

37. L. C. Berardi and W. H. Martinez, Gossypol source versus biological activity. Proceedings of the Conference on Inactivation of Gossypol with Mineral Salts. National Cottonseed Products Association. Memphis (1966).

38. E. Eagle, A review of some physiological effects of gossypol and cottonseed pigment glands. J. Am. Oil Chem. Soc. 37:40 (1960).

39. A. J. Clawson, F. H. Smith, L. C. Osborne, and E. R. Barrick, Effect of protein source, autoclaving, and lysine supplementation on gossypol toxicity. J. Anim. Sci. 20:547 (1961).

40. F. Hale, C. M. Lyman, and H. A. Smith, Use of cottonseed meal in swine rations. Bull. 898 Tex. Agric. Exp. Stn. (1958).

41. W. S. Harms and K. T. Holly, Hypoprothrombinemia induced by gossypol. Proc. Soc. Exp. Biol. Med. 77:297 (1951).

42. H. N. Ramaswamy and R. T. O'Connor, Spectroscopic properties of some metal complexes of gossypol. Appl. Spectrosc. 24:50 (1970).

43. H. N. Ramaswamy and R. T. O'Connor, Metal complexes of gossypol. J. Agric. Food Chem. 17:1406 (1969).

44. J. E. Braham, R. Jarquin, R. Bressani, J. M. Gonzalez, and L. G. Elias, Effect of gossypol on the iron-binding capacity of serum in swine. J. Nutr. 93:241 (1967).

45. M. B. Abou-donia, C. M. Lyman, and J. W. Dieckert, Metabolic fate of gossypol: The metabolism of ^{14}C-gossypol in rats. Lipids 5:939 (1970).

46. J. A. Buitrago, A. J. Clawson, and F. H. Smith, Effects of dietary iron on gossypol accumulation in and elimination from porcine liver. J. Anim. Sci. 31:554 (1970).

47. T. R. Shieh, E. Mathews, R. J. Wodzinski, and J. H. Ware, Effect of calcium and phosphate ions on the formation of soluble iron-gossypol complex. J. Agric. Food Chem. 16:208 (1968).

48. E. J. Conkerton and V. L. Frampton, Reactions of gossypol with free epsilon-amino groups of lysine of proteins. Arch. Biochem. Biophys. 81:130 (1959).

49. C. M. Lyman, B. P. Baliga, and M. W. Slay, Reactions of proteins with gossypol. Arch. Biochem. Biophys. 84:486 (1959).

50. J. N. Tone and D. R. Jensen, Effect of ingested gossypol on the growth performance of rats. Experientia 26:970 (1970).

51. F. H. Smith and A. J. Clawson, Effects of dietary gossypol on animals. J. Am. Oil Chem. Soc. *47*:443 (1970).
52. C. M. Lyman, J. T. Cronin, M. M. Trant, and G. V. Odell, Metabolism of gossypol in the chick. J. Am. Oil Chem. Soc. *46*:100 (1969).
53. C. M. Cater and C. M. Lyman, Effect of bound gossypol in cottonseed meal on enzymic degradation. Lipids *5*:765 (1970).
54. L. A. Meksongee, A. J. Clawson, and F. H. Smith, The *in vivo* effect of gossypol on cytochrome oxidase, succinoxidase, and succinic dehydrogenase in animal tissues. J. Agric. Food Chem. *18*:917 (1970).
55. J. N. Roehm, D. J. Lee, and R. O. Sinnhuber, Accumulation and elimination of dietary gossypol in the organs of rainbow trout. J. Nutr. *92*:425 (1967).
56. F. W. Hill and K. Totsuka, Studies on the metabolizable energy of cottonseed meals for chicks, with particular reference to the effect of gossypol. Poult. Sci. *43*:362 (1964).
57. S. W. Rojas and M. L. Scott, Factors affecting the nutritive value of cottonseed meal as a protein source in chick diets. Poult. Sci. *48*:819 (1969).
58. C. R. Grau, E. Allen, M. Nagumo, C. L. Woronick, and P. A. Zweigart, A distinctive yolk component in the fresh eggs of hens fed gossypol. J. Agric. Food Chem. *2*:982 (1954).
59. J. E. Kefford and B. V. Chandler, The chemical constituents of citrus fruits. Advances Food Research, Suppl. 2. Academic Press, New York (1970).
60. R. W. Jones, M. G. Stout, H. Reich, and M. N. Huffman, Cytotoxic activities of certain flavonoids against zebra-fish embryos. Cancer Chemother. Rep. *34*:19 (1964).
61. M. G. Stout, H. Reich, and M. N. Huffman, Neonatal lethality of offspring of tangeretin-treated rats. Cancer Chemother. Rep. *36*:23 (1964).
62. A. H. Williams, Dihydrochalcones, p. 297. In Comparative phytochemistry, T. Swain (ed.). Academic Press, New York (1966).
63. A. B. Durkee and P. A. Poapst, Phenolic constituents in core tissues and ripe seed of McIntosh apples. J. Agric. Food Chem. *13*:137 (1965).
64. F. W. McKee and W. B. Hawkins, Phlorizin glucosuria. Physiol. Rev. *25*:255 (1945).
65. W. D. Lotspeich, Phlorizin and the cellular transport of glucose. Harvey Lect. *56*:63 (1960–61).
66. S. Babu, T. V. Madhavan, and K. R. Rao, Effect of phlorizin and related compounds on glucose excretion, kidney glycogen content and alkaline phosphatase activity of treated rats. Indian J. Med. Res. *55*:1226 (1967).
67. M. T. Tellez de Inon, Inhibition of mitochondrial ATPase by phlorizin. Acta Physiol. Lat. Am. *18*:268 (1968).
68. G. Stenlid, On the physiological effects of phlorizin, phloretin, and some related substances upon higher plants. Physiol. Plantarum *21*:882 (1968).
69. E. G. Uribe, Phloretin: An inhibitor of phosphate transfer and electron flow in spinach chloroplasts. Biochem. *9*:2100 (1970).
70. D. F. Diedrich, Is phloretin the sugar transport inhibitor in intestine? Arch. Biochem. Biophys. *127*:803 (1968).
71. Anonymous, Cathartic action. Br. Med. J. *4*(5633):723 (1968).
72. N. Taylor, Plant drugs that changed the world. Dodd, Mead, New York (1965).
73. D. G. Patel, S. S. Karbhari, O. D. Gulati, and S. D. Gokhale, Antipyretic and analgesic activities of *Aconitum spicatum* and *Cassia fistula*. Arch. Int. Pharmacodyn. *157*:22 (1965).

74. J. W. Fairbairn, The anthracene derivatives of medicinal plants. Lloydia 27: 79 (1964).
75. A. Stoll and B. Becker, Sennosides A and B, the active principles of senna. Prog. Chem. Org. Nat. Prod. 7:248 (1950).
76. R. Kinget, Studies in the field of drugs containing anthracene derivatives. 17. The quantitative determination of anthracene derivatives of Rhamnus purshiana bark. Lloydia 31:17 (1968).
77. R. P. Labadie, Anthracene derivatives in Rhamnus frangula. 1. The aglycones. Pharm. Weekbl. 105:189 (1970).
78. T. J. McCarthy, Distribution of glycosyl compounds in South African aloe species. Planta Med. 17:1 (1969).
79. E. Leistner and M. H. Zenk, Chrysophanol (1,8-dihydroxy-3-methylanthraquinone) biosynthesis in higher plants. Chem. Commun. (5):210 (1969).
80. J. W. Fairbairn and M. J. R. Moss, Relative purgative activities of 1,8-dihydroxyanthracene derivatives. J. Pharm. Pharmacol. 22:584 (1970).
81. E. A. Kean, Rhein: An inhibitor of mitochondrial oxidations. Arch. Biochem. Biophys. 127:528 (1968).
82. E. A. Kean, Inhibitory action of rhein on the reduced nicotinamide adenine dinucleotide-dehydrogenase complex of mitochondrial particles and on other dehydrogenases. Biochem. Pharmacol. 19:2201 (1970).
83. E. A. Kean, M. Gutman, and T. P. Singer, Rhein, a selective inhibitor of the DPNH-flavine step in mitochondrial electron transport. Biochem. Biophys. Res. Commun. 40:1507 (1970).
84. E. Haslam, Chemistry of vegetable tannins. Academic Press, New York (1966).
85. E. M. Boyd, K. Bereczky, and I. Godi, The acute toxicity of tannic acid administered intragastrically. Can. Med. Assoc. J. 92:1292 (1965).
86. F. W. Blumenberg and F.-J. Kessler, Untersuchungen über die Resorbierbarkeit oral zugeführten Tannins. Arzneimittel-Forsch. 10:742 (1960).
87. B. Korpássy, Tannins as hepatic carcinogens. Prog. Exp. Tumor Res. 2:245 (1961).
88. W. Rewerski and S. Lewak, Einige pharmakologische Eigenschaften der aus Weissdorn (Crataegus oxyacantha) isolierten Flavan-Polymeren. Arzneimittel-Forsch. 17:490 (1967).
89. K. S. Kirby, Induction of tumours by tannin extracts. Br. J. Cancer 14:147 (1960).
90. V. Raghava and H. K. Baruah, Arecanut: India's popular masticatory—History, chemistry, and utilization. Econ. Bot. 12:315 (1958).
91. D. Schmahl, Krebserzeugung durch Naturstoffe. Dtsch. Med. Wochenschr. 89:575 (1964).
92. J. F. Morton, Tentative correlations of plant usage and esophageal cancer zones. Econ. Bot. 24:217 (1970).
93. M. L. Janower, L. L. Robbins, and D. E. Wenlund, A review of the use of tannic acid in patients with ulcerative colitis. Radiology 89:42 (1967).
94. F. F. Zboralske, P. A. Harris, S. Riegelman, O. N. Rambo, and A. R. Margulis, Toxicity studies on tannic acid administered by enema. 3. Studies on the retention of enemas in humans. 4. Review and conclusions. Am. J. Roentgen. 96:505 (1966).
95. Anonymous, A reprieve for tannic acid on the way? Food Cosmetol. Toxicol. 5:244 (1967).
96. Anonymous, Tannic acid again. Food Cosmetol. Toxicol. 7:364 (1969).

97. S. Mitjavila, G. De Saint-Blanquat, and R. Derache, Effet de l'acide tannique sur l'absorption intestinale chez le souris. Food Cosmetol. Toxicol. *8*:27 (1970).

98. M. S. Weinberg, R. E. Goldhamer, and S. Carson, Acute oral toxicity of various drugs in newborn rats after treatment of the dam during gestation. Toxicol. Appl. Pharmacol. *9*:234 (1966).

99. R. K. Boler, J. S. Broom, and R. B. Arhelger. Ultrastructural renal alterations following tannic acid administration to rabbits. Am. J. Pathol. *49*:15 (1966).

100. A. A-B. Badawy, A. E. White, and G. H. Lathe, The effect of tannic acid on the synthesis of protein and nucleic acid by rat liver. Biochem. J. *113*:307 (1969).

101. J. K. Reddy, M. Chiga, C. C. Harris, and D. J. Svoboda, Polyribosome disaggregation in rat liver following administration of tannic acid. Cancer Res. *30*: 58 (1970).

102. E. G. C. Clark and E. Cotchin, A note on the toxicity of the acorn. Br. Vet. J. *112*:135 (1956).

103. B. J. Camp, E. Steel, and J. W. Dollahite, Certain biochemical changes in blood and livers of rabbits fed oak tannin. Am. J. Vet. Res. *28*:290 (1967).

104. G. V. N. Rayudu, R. Kadirvel, P. Vohra, and F. H. Kratzer, Effect of various agents in alleviating the toxicity of tannic acid for chickens. Poult. Sci. *49*: 1323 (1970).

105. A. N. Booth and T. A. Bell, Physiological effects of sericea tannin in rats. Proc. Soc. Exp. Biol. Med. *128*:800 (1968).

106. J. Bichel and A. Bach, Investigation on the toxicity of small chronic doses of tannic acid with special reference to carcinogenicity. Acta Pharmacol. Toxicol. *26*:41 (1968).

107. Z. Glick and M. A. Joslyn, Food intake depression and other metabolic effects of tannic acid in the rat. J. Nutr. *100*:509 (1970).

108. P. Handler and R. D. Baker, The toxicity of orally administered tannic acid. Science *99*:393 (1944).

109. P. Vohra, F. H. Kratzer, and M. A. Joslyn, The growth depressing and toxic effects of tannins to chicks. Poult. Sci. *45*:135 (1966).

110. J. K. Conner, I. S. Hurwood, H. W. Burton, and D. E. Fuelling, Some nutritional aspects of feeding sorghum grain of high tannin content to growing chickens. Aust. J. Exp. Agric. *9*:497 (1969).

111. M. Tamir and A. Alumot, Carob tannins—Growth depression and levels of insoluble nitrogen in the digestive tract of rats. J. Nutr. *100*:573 (1970).

112. Z. Glick and M. A. Joslyn, Effect of tannic acid and related compounds on the absorption and utilization of proteins in the rat. J. Nutr. *100*:516 (1970).

113. G. V. N. Rayudu, R. Kadirvel, P. Vohra, and F. H. Kratzer, Toxicity of tannic acid and its metabolites for chickens, Poult. Sci. *49*:957 (1970).

114. D. K. Potter and H. L. Fuller, Metabolic fate of dietary tannins in chickens. J. Nutr. *96*:187 (1968).

115. M. A. Joslyn and Z. Glick, Comparative effects of gallotannic acid and related phenolics on the growth of rats. J. Nutr. *98*:119 (1969).

116. F.-W. Blumenberg and R. Dohrmann, Über den Ausscheidungsmechanismus oral zugeführter Gallussäure. Arzneimittel-Forsch. *10*:109 (1960).

117. W. S. Mueller, The significance of tannic substances and theobromine in chocolate milk. J. Dairy Sci. *25*:221 (1942).

118. E. C. Bate-Smith, Flavonoid compounds in foods. Adv. Food Res. 5:261 (1954).
119. W. Pearson, Flavonoids in human nutrition and medicine. J. Am. Med. Assoc. 164:1675 (1957).
120. J. J. Willaman, Some biological effects of the flavonoids. J. Am. Pharm. Assoc. Sci. Educ. 44:404 (1955).
121. Anonymous, Today's drugs—Vitamin P. Br. Med. J. No. 5368:235 (1969).
122. Y. Nakagawa, M. R. Shetlar, and S. H. Wender, Physiological effects of commercial rutin samples on rats. Life Sci. 4:753 (1965).
123. O. K. Kabiev and S. M. Vermenichev, O protivoopukholevykh svoistvakh 3,5-diglikozid-tsianidina. Vopr. Onkol. 16(8):60 (1970).
124. H. Pourrat, P. Bastide, P. Dorier, A. Pourrat, and P. Tronche, Preparation and therapeutic activity of some anthocyanin glycosides. Chem. Ther. 2:33 (1967).
125. M. K. Horwitt, Observations on behavior of the anthocyan pigment from Concord grapes in the animal body. Proc. Soc. Exp. Biol. Med. 30:949 (1933).
126. R. Alfieri and P. Sole, Influence des anthocyanosides administrés par voie oro-perlinguale sur l'adapto-électroretinogramme (AERG) en lumière rouge chez l'homme. C. R. Soc. Biol. 160:1590 (1966).
127. R. Wegmann, K. Maeda, P. Tronche, and P. Bastide, Effets des anthocyanosides sur les photorecepteurs. Aspects cytoenzymologiques. Ann. Histochim. 14:237 (1969).
128. V. Demole, Toxicité, résorption, élimination de la flavone synthétique. Helv. Physiol. Acta 20:93 (1962).
129. N. P. Das and L. A. Griffiths, Studies on flavonoid metabolism. Metabolism of (+)-[14C]-catechin in the rat and guinea pig. Biochem. J. 115:831 (1969).
130. C. W. Deyoe, L. E. Deacon, and J. R. Couch, Citrus bioflavonoids in broiler diets. Poult. Sci. 41:1088 (1962).
131. T. O. M. Nakayama and C. O. Chichester, Astringency of persimmons. Nature 199:72 (1963).
132. V. L. Singleton and P. Esau, Phenolic substances in grapes and wine and their significance, Adv. Food Res., Suppl. 1, p. 282. Academic Press, New York (1969).
133. K. Heintze, Untersuchungen über die Vitamin P-wirksam Flavonoidverbindungen und ihre Bedeutung in Pflanzlichen Lebensmitteln. Dtsch. Lebensm.-Rundsch. 61:309 (1965).
134. A. Porot, Les toxicomanies, étude medico-sociale. Libraire Ferraris, Algiers. (1945).
135. P. Stocks, Cancer mortality in relation to national consumption of cigarettes, solid fuel, tea, and coffee. Br. J. Cancer 24:215 (1970).
136. P. Budowski and K. S. Markley, The chemical and physiological properties of sesame oil. Chem. Rev. 48:125 (1951).
137. I. Pekker and E.-A. Schäfer, Vergleich von enteraler und perkutaner Resorption von Cumarin. Arzneimittel-Forsch. 19:1744 (1969).
138. J. Pütter, Resorptionsuntersuchung an Salicylaten. 2. Die percutane Resorption von Salicylsäure-2'-hydroxyläthylester bei äusserlicher Anwendung. Arzneimittel-Forsch. 20:1721 (1970).
139. A. R. Cooke, Aspirin, ethanol and the stomach. Australas. Ann. Med. 19:269 (1970).
140. R. K. Boutwell, Phenolic compounds as tumor-promoting agents, p. 120. In Phenolic compounds and metabolic regulation, B. J. Finkle and V. C. Runeckles (eds.). Appleton-Century-Crofts, New York (1967).

141. B. L. Van Duuren, A. Sivak, L. Langseth, B. M. Goldschmidt, and A. Segal, Initiators and promoters in tobacco carcinogenesis. Nat. Cancer Inst. Monogr. *28*:173 (1968).

142. H. E. Kaiser, Cancer-promoting effects of phenols in tea. Cancer *20*:614 (1967).

143. E. B. Higman, I. Schmeltz, and W. S. Schlotzhauer, Products from the thermal degradation of some naturally occurring materials. J. Agric. Food Chem. *18*: 636 (1970).

144. P. Issenberg, M. R. Kornreich, and A. O. Lustre, Recovery of phenolic wood smoke components from smoked foods and model systems. J. Food Sci. *36*: 107 (1971).

145. T. Fujita and M. Nakajima, The correlation between physiological activity and physicochemical property of the substituted phenols. Residue Rev. *25*:319 (1969).

146. M. Wahlqvist, I. M. Nilsson, F. Sandberg, S. Agurell, and B. Granstrand, Metabolism of cannabis. 4. Binding of Δ^1-tetrahydrocannabinol to human plasma proteins. Biochem. Pharmacol. *19*:2579 (1970).

147. A. I. Sandler, Interactions of oral coumarin anticoagulants with other drugs. Drug Intel. Clin. Pharm. *4*:146 (1970).

148. R. A. O'Reilly and G. Levy, Pharmacokinetic analysis of potentiating effect of phenylbutazone on the anticoagulant action of warfarin in man. J. Pharm. Sci. *59*:1258 (1970).

149. J. C. Byck and C. R. Dawson, Assay of protein-quinone coupling involving compounds structurally related to the active principle of poison ivy. Anal. Biochem. *25*:123 (1968).

150. N. R. Moudgal, E. Raghupathy, and P. S. Sarma, Studies on goitrogenic agents in foods. J. Nutr. *66*:291 (1958).

151. E. Jeney, Review and new data on the goitrogenic properties of flavonoids, Kiserl. Orvostud. *20*:514 (1968) (Trans.)

152. R. S. Cole, Light-induced cross-linking of DNA in the presence of a furocoumarin (psoralen). Studies with phage *Lambda, Escherichia coli,* and mouse leukemia cells. Biochim. Biophys. Acta *217*:30 (1970).

16 David W. Fassett

OXALATES*

Although oxalates have long been known to occur in nearly all forms of living matter, it is of interest to note that certain families and species of plants contain relatively large amounts of this substance, mainly as the soluble sodium or potassium salts or the insoluble calcium salts. The name is attributed to its occurrence in the plant *Oxalis* (wood sorrel).

The earliest interest in the toxicity of oxalates arose because of instances of severe or fatal human poisoning following the eating of large quantities of the leaves of certain plants (e.g., rhubarb) known to contain relatively large amounts of oxalates. Accidental ingestion of oxalic acid as a pure chemical was also known to produce severe corrosive and other toxic effects; hence, the conclusion was drawn that the acute poisonous effects of ingesting high-oxalate-content plants were probably related to that property.

The occurrence of calcium oxalate in the majority of cases of human kidney stones led to concern with the role of ingested oxalate in their formation. The insolubility of calcium oxalate occasioned many studies of the significance of ingestion of plant oxalates on calcium absorption and of the possibility that calcium deficiency might result from the oxalate content of foods. An attempt will be made in this chapter to evaluate the evidence for the role of plant oxalates in the production of toxic

* Literature reviewed through January 1972.

346

effects or disease in man and animals. Two recent general reviews of plant oxalates and their biochemistry and toxicity have appeared since the first edition of this book, and these provide additional sources of information.[1,2]

CHEMISTRY AND ANALYTICAL METHODS

Oxalic acid, HOOC-COOH, is the simplest of the dicarboxylic acids. It is a crystalline, white solid, soluble in water to about 10% at 20 °C. It is a strong acid (with a pK_1 of 1.46 and a pK_2 of 4.40) and commonly exists as a dihydrate. The neutral salts such as Na or K are readily water soluble, while the alkaline earth or metal salts are less soluble. The calcium salt is insoluble at neutral or alkaline pH but becomes soluble in acid.

Oke[1] has studied the effects of cations and of salts, amino acids, carbohydrates, and oxyacids on the solubility of calcium oxalate. The oxyacids tend to increase the solubility and to shift the pH at which precipitation occurs toward the basic side. Citric and tartaric acids are very effective.

Ester and amide formations occur as do other reactions of carboyxlic acids. The carbon–carbon bond is readily oxidized; heating of oxalic acid causes loss of CO_2 and the formation of formic acid and carbon monoxide.[3,4]

A variety of analytical methods is available for oxalates,[1] and many are based on isolation of the oxalate as the calcium salt followed by oxidation. In a detailed study of the conditions of precipitation of calcium oxalate (CaC_2O_4) from urine (using ^{14}C oxalate to check recoveries), it was found that water saturated with the bactericide pentachlorophenol and with CaC_2O_4 helped to prevent losses during washing of the precipitate. A known quantity of sodium oxalate ($Na_2C_2O_4$) added to urine before precipitation, and the use of a ^{14}C isotope-determined correction factor, improved the results.[5] The isolation from plants by means of an HCl extraction followed by ether extraction and evaporation has been used to determine total oxalate content.[6] Prolonged treatment with hot acid may give high results from conversion of other compounds to oxalates.[7]

It is possible to determine oxalic acid colorimetrically by reduction to glycolic acid with magnesium and development of color with 2,7-dihydroxynaphthalene.[8] The relatively high amounts present in plants have made the use of classical analytical methods generally feasible. However, considerable care is needed in applying them to mammalian tissues, where the quantities are much lower. The use of more modern methods, such as the formation of trimethyl silyl esters and determination by gas chromatography, may allow more certain determination of the identity of oxalates in body fluids and urine.[9] A fluorimetric method for determination in blood and urine has been described based on isolation of the calcium salt, reduction to glyoxylate, and formation of a fluorescent complex with ascorbic acid.[10]

OCCURRENCE OF OXALIC ACID IN PLANTS

A very large literature exists on the distribution of oxalates in the plant kingdom.[1,2] Generally, the highest levels are found in the families Polygonaceae (*Rheum, Rumex*), Chenopodiaceae (*Spinacia, Beta, Atriplex*), Portulacaceae (*Portulaca*), Ficoidaceae (*Tetragonia*). Some of the common plant foods containing appreciable oxalates (fresh-weight basis) are: spinach, 0.3–1.2%; rhubarb, 0.2–1.3%; beet leaves, 0.3–0.9%; tea, 0.3–2.0%; and cocoa, 0.5–0.9%. Most of the fruits and vegetables commonly used as food in the United States contain far less oxalate, perhaps one tenth the above amounts or less (e.g., lettuce, celery, cabbage, cauliflower, turnips, carrots, potatoes, peas, and beans).

One of the plants with the highest known oxalate content is *Halogeton glomeratus* (Chenopodiaceae), which grows in many parts of the western United States in cold, arid areas. This plant contains as much as 30% dry weight of oxalate. It is present almost entirely as the sodium salt. Another high oxalate plant is *Oxalis cernua* (Oxalidiaceae), which grows in parts of Australia and in southern Italy. This plant, which has the oxalate as the potassium acid salt, has a sap pH of about 2. Halogeton has a sap pH of about 6. Both of these plants have caused injury in sheep and cattle.[11] Maymone *et al.*[12] have made extensive studies of the metabolism of oxalates in ruminants fed large quantities of *Oxalis*.

The distribution of oxalates varies with families, but generally the leaves are higher in oxalate content than the stalks. The ratio of oxalate to calcium content also varies widely; it is possible to class plants in three groups: (a) those with an oxalate–calcium ratio of 2 : 7 (e.g., spinach, beet leaves, rhubarb, cocoa); (b) those with a ratio about 1 (e.g., potatoes, gooseberries); and (c) those with a ratio less than 1 (e.g., lettuce, cabbage, peas). Many kinds of mushrooms and molds also produce oxalates, e.g., *Aspergillus niger, Mucor, Boletus sulfurens, Sclerotina.*[13]

The biosynthesis of oxalates in plants has been the subject of much conjecture and some work. It seems clear that oxalates are an end product and tend to accumulate in plants. Some plant species accumulate certain organic acids only in the dark; these acids, e.g., malic and citric, are then used during photosynthesis. Generally, oxalates tend to increase during the life of the plant, although there may be a decrease later on as the plant ages.

Studies have been made of the effect of light on the synthesis of oxalate in spinach.[14] Seedlings kept in the dark had lower total oxalates than those grown in 12-h light and dark periods, indicating a photosynthetic process in oxalate formation. Also, spinach plants treated with 12-h dark and light periods, followed by 72 h of darkness, showed little further change in oxalate level, indicating that utilization was unlikely. Low temperatures increased oxalate formation as did treatment with cations.

One possible function of oxalic acid may be to act as a buffer system. In the case of beets, the addition of calcium and nitrates increased the amount of insoluble oxalate. However, some evidence was found for limited metabolism of ^{14}C-labeled oxalate by beet tissue disks. The accumulation of oxalate appeared to be related to nitrate assimilation and cation–anion imbalance.[15]

Oxalate almost certainly arises from some part of carbohydrate metabolism, e.g., from formation of glycolic acid and subsequent oxidation to glyoxylic and oxalic acid. A glycolic acid oxidase is present in spinach.[16] Another possibility is the splitting of oxalacetic acid; small amounts may be formed from purine or ascorbic acid metabolism.

An interesting recent report indicates that some organisms, e.g., *Aspergillus niger,* can adapt certain enzymic activities to produce more oxalate.[17] Normally, *A. niger* produces little oxalate in submerged culture but is able to form large amounts on a nitrogen-free carbohydrate medium. A lag period of some hours occurs when the organism is first transferred to such a medium. Increased activity of pyruvate carboxylase and oxaloacetate hydrolase was noted, and substrates were used up in both sets of conditions. Mechanisms such as this may play a role in determining oxalate production in other organisms.

METABOLISM IN MAN AND ANIMALS

Two recent comprehensive references on the metabolism of oxalate should be consulted for the details of this complex subject.[18,19] It has been recognized since 1838 that man excretes varying amounts of calcium oxalate crystals in the urine. The excretion is now known to vary in normal children and adults from about 6 to 45 mg/day, with a mean of about 20 mg/day, expressed as oxalic acid.

About one third of urinary oxalate is thought to be derived from ascorbic acid, and similar amounts are derived from glycine. A few milligrams come from dietary oxalate and possibly from precursors in vegetables such as glycolic or glyoxylic acids. Serum values have a mean of about 450 μg/100 ml (fluorimetric method), but the values may be lower (140 μg/100 ml plasma) with other analytical methods. About 45 μg/day are excreted in the feces. The content in tissues varies from about 60 μg/100 g (wet weight) in brain to 400 μg/100 g in the kidney. The turnover of the miscible pool is rapid (25–50 mg/day).

The absorption from the gut is only 1–6% if the oxalate is given with meals, but under fasting conditions 30–50% of a tracer dose may be absorbed and excreted in the urine. It is clear that in various mammalian species, ingested or injected oxalate is not broken down but is excreted unchanged in the urine or feces. Bacterial degradation in the rumen of cattle and sheep may allow the safe ingestion of quantities that would be hazardous for other species.[11]

A metabolic, genetically determined disease occurs in which much larger amounts of endogenous oxalates occur, producing renal stones and deposits of calcium oxalate in other tissues. Oxalates and glycolates are greatly increased in the urine along with slight increases in glyoxylic acid. It is thought that the basic defect is an inability to transaminate glyoxylate from glycine; this results in increased formation of glyoxylate from glycolates and hence in oxalic acid[18]:

$$\begin{array}{c} \text{glycolate} \\ \Updownarrow \\ \text{glycine} \xrightarrow{\hspace{0.3em}\not{\hspace{0.2em}}\hspace{0.3em}} \text{glyoxylate} \longrightarrow \text{oxalate} \\ \text{block in} \\ \text{transaminase} \end{array}$$

Studies of patients with urinary stones show that most excrete normal quantities of oxalic acid; some increase may be noted when the urine also contains more calcium. The urine is supersaturated with respect to oxalates, but other compounds in the urine may act as stabilizers. The role of exogenous oxalates in the production of renal stones seems doubtful in most cases.

ACUTE TOXIC EFFECTS

For many years case reports have appeared in textbooks and in the literature of acute poisoning from ingestion of oxalate-containing plants, particularly those in the Polygonaceae family and particularly the species rhubarb (*Rheum rhaponticum* L.) and sorrel grass (*Rumex acetosa*

L.). Because of the fact that these plants are known to contain a somewhat higher oxalate content than most other foods, the cause of the symptoms has almost invariably been attributed to this factor. A number of textbooks on poisoning or poisonous plants discuss the role of oxalic acid.[20-26] Symptoms are said to be similar to those noted in human beings ingesting oxalic acid, and the authors stress the occurrence of corrosive effects in the mouth or intestinal tract, and of gastric hemorrhage, renal colic or hematuria, and sometimes convulsions. Other authors have expressed doubt as to the role of oxalate content in rhubarb poisoning. For example, Sollmann[27] doubts if the oxalate content of rhubarb leaves is responsible for the poisoning. Locket[28] states that fatal poisoning by rhubarb leaves is probably mythical and that a person would need to eat some 4 kg of rhubarb to get the lowest recorded fatal dose of oxalic acid. Drill[29] mentions that the oxalate content of vegetables such as rhubarb and spinach has no "significance unless an unlikely degree of indulgence . . . is assumed." He points out that this may not be the case in cattle eating very large quantities of vegetable matter.

Although there is no question that the ingestion of sufficient (about 5 g or more) oxalic acid as crystals or in solution by human beings can be fatal, with associated corrosive gastroenteritis, shock, convulsive symptoms, low plasma Ca, high plasma oxalates,[30] and renal damage,[31] a careful examination of some of the alleged cases of oxalate poisoning from rhubarb allows some question as to the etiology. A case that has been repeatedly quoted is that reported by Robb.[32] This report, published in 1919, is a brief letter to the editor of the *Journal of the American Medical Association.* A housewife had prepared rhubarb for supper by frying some of the leaves for greens and by boiling the stalks. The husband ate the stalks but only a small quantity of the leaves. Some 12 h later the housewife developed cramp-like abdominal pains and by about 50 h after ingestion of the rhubarb she developed symptoms of shock, vomited a brownish fluid, and aborted a 6-week-old fetus. The woman died some hours later, and it was mentioned that there was some bleeding from the nose after death. The husband appeared to have few symptoms except for feeling weak and dizzy the day following ingestion of the rhubarb. There was no postmortem examination nor was there any analysis of the ingested plant. No mention was made of oxalate crystals in the urine or of any disturbance of kidney function. No description was given of corrosive effects in the mouth.

A more recent case is that reported by Tallqvist and Väänänen[33] of the death of a child from oxalic acid poisoning caused by eating rhubarb leaves. In this instance a 5-yr-old girl, along with other children in an orphanage, was said to have eaten some raw rhubarb stalks and in addition had been fed some rhubarb leaves by her friends. There was no evidence as to the quantity of leaves or stalks ingested. No immediate symptoms were reported, but later in the same day the child became drowsy and would not eat. She eventually vomited a dark material; she was treated with sedatives and developed coma and some reduction in urinary output. No oxalate crystals in the urine were mentioned, but it was stated that a qualitative oxalic acid test was strongly positive. No postmortem examination was done. Death, however, was definitely attributed to oxalic acid in the rhubarb leaves and stalks.

A second case was mentioned of a 4-yr-old girl with abdominal pain and vomiting the day after eating raw rhubarb. Vomiting persisted for some 5 days, following which the patient was hospitalized. It was established that uremia and anuria were present. An increase in potassium in the blood was noted, but the blood calcium was not determined. At autopsy this patient showed the typical picture of a lower nephron nephrosis, but no oxalate crystals were found. The authors consider the etiology of this case as not being clearly established.

Certainly neither of these cases appeared to fit the typical picture of a corrosive gastroenteritis that is known to follow ingestion of oxalic acid. Furthermore, it is rather doubtful that oxalic acid exists in the free form in plants.[34] The oxalates exist in vegetables such as spinach and rhubarb principally as the calcium or potassium salts. An extensive review by Jeghers and Murphy[35] on oxalate metabolism indicates that the oxalate content of spinach is actually not very different from that in rhubarb. It is thus apparent that the difference in oxalate content between rhubarb leaves or stalks and other common foods, such as spinach, is scarcely sufficient to establish rhubarb as a poison. Furthermore, the form in which the oxalate is present seems unlikely to be capable of causing a corrosive tissue change.

There seems to be a scarcity of experimental work on this subject. Tanner and Tanner,[25] however, quote a report by Maue[36] that he and five other individuals repeatedly ate cooked rhubarb leaves without effect and that these leaves contained 0.4% oxalate. Maue believed oxalates were not responsible for previously reported illnesses.

Although it is possible that, as stated by Locket,[28] some of the reports of poisoning from rhubarb leaves are coincidental, there does seem to be a certain amount of evidence that rather severe symptoms have been produced at times from this source. It is somewhat remarkable that toxicologists have not generally considered the role that might be played by various toxic anthraquinone derivatives present in these species[34] (see Chapter 15). In a recent monograph,[37] there is considerable discussion of the chemistry of the anthraquinone type of purgative, and it has been pointed out that these compounds may exist in both the roots and stems of species such as rhubarb or sorrel grass. It has also been found that the glycoside is probably the active form of the compound and that the reduced form of the quinone may be oxidized on storage. It therefore seems possible that these substances may have been involved in some of the cases.

A recent report by Streicher[38] makes this suggestion. In this instance a 6-yr-old girl and her 4-yr-old brother ate the stems and leaves of raw rhubarb in quantities varying from 20 to 100 g. Both developed profuse vomiting within 2 h and eventually developed slight icterus and enlargement of the liver. The girl developed a renal insufficiency and a 4+ albumin in the urine. It is significant that no oxalates were present in the urine in this case. Recovery followed extracorporeal hemodialysis. Streicher suggests that these cases could scarcely have been attributed to oxalates, since the ingestion of the latter would have been of the order of only 0.2–0.8 g. He points out that 200 g of rhubarb stalk, 300 g of red beets, 150 g of celery, or 200 g of spinach would have furnished the same amount of oxalate as that eaten by the girl.

It was also stated in this paper that the anthraquinone glycosides are present in the leaves, especially in the early summer, and that in their fresh state they are extremely irritating. The content of anthraquinones could be as high as 0.5–1% of the weight of the fresh leaf. A study with human volunteers by Schmid[39] showed that 10–20 g of fresh rhubarb leaves caused immediate vomiting. Streicher proposes that the highly irritating reduced forms of the anthraquinone glycosides are likely to be absorbed readily and are probably responsible for toxic effects in the liver and kidney.

Another example of confusion as to the etiology of the toxic effects of an oxalate-containing plant is discussed in a recent study of the toxic principle in *Dieffenbachia,* an ornamental plant.[40] The juice of this plant has been known for centuries to cause a severe local irritation in the mouth, the cause allegedly being its content of calcium oxalate crystals. The mechanism was shown to be due to the presence of a labile protein-like substance that was capable of causing histamine release.

There has been much interest in the nature of the toxic effects in sheep and cattle grazing on plants containing very high levels of oxalates, such as *Halogeton glomeratus* and *Oxalis cernua.* The ability of the rumen organisms to metabolize oxalates appears to be limited; if the intake is sufficient, both acute and chronic effects occur.[12,41]

James[41] considers that there are three syndromes following excessive oxalate ingestion in ruminants: the first related to acute hypocalcemia, the second to vascular damage to the gut but no hypocalcemia, and the third to gradual renal insufficiency from calcium oxalate deposits. Cattle are less frequently involved than sheep, perhaps due to their grazing patterns. Abnormalities in some serum enzymes—e.g., serum glutamic oxalacetic transaminase (SGOT), serum glutamic pyruvic transaminase (SGPT), and lactic acid dehydrogenase (LDH)—have been observed in sheep.[42]

The evidence for oxalate as the cause of ruminant toxicity from grazing on *Halogeton* and similar plants seems reasonable. However, no studies were found in which an effort was made to uncover other toxic principles in these plants.

It is obvious from this review of the literature that, in spite of many reports of human poisoning attributed to oxalic acid in plants, those cases described in any detail bear little, if any, resemblance to those known to have occurred from the chemical oxalic acid. There seems to be little evidence for a corrosive action on the mouth, esophagus, or stomach. The onset of symptoms seems to be delayed, and there is no apparent uniformity regarding the matter of oxaluria. A review of inquiries at the National Clearinghouse for Poison Control Centers[43] shows 18 reported episodes of eating of rhubarb leaves in the years 1959 through 1964; no fatalities occurred, and only five instances of nonspecific symptoms such as vomiting, diarrhea, or abdominal cramps were reported. It is possible that oxalates may play a role in some cattle poisoning, but it appears much more likely that toxic anthraquinone glycosides may have been involved in human cases. Seasonal variations in glycoside content and alterations during cooking would seem to be important variables in the toxic actions. Additional toxicologic work is needed to clarify the nature of any toxic principles in rhubarb leaves and in other species of Polygonaceae.

CHRONIC EFFECTS

With regard to chronic effects of oxalate-containing foods in human nutrition, there are a number of reports in the literature dealing with this subject. The principal question raised is whether there are any practical circumstances in which the oxalic acid content of food would sufficiently affect calcium metabolism to produce a deleterious effect. The same question has also been raised with the phosphate and phytate content of the diet, and considerations have also been given to other organic acids such as citric, malic, tartaric, and benzoic in relation to the possibility of influencing calcium metabolism. The role of oxalates was reviewed by Jeghers and Murphy[35] and also discussed briefly in a review by Nicolaysen et al.[44]

It is difficult to discuss the possible effect of oxalates in foods without some consideration of modern concepts of calcium metabolism and calcium homeostasis. There seems to be general agreement[45,46] that man and a number of other animals have an extraordinary ability to adapt to widely varying intakes of calcium without the production of deleterious effects. In many parts of the world the daily intake of calcium is perhaps half or less than that occurring in the United States, and yet the evidence for a true calcium deficiency is not readily apparent. It is also obvious that the dietary content of vitamin D has a major effect on the uptake of calcium from the intestinal tract. In addition, it is known that the efficiency of absorption of calcium may be greater in individuals on a low-calcium diet than in those with high intake. The higher percentage of absorption of calcium in the young growing individual is, of course, well known. Whether a borderline calcium deficiency in older individuals is related to the general tendency to osteoporosis is uncertain; there seems to be no clear evidence that calcium deficiency is involved, although theoretically this is possible. In general, it is apparent that, because of the very large storage of available calcium in the bony structure of the body, many species, including man, adapt very successfully to widely varying levels of calcium intake, provided certain diseases are not present and vitamin D intake is adequate for that species.

One of the earlier and more comprehensive reports on studies of the possible effect of oxalic acid in food is that by Kohman.[47] This article reported an extensive study of the calcium and oxalate content of a wide variety of foods, and it was pointed out that there was no necessary relationship between the calcium and oxalate content. Some foods, such as spinach, although having a high calcium content, have a sufficiently high oxalate content to interfere with the absorption of the contained calcium and with other dietary calcium as well. In this experiment, 21-day-old rats were fed a basal diet of roast beef, peas, carrots, and sweet potatoes; the calcium content was only 0.093%. To this diet was added about 5–8% of various greens containing sufficient calcium to raise the total calcium level to about 0.22%. Dietary feeding was continued for a period of 21 days. Under these conditions the addition of spinach having an oxalate content of about 0.9% and a calcium content of 1.25% on a dry-weight basis caused interference with growth and bone formation. On the other hand, if the rats were fed greens containing fairly high calcium levels (2–4% dry weight) but a low oxalate content (0.14% dry weight), e.g., turnip greens, kale, mustard greens, and collards, they showed good growth and bone formation. If additional calcium carbonate was added to the spinach supplement in the diet, then growth and bone formation were comparable to those obtained on a greens diet low in oxalates. When the dietary feeding period was continued until the rats were 90 days of age, the group on the spinach diet had obvious bone difficulties, including dental abnormalities and soft pliable bones. It seems probable from the results of this experiment that the animals may have been on a diet borderline in vitamin D as well as very low in calcium.

On the other hand, MacKenzie and McCollum[48] did not produce serious effects in the rats at an oxalate concentration in the diet of 2.5% unless there was also a deficiency of calcium, phosphorus, or vitamin D. For example, on a 1.7% potassium oxalate diet, containing 0.35% calcium and 0.35% phosphorus, some slowing of growth and of bone formation was noted. If vitamin D intake was optimum and the calcium and phosphorus contents of the diet were 0.6% and 0.7%, respectively, then the presence of 0.9% potassium oxalate did not affect growth or percent bone ash in a period of 10 weeks. The 2.5% level of potassium oxalate did, however, cause a somewhat lower bone ash but caused no growth effects. It was concluded that it would be impossible for a person with an adequate calcium intake to ingest enough oxalate from foods in a normal diet for it to be harmful; if, however, there was borderline intake of calcium plus a high oxalate intake, calcium deficiency might result.

One of the most extensive experimental studies of the chronic toxicity of oxalic acid is that by Fitzhugh and Nelson.[49] In this case, addition of oxalic acid to the diets of rats at levels varying from 0.1 to 1.2% caused no significant effects over the entire 2-yr period of the experiment. No mention was made of any type of bone deformity. While the calcium content of the diet was not specifically stated, it is believed that the diet consisted of a standard laboratory chow, which usually contains calcium in considerable amounts (probably 1.5%). In any event, the conclusion could be drawn that, under the circumstances of this experiment, even massive quantities of oxalic acid produced no toxicity.

Another pertinent study is that by Nicolaysen *et al.,* in which rats were placed on a vitamin D-free diet containing 0.5% calcium and 0.5% phosphorus.[50] When 0.5% sodium oxalate was added to this diet, some resorption of calcium from bones was noted, and a negative balance occurred. However, if vitamin D was added to the diet, there was a large increase in uptake of calcium—even in the presence of the sodium oxalate. In other words, the vitamin D-fed rats adapted their calcium absorption when vitamin D was present to meet the deficiency encountered by reason of the presence of oxalates in the diet.

Since calcium requirements vary considerably in different species,[51] it is difficult to predict the effect of food oxalate on human calcium metabolism. For example, in the young male adult of various species, requirements for calcium in terms of mg/kg/day are stated to be as follows: man, 12; cattle, 22; dog, 260; monkey, 155; rat, 160; and mouse, 900. While there may be some question as to the validity of the very high values for dogs and mice, it is evident that several species require 10 times as much calcium on a body-weight basis as does man.

Some of the more important human studies on calcium metabolism or on the effects of oxalate on human calcium metabolism are pertinent to this discussion. Extensive long-term calcium balance studies were carried out by Malm[45] over periods of 70–812 days with carefully controlled calcium intake levels of 937 mg/day and 459 mg/day. The results showed remarkable adaptation of most individuals to this drastic restriction in calcium intake, although the length of time for this to occur varied considerably between individuals. The adaptation was probably achieved primarily through an increase in absorption efficiency in the intestine as well as through some reduction in urinary calcium excretion. It seems likely, therefore, in view of this comprehensive study, that food oxalates would have to reduce calcium availability more than half in order to cause deleterious effects.

Another human study was that by Johnston *et al.*[52] Six college women, 21 yr of age, were placed for a 4-week period on a basal diet containing 820 mg of calcium/day. During a second 4-week period, 120 g of spinach was added daily to the diet. The spinach provided an added amount of calcium equivalent to 160 mg and had an oxalic acid content of 0.6 g. The diet was adequate but probably provided a relatively low vitamin D intake. During a third 4-week period, the time of feeding the spinach was changed from morning to night; the milk in the diet was not taken in conjunction with the spinach. Aside from an increase in fecal output of calcium (more or less equivalent to the calcium content in the spinach), no significant changes were noted in calcium balance. Urinary output showed no significant effect. All the subjects had a small negative balance throughout the entire period, including the first 4-week control period.

A second human study of the effect of spinach is that by Bonner *et al.*[53] Ten children, 5–8 yr of age, were put on a control diet for 7 months prior to the beginning of the study. During the experimental periods, the children received the basal diet plus 100 g of canned spinach daily. This amount of spinach contained 0.7 g of oxalic acid and contributed 5–7% of the calcium of the basal diet. After a 25-day period on the basal diet, there was a 15-day period on the basal diet plus spinach, followed by a 5-day period in which oxalic acid and calcium equivalent to the amount in spinach were added to the basal diet. Nitrogen, calcium, and phosphorus were measured in the urine and feces. The results of this careful experiment showed no effect on the storage of any of the elements (including calcium) as a result of the spinach feedings. Although the results were variable in the oxalate–calcium portion of the feeding study, there was no significant deleterious effect. In general, the conclusion was reached that this very intensive treatment with spinach caused no obvious alteration in calcium metabolism or balances in the children.

Finally, an interesting study by Brune and Bredehorn,[54] carried out in the pig, was concerned with the ability of that animal to utilize some of the calcium from calcium oxalate added to the diet. Calcium oxalate (20 g) was added to the diet daily for 155 days. The diet was low in both calcium and oxalate. Surprisingly, 76% of the 20 g could not be accounted for in the feces. The assumption was made that bacterial degradation might have occurred in the intestine, making the calcium available. There was also no increase in the oxalate in the urine, and no toxic symptoms were noted. Of even more significance, the authors gave calcium oxalate-^{14}C by mouth and noted the rapid appearance of carbon dioxide-^{14}C in expired air. Studies were also made with calcium oxalate containing [45]Ca. These studies indicated that 15% of the total calcium oxalate was degraded during its passage through the gastrointestinal tract. Balance studies indicated definite absorption of a considerable portion of calcium from calcium oxalate in this species.

Considering the above experimental data in relation to modern understanding of calcium metabolism and homeostasis, as well as the relatively low intake per day of the high-oxalate-containing vegetables,[55] the concern expressed by Kohman[47] regarding the possible hazardous effects of ingesting oxalate-containing vegetables seems unwarranted. The generally high calcium and vitamin D intakes in the United States seem to provide further assurance that no deleterious effects are resulting from such sources. It would seem to require a rather improbable combination of circumstances—a very high intake of oxalate-containing food plus a simultaneously low calcium and vitamin D intake over a prolonged period—for chronic toxic effects to be noted.

SUMMARY

Biochemical studies in recent years have clarified to a considerable extent the biosynthetic mechanisms for oxalate production in living matter. In both plants and animals, it appears to be principally an end product of metabolism, and in mammals at least is excreted unchanged in the urine. Oxalate is very poorly absorbed under nonfasting conditions in humans, and urinary oxalate arises principally from endogenous sources; ascorbic acid and glycine–glycolate metabolism furnish the bulk.

Continued re-examination of the possibility of calcium deprivation from dietary oxalate interference with calcium absorption provides little evidence that this is a significant problem. The metabolism of orally ingested calcium oxalate in the human probably needs further study, since there may be some possibility of bacterial oxalate decomposition in the gut.[54] The effect of dietary oxalate on the absorption of other essential metals (e.g., zinc) has had relatively little attention, nor is there any evidence regarding possible interactions of oxalates with other chelating agents such as phytates (see Chapter 17).

The cause of acute toxic effects of rhubarb leaves and similar plants in humans needs further study, since there is a strong possibility that toxic agents other than oxalates may be the principal cause of symptoms. The current fad for ingestion of enormous quantities of ascorbic acid as a cold preventive should be examined as to the possibility of producing undesirably large increases of urinary oxalate.

There appears little doubt that if the intake from forage exceeds the capacity of rumen decomposition, sheep and cattle may develop serious acute and chronic symptoms accompanied by deposition of calcium oxalate crystals in various tissues. Although other toxic principles in plants such as *Halogeton* have not been entirely ruled out, the evidence points to an extreme oxalate absorption as the causative agent. This is perhaps the sole example of a well-documented toxic effect of naturally occurring oxalates in animals or man.

REFERENCES

1. O. L. Oke, Oxalic acid in plants and in nutrition, p. 262. World review of nutrition and dietetics, *10*. S. Karger, Basel (1969).

2. I. Gontzea and P. Sutzescu, Natural antinutritive substances in foodstuffs and forages, C. Maugsch (trans.). S. Karger, Basel (1968).

3. P. Karrer, Organic chemistry. Elsevier Publishing Co., New York (1950).

4. L. S. Fieser and M. Fieser, Organic chemistry. 3rd ed. Reinhold, New York (1956).

5. G. C. Koch and F. M. Strong, Determination of oxalate in urine, Anal. Biochem. *27*:162 (1969).

6. J. C. Andrews and E. T. Viser, Oxalic acid content of some common foods. Food Res. *16*:306 (1951).

7. P. M. Zarembski and A. Hodgkinson, The determination of oxalic acid in food. Analyst *87*:698 (1962).

8. B. Niedieck, Eine Schnellmethode zur Gesamtoxalatbestimmung in Blattge-
    müsen. Züchter *29*:184 (1959).
9. C. E. Dalgliesh, E. C. Horning, M. G. Horning, K. L. Knox, and K. Yarger, A
    gas-liquid chromatographic procedure for separating a wide range of metabo-
    lites occurring in urine or tissue extracts. Biochem. J. *101*:792 (1966).
10. P. M. Zarembski and A. Hodgkinson, The fluorimetric determination of oxalic
    acid in blood and other biological materials. Biochem. J. *96*:717 (1965).
11. L. F. James, Locomotor disturbance of cattle grazing: *Halogeton glomeratus*.
    J. Am. Vet. Assoc. *156*:1310 (1970).
12. B. Maymone, M. Tiberio, M. Dattilo, and A. Giacomini, The metabolism of
    oxalic acid in ruminants given exclusive and prolonged alimentation of
    Oxalis cernua Thunb. Ann. Sper. Agrar. *16*:515 (1962).
13. B. J. Wilson and C. H. Wilson, Oxalate formation in moldy feedstuffs as a pos-
    sible factor in livestock toxic disease. Am. J. Vet. Res. *22*:961 (1961).
14. J. W. Kitchen, E. E. Burns, and R. Langston, The effects of light, temperature
    and ionic balance on oxalate formation in spinach. Proc. Am. Soc. Hortic. Sci.
    85:465 (1964).
15. K. W. Joy, Accumulation of oxalate in tissues of Sugar-beet, and the effect of
    nitrogen supply. Ann. Bot. *28*:689 (1964).
16. J. S. Fruton and S. Simmonds, General biochemistry. 2nd ed. Wiley, New York
    (1958). P. 520.
17. W. E. Jefferson and J. L. Harrison, Adaptive changes in enzymic activities
    associated with oxalate production in *Aspergillus niger*. Fed. Proc. *30*, Part II:
    1167 (1971).
18. J. B. Wyngaarden and T. D. Elder, Primary hyperoxaluria and oxalosis. In The
    metabolic basis of inherited disease, 2nd ed., J. B. Stanbury, J. B. Wyngaarden
    and D. S. Frederickson (eds.). McGraw-Hill, New York (1966). Pp. 189–212.
19. A. Hodgkinson and P. M. Zarembski, Oxalic acid metabolism in man: A review.
    Calc. Tiss. Res. *2*:115 (1968).
20. G. M. Dack, Food poisoning, University of Chicago Press, Chicago (1943). Pp.
    55–56.
21. E. B. Dewberry, Food poisoning, Leonard Hill, London (1959). Pp. 188–189,
    245–246, and 248.
22. R. H. Dreisbach (ed.), Handbook of poisoning: Diagnosis and treatment, 3rd ed.
    Lange Medical Publications, Los Altos, Calif. (1961).
23. K. F. Maxcy, pp. 918–919. In Preventive medicine and public health, M. J.
    Rosenau (ed.). Appleton-Century-Crofts, New York (1956).
24. W. C. Muenscher, Poisonous plants of the U.S. Macmillan, New York (1957).
    P. 67.
25. F. W. Tanner and L. P. Tanner, Food borne infections and intoxications. 2nd
    ed. Garrard Press, Champaign, Ill. (1953). Pp. 157–160.
26. J. M. Watt and M. G. Breyer-Brandwijk, The medicinal and poisonous plants of
    southern and eastern Africa. 2nd ed. Livingstone, Edinburgh (1962).
27. T. Sollmann, A manual of pharmacology and its applications to therapeutics
    and toxicology. 8th ed. Saunders, Philadelphia (1957).
28. S. Locket, Clinical toxicology. Mosby, St. Louis (1957).
29. V. A. Drill (ed.), Pharmacology in medicine. 2nd ed. McGraw-Hill, New York
    (1958).
30. P. M. Zarembski and A. Hodgkinson, Plasma oxalic acid and calcium levels in
    oxalate poisoning. J. Clin. Path. *20*:283 (1967).

31. M. N. Gleason, R. E. Gosselin, and H. C. Hodge (eds.), Clinical toxicology of commercial products. Williams & Wilkins, Baltimore (1963).
32. H. F. Robb, Death from rhubarb leaves due to oxalic acid poisoning. J. Am. Med. Assoc. *73*:627 (1919).
33. H. Tallqvist and I. Väänänen, Death of a child from oxalic acid poisoning due to eating rhubarb leaves. Ann. Paediatr. Fenn. *6*:144 (1960).
34. C. Wehmer, Die Pflanzenstoffe, Vol. 1. Gustav Fischer, Jena (1929).
35. H. Jeghers and R. Murphy, Practical aspects of oxalate metabolism. N. Engl. J. Med. *233*:208 (1945).
36. G. Maue, Über die Inhaltsstoffe der Rhabarberblätter. Z. Unters. Nahr. Genuss. *40*:345 (1920).
37. J. W. Fairbairn (ed.), The pharmacology of plant phenolics. Academic Press, London (1959).
38. E. von Streicher, Akutes Nierenversagen und Ikterus nach einer Vergiftung mit Rhabarberblattern. Dtsch. Med. Wochenschr. *89*:2379 (1964).
39. W. Schmid, Assay of anthraglycoside drugs. Use of the leaves of medicinal and edible rhubarb. Dtsch. Apoth.-Ztg. *91*:452 (1951).
40. F. W. Fochtman, J. E. Manno, C. L. Winek, and J. A. Cooper, Toxicity of genus *Dieffenbachia*. Toxicol. Appl. Pharmacol. *15*:38 (1969).
41. M. P. James, A. A. Seawright, and D. P. Steele, Experimental acute ammonium oxalate poisoning of sheep. Aust. Vet. J. *47*:9 (1971).
42. L. F. James, Serum, electrolyte, acid-base balance and enzyme changes in acute *Halogeton* poisoning in sheep. Can. J. Comp. Med. *32*:539 (1968).
43. J. J. Crotty, National Clearinghouse for Poison Control Centers, Washington, D.C., personal communication.
44. R. Nicolaysen, N. Eeg-Larsen, and O. J. Malm, Physiology of calcium metabolism. Physiol. Rev. *33*:424 (1953).
45. O. J. Malm, Adaptation to alterations in calcium intake, p. 143. In The transfer of calcium and strontium across biological membranes, R. H. Wasserman (ed.). Academic Press, New York (1963).
46. R. H. Wasserman (ed.), The transfer of calcium and strontium across biological membranes. Academic Press, New York (1963).
47. E. F. Kohman, Oxalic acid in foods and its behavior and fate in the diet. J. Nutr. *18*:233 (1939).
48. C. G. MacKenzie and E. V. McCollum, Some effects of dietary oxalate on the rat. Am. J. Hyg. *25*:110 (1937).
49. O. G. Fitzhugh and A. A. Nelson, The comparative chronic toxicities of fumaric, tartaric, oxalic and maleic acids. J. Am. Pharm. Assoc. Sci. Ed. *36*:217 (1947).
50. Anonymous, Calcium metabolism in rats. Nutr. Rev. *16*:148 (1958).
51. W. S. Spector (ed.), Handbook of biological data. W. B. Saunders, Philadelphia (1956). P. 196.
52. F. A. Johnston, T. J. McMillan, and G. D. Falconer, Calcium retained by young women before and after adding spinach to the diet. J. Am. Diet. Assoc. *28*:933 (1952).
53. P. Bonner, F. C. Hummel, M. F. Bates, J. Horton, H. A. Hunscher, and I. G. Macy, The influence of a daily serving of spinach or its equivalent in oxalic acid upon the mineral utilization of children. J. Pediatr. *12*:188 (1933).
54. H. Brune and H. Bredehorn, On the physiology of bacterial degradation of calcium oxalate and the ability to utilize calcium from calcium oxalate in the pig.

Z. Tierphysiol. Tierernähr. Futtermittelk. *16*:214 (1961); Chem. Abstr. *56*: 5190a (1962).

55. U.S. Department of Agriculture, Food consumption of households in the United States. Household Food Consumption Survey 1955, Rep. No. 1. Washington, D.C. (1956).

17 Donald Oberleas

PHYTATES*

CHEMISTRY

Phytate was first encountered as early as 1872 by Pfeffer. Early chemical studies[3] led to the opinion that it was an "inosite hexaphosphate," but the exact structure (Figure 1a) was not firmly established until recently.[26] The proper chemical designation of phytic acid is *myo*-inositol 1,2,3,4,5,6-hexakis(dihydrogen phosphate).[25] Dodecasodium phytate in the crystal unexpectedly has the conformation with five phosphate groups axial and one equatorial[6] (Figure 1b). Dehydration of the sodium salt yields an amorphous hexasodium salt of inositol tri-pyrophosphate.[26] Nine stereoisomeric inositols are possible, two optically active and seven *meso* forms. Only *myo*-inositol hexaphosphate has been isolated from plants, whereas *neo-, chiro-,* and *scyllo*-inositol hexaphosphates have also been isolated from soils.[11] The latter forms probably represent the influence of microorganisms in different soil types. Inositol phosphates with fewer phosphate groups, namely mono-, di-, and tri-esters,[10] are common components of complex lipids in animals, but the hexaphosphate has not been encountered in animal tissue. *Myo*-inositol 1,3,4,5,6-pentaphosphate occurs in avian and reptilian erythrocytes.[26]

* Literature reviewed through June 1971.

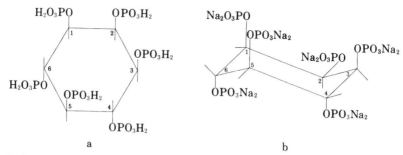

FIGURE 1 (a) Structure and configuration of phytic acid, *myo*-inositol 1,2,3,4,5,6-hexa-kis(dihydrogen phosphate); (b) conformation of crystalline hydrated sodium phytate.

OCCURRENCE

Toxicologically, only the phytate found in plant foodstuffs is of nutritional importance and, thus, will be the focus of this review. DeTurk *et al.*[15] have studied the metabolism of phosphorus in corn grain from pollination to maturity. Phytate was not present in the leaves, stems, tassel, or cob of the corn plant. Nor was phytate synthesized by rudimentary kernels formed in unpollinated plants. Synthesis of phytate in seeds began at about 3 weeks after pollination and increased to maturity. This work was later extended by Earley and DeTurk[16] and confirmed recently by Asada *et al.*[5] with rice and wheat. Asada further showed that the phytate content of rice was increased by phosphate fertilization. In mature cereal grains, phytate contributes 60–80% of the total phosphorus. Phytate has also been demonstrated in roots and tubers.[29,41] These results indicate that the presence and concentration of phytate depend largely on the portion of plant consumed and its stage of maturity at harvest. As examples, lettuce, onions, mushrooms, celery, and spinach are devoid of phytate; green beans, carrots, and broccoli have only a trace; potatoes, sweet potatoes, and artichokes contain moderate amounts; and cereals, nuts, and legumes contain larger portions of phytate. Fruits such as citrus, apples, pineapple, bananas, and prunes are devoid of phytate, whereas blackberries, strawberries, and figs contain small to moderate amounts.[7,29,35,41]

The phytate of plant seeds is contained primarily in the bran and germ. In corn phytate is exclusively in the germ and constitutes up to 6% of the germ dry matter.[40] Ferrel *et al.*[17] have shown that much of the phytate goes into the by-products of flour milling and may become concentrated in high-protein flours prepared by remilling selected by-products. The location of phytate in legume seeds has not been determined; however, recent evidence by Fontaine *et al.*[18] and Smith and Rackis[45] indicates that phytate is associated with protein. Therefore, any process that utilizes solution and isoelectric reprecipitation would concentrate the phytate into the resulting product.

Phytase is also present in the mature seeds but appears to have little, if any, effect on the phytate in the dry or dormant seed. Glass and Geddes[19] showed increased inorganic phosphorus and decreased phytate in wheat stored at increased moisture content and temperature. They suggested using high levels of inorganic phosphorus to indicate a sample stored under poor conditions. Even in the seed germinating under ideal conditions, 72–120 h are required for the complete disappearance of phytate.[1] Destruction of phytate during cooking is dependent on several factors. Rye contains a more active phytase than other cereal grains; therefore, Hoff-Jorgensen *et al,*[23] by using rye and leavening, were able to hydrolyze most of the phytate while bread was being made. deLange *et al.*[14] showed that bread made from 80% extraction flour destroyed more phytate than 90 or 100% extract flours. They further reported that pH and concentration of ionizable calcium were important factors. Reinhold[42] has shown that leavening of bread by yeast may be important in decreasing the phytate content. Bread made without leavening had 50% more phytate than leavened bread.

DETERMINATION

Methods for analysis of phytate have been recently reviewed.[38] There are no specific reagents that identify phytate, nor does it have a characteristic absorption spectrum. Instead, one is dependent upon estimating inositol or phosphate, or upon establishing a stoichiometric relationship between phytate and some cation that can be measured easily. The most common methods used are derived from that of Heuber and Stadler.[22] Their method was based on the principle that phytate forms an insoluble complex with ferric ion in dilute acid and presumably is the only phosphate compound with that property. It has since been shown that other inositol polyphosphates may also be precipitated under these conditions, and at least a trace of inorganic phosphate will also coprecipitate under these conditions. A fairly reliable method may be patterned after that of Earley and DeTurk,[16] as modified by Oberleas,[34] or after that of deLange.[14] In addition, the latter method may be modified by quantitative estimation of iron in the precipitated ferric phytate by dissolving in concentrated HCl or H_2SO_4 followed by atomic-absorption analysis. Variability of 10% has been recorded for the phytate content of the same foodstuffs when analyzed by various laboratories over several years and with slight variations in methodology.[7,29,35,41] Appropriate modification of the above techniques permits detection of less than 1 mg of phytate in a sample, with variation of less than 10%. These methods are quite adequate for the determination of phytate within limits of nutritional or toxicologic significance.

METAL COMPLEXES

Phytate is a strong acid that forms a wide variety of salts with several heavy metals. Whether or not a particular salt is formed is dependent on pH as well as on the presence of secondary cations, among which calcium has been most prominently mentioned. For example, phytate quantitatively precipitates zirconium, thorium, titanium, and uranium in 6 N acid.[2,43] Ferric and scandium phytates are least soluble in dilute acid and dissociate in concentrated acid or dilute alkali.[8] Zinc and copper phytates are least soluble at pH values between 4 and 7; calcium, magnesium and barium phytates form best under slightly alkaline conditions.[35,36] Maddaiah et al.[28] and Vohra et al.[47] have recently studied titration curves of phytate as the free acid and as the sodium salt in the presence of single divalent cations. At pH 7.4 phytate formed complexes with metals in the following decreasing order: $Cu^{++} > Zn^{++} > Co^{++} > Mn^{++} > Fe^{+++} > Ca^{++}$.

An important factor in the precipitation of phytate as its salts is the synergistic effect of two or more cations, which, when present simultaneously, may act together to increase the quantity of metallic phytate precipitated. (See Figure 2.) This phenomenon has been demonstrated only for zinc and calcium[34-36] and for copper and calcium.[24] Under the conditions represented in Figure 2, for example, doubling the molar proportion of calcium present increased the percentage of calcium and zinc recovered in the phytate precipitate from 63 to 84% and from 67 to 97%, respectively. Interestingly, at pH 6 there is maximum precipitation of zinc phytate or of zinc–calcium phytate; pH 6 is also the approximate pH of the duodenum, where most of the absorption of these divalent cations occurs. The copper, calcium, and phytate curves (Figure 3) show a similar phenomenon; however, a smaller portion of copper and of calcium was precipitated at pH 6. This same relationship was observed when only traces of zinc were used.[34-36]

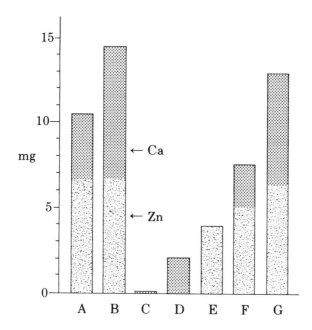

FIGURE 2 The synergistic relationship between zinc, calcium, and phytate. A and B represent the quantities of calcium and zinc added to a phytate solution at 1 : 1 : 1 molar ratios and 2:1:1 molar ratios, respectively. C and D represent quantities of calcium precipitated at 1:1 and 2:1 molar ratios of calcium : phytate. E shows the amount of zinc precipitated at 1:1 molar ratio zinc : phytate. F and G show amounts of calcium and zinc precipitated with calcium : zinc : phytate at 1:1:1 and 2:1:1 molar ratios, respectively, and demonstrate a synergistic effect. All measurements were made at pH 6.[34-36]

EFFECT ON NUTRITIONAL AVAILABILITY OF ELEMENTS

A great deal of attention has been given to the effect of phytate in foods in decreasing calcium absorption in the gut.[9,20] Calcium absorption is influenced not only by dietary phytate but also by vitamin D, lipids, and other dietary factors. If vitamin D is limiting in the diet, calcium absorption will be less efficient and the phytate effect will appear more pronounced.[21,30] Foodstuffs that have a calcium : inorganic phosphate ratio between 1:1 and 2:1, and that have adequate amounts of calcium, phosphate, and vitamin D, are not likely to be rachitogenic even though much calcium may be bound by phytate.

Phytate should not be considered a source of available phosphate for monogastric animals or man.

Decreased iron availability has also received much attention. Iron ab-

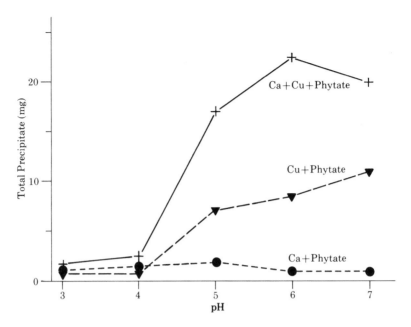

FIGURE 3 The amount of precipitate formed by equimolar ratios of copper and/or calcium and phytate. Formation of blue copper hydroxide at higher pH's was not apparent in the presence of phytate. (Methodology was the same as described in Oberleas *et al.*[36])

sorption depends on body-iron stores, amount and chemical form ingested, ascorbic acid, and other interrelated factors.[46] As noted above, ferric phytate is least soluble in dilute acid, so that it is insoluble in the stomach but becomes dissociated at the pH of the duodenum and forms ferric hydroxide.[4] Recent studies by Koepke and Stewart[27] and by Murray and Stein,[32,33] together with the isolation and characterization of gastroferrin by Multani *et al.*[31] indicate that phytate decreases iron availability by decreasing the complexing of iron with gastroferrin in the stomach. Only after thorough washing with EDTA has a phytate containing protein been shown to cause iron deficiency.[13]

The effect of phytate in decreasing zinc availability is logical in view of the work of Vohra *et al.*,[47] Maddaiah *et al.*,[28] and Oberleas *et al.*,[34-36] which indicated that zinc forms a very insoluble salt of phytate at pH values found in the upper small intestine and appears to be most readily affected by the phytate–calcium synergism. Therefore, under present nutritional policy in which zinc cannot be supplemented to human foodstuffs, zinc can easily become the first limiting nutrient. The reluctance on the part of many nutritionists to supplement adequate zinc in experimental diets has resulted in the belief that plant-seed proteins are inferior—when in fact they may be quite comparable—to animal proteins.[37] By varying the dietary ratios of zinc, calcium, and phytate, it is possible to produce a gradient of severities of zinc deficiency.[39]

Other polyphosphates, namely, hexametaphosphate, acid pyrophosphate, and tripolyphosphate, have been shown similarily to affect zinc availability.[48] Though these polyphosphates are not present in natural foodstuffs, they enter the human food chain in processed foods.

Davis *et al.*[12] have shown that an isolated soybean protein that contains phytate reduces the availability of manganese and copper in the chick. Seelig[44] has reported that phytate also decreases magnesium availability and that magnesium deficiency may be possible if conditions are appropriate.

These results indicate that a compound such as phytate that complexes with such a broad spectrum of metals may produce a wide variety of deficiences depending on which element first becomes limiting under specified dietary conditions. They further point out the fallacy of depending only on chemical concentrations to specify levels of trace elements needed in a nutritionally adequate diet.

The effect of phytate on zinc and calcium balances in human subjects was recently demonstrated by Reinhold *et al.*[49]

REFERENCES

1. H. G. Albaum and W. W. Umbreit, Phosphorus transformation during the development of the oat embryo. Am. J. Bot. *30*:553 (1943).
2. I. P. Alimarin and L. Z. Zozel, Determination of zirconium with phytin. Inst. Abschei Neorg. Khim. *3*:114 (1957). Chem. Abstr. *52*:2659b (1958).
3. R. J. Anderson, A contribution to the chemistry of phytin. J. Biol. Chem. *17*:171 (1914).
4. Anonymous, Effect of phytate on iron absorption. Nutr. Rev. *25*:218 (1967).
5. K. Asada, K. Tanaka, and Z. Kasai, Formation of phytic acid in cereal grains. Ann. N.Y. Acad. Sci. *165*:801 (1969).
6. G. E. Blank, J. Pletcher, and M. Sax. The structure of *myo*-inositol hexaphosphate dodecasodium salt octatriacontahydrate: A single crystal x-ray analysis. Biochem. Biophys. Res. Comm. *44*:319 (1971).
7. H. P. Averill and C. G. King, The phytin content of foodstuffs. J. Am. Chem. Soc. *48*:784 (1926).
8. G. Beck, The biochemistry of scandium and its precipitation as phytate. Mikrochem. Mikrochim. Acta *34*:62–66 (1948); Chem. Abstr. *42*:8703 (1948).
9. H. M. Bruce and R. K. Callow, Cereals and rickets. The role of inositolhexaphosphoric acid. Biochem. J. *28*:517–528 (1934).
10. J. J. Burns and A. H. Conney, Water soluble vitamins, part I (ascorbic acid,

nicotinic acid, vitamin B_6, biotin, inositol). Ann. Rev. Biochem. *29*:430 (1960).

11. D. J. Cosgrove, The chemistry and biochemistry of inositol polyphosphates. Rev. Pure Appl. Chem. *16*:209 (1966).

12. P. N. Davis, L. C. Norris, and F. H. Kratzer, Interference of soybean proteins with the utilization of trace minerals. J. Nutr. *77*:217 (1961).

13. P. N. Davis, L. C. Norris, and F. H. Kratzer, Iron deficiency studies in chicks using treated isolated soybean protein diets. J. Nutr. *78*:445 (1963).

14. D. J. deLange, C. P. Joubert, and S. F. M. duPreez, Determination of phytic acid and factors which influence its hydrolysis in bread. Proc. Nutr. Soc. S. Afr. *2*:69 (1961).

15. E. E. DeTurk, J. R. Holbert, and B. W. Hawk, Chemical transformations of phosphorus in the growing corn plant with results on two first generation crosses. J. Agric. Res. *46*:121–141 (1933).

16. E. B. Earley and E. E. DeTurk, Time and rate of synthesis of phytin in corn grain during the reproductive period. J. Am. Soc. Agron. *36*:803 (1944).

17. R. E. Ferrel, E. L. Wheeler, and J. W. Pence, Phytic acid in millfeed by-products. Cereal Sci. *14*:110 (1969).

18. T. D. Fontaine, W. A. Pons, and W. G. Irving, Protein-phytic acid relationship in peanuts and cottonseed. J. Biol. Chem. *164*:487 (1946).

19. R. L. Glass and W. F. Geddes, Inorganic phosphorus content of deteriorating wheat. Cereal Chem. *36*:186 (1959).

20. R. S. Harris and J. W. M. Bunker, The phytin phosphorus of the corn component of a rachitogenic diet. J. Nutr. *9*:301 (1935).

21. D. C. Harrison and E. Mellanby, Phytic acid and the rickets-producing action of cereals. Biochem. J. *33*:1660 (1939).

22. W. Heuber and H. Stadler, Uber eine Titrationmethode zur Bestimmung des Phytins. Biochem. Z. *64*:422 (1914).

23. E. Hoff-Jorgensen, O. Anderson, and G. Nielsen, The effect of phytic acid on the absorption of calcium and phosphorus. Biochem. J. *40*:555 (1946).

24. R. Hunter, D. Oberleas, and B. L. O'Dell, unpublished data (1963).

25. IUPAC-IUB, The nomenclature of cyclitols. Eur. J. Biochem. *5*:1 (1968).

26. L. F. Johnson and M. E. Tate, Structure of "phytic acids." Can. J. Chem. *47*: 63 (1969).

27. J. A. Koepke and W. B. Stewart, Role of gastric secretion in iron absorption. Proc. Soc. Exp. Biol. Med. *115*:927 (1964).

28. V. T. Maddaiah, A. A. Kurnick, and B. L. Reid, Phytic acid studies. Proc. Soc. Exp. Biol. Med. *115*:391 (1964).

29. R. A. McCance and E. M. Widdowson, Phytin in human nutrition. Biochem. J. *29*:2694 (1935).

30. E. Mellanby, A story of nutritional research, Williams & Wilkins, Baltimore (1950). P. 395.

31. J. S. Multani, C. P. Cepurneek, P. S. Davis, and P. Saltman, Biochemical characterization of gastroferrin. Biochemistry *9*:3970 (1970).

32. J. Murray and N. Stein, The effect of antigastric mucosal antibodies on iron absorption in experimental achylia gastrica. Proc. Soc. Exp. Biol. Med. *133*:86 (1970).

33. J. Murray and N. Stein, Gastric secretions and iron absorption in rats. In Trace element metabolism in animals, p. 321. C. F. Mills (ed.). Livingstone, Edinburgh (1970).

34. D. Oberleas, Dietary factors affecting zinc availability. PhD Dissertation, University of Missouri (1964).
35. D. Oberleas, M. E. Muhrer, and B. L. O'Dell, The availability of zinc from foodstuffs, p. 225. In Zinc metabolism, A. S. Prasad (ed.). Charles C Thomas, Springfield, Ill. (1966).
36. D. Oberleas, M. E. Muhrer, and B. L. O'Dell, Dietary metal-complexing agents and zinc availability in the rat. J. Nutr. *90*:56 (1966).
37. D. Oberleas and A. S. Prasad, Growth as affected by zinc and protein nutrition. Am. J. Clin Nutr. *22*:1304 (1969).
38. D. Oberleas, The determination of phytate and inositol phosphates, p. 87. In Methods of biochemical analysis, Vol. 20, D. Glick (ed.). Wiley, New York (1971).
39. D. Oberleas, D. F. Caldwell, and A. S. Prasad, Trace elements and behavior. In International review of neurobiology, C. C. Pfeiffer and J. Smythies (eds.). Supplement 1, Academic Press, New York, p. 83 (1972).
40. B. L. O'Dell, Effect of dietary components upon zinc availability. Am. J. Clin. Nutr. *22*:1315 (1969).
41. O. L. Oke, Phytic acid-phosphorus content of Nigerian foodstuffs. Indian J. Med. Res. *53*:417 (1965).
42. J. G. Reinhold, High phytate content of rural Iranian bread: A possible cause of human zinc deficiency. Am. J. Clin. Nutr. *24*:1204 (1971).
43. D. I. Ryabchikov, V. K. Belyaeva, and A. M. Ermakov, Use of phytic acid in the analytical chemistry of thorium. Zh. Anal. Khim. *11*:658 (1956); Chem. Abstr. *51*:7940e (1957).
44. M. S. Seelig, The requirement of magnesium by the normal adult. Am. J. Clin. Nutr. *14*:342 (1964).
45. A. K. Smith and J. J. Rackis, Phytin elimination in soybean protein isolation. J. Am. Chem. Soc. *79*:633 (1957).
46. E. J. Underwood, Trace elements in human and animal nutrition. 3rd ed. Academic Press, New York (1971). P. 26.
47. P. Vohra, G. A. Gray, and F. H. Kratzer, Phytic acid-metal complexes. Proc. Soc. Exp. Biol. Med. *120*:447 (1965).
48. P. Vohra and F. H. Kratzer, Influence of various phosphates and other complexing agents on the availability of zinc for turkey poults. J. Nutr. *89*:106 (1966).
49. J. G. Reinhold, K. Nasr, A. Lahimgarzadeh, and H. Hedayati, Effects of purified phytate and phytate-rich bread upon metabolism of zinc, calcium, phosphorous and nitrogen in man. Lancet *I*:283 (1973).

18 Benjamin J. Wilson and
A. Wallace Hayes

MICROBIAL TOXINS*

INTRODUCTION

Although microorganisms are sometimes considered simple examples of plant and animal life, their impact on higher biotic forms, including man, has been remarkable. This relationship has led to the categorizing of microbes as either beneficial or harmful (or at times both). In any case it is, in the final analysis, largely through the metabolic or biochemical features of the microbial cell that its favorable or detrimental characteristics are expressed. This is as true of strict parasites that invade host cells as it is of saprophytes, which form either useful or undesirable chemical substances on nonliving materials.

This chapter will deal mainly with some of the better documented toxigenic bacterial and fungal organisms that sometimes find their way into the food supplies of man and animals and there elaborate one or more toxic substances. This situation occurs where a food provides suitable substrates and where physical conditions (time, temperature, pH, moisture, and gaseous elements) are also propitious for both microbial growth and toxin biosynthesis.

* Literature reviewed to July 1, 1972.

BACTERIAL TOXINS CONTAMINATING FOODS OF MAN

This category of toxins emanates from bacteria that include species of the genera *Staphylococcus, Clostridium,* and other less important organisms. Members of the genus *Salmonella* produce their effects through proliferation in the host's intestinal tract and, occasionally, the invasion of various body tissues. The bacterial toxins to be discussed in this chapter, however, are the two most important representatives from species that grow (reproduce repeatedly) in contaminated foods and form toxic metabolites of complex chemical structure. They are, respectively, the causative agents of common food poisoning emanating from enterotoxin-producing staphylococci and the rare, but often fatal, intoxication known as botulism caused by *Clostridium botulinum.* The reader is referred to a series of monographs edited by Riemann in 1969[1] for details on other types of bacterial food toxins as well as infectious types of bacteria conveyed by foods.

Staphylococcus Enterotoxins

The acute illness caused by staphylococcus enterotoxins is fairly common in the United States and in other countries of the world, although the officially reported incidence of salmonellosis in this country is now much greater than enterotoxin poisoning.[2,3]

Symptoms of staphylococcus food poisoning begin 1–6 h after ingestion of contaminated foods and consist initially of salivation, nausea, and pallor followed by vomiting, retching, abdominal cramping, and diarrhea. Prostration may occur in severe cases, and supportive therapy such as intravenous fluids and electrolytes may be indicated. The acute phase will usually subside after a few hours, although the patient may feel weak for another day or two. Fatalities are rare and have occurred most often when supportive treatment was not provided.[4]

Only certain strains of *Staphylococcus aureus* produce enterotoxin, the principal if not the sole agent causing this particular food poisoning. Several other recognized toxins with different activities may be formed by the bacterium. This organism is a gram-positive, spherical cell that characteristically forms grape-like clusters as the cells divide in all planes. As an infectious bacterium of man, it is capable of causing diseases varying in severity from minor skin infections to a bacteremia with large suppurative lesions of various internal organs. Man is considered the main reservoir of enterotoxic staphylococci. They are frequent inhabitants of the skin and mucosal surfaces of the upper respiratory tract. In fact, the nasal passages constitute the principal sites of bacterial multiplication from which the organisms can be transferred readily to food by sneezing. Food handlers with skin lesions or contaminated hands may also carry out the inoculation of food.

Foods most frequently involved in outbreaks of enterotoxin poisoning are cooked protein-containing items. Ham, poultry, and beef frequently convey the toxin, and cream-filled pastry, fish, shellfish, potato salad, macaroni salad, and products of eggs and milk are other preparations likely to be involved.[5]

Following introduction of the organism into food, a period of several hours at room temperature or somewhat higher is necessary for the organism to multiply and elaborate toxins. The optimal incubation temperature is 35–37 °C (95–99 °F), but small amounts of enterotoxin have been detected after experimental incubation of cultures at 16 and 20 °C (61 and 60 °F).[6] Sometimes large masses of food placed under refrigeration cool so slowly that bacterial growth and toxin formation may have ample time to occur.

Most outbreaks of staphylococcus food poisoning reported in 1967 and 1968 emanated from food served in restaurants, schools, and medical institutions. A smaller number came from home-cooked food, and a few originated from food prepared in food processing plants.[5] Most outbreaks that occur in individual homes are probably not reported.

The fact that few people die from staphylococcus food poisoning favored an early belief that the toxic principle was probably not a potent substance. Also, the marked variations noted among people consuming nearly equal quantities of incriminated food suggested great differences in susceptibility among individuals. The latter observation has been confirmed in subsequent experiments. Work with the purified toxin, however, has established its high toxicity for both man and susceptible experimental animals. Fascinating historical accounts of research that led gradually to recognition of the bacterial agent and eventually to the nature of the toxic substance causing staphylococcus food poisoning are contained in accounts by Barber[7] and Dack[4]; in several of the early research reports by Surgalla, Bergdoll, and Sugiyama, working at the Food Research Institute, University of Chicago; and in work by Casman of the U.S. Public Health Service (see references 4 and 20).

The name enterotoxin was derived from the Latin word *enterus* (gut). Enterotoxin exerts considerable adverse effect on the intestinal mucosa,[8–13] and the irritative phenomena occurring there are undoubtedly responsible in large measure for the intestinal contractility and diarrhea so characteristic of the intoxication.[13] Denervation studies indicate that the emetic receptors for enterotoxin are in the abdominal viscera.[14] Several other biological effects of the toxin, such as leucocytosis[15] and reticuloendothelial system response,[16] are similar to the actions of the endotoxin of gram-negative organisms.[17] The role of other toxins that are formed simultaneously in foods by the staphylococcus remains unknown.[18] Also, the specific mechanisms of the intoxication in man have not been studied, since attacks infrequently require hospitalization, and recovery is generally uneventful.

At present five principal types of enterotoxins have been described. They are distinguished by immunological properties and are designated A, B, C, D, and E. The C category contains two subtypes, C_1 and C_2, which differ somewhat in chemical properties. Type B was the first to be purified,[19] and most experimental toxicity data have been derived from work with this enterotoxin. Relatively little information exists on types D and E, which were the latest to be identified. It seems likely that other immunological types will eventually be recognized, since toxins not identical with any of the foregoing types have been detected.[20] A simple *in vitro* test that identifies enterotoxigenic strains is not available.

All enterotoxins purified to date appear to be simple proteins that contain relatively high amounts of lysine, aspartic acid, glutamic acid, and tyrosine among the 18 different amino acids making up the peptide chain. Detailed amino acid analyses of enterotoxin B have revealed a total of 239 amino acid residues, and their respective order in the toxin molecule has been established.[21–23] However, the amino acid identity, sequence, and chain conformation responsible for toxicity remain to be determined. Similar studies are currently in progress on other enterotoxin types.[24]

Enterotoxin has been characterized as a relatively heat-stable material, since toxin developed in foods could resist cooking processes. It is possible that a food contains enterotoxin but not viable staphylococci. Data on partially or totally purified enterotoxins also confirms that heating to 100 °C for several minutes fails to destroy their activity completely. The influence of various other potentially adverse factors is reviewed by Dack[25] and Bergdoll.[26]

The emetic or vomiting dose (ED$_{50}$) of purified enterotoxins administered by stomach tube to the rhesus monkey is about 5 µg (0.9 µg/kg body weight). Smaller quantities are required with parenteral challenge (0.1 µg/kg IV).[19] Infrequent human volunteer toxicity studies made with crude toxin, culture broths, or toxin-bearing foods have shown that man is one of the most susceptible species to the action of enterotoxin. This was confirmed in a small group of volunteers who were fed an aqueous solution of enterotoxin B preparation of 50% purity.[27] In this experiment a dose of 50 µg produced typical symptoms in all three subjects. This suggests that a dose of 20–25 μg of pure B toxin or 0.4 μg/kg should cause typical enterotoxin poisoning in these persons. It indicates also that man may be two or more times as susceptible to enterotoxin as the rhesus monkey, which currently is the best animal for toxicity assays using intragastric administration.

The lack of a sensitive and specific assay method for enterotoxins was responsible for slow progress of early research on this problem. The simultaneous production by the staphylococcus of several other metabolites that are toxic when injected parenterally led initially to many erroneous reports concerning the nature of the enterotoxic principle. As previously indicated, the rhesus monkey is the only reliable assay animal known other than more costly primates[28] and man. Toxin solution is administered to monkeys by stomach tube, and the animals must be closely observed for 5 to 6 h for emesis and other signs of the intoxication. Diarrhea alone is not affirmative evidence for the toxin, whereas vomiting in two or more out of a group of six animals, with or without diarrhea, at any time during observation is considered a positive reaction. Because of costs involved in the purchase and maintenance of monkeys and the fact that they may rapidly develop resistance to toxin,[29] other animal assay methods are greatly needed.

The eventual development of immunological methodology for the qualitative and quantitative assay of enterotoxins facilitated the bioproduction, extraction, and purification of enterotoxin B and subsequently discovered types. These assays are based on the specific serological reactivity of the toxic proteins with antibodies produced by injecting purified toxin (or toxoid) into rabbits.[30] The specificity of the immunological methods depends on the antiserum having antibodies that react with enterotoxin only. The enterotoxin–antibody reaction may be evidenced by the precipitin, hemagglutination inhibition, or reversed passive hemagglutination reactions.

The precipitin reaction can be quantitated by the single gel diffusion tube (Oudin method).[31,32] The double gel diffusion tube,[33] the Ouchterlony plate, and a microslide method[34,35] are useful for detection of very small quantities (0.1 μg/ml) of specific enterotoxin. Fluorescein isothiocyanate has been used to tag antibody attached to enterotoxin in order to render the toxin–antibody reaction more easily detectable.[36] Reversed passive hemagglutination has been reported capable of detecting as little as 0.0007 μg enterotoxin B.[37]

Some of the foregoing techniques of enterotoxin detection and quantitation have been applied to naturally and experimentally contaminated foods with partial success. Preliminary concentration procedures are necessary, depending on the amount of toxin present, and antiserum to the specific enterotoxin must be available. Since there is evidence that other, as yet unidentified, enterotoxins exist, these methods cannot be considered all-inclusive.

McGann and associates[38] have demonstrated the presence of antibody to enterotoxin B in 70% of 191 human serum samples from the eastern United States using hemagglutination of ovine erythrocytes coupled to enterotoxin B, whereas only 30% of the sera had precipitins. Repeated parenteral exposure of monkeys to toxin was required to elicit titers of antibody observed in human sera. Resistance to high doses by parenteral challenge in monkeys was related to the presence of precipitins in the serum.

In addition to experimental enterotoxin production in foods, relatively large quantities of toxin for investigative work may be obtained using a variety of bacteriological culture methods that favor optimal growth of specific enterotoxigenic *S. aureus* strains. Although toxin may be formed in cultures grown in chemically defined solutions containing various amino acids, maximum growth of the cocci and enterotoxin production are obtained in media containing protein hydrolysates, glucose, and traces of certain vitamins. Keeping the medium as simple as possible, however, facilitates subsequent enterotoxin extraction and purification. Specific methods applicable to these purposes are reviewed, along with many other aspects of enterotoxin research, by Bergdoll.[39]

Botulinum Toxins

Botulism is a rare food-borne disease, known throughout the world, that afflicts man and several animal species with a high fatality rate. It results from the contamination of food materials by any one of a specific group of spore-forming bacteria, found in the soil and aquatic environments, followed by anaerobic growth of the organism and elaboration of potent neurotoxins. Almost all warm-blooded animals are susceptible to the toxic effects, although natural outbreaks of the disease have been documented in a relatively small number of species.

Signs and symptoms of botulism are sometimes noted 2–4 h after one eats toxin-contaminated food, but typically they appear within 12–36 h. In one documented case the first symptoms were not noted until 108 h after the fatal meal.[40] In general, the earlier the first symptoms appear, the greater likelihood of a fatal outcome.

Nausea and vomiting may herald the disease onset. Vomiting can be an important means of reducing the amount of toxin that is available for absorption. The subsequent symptoms and signs result from paralysis of various muscles related to effects of the toxin at the neuromuscular junction. Double vision (diplopia) often occurs early and is considered one of the most important pathognomonic manifestations of botulism. Drooping eyelids, dilated pupils, and a loss of light reflex with photophobia are usually observed. The patient exhibits lassitude, marked fatigue, and sometimes dizziness. Difficulty in swallowing is an early symptom due to the paralyzing action of the toxin on the pharyngeal muscles. This may also lead to a peculiar nasal distortion of the voice (dysphonia), and orally administered fluids may be regurgitated through the nose and mouth. The tongue and throat become inflamed due to the patient's inability to swallow secretions. Muscles of the neck are weakened so that the patient cannot raise his head from the pillow. There is usually no elevation of body temperature. Often the mental faculties remain lucid until death, which may be attributed to respiratory paralysis, although some patients have died following sudden cardiac arrest. Death is likely to occur 3–6 days after eating the poisoned food. Recovery, in those who are so fortunate, is prolonged, with considerable muscle weakness as a residual effect.

The mortality rate in botulism has varied according to the immunological type of toxin involved but reached 65% in the United States during the years 1899–1949. Although the disease is quite likely to maintain a high fatality rate, early recognition, prompt administration of type-specific antiserum, and adequate supportive therapy will increase the patient's chances for survival. Data obtained in more recent years (1940–1969) show a declining mortality rate that was less than 30% from 1960 to 1969.[41]

The causative agent of botulism is the gram-positive, anaerobic bacillus, *Clostridium botulinum.* This species constitutes a group of endospore-forming bacteria. The endospore is a heat-resistant structure, the dormant form of the organism that, under suitable growth conditions, will germinate to form the rod-shaped organism or vegetative stage. The latter form is then capable of active proliferation and exotoxin formation in suitable substrates such as canned foods or other products that have the required low oxygen tension. The endospore is usually not killed at the normal boiling point of water, 100 °C (212 °F), which would destroy the rod-shaped vegetative bacillus. Moist heat at temperatures attainable above atmospheric pressure is usually required for spore inactivation. Thus in canning and in similar food preservation methods the enclosed food must be subjected to temperatures considerably above 100 °C (115–120 °C, 230–250 °F) for several minutes to assure destruction of all spore-forming bacteria present, including *Clostridium botulinum.*

There are six types of botulinum bacilli presently recognized; these are designated with the capital letters A through F. Almost all typed cases of human botulism in the United States have been due to types A, B, and E. Each type produces a specific neurotoxin that causes typical botulism but differs from the others in immunological properties. Thus, each type toxin (or toxoid), when injected repeatedly into an animal such as a horse, causes the appearance of antibodies in the serum capable of neutralizing only the toxin type needed to obtain the antitoxin. For effective disease therapy it is therefore essential to ascertain the type of toxin involved and to use the appropriate specific antiserum or an inclusive polyvalent antiserum mixture. A polyvalent antiserum containing types A, B, and E antitoxins is now available from the Center for Disease Control, Atlanta, Georgia.

Types A and B *Cl. botulinum* are widespread soil organisms. In the United States, A has been noted more often in states west of the Mississippi River, and type B has been detected more frequently in the eastern United States as well as in Europe. Type E is encountered in lake mud or coastal sediment and is therefore likely to contaminate fish and other marine life. This type of botulinum toxin is discussed in Chapter 19. Type F was recently discovered,[41,42,43] and only a few human cases have been described. Type C and D intoxications are important diseases of certain animals, but conclusively proven human cases are not known. Possibly other toxin types eventually will be discovered.

Many foods support botulinum toxin production. These include many different canned fruits and vegetables, including beans, spinach, tomatoes, beets, and olives; cheese spreads, pot pies, smoked and canned fish, and meats also have been implicated. Since the 1930's, outbreaks of botulism have been caused for the most part by home-preserved or otherwise home-prepared foods in which the heat treatment used, if any, was insufficient to kill the endospores present as natural contaminants. To assure complete spore inactivation one must apply steam under pressure to reach and maintain temperatures up to 121 °C (250 °F) for a period of 10–15 min for foods that are to be preserved, especially those that may provide areas of relative anaerobiosis that would favor growth and toxin formation of *Cl. botulinum*. Large volumes of food require relatively longer periods of heating in order to permit the interior of a food mass to reach the desired temperature. Acidic food products are rarely involved in this type of food poisoning since toxin formation is generally not possible at a pH below 4.5. However, the toxin, once formed, is more stable in acidic solutions.

Growth of *Cl. botulinum* in foods will often lead to off-flavors and odors in preserved food that may cause its rejection. However, unfavorable organoleptic qualities may be slight or may be masked by natural or added food flavors. Since the botulinum toxins are heat-labile proteins, any questionable foods should be heated uniformly at 100 °C (212 °F) for at least 10 min before eating or even tasting. This procedure will readily destroy toxin, but any spores present may still remain viable.

Botulinum toxin can develop within 2–3 days under optimal conditions on suitable food substrates. However, one cannot be assured that refrigerator temperatures will always inhibit toxin production. Reports indicate that types A and B toxin may be formed in the range of 10–50 °C.[44] Most experimental toxin production is carried out at 20–30 °C. Type E toxin usually can be formed at temperatures lower than those promoting toxin formation by other types.

In addition to the factors of pH and temperature, available moisture (as influenced by the concentrations of salt and sugar in foods) also must be considered in toxin elaboration. For example, 10% sodium chloride and 50% sucrose are the respective salt and sugar concentrations that prevent growth of *Cl. botulinum.*[45] The toxinogenesis of different *Cl. botulinum* types varies with the particular food (i.e., the substrate) as well as with environmental factors.[45,46]

The exotoxins of *Cl. botulinum* are simple proteins whose exact molecular weights have been the subject of much investigation. Crystalline type A toxin was first shown to have a molecular weight of close to a million units.[47] However, it contained both toxic and hemolytic components. Recent studies suggest the toxic moiety has a molecular weight of 150,000.[48] Smaller toxic units for types A, B, and E have been reported by only one group of workers.[49-52]

The botulinum toxins have been termed appropriately "the most poisonous poisons."[53] Crystalline preparations of pure type A toxin contain approximately 3.0×10^{10} mouse IP LD_{50} units/g. Assuming equal human susceptibility, about 2 µg of pure toxin would be lethal.

The active sites on the toxin molecule are not known. Some studies have indicated a special role for tryptophan in the toxicity of type A,[54] although the fluorescent properties of the toxin, probably due to tryptophan, are not related to the toxicity.[55] If certain free amino groups of the toxin are acetylated or removed by deamination with nitrous acid, all activity is lost.[56,57] Type E toxin is readily detoxified when exposed to alkaline conditions of pH about 9 or above.

The search for information on the mechanism of action for botulinum toxin continues.[58-60] The principal action on ganglia of the autonomic nervous system, on other cholinergic receptors, and on peripheral motor end plates in voluntary muscle consists of inhibition of acetylcholine release and a resultant blocking of neural transmission with manifestations of muscular paralysis.[61-63] Paralysis of the muscles of respiration is considered the ultimate cause of death, although there may be a marked general debilitation as a result of widespread neurological involvement.[64] Muscles innervated by affected nerves tend to undergo reversible degenerative changes.

The toxins can be detected in foods and clinical specimens by injecting extracts intraperitoneally into mice. In this animal the typically fatal paralytic disease may be evident as early as 3 h or as late as 96 h after injection. A duplicate sample extract that has been heat inactivated should produce no effect. All animals should be held 96 h before a negative report is given. Mice receiving specific antitoxin or polyvalent antiserum are protected from injected toxin. Sakaguchi *et al.*[65] have developed a rapid assay for type E toxin in foods by injecting intravenously 0.1 ml of serial dilutions of a food extract into mice and measuring the time of death. A death time of 20 min indicates 10^5 mouse IP LD$_{50}$ units; one of 50 min indicates 1.7×10^3 mouse IP LD$_{50}$ units. If five mice are injected with each of five serial twofold dilutions, the fiducial limits of the toxicity should be about ±30%. A standardized reference toxin is used for comparison. Details of appropriate laboratory methods are given in Chapter XI of Riemann[1] and in a publication by the Food Protection Committee.[238]

As indicated earlier, botulinum toxins are heat-labile substances that, depending on the toxin type and environmental factors, can be detoxified by heating at 80–100 °C (176–212 °F) for approximately 10 min. In general, increments in holding temperature or pH tend to hasten their inactivation. The toxins are quite resistant to ionizing radiation. Formaldehyde treatment eliminates toxicity without destroying specific antigenicity; therefore, the resulting toxoid can be used for antiserum production in horses. There is evidence that crude toxin in foods is more resistant to adverse influences than purified toxins, and this factor should be considered in assessing naturally occurring toxin in foods. Storage of crude type A toxin in cheese at 30 °C for 2 months did not result in much reduction in activity.[44] It is significant from the public health viewpoint, however, that standard chlorination treatment of water supplies is effective in inactivating toxin that might be added with criminal intent to potable water sources.

FUNGUS TOXINS (MYCOTOXINS)

Fungus toxins is a broadly inclusive term encompassing all toxic metabolites of true fungi (Eumycetes). Those toxic for animals, and presumably man, are referred to as mycotoxins, and the diseases they produce (usually through ingestion of contaminated foods) are referred to as mycotoxicoses.

The first such disease known to affect man was related to ergot development on cereal grains caused by infection by the parasitic fungus *Claviceps purpurea*. The great impact of ergotism as an affliction of many people in centuries past has been recorded in various historical accounts of extensive outbreaks of the disease once called "St. Anthony's Fire."[66] The later recognition of ergot from infected rye as a complex mixture of pharmacologically active alkaloids led to the therapeutic use of both the crude product and its purified components for a variety of applications ranging from induction of parturition to the treatment of migraine headaches.[67]

Ergot contamination of foods destined for human consumption seldom occurs to any extent in civilized countries today. The last notable outbreak in man attributed to ergot occurred in Pont St. Esprit, France, in 1951.[68] However, considerable controversy still exists today as to whether this local epidemic, traced to a certain batch of commercial flour, was due to ergot, to mercury contamination,[69] or perhaps to both agents.

Although the word *mycotoxin* might also include mushroom poisons, it is usually restricted to the filamentous fungi, commonly called molds, that are often both parasitic and saprophytic in nature. These fascinating microorganisms are widely distributed over the earth's surface. In addition to their sexual reproductive cells, they also form more numerous asexual structures (spores, conidia, etc.), which are produced by the millions and readily find their way onto everything contacted and ingested by man and animals.

The utility of mold metabolism in biotic cycling of waste materials is readily recognized and welcomed, but molds' indiscriminate and omnivorous habits of destroying apparel, food, and certain building materials (to mention only a few objects of attack) are seen as undesirable properties that must be controlled.

For countless centuries the organoleptic changes in foods due to mold growth have been recognized. Some of these changes are desirable in that a pleasing flavor is imparted to the food, as in roquefort and camembert cheeses. In most instances, however, molds cause unwanted changes in foods, including textural decomposition along with unpleasant odors and tastes. Such changes are usually sufficient to prevent food consumption by man and animals unless they are subjected to conditions of starvation.

The often asked question "Will moldy food hurt you?" had not been clearly answered until the unfortunate experiences with molded grain in

Russia during World War II[70] and subsequent experimental work in the
1950's, which gave a qualified but affirmative answer applicable to both
man and animals. Grain that had overwintered in the fields of certain
areas of Russia, because of a lack of farm manpower, was believed re-
b) sponsible for a disease syndrome known as alimentary toxic aleukia
(ATA). In this condition a toxic depression of blood-forming cells in
the bone marrow was a prominent feature. This disease (stachybotryotoxicosis) was seen as an affliction of livestock—especially horses—in the
U.S.S.R. due to consumption or contact with hay containing growth of
c) the black fungus *Stachybotrys atra*. A peculiar disease called Kaschin-
Beck or Urov disease, which affects the long bones and joints of children
and adolescents, also was attributed to fungus toxins, but some doubt
apparently exists on this point at present.

Although farmers and veterinarians in the United States have recognized for several decades that moldy feed was seemingly responsible for
illness or death in livestock, reports giving acceptable experimental proof
of fungus causation were lacking in agricultural and scientific publications until the 1950's. The experiments of Forgacs, Carll, and other
workers in this country demonstrated clearly for the first time that certain species of common molds can elaborate substances on foodstuffs
with a variety of toxic effects ranging from dermal necrosis to liver
damage and body hemorrhages, often with acute lethality.[71] Their
studies constituted the beginning of an eventual expansion of scientific
endeavors leading to the discovery of many new mold metabolites that
have since been found to be potent agents of disease. In retrospect, these
developments should have been anticipated in view of earlier work in
this century leading to isolation of several antibiotic mold metabolites
that proved therapeutically unacceptable because of marked animal
toxicity.[72,73]

The prevalence of mycotoxins is now recognized in many areas of the
world. Although domestic animals and livestock are more often the victims of mycotoxic diseases than man, there is mounting evidence that
humans, especially in more primitive societies, are also ingesting significant amounts of such deleterious substances,[74-76] which may account
for a high incidence of liver disease and other conditions.

A) The ubiquity of fungi satisfies an initial requisite (an inoculum) in a
sequence of events leading to mycotoxin contamination of foods. Fortunately, however, not all species are toxigenic, nor are all strains of
toxigenic isolates comparable in this capacity. Excessive contamination
and growth of fungi in foods are usually indicated by off-flavors and
odors, but this is not invariably the case. Hunger on the part of an animal may help to overcome its aversion to objectionable properties of

such foods. Visual inspection by man may not detect the presence of small amounts of fungal growth on his food.

(B) The second and limiting factor in the contamination sequence is sufficient moisture in the food, permitting spore germination and mycelial growth with toxin biosynthesis. The critical amount of moisture varies somewhat with the particular food material, but once the value is reached or exceeded, growth and toxin formation can then occur over a relatively wide range of temperatures varying from below 0 °C (32 °F), for certain fungi, to 30 °C (86 °F) or slightly higher for others. For most toxigenic species, however, the optimal range is 15–25 °C (59–77 °F).

(C) Not all foods serve as suitable substrates for the formation of any given toxin, although the growth of mold may be luxuriant. In some instances, where a microorganism has the metabolic capacity to synthesize more than one toxic substance, a particular food may favor the formation of only one or two of the compounds.[77] The time required for initial toxin formation may be only a few days after growth commences, but quantities often will reach a maximum when incubation is conducted experimentally for 2–3 weeks.

As chemical compounds, the mycotoxins vary considerably in structure and properties, and belong to several different chemical groups. Most of those presently recognized are relatively heat-stable, nonvolatile compounds capable of producing diseases of an acute or chronic nature when ingested with food. Some substances, such as aflatoxin, are secreted into the milk by lactating animals and are theoretically capable of affecting other animals or man consuming this product.

The range of toxic effects attributed to known mycotoxins is broad, and different organ systems may be affected characteristically by a particular toxin. The pathological effects include dermal and ocular irritation, diuretic effects, liver damage (sometimes followed by neoplasia) (see also Chapter 23), widespread body hemorrhages, neurotoxic actions, hormonal stimulation, teratogenic and mutagenic phenomena, uterotrophic and anabolic aberrations (see also Chapter 24), and cerebral necrosis.[78] A special type of dermal toxicity is exemplified by the coumarin compounds (psoralens) that are produced in the pink rot lesion of celery infected with *Sclerotinia sclerotiorum*. These phototoxic substances are discussed in Chapter 25. In the foregoing manifestations, species variation in susceptibility may be considerable in that µg quantities may be sufficient toxin to kill one species, although another will be resistant to much higher levels of the same material.

Recognized mycotoxins may be detected or assayed using both chemical and biological (including toxicological) tests. Availability of authentic pure material as a control aids immeasureably in the identification. Thin-layer chromatography (TLC) procedures are usually simply applied; for the highly fluorescing toxins, especially, they give reliable presumptive evidence for identification, which may be confirmed by spectral data and conventional chemical tests. Toxicological determinations are, of course, generally less specific but may add confirmatory information.

It is impossible here to discuss or even mention all of the fungus metabolites that might qualify as food mycotoxins. Instead, only a few of the more significant ones, particularly some that have been incriminated in food disease outbreaks, will be considered. It should be emphasized that many species capable of producing identifiable toxins have been isolated from foodstuffs in various countries, although most food surveys have not included analyses for the toxic metabolites.

Aflatoxins

The aspergilli are fascinating organisms both to the mycologist interested in morphological taxonomy and to natural-products chemists, who have found them to be sources of many biologically active metabolites. The widespread geographical distribution of these organisms and their presence on several foods as "storage fungi" make them of much concern to scientists, especially food technologists, throughout the world.

Although many mycotoxins are now attributed to species of aspergilli, none outranks the aflatoxins in importance and research interest. An appreciable body of information on these compounds has appeared in print since their discovery about 12 yr ago. A significant portion of these data is briefly surveyed in this section.

The word *aflatoxin* is used in a generic sense to designate some 10 or more brightly fluorescing furanocoumarin compounds of which aflatoxin B_1 is a prototype. They are hepatotoxic–carcinogenic metabolites of *Aspergillus flavus* and of closely related fungi that grow on many different foodstuffs when sufficient moisture is present.

The first aflatoxins were discovered in the early 1960's after the occurrence of disease outbreaks among poultry in England.[79] In 1960 thousands of turkey poults died in that country with severe liver lesions. Intensive research showed that the "turkey x disease" was caused neither by a pesticide nor by a plant alkaloid; it was traceable to another substance contaminating the Brazilian groundnut meal used in formulating the poultry rations. A single feed manufacturing company was shown to be the common supplier of the peanut meal involved in these disease outbreaks. British mycologists found dead fungal hyphae associated

Aflatoxin B₁

only with toxic meal,[80] and in 1961 another group of investigators isolated a common mold, *Aspergillus flavus*, from toxic peanut meal that had been involved in the initial turkey epizootic.[81] They grew the mold on sterile, nontoxic groundnuts and were able to reproduce the toxic syndrome in duckling feeding trials. Contaminated peanut meal fed to rats also was found to produce primary hepatomas.[82]

Thin-layer chromatography revealed that there were at least four related compounds responsible for acute toxicity and liver carcinogenicity of several species. The name, aflatoxin, relating the toxic material to its biological source, *Aspergillus flavus*, was derived by the Interdepartmental Working Party on Groundnut Toxicity Research in England.[83]

Liver carcinomas in trout also were traced to food sources.[84] It was found that naturally contaminated fish-food components, as well as regular fish diet experimentally contaminated with aflatoxin, produced liver cancer when fed to trout. Rainbow trout were more sensitive to aflatoxin than to dimethylnitrosamine,[85] a well-known carcinogen.

Several toxic conditions of animals associated with groundnut meal appeared in the literature prior to 1961. For example, French investigators in 1957 reported diseases in guinea pigs that were dietary in nature.[86,87] The diets contained approximately 15% groundnut meal, which in retrospect is believed to have been contaminated with aflatoxin or another mycotoxin. In addition, fungus contamination of corn in the United States in the 1950's was reported as the cause of hepatitis in swine and in dogs.[88,89] Later work showed a correlation between several of these outbreaks and aflatoxin contamination of corn.[90]

Most reports mention only members of the *Aspergillus flavus* group, particularly *A. flavus* and *A. parasiticus*, as sources of aflatoxin. A few investigators, however, have suggested that other species of *Aspergillus* and certain members of the genus *Penicillium* and other genera also produce these metabolites.[91-94] Biochemical relationships among diverse species of microorganisms, as evidenced by formation of common toxic metabolites, are well known. However, failure by certain workers to detect aflatoxin in the specific cultures of penicillia and aspergilli, earlier reported to be aflatoxin producers, indicates that only the *A. flavus* group can presently be certified as sources of these mycotoxins.[95] In addition to this report, studies by three other groups[96-98] also have failed to demonstrate fungi other than *A. flavus* or *A. parasiticus* that produce aflatoxin. Several possible pitfalls in analytical techniques that may result in false positive aflatoxin findings have been noted.[95] They include: (1) residual contamination of glassware and instruments with aflatoxin solution, (2) inadvertent use of food materials previously contaminated with aflatoxin (for example, commercial peanut meal) as substrates for fungus cultures, (3) undetected contamination of aflatoxin-negative fungus cultures with aflatoxigenic species, and (4) misidentification of fluorescent spots on thin-layer chromatograms.

Table 1 shows the number of aflatoxigenic *A. flavus* cultures isolated from certain foods. Other foods found naturally contaminated with the toxin include corn, barley, cassava, cottonseed meal, peanuts, peanut meal, peas, rice, soybeans, wheat, and sorghum seed. Experimentally, aflatoxins have been produced by growing *A. flavus* in many foods, including cereal grains, fruits, certain meats, cheddar cheese, various prepared foods, and spices.[99] Toxigenic isolates are components of the soil, air, seed, and forage microflora throughout the world. Isolates vary widely in the amount of aflatoxin produced experimentally on natural substrates, and individual species vary in their ability to biosynthesize the different aflatoxins. Several studies indicate that repeated transfers

TABLE 1 Incidence of Aflatoxigenic Isolates of *Aspergillus flavus* from Various Foods

Origin of Isolates	Country	Investigators	Reference	Substrates	Number of Isolates Surveyed	Toxic
Peanuts	U.K.	Austwick and Ayerst	80	NM[a]	59	11
Peanuts	U.K.	Codner *et al.*	102	Peanuts	6	6
Peanuts	United States	Armbrecht *et al.*	100	Grains, NM	10	7
Peanuts	U.K.	Wallbridge	103	NM	43	32
Peanuts	India	Sreenivasamurthy *et al.*	104	Peanuts	150	4
Grains, legumes	S. Africa	Scott	105	Corn	10	6
Peanuts, soil	Israel	Borut and Joffe	106	Peanuts	330	235
Peanuts	India	Rao *et al.*	107	Peanuts	29	6
Rice	United States	Boller and Schroeder	108	Peanuts, rice	284	268
Peanuts, grains	United States	Diener and Davis	109	Peanuts, NM	44	35
Koji (Japan)	United States	Hesseltine *et al.*	110	NM	53	0
Spanish peanuts	United States	Taber and Schroeder	111	Peanuts, rice	213	107
					1,231	711

[a] Nutrient medium.

on synthetic media may reduce the aflatoxigenic capacity of an isolate.[100,101]

A number of well-defined factors predispose to *A. flavus* contamination and potential aflatoxin production. Reports from various countries suggest that aflatoxin contamination of foods is a widespread occurrence.[112] Several investigators have found that contamination of peanuts occurs most often after nuts are lifted from the ground, during the drying period.[113-115] Mechanical damage in harvesting or damage by insects, as well as improper drying and storage, are also important events favoring contamination and toxin production.[113] Investigators at Auburn University have reported the optimal temperature and time for aflatoxin production by *A. flavus* on sterilized peanuts to be 25 °C (77 °F) for 7–9 days.[109] Safe storage for groundnuts requires an atmosphere with less than 70% relative humidity. Similar observations for rice storage have been noted.[116] Most fungi are highly aerobic and require at least 1% oxygen for growth.

Considerable work has led to development of reliable assay procedures for the aflatoxins, most of which are based on physicochemical and biological assays. Since the aflatoxins are intensely fluorescent when exposed to long-wave ultraviolet illumination, extremely low amounts (0.0001 μg) of B_1 can be measured by these methods. Many procedures have been developed employing variations in chromatographic techniques. One general procedure for the isolation and separation of the four most common aflatoxins (B_1, B_2, G_1, and G_2) follows: A suspected food material is subjected to primary extraction followed by purification using thin-layer or column chromatography. Concentrated chloroform solutions of partially purified aflatoxin extracts are spotted on high-resolution silica gel thin-layer plates, and the plates are developed first with diethyl ether and then with chloroform : methanol (95 : 5) to separate the fluorescent aflatoxins. Estimation of quantities can be made visually by comparison with spots containing known concentrations of aflatoxins, or preferably by fluorodensitometric measurements. The identification of individual aflatoxins in sample extracts is customarily based on R_f values and colors of the fluorescent spots when extract samples, aflatoxin standards, and extract samples containing an internal aflatoxin standard are chromatographed on the same thin-layer plate. Chemical derivatives of aflatoxin B_1 may be used for confirmatory identification.[117,118] Doubtful results may be resolved when necessary by use of infrared and other spectral data.

Additional information on practices for handling, storage, processing, and testing of peanuts officially recommended by the National Peanut Council and other authorities has been published.[119,120]

When aflatoxin contamination is suspected by T L C analysis, a biological assay (i.e., duckling tests) may be used for additional confirmation. Aflatoxin poisoning in ducklings is characterized by loss of appetite, lethargy, and wing weakness. Early induction of bile ductule cell proliferation in the duckling liver is a characteristic reaction to repeated nonlethal doses.[121] In addition to the duckling assay, other procedures involving genetic effects of aflatoxin have been developed, including bacterial cultures and mammalian cell cultures.[122,123]

The aflatoxins have closely related structures and form a unique group of highly oxygenated, heterocyclic compounds.[124] The chemical characteristics of the four principal aflatoxins and the several minor aflatoxins were determined by different investigators.[124-128] Formulas for the various aflatoxins and some of their derivatives are presented in Figure 1. A list of physical properties of the aflatoxins is shown in Table 2. X-ray crystallography has confirmed the structure of aflatoxins B_1 and G_1.[129,130] The absolute configuration of aflatoxin B_1, and hence B_2, has been demonstrated by degrading aflatoxin B_1 to an optically active aliphatic acid whose absolute stereochemistry was known.[131] Racemic aflatoxin B_1 has been synthesized in 12 steps from phloroglucinol.[132] Because of the increasing complexity of nomenclature for the various aflatoxins, a system based on the linear difuran structure of these metabolites has been suggested.[133] Thus, aflatoxin B_1 would be 6-methoxydifurocoumarone, and aflatoxin G_1, 6-methoxydifurocoumarolactone.

A hypothetical pathway for the biosynthesis of aflatoxins, consonant with the distribution of labels in aflatoxin molecule from $1\text{-}^{14}C$ and $2\text{-}^{14}C$ acetates and from methyl-^{14}C methionine, has been proposed.[134] The carbon skeleton is derived from acetate with a single intermediate polyacetate chain.

The day-old duckling is the most sensitive animal to aflatoxin toxicity. Guinea pigs, rats, and dogs also are susceptible, but sheep and mice are somewhat resistant to the toxin. The respective oral 7-day LD_{50} values for day-old ducklings of 50-g body weight according to Carnaghan *et al.*[135] are: B_1, 18.2 µg (5% fiduciary limits 14.0–23.8 µg); B_2, 84.8 µg (65–110 µg); G_1, 39.2 µg (27.1–56.7 µg); and G_2, 172.5 µg (158–188 µg). Older animals are more resistant.[136] The acute oral LD_{50} values of B_1 for several additional animals have been established[121]: rat, 5.5–7.4 mg/kg; guinea pigs, 1.4 mg/kg; dogs, 1 mg/kg; hamsters, 10.2 mg/kg; mice, 9 mg/kg; and trout 0.5–1.0 mg/kg. Data primarily from rats and trout have demonstrated the carcinogenic response of aflatoxin B_1; the teratogenic effect has been demonstrated in hamsters, and a mutagenic response has been suggested by the induced chromosome abnormalities in plants and animal cells.[122]

The day-old ducking oral LD_{50} values reported for other aflatoxins

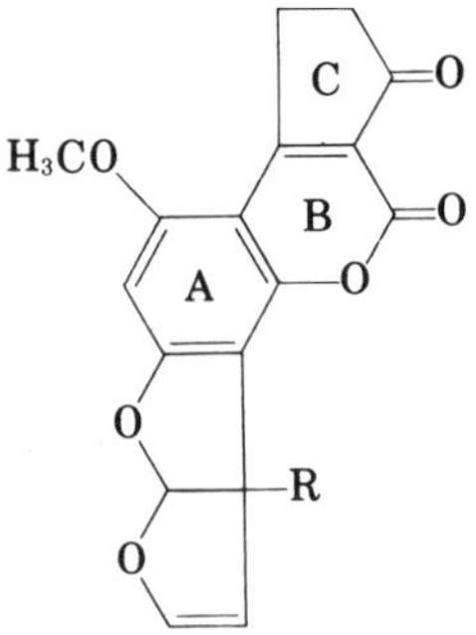

Aflatoxin B₁, R = H
Aflatoxin M₁, R = OH
Aflatoxin P₁, same as
B₁, except CH₃O on
ring A replaced by OH

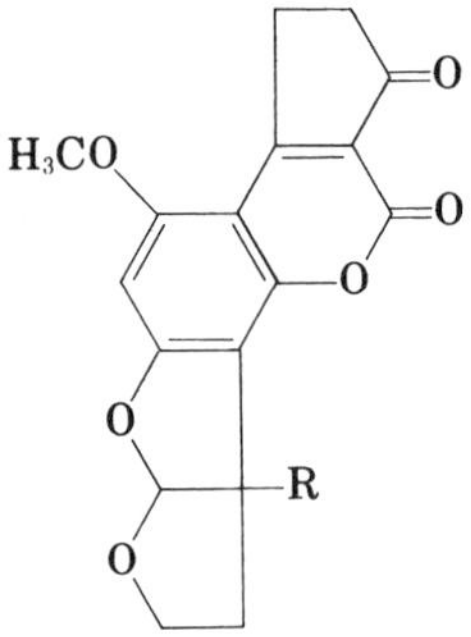

Aflatoxin B₂, R = H
Aflatoxin M₂, R = OH

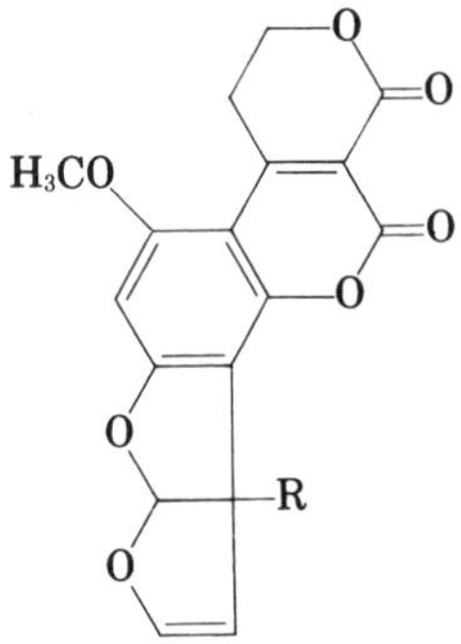

Aflatoxin G₁, R = H
Aflatoxin GM₁, R = OH

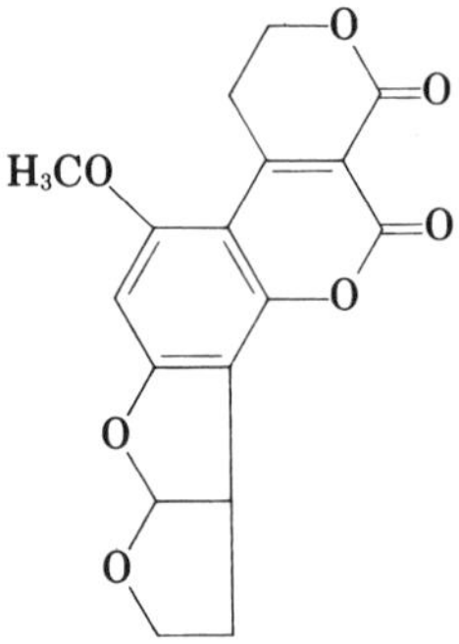

Aflatoxin G₂

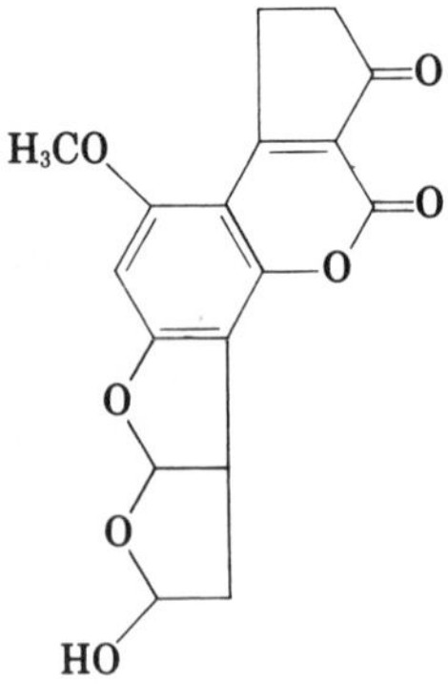

Aflatoxin B₂ₐ

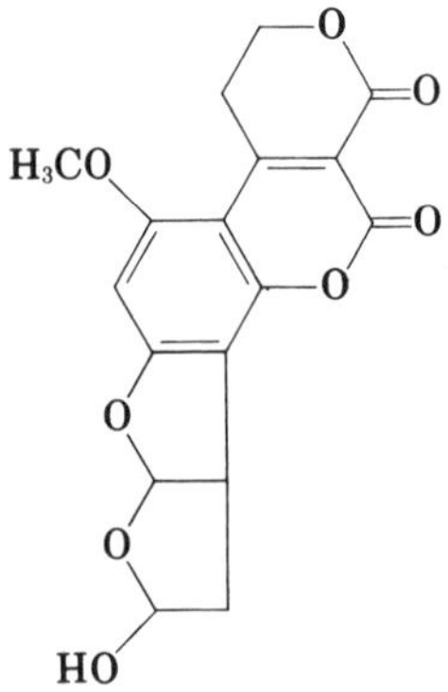

Aflatoxin G₂ₐ

FIGURE 1   Structures of aflatoxins.

TABLE 2 Physical Properties of Aflatoxins

Afla-toxin	Mol. Formula	Mol. Weight	Melting Point (°C) (Decomp.)	$[\alpha]$ CHCl$_3$ D	Maximum Fluorescence Emission (nm)	R$_f^a$	UV Absorption λ_{max}. EtOH (Extinction Coefficient)		
B$_1$	C$_{17}$H$_{12}$O$_6$	312	268–269	−558 (C 0·101)	425	0·56	233 (25,600)	265 (13,400)	360 (21,800)
B$_2$	C$_{17}$H$_{14}$O$_6$	314	286–289	−430 (C 0·100)	425	0·53	222 (17,000)	265 (11,000)	362 (20,800)
G$_1$	C$_{17}$H$_{12}$O$_7$	328	244–246	−556 (C 0·133)	450	0·48	243 (11,500)	264 (10,000)	362 (16,100)
G$_2$	C$_{17}$H$_{14}$O$_7$	330	237–240	−473 (C 0·084)	450	0·46	214 (28,100)	265 (11,600)	362 (20,900)
M$_1$	C$_{17}$H$_{12}$O$_7$	328	299	−280^b	425	0·40	226 (23,100)	265 (11,600)	357 (19,000)
M$_2$	C$_{17}$H$_{14}$O$_7$	330	293	–	425	0·30	221 (20,000)	264 (10,900)	357 (21,000)
B$_{2a}$	C$_{17}$H$_{14}$O$_7$	330	–	–	–	0·13	–	265 (10,100)	363 (20,200)
G$_{2a}$	C$_{17}$H$_{14}$O$_8$	346	–	–	–	–	–	–	–
GM$_1$	C$_{17}$H$_{12}$O$_8$	344	276	–	–	–	235 (21,200)	262 (16,300)	358 (12,000)
B$_3$	C$_{16}$H$_{14}$O$_6$	302	217	–	–	–	229 (10,000)	262 (7,550)	358 (9,350)

^{a} Silica gel G 0·25-mm-thick layer, chloroform : methanol (97 : 3).
^{b} In dimethylformamide.

are as follows: M$_1$, 16 μg; M$_2$, 61.4 μg. B$_{2a}$ and G$_{2a}$ were without effect when given at 1,200 and 1,600 μg, respectively, to ducklings.[121]

A detailed study of dose-response relationships of aflatoxin B as a carcinogen has been carried out by investigators at the Massachusetts Institute of Technology.[137] The cancer-inducing potency of aflatoxin B$_1$ relative to other carcinogens is striking. (See Chapter 23.) Early studies of tumor induction by approximately 10 μg aflatoxin B$_1$/day prompted the conclusion that this toxin is the most potent natural hepatocarcinogen known.[138] High incidence of tumors was obtained in rats fed only 0.2 μg/day for 476 days.[137] Continuous low-level feeding of toxin "sensitizes" liver cells to additional toxic insults, culminating in a cancerous state.

These observations may be significant in evaluating the potential human health hazard associated with prolonged aflatoxin ingestion.

Cancer development in rats following ingestion of a diet containing
15 ppb/day aflatoxin B_1 for 476 days also related to natural food contamination levels of the toxin, since many contamination reports fall
into the ppb range. Most analyses for natural aflatoxin contamination
have a lower detection limit of 1–10 ppb. The term *aflatoxin-free* applied to foods may be misleading, since feeding levels below 15 ppb may
produce tumors if an appropriate induction period is utilized. Further
studies on the long-range effect of feeding material contaminated with
less than 15 ppb aflatoxin B_1 are required before any acceptable tolerance level can be considered.

Crystalline aflatoxin is fairly stable and tends to resist detoxification.
The photodecomposition of aflatoxin is known to occur at fairly low
light levels.[139] Some of the unidentified products have about the same
UV absorption spectrum and a very similar fluorescence spectrum as
aflatoxin B_1. Studies on light-exposed DNA–aflatoxin mixtures have
shown that photodegradation of aflatoxin can occur in the course of
routine laboratory manipulations.[140] UV light affects pure toxin but
appears to have no effect on contaminated agricultural products.[141] In
one study, samples of naturally contaminated hepatotoxic corn, held in
sealed containers for 8 yr at room temperature, contained significant
amounts of aflatoxins.[90] Gamma radiation (2.5 megarads) does not reduce the toxicity of contaminated agricultural products. Although aflatoxin B_1 is fairly heat stable, a reduction of aflatoxin B_1 in peanut meal
from 7,000 to 340 $\mu g/kg$ was produced by autoclaving the moist meal
(60% moisture content) at 15 lb pressure (120 °C) for 4 h.[141] Pure aflatoxin B_1 was converted to nonfluorescent products when autoclaved
under similar conditions, and toxicity was reduced in duckling feeding
tests.[142] This was confirmed in rat-feeding studies also.[143] Several reagents (including ammonia, methylamine, hydrogen peroxide, and
ozone) reduce toxin levels significantly when added to contaminated
agricultural commodities.[144] However, the chemistry of this detoxification has not been established.

The metabolic fate of aflatoxin in animals is incomplete, but important work has been done on this problem.[145] Two metabolic conversion
products of aflatoxin B_1 have been described. Aflatoxin M_1 was found
in milk, excreta, liver, and in contaminated peanuts.[136] O-demethyla-
tion of aflatoxin B_1 was noted to occur in rats, and very recently a new
metabolite from this reaction (aflatoxin P_1, a phenolic derivative of B_1)
was isolated from the urine of monkeys injected intraperitoneally with
radioactive B_1 in dimethyl sulfoxide. The compound was excreted
principally as a glucuronide.[146] Unlike aflatoxin M_1 and M_2, this compound is nontoxic. Aflatoxins B_2, G_1, and G_2 apparently undergo a

similar fate, but less is known about their metabolism than is the case with aflatoxin B_1. Derivatives (predominantly M_1 and M_2) appear in the urine, feces, and milk of rats following oral administration. Most aflatoxin excretion occurs via the biliary and fecal routes within 24 h after administration. Much of the remainder apparently is excreted in the urine, although a significant portion of labeled carbon from the methoxy group attached to the ring is excreted as CO_2 in the expired air of toxin-fed rats.[145]

The biological activity of aflatoxin has been investigated in animals,[147] tissue cultures,[148-150] plants,[151,152] insects,[153,154] and a variety of microorganisms.[123,155] On the basis of current information, it is impossible to formulate a sequence of biochemical events clearly defining aflatoxin effects. Most studies have involved changes in liver tissue during relatively short periods following the *in vivo* or *in vitro* incubation with toxin. In recent studies in which crystalline preparations of aflatoxin B_1 were administered to rats, a rapid and marked inhibition of DNA and RNA synthesis in the liver—through inhibition of the respective polymerases—has been observed. Inhibition of nucleic acid polymerase action could result either from direct action of aflatoxin with the enzymes or from an aflatoxin–DNA binding that modifies the DNA template, at least in chromatin-containing preparations.[156] The mode of action in avian species appears to involve lipid metabolism prior to affecting RNA metabolism.

There is little direct evidence as to the susceptibility of man to aflatoxins. However, much information is accumulating from experimental animal work and from *in vitro* human-tissue-culture studies. In addition, various geographical and concomitant environmental factors provide only presumptive evidence that the relatively high incidence of hepatitis and primary hepatoma in certain developing countries is associated with environmental exposure to toxins rather than being primarily genetic in origin.[156-161]

Several investigators have reported the presence of aflatoxin or one of its metabolites in human urine and milk of individuals in India.[75] Aflatoxin M_1 has been detected in peanut butter samples and in the urine of Filipinos who had eaten contaminated peanut butter.[76]

Other Aspergillus Toxins

Oxalic acid, $H_2C_2O_4$, the simplest dicarboxylic acid, has long been recognized as a metabolite of *A. flavus* as well as of *A. niger, A. chevalieri,* and certain species of *Penicillium.* The presence of cations, especially Ca^{++}, in culture media favors the accumulation of oxalate as soluble or insoluble salts.[162] Oxalate may also be formed by mold contaminants growing on cereal grains and other foods. Quantities sufficient to precipitate a large amount of the available calcium may be formed on several products,[163] but the quantity produced on corn is very low. Oxalate may be readily extracted from foods, precipitated as the calcium salt, and titrated using potassium permanganate titration.

Oxalate as the free acid or as water-soluble salts is toxic when ingested in large quantities. Gastric irritation is caused by direct contact, and after absorption the serum levels of calcium are reduced, causing tetany, convulsions, and death. Abnormal oxalate formation in man may cause deposition of insoluble calcium oxalate crystals in various tissues (especially in kidney tubules, causing severe kidney damage).

The likelihood of mold-produced oxalate being a problem in human food seems quite remote in view of the normal tolerance by man of high-oxalate foods such as spinach and rhubarb. (See Chapter 16 for a discussion of oxalate as a potential food toxin.) The possibility of oxalate serving as a toxic factor in moldy-feed diseases of animals, such as winter tetany,[164] has not yet been demonstrated.

Kojic acid has been known for several decades as a metabolite of several fungi and some bacteria.[72] It is produced in appreciable quantities on moist sweet corn experimentally inoculated with *A. flavus* but has been detected only as traces in moldy samples from the field.[77] It was first isolated from koji, the starter used in fermentation of certain Oriental foods. Kojic acid is classified as a convulsant, but relatively large quantities are required to produce severe intoxication or death in animals. Kojic acid is soluble in water and in alcohol; it may be extracted readily and detected colorimetrically using ferric chloride to produce a nonspecific wine-colored reaction. It may be quantitated gravimetrically as the insoluble copper kojate salt.[77]

Interestingly, a pharmaceutical company that had developed efficient bioproduction methods for kojic acid has recently employed the compound as starting material in the development of a food flavor enhancer. The product, ethyl maltol, has been given the trade name Veltol plus® (Charles Pfizer Company, Data Sheet No. 635).

Certain strains of *A. flavus*, including aflatoxin producers, also form small quantities of at least one tremorgenic–convulsant metabolite that has not yet been well characterized.[165] This unusual toxin is a neutral compound having a molecular weight of 501 or more. It contains nitrogen and has a condensed atomic arrangement. Corn and various other moist foods are suitable substrates for toxin production, but the extractable yields of crystalline toxin are small.

Small quantities of the purified tremorgen fed or injected intraperitoneally into mice cause several behavioral changes, including a pronounced trembling that sometimes persists for 3 days. Larger doses cause the initial trembling to be replaced abruptly by convulsive seizures that may prove fatal.

The toxin may be extracted from the contaminated foods with several organic solvents and may be detected on thin-layer plates using phosphomolybdic acid or *m*-dinitrobenzene spray reagents.[72] The neurotoxic response in animals to this toxin is quite similar to that obtained with a tremorgenic–diuretic toxin from *Penicillium crustosum* and related species (see below). Low yields of *A. flavus* tremorgen have hampered detailed toxicity studies.

South African workers first isolated ochratoxin A as a metabolite of *A. ochraceus* grown on maize.[166] It has been identified also as a metabolite of *Penicillium viridicatum*[167] and has been detected as a natural contaminant of foods in the United States and Japan.[168]

Ochratoxin A is a greenish blue fluorescing compound, as are the less toxic ochratoxins B and C that may accompany it. It produces liver damage in experimental animals at low doses, but no natural outbreaks of disease have been attributed to this compound. Standard methods for ochratoxin detection and quantitation in commodities have been developed by U.S. Food and Drug Administration scientists using TLC.[169]

Sterigmatocystin is a hepatic–carcinogenic metabolite of *Aspergillus nidulans, A. versicolor*, and *Bipolaris* species. Its chemical structure has features resembling those of aflatoxin.[170,171] While these fungi are often found as food contaminants, sterigmatocystin contamination under natural conditions has not been reported. The hepatotoxicity and carcinogenic potency of sterigmatocystin are less than those of aflatoxin B_1. *O*-methyl sterigmatocystin[172] and hydroxy-*O*-methylsterigmatocystin ("aspertoxin") have also been isolated as metabolites of *A. flavus*.[172,173] These substances appear as fluorescent spots on thin-layer plates and presumably can be quantitated by fluorimetric or spectrometric methods.

Abbreviated data on the foregoing substances and certain other *Aspergillus* toxins are listed in Table 3.

Myctotoxins from Penicillium

The genus *Penicillium*, like *Aspergillus*, includes numerous species that are both common contaminants of foods and sources of interesting toxic metabolites. Some of these toxins are antibiotic substances that were screened for therapeutic usefulness long before the mycotoxin concept was defined. Certain ones are mentioned among the carcino-

TABLE 3 Aspergillus Toxins

Toxin and Biological Source	Formula	Physical Properties	Toxic Reaction $(LD_{50})^a$	Foods Naturally Contaminated with Mycotoxin	Foods Supporting Experimental Production	Remarks	References
Sterigmatocystin A. versicolor A. nidulans Bipolaris sp.	See Structure I below R = H R^1 = H	Pale, yellow needles	Degenerative liver and kidney changes 65 mg/kg IP, (R) 120 mg/kg oral, (R) 800 mg/kg oral, (M)	None reported	Maize meal	Carcinogenic; histopathology differs from that due to aflatoxin; 1/250 activity of aflatoxin	170,171, 175
O-methyl sterigmatocystin A. versicolor A. flavus	Above R = CH$_3$ R^1 = H	Crystals; Yellow fluorescence; m.p. 265 °C	Not reported	Not reported	Not reported		172
Aspertoxin A. flavus	Above R = CH$_3$ R^1 = OH	Blue fluorescence on TLC; tiny, colorless crystals; decomposes at 240–280 °C	Toxic to chick embryos and zebra fish larvae 0.7 µg in embryonated eggs	None reported	Shredded wheat	Separated from aflatoxins on TLC (less fluorescent than aflatoxins)	173,174

Toxin / Organism	Structure	Properties	Toxicity / LD	Natural occurrence	Substrate	Remarks	References
Ochratoxin A *A. ochraceus* and perhaps other organisms	See Structure II below	White crystals from benzene; blue green fluorescence on TLC; m.p. 89–95 °C	Hepatotoxic and nephrotoxic; also causes enteritis 20–22 mg/kg oral (R)	Corn	Corn, wheat, rice, peanut, soybeans, etc.	Organism found in soil, moist cereals, legumes, and spices	166,167 176,177
Oxalate *A. flavus* *A. niger*, etc.	See Structure III below	Water-soluble crystals	Esophagogastric irritation, tetany, calcium oxalate crystals in kidneys	Found as normal constituent of many food plants	Wheat, oats, hay	Calcium salts are water insoluble	162,163
Aspergillic acid (and related compounds) *A. flavus* *A. sojae*, and other fungi.	See Structure IV below	Yellow crystals; deoxy compounds; fluorescence; m.p. 97–99 °C	Acute death, mechanism unknown 150 mg/kg IP, (M)	None reported	Soybeans and wheat	Several Japanese fermentation strains produce aspergillic acid and numerous related pyrazine compounds	72,178
Kojic acid *A. flavus* and several other fungi and bacteria	See Structure V below	Nearly colorless, water-soluble crystals	Convulsant (large doses required) 250 mg/kg IP (M)	Small amounts in corn heavily contaminated with *A. flavus*	Corn, koji	Nonspecific red color with ferric chloride; forms insoluble copper kojate crystals used for gravimetric quantitation	72,179 180

TABLE 3 (Continued)

Toxin and Biological Source	Formula	Physical Properties	Toxic Reaction $(LD_{50})^a$	Foods Naturally Contaminated with Mycotoxin	Foods Supporting Experimental Production	Remarks	References
Tremorgenic toxin, A. flavus	Unknown	Colorless microcrystals; m.p. 234 °C	Sustained trembling, convulsions, diuresis	None reported	Corn, oats, rice, potato–milk solid mixture	Neutral compound containing nitrogen; molecular weight 501 or more	165,181

[a] Letter following LD_{50} designates the experimental animals as follows: D = duckling; R = rat; M = mouse.

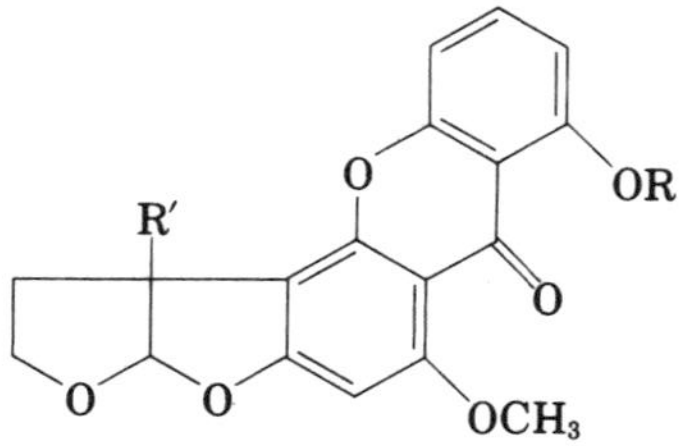

STRUCTURE I

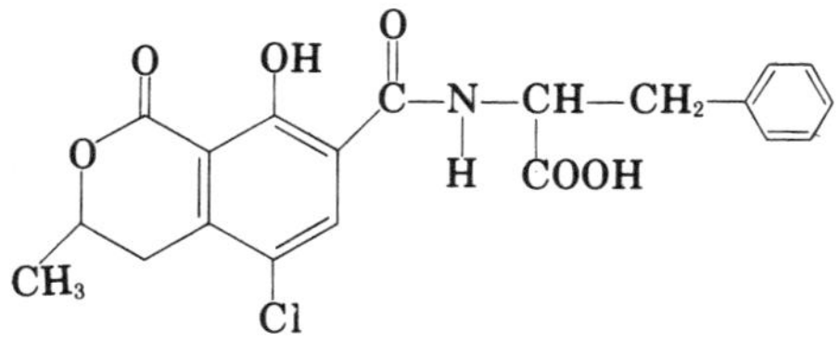

STRUCTURE II

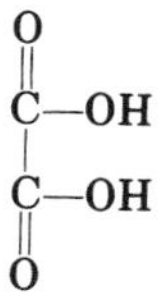

STRUCTURE III

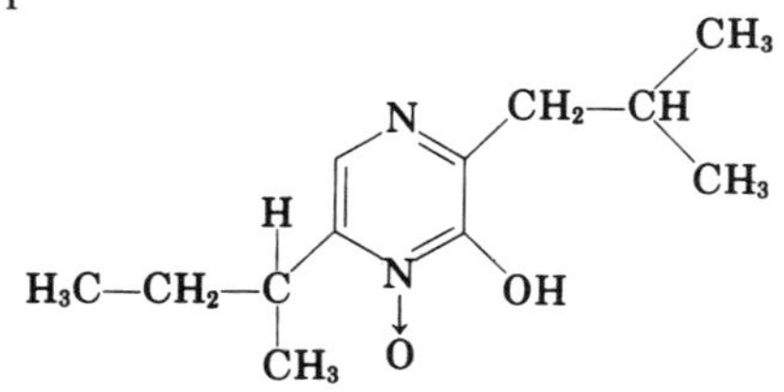

STRUCTURE IV

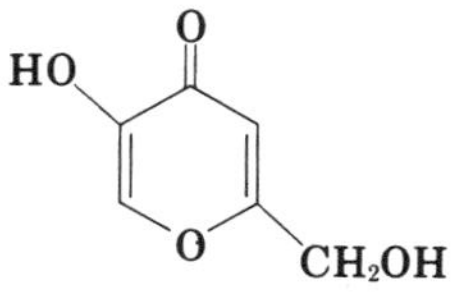

STRUCTURE V

398

genic agents in Chapter 23; others are included as toxic peptides in Chapter 5.

Reports on toxins derived from penicillia have come from various parts of the world. For example, Japanese workers have noted several toxigenic species as frequent isolates from molded foods in that country and have identified several new mycotoxins.[168] In addition to cyclochlorotine and luteoskyrin (discussed briefly in Chapters 5 and 23), citrinin and citromycetin, both previously recognized renal toxins, and citreoviridin, a neurotoxic, yellow compound, are metabolites of fungi associated with yellowed rice imported by Japan.[182]

South African workers have described cyclopiazonic acid, a neurotoxic compound,[183,184] whereas English and American scientists have studied several other penicillium metabolites, including a few previously recognized antibiotic compounds.[73]

An unusual and potent neurotoxin having other physiological effects has been isolated from foods contaminated with *Penicillium cyclopium* and closely related species that are frequent contaminants of foods.[181] Lethal disease outbreaks in animals have been attributed to feedstuffs heavily contaminated with the fungi. This toxin has been termed tremorgenic–diuretic toxin (trivial name: penitrem A) because of its potency in causing sustained trembling or convulsions and a diuresis in which glucose and electrolytes are hyperexcreted in the urine. Other unusual effects noted include a rapidly developing hyperglycemia and liver glycogen accumulation in fasted rats. This toxin may be formed on food stored at temperatures as low as 39 °F (4 °C), although the largest quantities are attained at about room temperature, 77 °F (25 °C). Several workers are currently studying the chemical structure of this compound and the mechanisms of its toxicity.

The *P. cyclopium–viridicatum* group of fungi also form the antibiotic viridicatin and related compounds whose toxic properties as yet have not been carefully studied.[185,186]

Viridicatin

Two potent liver toxins, rubratoxins A and B, have been isolated as major metabolites of certain strains of *Penicillium rubrum*[187,188] and

P. purpurogenum.[189] These organisms are frequent isolates from soil and food materials. The first toxigenic *P. rubrum* isolate studied came from feed involved in toxic hepatitis of livestock. Although the organism can produce its toxic factor(s) on several food materials, rubratoxins have not been specifically identified in feeds from recent naturally occurring intoxications, nor have recent cases of poisonings attributable to these toxins been reported.

The acidic, crystalline rubratoxins are primarily toxic to the liver and often cause hemorrhages in various visceral organs.[88] They are not carcinogenic when fed for long periods to the rat. Weak antimicrobial activity has been reported.[190]

Rubratoxins are not easily detected in foods, and this may account in part for a lack of reports implicating the toxins in disease outbreaks. A colorimetric method for quantitating isolated rubratoxin A has been developed based on the yellow color developed when the A toxin is heated with 1 N NaOH.[191]

Table 4 lists several penicillium toxins that either have been involved in disease outbreaks or are formed by prominent isolates from foods. The isolated organisms are grown experimentally on moistened food substrates. Several other penicillium metabolites are discussed in more detail in various review articles.[73,192]

Fusarium Toxins

Fusarium toxins make up a diverse group of relatively potent compounds allegedly responsible for both human and animal diseases; they are also toxic to fungus-parasitized plants. Although the fusaria have in the past been better known as plant pathogens than as sources of mycotoxins, recently conducted research has shown that newly identified toxins may have been responsible for debilitation and death of animals consuming damaged grain.[203,204]

Among the bizarre diseases due to fusarium toxins is the vulvovaginitis in swine caused by feeding grain contaminated with zearalenone from *Fusarium graminearum.*[205] *Fusarium tricinctum* and other species form trichothecenes, which cause severe dermal irritation when applied to the skin of experimental animals[206,207] and are lethal when fed or injected. Laboratory workers frequently suffer serious dermal reactions from inadvertent contact with pure toxins or extracts containing these compounds. A butenolide, formed by several fusaria, may yet prove to be the cause of a peculiar necrotizing disease of cattle known as "fescue foot."[203] *Fusarium moniliforme* has recently been identified as a pathogen of corn in Egypt. Consumption of the grain by donkeys causes a fatal disease characterized by massive necrotic lesions in the white matter of one or both brain hemispheres.[208,209] The causative chemical agent is currently being sought.

Soviet scientists have implicated species of *Fusarium*, as well as other fungus contaminants of grain overwintered in the field, as causative agents of a human disease known as alimentary toxic aleukia (ATA).[210] This disease may progress in four clinical stages from local irritation of mucous membranes of the oral cavity and pharynx (occurring shortly after eating contaminated cereal products) to a hemorrhagic diathesis with anemia and severe leukopenia, which develop upon continued ingestion of toxic food.

Although several toxic compounds have been obtained as metabolites of fungi isolated from contaminated grain, the types of toxic responses to the trichothecenes (Table 5), along with other lines of evidence, suggest that ATA may have been caused by one or more of these compounds.

A compilation of data pertaining to various fusarium toxins is found in Table 5. A review of information on the trichothecenes has been written by Bamburg and Strong.[214]

The genus *Tricothecium* includes toxigenic species that form tricothecenes closely related to those from *F. trincinctum* and other fusaria. *Tricothecium roseum* produces trichothecin, which has an LD_{50} of 300 mg/kg for mice. *Trichoderma viride* forms the closely related

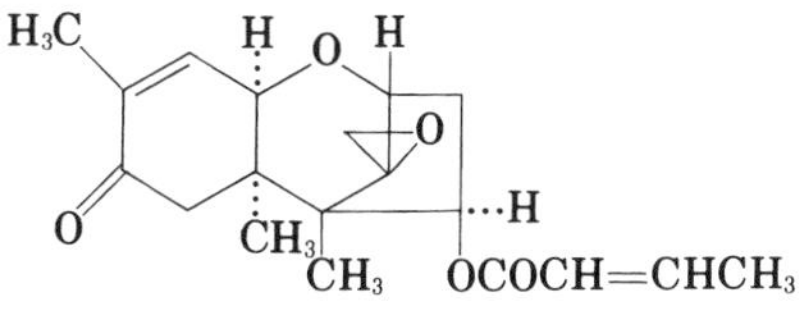

Trichothecin

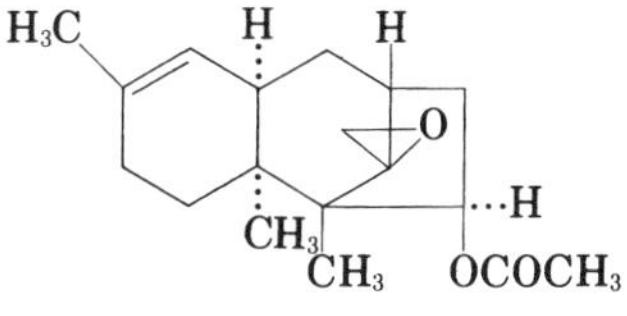

Trichodermin

trichodermin. Representative "scirpene" metabolites of several fungi, including species of *Myrothecium*, are listed in a paper by Saito *et al.*[214,215]

Other Fungus Toxins

A considerable number of other fungus species have been identified as actual or potential toxigenic contaminants of foods used both by animals and man. A few of the more outstanding ones are mentioned here.

Among Russian reports of intoxications attributed to fungi are two important fungus toxins that have been prominently mentioned in litera-

TABLE 4 Penicillium Toxins

Toxin and Biological Source	Formula	Physical Properties	Toxic Reaction (LD$_{50}$)[a]	Foods Naturally Contaminated with Mycotoxin	Foods Supporting Experimental Production	Remarks	References
Rubratoxins P. rubrum P. purpurogenum	See Structure I below A, R=HOH B, R=O	Acidic, colorless crystalline compounds; rubratoxin A m.p. 214 °C; rubratoxin B m.p. 168–170 °C	Body hemorrhages; liver necrosis and kidney hemorrhage Rubratoxin A 6.6 mg/kg IP(M) Rubratoxin B 400 mg/kg oral (M) 3.0 mg/kg IP (M)	Corn	Corn, wheat, rice, oats, rye seed, and timothy hay	These toxins affect several animal species causing liver damage and body hemorrhages; they are not carcinogenic	88,187 188,189 193
Patulin P. urticae P. expansum A. giganteus A. flavus	See Structure II below	Rectangular, colorless, water-soluble crystals; m.p. 111–112 °C	Local eye irritation; neurotoxin; marked pathological changes in visceral organs 10 mg/kg SC (M)	Rice, apple juice	Animal feeds	Antimicrobial and phytotoxic properties; considered carcinogenic	194,195 196
Puberulum toxin P. puberulum	Unknown; contains nitrogen	Acidic compound; green fluorescence; m.p. 200 °C	Ataxia, anoxia; acutely lethal	Unknown	Wheat, corn peanuts, millet, and oats	Red ferric chloride test; antibiotic action against gram-positive organisms	197

402

Toxin / organism	Structure	Physical properties	Toxicity; LD$_{50}$			Remarks	Ref.
Cyclopiazonic acid P. cyclopium	See Structure III below	Crystalline; monobasic acid, insoluble in aqueous solvents at pH below 7.0	Acute neurotoxicity and lethality; subacute effect on cells of kidney, pancreas, and liver 2.3 mg/kg IP (R)	None reported	Grains, maize meal	P. cyclopium; principal cause of decay in stored garlic; organism is frequent contaminant of foods	183,184
Tremorgenic toxin P. cyclopium group	Not yet determined	Fibril-like micro crystals; acid unstable; m.p. 180–200 °C, decomp.	Acute neurotoxicity, sustained trembling and convulsions; diuretic; lethal 2.5 mg/kg IP (M)	Corn, mixed animal feeds	Several food materials	Differs from cyclopiazonic acid; green spot with ferric chloride on TLC	181
Penicillic acid Several Penicillium species	See Structure IV below	Soluble in water; m.p. 83-84 °C	Convulsions, coma and death 250 mg/kg IV (M)		Corn	One of the first mycotoxins discovered; acidic reaction by Congo red	198,199 200
Citrinin P. citrinum P. citreviride A. terreus	See Structure V below	Yellow, fluorescent, water-insoluble crystals; m.p. 170 °C	Nephrotoxin 35 mg/kg SC (M)	Rice	Rice, corn	Citrinin proved too toxic to be used therapeutically as an antibiotic	201

403

TABLE 4 (*Continued*)

Toxin and Biological Source	Formula	Physical Properties	Toxic Reaction (LD$_{50}$)[a]	Foods Naturally Contaminated with Mycotoxin	Foods Supporting Experimental Production	Remarks	References
Citreoviridin *P. citreoviride* (*P. toxicarum*) *P. ochrosalmoneum*	See Structure VI below	Yellow needles; m.p. 107–111 °C	Damage to central nervous system; progressive paralysis of ascending type ~20 mg/kg SC (M)	Rice (?)	Rice	*P. citreoviride* was the first toxic fungus found in molded rice; toxicity inactivated by ultraviolet rays or 2 days sunlight	182,202

[a] Letter following LD$_{50}$ designates the experimental animal as follows: D = duckling; R = rat; M = mouse.

404

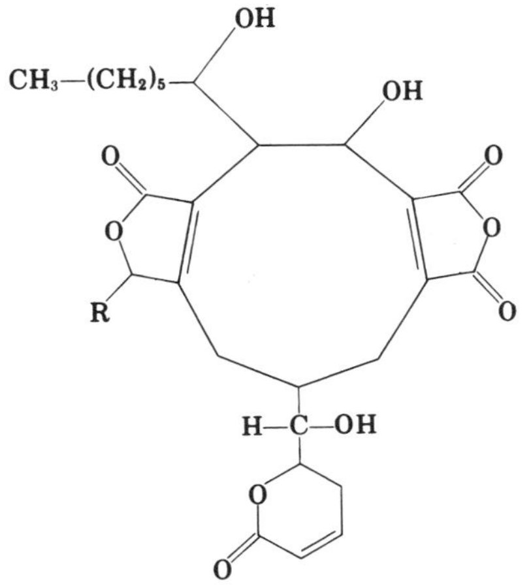

STRUCTURE I

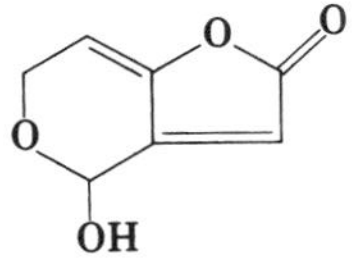

STRUCTURE II

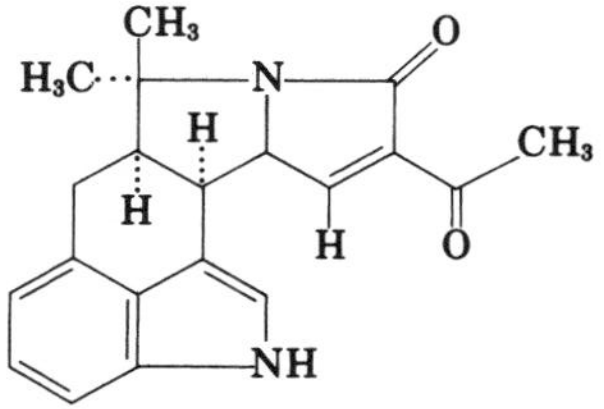

STRUCTURE III

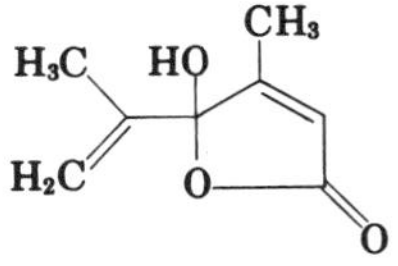

STRUCTURE IV

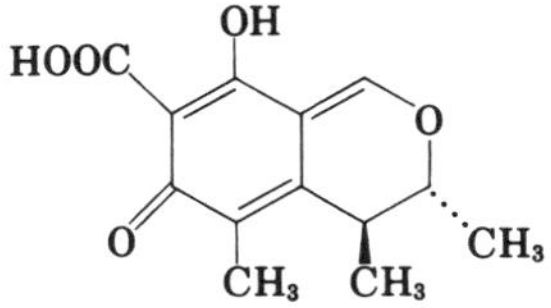

STRUCTURE V

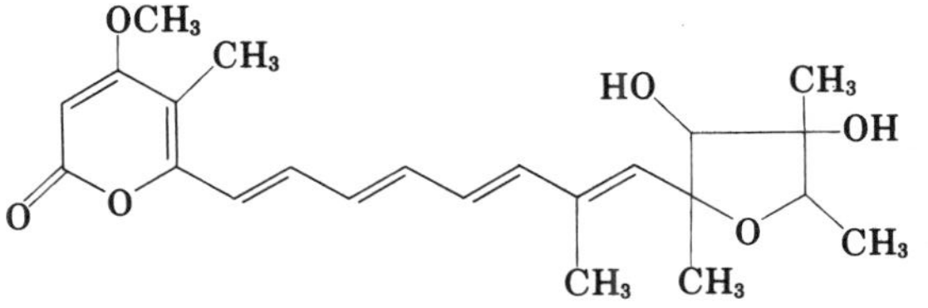

STRUCTURE VI

405

TABLE 5 Fusarium Toxins

Toxin / Biological Source	Formula	Physical Properties	Toxic Reaction $(LD_{50})^a$	Foods Naturally Contaminated with Mycotoxin	Foods Supporting Experimental Production	Remarks	References
Diacetoxyscirpenol F. scirpi F. tricinctum	See Structure I below $R_1, R_2, R_3 = H$ $R_4, R_6 = OAc$ $R_5 = OH$	Colorless crystals soluble in polar organic solvents; m.p. 161–162 °C	Direct skin irritation, marked cellular damage to several tissues by inhibition of DNA and protein synthesis; 0.75 mg/kg IP(R) 7.3 mg/kg oral (R)	Millet, wheat, oats, rye, buckwheat, corn	Wheat	Most potent skin irritant of trichothecenes isolated from fungi	204,207, 211,214
T-2 toxin F. tricinctum F. nivale	Above $R_1, R_3 = H$ $R_2 = 3$-methyl-butyryl oxy $R_4, R_6 = OAc$ $R_5 = OH$	White crystals soluble in polar organic solvents; m.p. 150–152 °C.	Similar to above 4.0 mg/kg oral (R)	Fescue, corn, other cereals	Grits, rice, oats, sorghum, wheat, fescue, cranberries	May be associated with "fescue foot" of cattle	203,213
Nivalenol F. nivale (atypical strain of F. tricinctum)	Above $R_1 = O$ $R_3, R_4, R_5, R_6 = OH$	White rectangular crystals; m.p. 222–223 °C	Similar to above 4.1 mg/kg IP (M)	Rice	Wheat, rice	Suppresses DNA and protein synthesis of HeLa cells; no microbial activity	206,215
Fusarenone F. nivale	See Structure II below	Water-insoluble, white powder; m.p. 78–80 °C	Inhibits protein synthesis—injures hematopoietic cells; 3.56 mg/kg IP (M)	Cereal grains, rice	Rice		212,215, 216

406

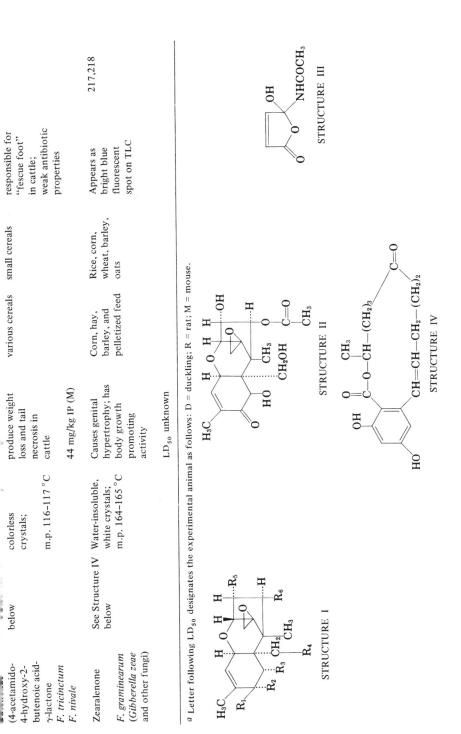

(4-acetamido-4-hydroxy-2-butenoic acid-γ-lactone) F. tricinctum F. nivale	below	colorless crystals; m.p. 116–117 °C	produce weight loss and tail necrosis in cattle 44 mg/kg IP (M)	various cereals	small cereals	responsible for "fescue foot" in cattle; weak antibiotic properties
Zearalenone F. graminearum (Gibberella zeae and other fungi)	See Structure IV below	Water-insoluble, white crystals; m.p. 164–165 °C	Causes genital hypertrophy; has body growth promoting activity LD$_{50}$ unknown	Corn, hay, barley, and pelletized feed	Rice, corn, wheat, barley, oats	Appears as bright blue fluorescent spot on TLC	217,218

a Letter following LD$_{50}$ designates the experimental animal as follows: D = duckling; R = rat; M = mouse.

STRUCTURE I

STRUCTURE II

STRUCTURE III

STRUCTURE IV

ture emanating from that country. Stachybotryotoxicosis is a disease, occurring in man and animals, whose manifestations depend on the extent and type of exposure to contaminated materials. Farmers inhaling dust from hay or straw contaminated with the black conidiated fungus *Stachybotrys atra* (*alternans*) may experience considerable dermal and upper respiratory tract irritation. Animals that consume large quantities of contaminated foods suffer liver damage along with extensive irritation and hemorrhages of internal organs. The disease in animals is likely to be fatal. A more chronic form produced by continued intake develops in stages in which elements of the hemotopoietic system are depressed with accompanying physical signs secondary to this toxic reaction.[219]

The toxic principles of *Stachybotrys atra*, stachybotryotoxins A and B, have reportedly been isolated as noncrystalline substances having complex chemical structures. Very little specific information considered reliable has been published on the chemistry of the toxins.[220]

Members of the genus *Alternaria* are very frequently isolated from stored grain.[221] Several species are sources of toxins that may be formed on food materials and could account for the toxicity of experimentally contaminated grain.[221,222] Some species are well-recognized pathogens of such plants as tobacco, pears, tomatoes, and ornamental flowers. Alternariol, alternariol monomethyl ether, and altenuene have been noted and described as toxic antimicrobial metabolites of *A. tenuis.*[223,224]

Alternariol, R = H
Alternariol Monomethyl Ether, R = CH₃

Altenuene

Reports on extracts from *Alternaria* cultures, which are toxic for tissue culture cells and laboratory animals[221] as well as *Alternaria*-contaminated feed toxic to chicks, have been reported, but the toxic principles are unknown.[222]

For additional summarized information on mycotoxins the reader is referred to an extended review by Herzberg and recent books edited by Riemann[1] and Goldblatt.[226]

TOXIC METABOLITES PRODUCED BY THE SWEET POTATO

The toxicity of mold-damaged sweet potatoes for farm animals has been documented repeatedly in the United States, Japan, and other countries.[227] An abundant supply of black-rotted sweet potatoes following World War II provided the necessary raw materials for Japanese investigators studying their toxic properties. This research led to isolation of several metabolites, most of which contained a furan moiety with attached side chain at the 3- or β-position.[228] These substances, which are formed by the sweet potato tuber largely in response to microbial or insect attack, apparently represent products of an altered metabolism.[229] Some investigators claim the compounds possess antifungal activity.[230]

One of the most abundant of these substances is an oil called ipomeamarone, a steam-distillable furanosesquiterpenoid. Like many of the furan metabolites, this substance is Ehrlich reagent*-positive, giving

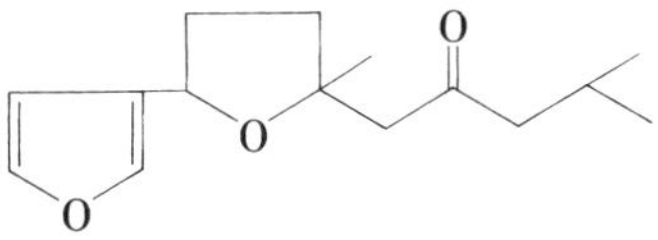

Ipomeamarone

an initial pink color that turns very dark gray. Ipomeamarone produces liver necrosis in mice and other animals when fed or injected intraperitoneally.[231] An IP LD$_{50}$ of 230 mg/kg has been reported by Japanese investigators.[228] Ipomeamarone is the enantiomer of ngaione, a levorotatory oil that appears as a normal metabolite in the leaves and twigs of the Ngaio tree and several shrubs in Australia and New Zealand.[232]

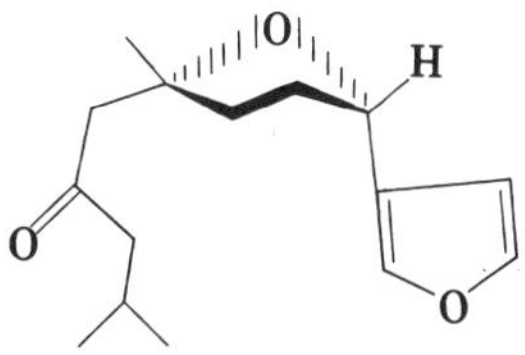

Ngaione

Ipomeamarone [(+)-ngaione] apparently has the I(R),4(S)-configuration.[233]

In recent American work, the hydroxy derivative of ipomeamarone, given the name ipomeamaronol, has also been isolated from moldy

p-Dimethylaminobenzaldehyde and hydrochloric acid.

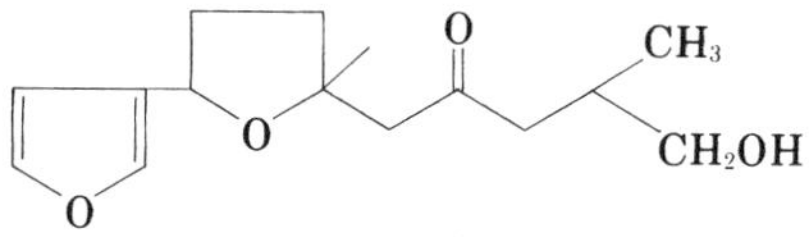

Ipomeamaronol

sweet potatoes.[234] It is hepatotoxic, but a measure of its potency has not yet been possible.

Other β-furans isolated from damaged sweet potatoes include β-furoic acid, ipomeanine, and batatic acid. The toxicity of these latter com-

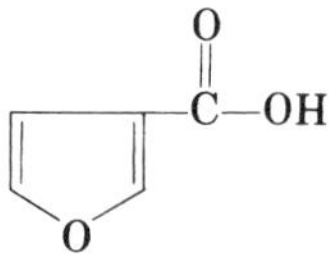

β-Furoic Acid 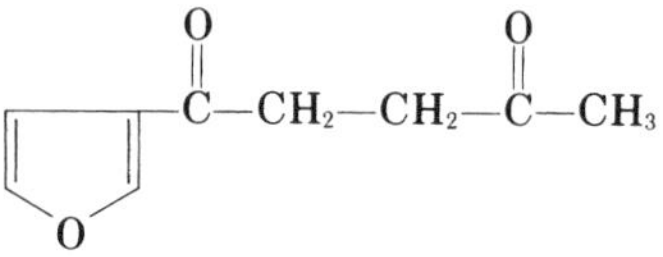   Ipomeanine

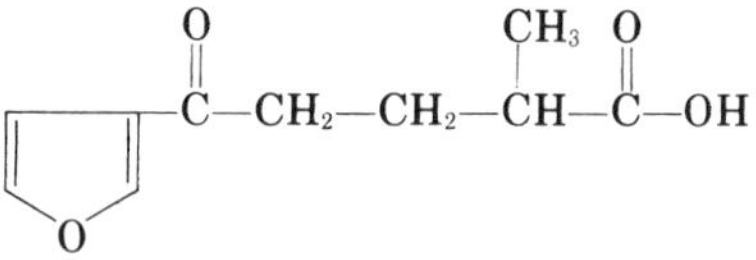

Batatic Acid

pounds has not been reported in the literature; however, recent studies have shown that ipomeanine is a potent toxin (unpublished observations by B. J. Wilson and M. R. Boyd).

In large-scale outbreaks of moldy sweet potato poisoning, especially among cattle, the predominant disease sign is not liver damage such as might be attributed to ipomeamarone. Rather, the animals develop lung edema and die from apparent asphyxia.[227] The extent of accompanying cellular changes in the lungs depends somewhat on the length of the animals' survival. This syndrome can be reproduced in mice by feeding them the ether-extracted material from moldy sweet potatoes. Lungs of the afflicted animals contain clear fluid surrounded by appreciable quantities of pleural fluid.

Very recent studies have demonstrated that this condition is caused by toxin(s) other than ipomeamarone or ipomeamaronol. In fact, two isomeric oils, 4-ipomeanol and 1-ipomeanol, have been isolated from certain kinds of mold-damaged sweet potatoes both naturally and artificially contaminated.[235]

4-Ipomeanol   1-Ipomeanol

These Ehrlich-positive compounds are related to ipomeanine, described earlier by Japanese scientists, as partial reduction products. Only 4-ipomeanol has been studied adequately to establish its lung toxicity. This compound has been synthesized using diethyl 3,4-furandicarboxylate as starting material.[236]

Most Japanese reports refer to the black-rot fungus, *Ceratocystis fimbriata*, being used to infect sweet potato slices for experimental production of ipomeamarone and related furanoterpenoids.[237] American workers have used a fungus isolate, *Fusarium solani javanicum,* obtained from naturally contaminated sweet potatoes, as an infectious agent causing rapid elaboration of the lung edema toxins, of ipomeamarone, and of ipomeamaronol by tuber slices. Significant quantities are obtained in about 6 days at 29 °C incubation. Several bacteria, yeast, other filamentous fungi, and different chemical compounds also have been studied briefly for their toxin-promoting properties. Preliminary work suggests the type of stimulating agent has an effect on the spectrum of compounds formed by injured sweet potato cells.[227]

A preliminary survey of slightly damaged sweet potatoes in several food markets and stores has demonstrated the four toxins in sweet potatoes having minor subcortical blemishes and discoloration. Quantitative analyses for ipomeamarone only showed surprisingly large quantities of this hepatotoxin 9–950 mg/root in selected sweet potatoes offered for sale).[231] Normal boiling or baking of the whole sweet potato does not eliminate its toxins if they are present in significant quantities. The importance of selecting only unblemished, sound sweet potatoes for animal feeding and human diets is certainly indicated. So far no reports of human intoxications due to sweet potatoes have been documented.

Authentic yams (*Dioscorea* species) obtained from West Africa and Puerto Rico did not contain any of the Ehrlich-reacting furanoterpenoids even when inoculated experimentally with molds capable of stimulating the sweet potato to form such compounds.

Since much of the research leading to new toxin discoveries is of very recent origin, it is expected that assessments of hazards associated with damaged sweet potato consumption can be made only after further study of the problem.

REFERENCES

1. H. Riemann (ed.), Food-borne infections and intoxications, Academic Press, New York (1969).
2. B. Aserkoff, S. A. Schroeder, and P. S. Brachman, Salmonellosis in the United States—A five-year review, Am. J. Epidemiol. *92*:13 (1970).
3. F. L. Bryan, The epidemiology of staphylococcal food poisoning, p. 1. In Symposium on staphylococci in foods. N.Y. State Agric. Exp. Stn., Geneva. Res. Circ. No. 23, April (1970).
4. G. M. Dack, Food poisoning, 3rd ed. University of Chicago Press, Chicago (1956). P. 122.
5. M. P. de Figueiredo, Staphylococci control and the food processor, p. 21. In Symposium on staphylococci in foods. N.Y. State Agric. Exp. Stn., Geneva. Res. Circ. No. 23, April (1970).
6. R. A. McLean, H. Lilly, and J. A. Alford, Effects of meat-curing salts and temperature on production of staphylococcal enterotoxin B. J. Bacteriol. *95*: 1207 (1968).
7. M. A. Barber, Milk poisoning due to a *Staphylococcus albus* occurring in the udder of a healthy cow. Philipp. J. Sci. Sect. B. *9*:515 (1913).
8. J. V. Prohaska, Role of staphylococcal enterotoxin in the induction of experimental ileitis. Ann. Surg. *158*:492 (1963).
9. S. E. Warren, H. Sugiyama, and J. V. Prohaska, Correlation of staphylococcal enterotoxins with experimentally induced enterocolitis. Surg. Obstet. Gynecol. *116*:29 (1963).
10. T. G. Merrill and H. Sprinz, The effect of staphylococcal enterotoxin on the fine structure of the monkey jejunum. Lab. Invest. *18*:114 (1968).
11. D. G. Sheahan, H. R. Jervis, A. Takeuchi, and H. Sprinz, The effect of staphylococcal enterotoxin on the epithelial mucosubstances of the small intestine of rhesus monkeys. Am. J. Pathol. *60*:1 (1970).
12. R. Sullivan, Effect of enterotoxin B on intestinal transport *in vitro*. Proc. Soc. Exp. Biol. Med. *131*:1159 (1969).
13. T. H. Kent, Staphylococcal enterotoxin gastroenteritis in rhesus monkey. Am. J. Pathol. *48*:387 (1966).
14. H. Sugiyama and T. Hayama, Abdominal viscera as site of emetic action for staphylococcal enterotoxin in the monkey. J. Infect. Dis. *115*:330 (1965).
15. H. Sugiyama and E. M. McKissic, Jr., Leucocytic response in monkeys challenged with staphylococcal enterotoxin. J. Bacteriol. *92*:349 (1966).
16. H. Sugiyama, E. M. McKissic, Jr., and M. S. Bergdoll, Sensitivity of thorotrast-treated monkeys to staphylococcal enterotoxin. Proc. Soc. Exp. Biol. Med. *113*:468 (1963).
17. H. Sugiyama, Endotoxin-like responses induced by staphylococcal enterotoxin. J. Infect. Dis. *116*:162 (1966).
18. J. A. Vick, F. Klein, C. R. Roberts, and R. Lincoln, Toxicity vs. purity in staphylococcal enterotoxin "B." Mil. Med. *135*:892 (1970).
19. E. J. Schantz, W. G. Roesller, J. Wagnan, L. Spero, D. Dunnery, and M. S. Bergdoll, Purification of staphylococcal enterotoxin B. Biochemistry *4*:1011 (1965).
20. M. S. Bergdoll, Enterotoxins, p. 287. In Microbial toxins, Vol. III, S. Kadis, A. Ciegler, and S. Ajl (eds.). Academic Press, New York (1970).
21. I. Y. Huang and M. S. Bergdoll, The primary structure of staphylococcal en-

terotoxin B. I. Isolation, composition and sequence of tryptic peptides from oxidized enterotoxin B. J. Biol. Chem. *245*:3493 (1970).

22. I. Y. Huang and M. S. Bergdoll, The primary structure of staphylococcal enterotoxin B. II. Isolation, composition, and sequence of chymotryptic peptides. J. Biol. Chem. *245*:3511 (1970).

23. I..Y. Huang and M. S. Bergdoll, The primary structure of staphylococcal enterotoxin B. III. The cyanogen bromide peptides of reduced and aminoethylated enterotoxin B, and the complete amino acid sequence. J. Biol. Chem. *245*:3518 (1970).

24. M. S. Bergdoll, I. Y. Huang, F. S. Chu, and C. Borja, The chemistry of bacterial toxins: The staphylococcal enterotoxins. J. South Afr. Chem. Inst. *22*: 599 (1969).

25. G. M. Dack, Food poisoning, 3rd ed. University of Chicago Press, Chicago (1956). Pp. 146–152.

26. M. S. Bergdoll, Enterotoxins, p. 294. In Microbial toxins, Vol. III, S. Kadis, A. Ciegler, and S. Ajl (eds.). Academic Press, New York (1970).

27. H. D. Raj and M. S. Bergdoll, Effect of enterotoxin B on human volunteers. J. Bacteriol. *98*:833 (1969).

28. B. J. Wilson, Comparative susceptibility of chimpanzees and *Macaca mulatta* monkeys to oral administration of partially purified staphylococcal enterotoxin. J. Bacteriol. *78*:240 (1959).

29. H. Sugiyama, M. S. Bergdoll, and G. M. Dack, Early development of a temporary resistance to the emetic action of staphylococcal enterotoxin. J. Infect. Dis. *111*:233 (1962).

30. S. J. Silverman, D. A. Espeseth, and E. J. Schantz, Effect of formaldehyde on the immunochemical and biological activity of staphylococcal enterotoxin B. J. Bacteriol. *98*:437 (1969).

31. M. J. Surgalla, M. S. Bergdoll, and G. M. Dack, Use of antigen–antibody reactions in agar to follow the progress of fractionation of antigenic mixtures. Application to purification of staphylococcal enterotoxin. J. Immunol. *69*: 357 (1952).

32. M. J. Surgalla, M. S. Bergdoll, and G. M. Dack, Staphylococcal enterotoxin: Neutralization by rabbit antiserum. J. Immunol. *72*:398 (1954).

33. M. S. Bergdoll, H. Sugiyama, and G. M. Dack, Staphylococcal enterotoxin. I. Purification. Arch. Biochem. Biophys. *85*:62 (1959).

34. E. P. Casman and R. W. Bennett, Detection of staphylococcal enterotoxin in food. Appl. Microbiol. *13*:181 (1965).

35. H. E. Hall, R. Angelotti, and K. H. Lewis, Quantitative detection of staphylococcal enterotoxin B in foods by gel-diffusion methods. Public Health Rep. *78*:1089 (1963).

36. C. Genigeorgis and W. W. Sadler, Immunofluorescent detection of staphylococcal enterotoxin B. II. Detection in foods. J. Food Sci. *31*:605 (1966).

37. S. J. Silverman, A. R. Knott, and M. Howard, Rapid, sensitive assay for staphylococcal enterotoxin and a comparison of serological methods. Appl. Microbiol. *16*:1019 (1968).

38. V. G. McGann, J. B. Rollins, and D. W. Mason, Evaluation of resistance to staphylococcal enterotoxin B: Naturally acquired antibodies of man and monkey. J. Infect. Dis. *124*:206 (1971).

39. M. S. Bergdoll, Enterotoxins, p. 278. In Microbial toxins, Vol. III, S. Kadis, A. Ciegler, and S. Ajl (eds.). Academic Press, New York (1970).

40. G. M. Dack, Food poisoning, 3rd ed. University of Chicago Press, Chicago (1956). P. 70.

41. E. J. Gangarosa, J. A. Donadio, R. W. Armstrong, K. F. Meyer, P. S. Brachman, and V. R. Dowell, Botulism in the United States, 1899–1969. Am. J. Epidemiol. 93:93 (1971).

42. V. Moller and I. Scheibel, Preliminary report on the isolation of an apparently new type of Cl. botulinum. Acta Pathol. Microbiol. Scand. 48:80 (1960).

43. J. M. Craig and K. S. Pilcher, Clostridium botulinum type F: Isolation from salmon from the Columbia River. Science 153:311 (1966).

44. H. Riemann, Food-borne infections and intoxications. Academic Press, New York (1969). P. 310.

45. H. Pivnick and H. Barnett, Effect of salt and temperature on toxinogenesis by Clostridium botulinum in perishable cooked meats vacuum-packed in air-impermeable plastic pouches. Food Technol. 19:140 (1965).

46. H. Pivnick and H. Bird, Toxinogenesis by Clostridium botulinum types A and E in perishable cooked meats vacuum packed in plastic pouches. Food Technol. 19:132 (1965).

47. C. Lamanna, H. W. Eklund, and O. E. McElroy, Botulinum toxin (Type A): Including a study of shaking with chloroform as a step in the isolation procedure. J. Bacteriol. 52:1 (1946).

48. B. R. Das Gupta, L. J. Berry, and D. A. Boroff, Purification of Clostridium botulinum type A toxin. Biochim. Biophys. Acta 214:343 (1970).

49. J. Gerwing, C. E. Dolman, M. E. Reichmann, and H. S. Bains, Purification and molecular weight determination of Clostridium botulinum type E toxin. J. Bacteriol. 88:216 (1964).

50. J. Gerwing, C. E. Dolman, and H. S. Bains, Isolation and characterization of a toxic moiety of low molecular weight from Clostridium botulinum type A. J. Bacteriol. 89:1383 (1965).

51. J. Gerwing, C. E. Dolman, D. V. Kason, and J. H. Tremaine, Purification and characterization of Clostridium botulinum type B toxin. J. Bacteriol. 91:484 (1966).

52. E. J. Schantz, Some chemical and physical properties of Clostridium botulinum in culture. Jap. J. Microbiol. 11:380 (1967).

53. C. Lamanna, The most poisonous poison. Science 130:763 (1959).

54. D. A. Boroff and B. R. Das Gupta, Study of the toxin of Clostridium botulinum. VIII. Relation of tryptophane to the biological activity of the toxin. J. Biol. Chem. 239:3694 (1964).

55. E. J. Schantz, D. Stefayne, and L. Spero, Observations on the fluorescence and toxicity of botulinum toxin. J. Biol. Chem. 235:3489 (1960).

56. E. J. Schantz and L. Spero. The reaction of botulinum toxin type A with ketene. J. Am. Chem. Soc. 79:1623 (1957).

57. L. Spero and E. J. Schantz, The reaction of botulinum toxin type A with nitrous acid. J. Am. Chem. Soc. 79:1625 (1957).

58. M. Cherington and D. W. Ryan, Treatment of botulism with guanidine. N. Engl. J. Med. 282:195 (1970).

59. E. H. Polley, J. A. Vick, H. P. Ciuchta, D. A. Fischetti, F. J. Macchitelli, and N. Montanarelli, Botulinum toxin, type A: Effects on central nervous system. Science 147:1036 (1965).

60. L. L. Simpson, F. de Balbian Verster, and J. T. Tapp, Electrophysiological

manifestations of experimental botulinal intoxication: Depression of cortical EEG. Exp. Neurol. *19*:199 (1967).

61. S. I. Zacks, M. V. Rhoades, and M. F. Sheff, The localization of botulinum A toxin in the mouse. Exp. Mol. Pathol. *9*:77 (1968).

62. L. W. Duchen and S. J. Strich, The effect of botulinum toxin on the pattern of innervation of skeletal muscle in the mouse. Q. J. Exp. Physiol. *53*:84 (1968).

63. L. L. Simpson, Effects of intraperitoneally injected botulinum toxin on rat cerebral cortex levels of acetylcholine. J. Neurochem. *15*:359 (1968).

64. W. Schaffner and M. G. Koenig, Botulism, Chapter 26, p. 1. In Tice's practice of medicine, Vol. III. Harper and Row, Hagerstown, Md. (1970).

65. G. Sakaguchi, S. Sakaguchi, and H. Kondo, Rapid bioassay for *Cl. botulinum* type E toxins by intravenous injection into mice. Jap. J. Med. Biol. *21*:369 (1968).

66. G. Barger, Ergot and ergotism. Guerney and Jackson, London (1931).

67. P. Brazeau, Drugs affecting uterine motility, p. 900. In The pharmacological basis of therapeutics.-4th ed. L. S. Goodman and A. Gilman (eds.). Macmillan, New York (1970).

68. Anonymous, Bread of madness infects a town. Life *31*:25 (September 10, 1951).

69. J. G. Fuller, The day of St. Anthony's fire. Macmillan, New York (1968).

70. V. I. Bilay (ed.), Mycotoxicoses of man and agricultural animals. Office of Tech. Ser., U.S. Dept. of Commerce, Washington, D.C. (1960). (English trans.)

71. J. Forgacs, Mycotoxicoses—The neglected diseases. Feedstuffs *34*(18):124 (1962).

72. B. J. Wilson, Miscellaneous aspergillus toxins, pp. 207–295. In Microbial toxins, Vol. VI, S. Kadis, A. Ciegler, and S. Ajl (eds.). Academic Press, New York (1972).

73. B. J. Wilson, Miscellaneous penicillium toxins., pp. 459–521. In Microbial toxins, Vol. VI, S. Kadis, A. Ciegler, and S. Ajl (eds.). Academic Press, New York (1972).

74. H. F. Kraybill and R. E. Shapiro, Implications of fungal toxicity to human health, p. 401. In Aflatoxin, L. A. Goldblatt (ed.). Academic Press, New York (1969).

75. P. Robinson, Infantile cirrhosis of the liver in India. Clin. Pediatr. *6*:57 (1967).

76. T. C. Campbell, J. P. Caedo, Jr., J. Bulatoo-Jayme, L. Salamat, and R. W. Engel, Aflatoxin M_1 in human urine. Nature *227*:403 (1970).

77. B. J. Wilson, Toxins other than aflatoxins produced by *Aspergillus flavus*. Bacteriol. Rev. *30*:478 (1966).

78. B. J. Wilson, Mycotoxins, p. 141. In The safety of foods. Avi, Westport, Conn. (1968).

79. W. P. Blount, Turkey X disease. Turkeys (J. Br. Turkey Fed.) *9*:52 (1961).

80. P. K. C. Austwick and G. Ayerst, Toxic products in groundnuts. Groundnut microflora and toxicity. Chem. Ind. (London) *2*:55 (1963).

81. K. Sargeant, A. Sheridan, J. O'Kelly, and R. B. A. Carnaghan, Toxicity associated with certain samples of groundnuts. Nature *192*:1096 (1961).

82. R. Schoental, Aflatoxins. Ann. Rev. Pharmacol. *7*:343 (1967).

83. Interdepartmental Working Party on Groundnut Toxicity Research, Toxicity

associated with certain batches of groundnuts. U.K. Agric. Res. (Counc., Dep. Sci. Ind. Res., Dep. Tech. Co-op. Med. Res. Counc., Minist. Agric., Fish. Food Progr. Rep. (1962).

84. H. Wolf and E. W. Jackson, Hepatoma in rainbow trout: Descriptive and experimental epidemiology. Science *142*:676 (1963).

85. M. F. Argus and C. Hoch-Ligeti, Comparative study of the carcinogenic activity of nitrosamines. J. Nat. Cancer Inst. *27*:695 (1961).

86. G. E. Paget, Exudative hepatitis in guinea pigs. J. Pathol. Bacteriol. *47*:393 (1954).

87. A. L. Stalker and D. L. McLean, The incidence of oedema in young guinea pigs. J. Anim. Tech. Assoc. *8*:18 (1957).

88. J. E. Burnside, W. L. Sippel, J. Forgacs, W. T. Carll, M. B. Atwood, and E. R. Doll, A disease of swine and cattle caused by eating moldy corn. II. Experimental production with pure cultures of molds. Am. J. Vet. Res. *18*:817 (1957).

89. W. S. Bailey and A. H. Groth, The relationship of hepatitis x of dogs and moldy corn poisoning of swine. J. Am. Vet. Med. Assoc. *134*:514 (1959).

90. B. J. Wilson, P. A. Teer, G. H. Barney, and F. R. Blood, Relationship of aflatoxin to epizootics of toxic hepatitis among animals in southern United States. Am. J. Vet. Res. *28*:1217 (1967).

91. F. A. Hodges, J. R. Zust, H. R. Smith, A. A. Nelson, B. H. Armbrecht, and A. D. Campbell, Mycotoxins: Aflatoxin isolated from *Penicillium puberulum*. Science *145*:1439 (1964).

92. M. M. Kulik and C. E. Holaday, Aflatoxin: A metabolic product of several fungi. Mycopathol. Mycol. Appl. *30*:137 (1967).

93. P. M. Scott, W. van Walbeek, and J. Forgacs, Formation of aflatoxins by *Aspergillus ostianus Wehmer*. Appl. Microbiol. *15*:945 (1967).

94. W. van Walbeek, P. M. Scott, and F. S. Thatcher, Mycotoxins from food-borne fungi. Can. J. Microbiol. *14*:131 (1968).

95. B. J. Wilson, T. C. Campbell, A. W. Hayes, and R. T. Hanlin, Investigation of reported aflatoxin production by fungi outside the *Aspergillus flavus* group. Appl. Microbiol. *16*:819 (1968).

96. F. W. Parrish, B. J. Wiley, E. G. Simmons, and L. Long, Jr., A survey of some species of *Aspergillus* and *Penicillium* for production of aflatoxins and kojic acid. U.S. Army, Natick Labs, Tech. Rep. Microbiol. *20* (1965).

97. P. B. Mislivec, H. J. Hunter, and J. Tuiet, Assay for aflatoxin production by the genera *Aspergillus* and *Penicillium*. Appl. Microbiol. *16*:1053 (1968).

98. C. W. Hesseltine, O. L. Shotwell, M. L. Smith, G. M. Shannon, E. E. Vandergraft, and M. L. Goulden. Laboratory studies of the formation of aflatoxin in forages. Mycologia *60*:304 (1968).

99. C. Golumbic and M. Kulik. Fungal spoilage in stored crops and its control, p. 319. In Aflatoxin, L. A. Goldblatt (ed.). Academic Press, New York (1969).

100. B. H. Armbrecht, F. A. Hodges, H. R. Smith, and A. A. Nelson, Mycotoxins. I. Studies on aflatoxin derived from contaminated peanut meal and certain strains of *Aspergillus flavus*. J. Assoc. Off. Anal. Chem. *46*:805 (1963).

101. P. deVogel, R. Van Rhee, and W. A. A. Blanche Koelensmid, A rapid screening test for aflatoxin synthesizing aspergilli of the flavus-oryzae group. J. Appl. Bacteriol. *28*:213 (1965).

102. R. C. Codner, K. Sargeant, and R. Yeo. Production of aflatoxin by the culture

of strains of *Aspergillus flavus-oryzae* on sterilized peanuts. Biotechnol. Bioeng. *5*:185 (1963).

103. A. Wallbridge. Behavior of different strains of *A. flavus* and related species. UNICEF Conference on Groundnut Toxicity Problems. Trop. Prod. Inst., London (1963). (Abstr.)

104. V. Sreenivasamurthy, H. Jayarman, and H. A. B. Parpia, Aflatoxin in Indian peanuts: Analysis and extraction, p. 251. In Mycotoxins in foodstuffs, G. N. Wogan (ed.). M. I. T. Press, Cambridge, Mass. (1965).

105. De B. Scott, Toxigenic fungi isolated from cereal and legume products. Mycopathol. Mycol. Appl. *2051*:213 (1964).

106. S. Y. Borut and A. Z. Joffe, *Aspergillus flavus* link aflatoxins and toxicity of groundnuts in Israel. Isr. J. Bot. *14*:198 (1965).

107. K. S. Rao, T. V. Madhavan, and P. G. Tulpule, Incidence of toxigenic strains of *Aspergillus flavus* affecting groundnut crop in certain coastal districts in India. Indian J. Med. Res. *53*:1196 (1965).

108. R. A. Boller and H. W. Schroeder, Aflatoxin producing potential of *Aspergillus flavus oryzae* isolated from rice. Cereal Sci. Today *11*:324 (1966).

109. U. L. Diener and N. D. Davis, Aflatoxin production by isolates of *Aspergillus flavus*. Phytopathology *56*:1390 (1966).

110. C. W. Hesseltine, O. L. Shotwell, J. J. Ellis, and R. D. Stubblefield, Aflatoxin formation by *Aspergillus flavus*. Bacteriol. Rev. *30*:795 (1966).

111. R. A. Taber and H. W. Schroeder, Aflatoxin-producing potential of isolates of *Aspergillus flavus-oryzae* group from peanuts (*Arachis hypogaea*). Appl. Microbiol. *15*:1099 (1967).

112. L. A. Goldblatt, Aflatoxin. Assoc. Food Drug Off. Q. Bull. U.S. *29*:58 (1965).

113. L. J. Ashworth, Jr., and B. C. Langley, The relationship of pod damage to kernel damage by molds in Spanish peanut. Plant Dis. Rep. *48*:875 (1964).

114. D. McDonald and C. Harkness, Growth of *Aspergillus flavus* and production of aflatoxin in groundnuts. II. Trop. Sci. *5*:143 (1963).

115. H. W. Schroeder and L. J. Ashworth, Jr., Aflatoxins in Spanish peanuts in relation to pod and kernel condition. Phytopathology *55*:464 (1965).

116. W. G. Sorenson, C. W. Hesseltine, and O. L. Shotwell, Effect of temperature on production of aflatoxin on rice by *Aspergillus flavus*. Mycopathol. Mycol. Appl. *33*:49 (1967).

117. P. J. Andrellos and G. R. Reid, Confirmatory tests for aflatoxin B. J. Assoc. Off. Agric. Chem. *47*:801 (1964).

118. E. V. Crisan and A. T. Grefig, The formation of aflatoxin derivatives. Contrib. Boyce Thompson Inst. *24*:3 (1967).

119. Voluntary code of good practices for purchasing, handling, storage, processing and testing of peanuts. 8th ed., National Peanut Council, August (1970).

120. C. J. Kensler and D. J. Natoli, Processing to insure wholesome products, p. 333. In Aflatoxin, L. A. Goldblatt (ed.). Academic Press, New York (1969).

121. G. N. Wogan, Chemical nature and biological effects of the aflatoxins. Bacteriol. Rev. *30*:460 (1966).

122. M. S. Legator, Biological effects of aflatoxin in cell culture. Bacteriol. Rev. *30*:474 (1966).

123. J. B. Wragg, V. C. Ross, and M. S. Legator, Effect of aflatoxin B_1 on the deoxyribonucleic acid polymerase of *Escherichia coli*. Proc. Soc. Exp. Biol. Med. *125*:1052 (1967).

124. T. Asao, G. Büchi, M. M. Abdel-Kader, S. B. Chang, E. L. Wick, and G. N. Wogan, Aflatoxins B and G. J. Am. Chem. Soc. *85*:1706 (1963).

125. T. Asao, G. Büchi, M. M. Abdel-Kader, S. B. Chang, E. L. Wick, and G. N. Wogan, The structures of aflatoxins B_1 and G_1. J. Am. Chem. Soc. *87*:882 (1965).

126. S. B. Chang, M. M. Abdel-Kader, E. L. Wick, and G. N. Wogan, Aflatoxin B_2: Chemical identity and biological activity. Science *142*:1191 (1963).

127. P. A. van Dorp, A. S. M. van der Zijden, R. K. Berrthuis, S. Sparreboom, W. O. Ord, K. de Jong, and R. Keuning, Dihydroaflatoxin B, a metabolite of *Aspergillus flavus*. Remarks on the structure of aflatoxin B. Rec. Trav. Chim. *82*:587 (1963).

128. C. M. Holzapfel, P. S. Steyn, and I. F. H. Purchase, Isolation and structure of aflatoxins M_1 and M_2. Tetrahedron Lett. *25*:2799 (1966).

129. K. K. Cheung and G. A. Sim, Aflatoxin G_1: Direct determination of the structure by the method of isomorphous replacement. Nature *201*:1185 (1964).

130. T. C. van Soest and A. F. Peerdeman, The crystal structures of aflatoxin B_1. I. The structure of the chloroform solvate of aflatoxin B_1 and the absolute configuration of aflatoxin B_1. Acta Cryst. *B26*:1940 (1970).

131. S. Brechbuhler, G. Büchi, and G. Milne, The absolute configuration of the aflatoxins. J. Org. Chem. *32*:2641 (1967).

132. G. Büchi, D. M. Foulkes, M. Kurono, G. F. Mitchell, and R. S. Schneider, The total synthesis of racemic aflatoxin B_1. J. Am. Chem. Soc. *89*:6745 (1967).

133. A. C. Waiss, M. Wiley, D. R. Black, and R. E. Lundin, 3-Hydroxy-6,7-dimethoxy difuroxanthone—A new metabolite from *Aspergillus flavus*. Tetrahedron Lett. 3207 (1968).

134. M. Biollaz, G. Büchi, and G. Milne, The biosynthesis of the aflatoxins. J. Am. Chem. Soc. *92*:1035 (1969).

135. R. B. A. Carnaghan, R. D. Hartley, and J. O'Kelley, Toxicity and fluorescent properties of the aflatoxins. Nature *200*:1101 (1963).

136. R. Allcroft and R. B. A. Carnaghan, Toxic products in groundnuts. Biological effects. Chem. Ind. (London) *12*:50 (1963).

137. G. N. Wogan and P. M. Newberne, Dose-response characteristics of aflatoxin B_1 carcinogenesis in the rat. Cancer Res. *27*:2370 (1967).

138. W. H. Butler and J. I. Clifford, The extraction of aflatoxin from rat liver. Nature *206*:1045 (1965).

139. P. J. Andrellos, A. C. Beckwith, and R. M. Eppley, Photochemical changes of aflatoxin B_1. J. Assoc. Off. Anal. Chem. *50*:346 (1967).

140. W. C. Neely, J. A. Lansden, and J. R. McDuffie, Spectral studies on the deoxyribonucleic acid-aflatoxin B_1 system. Binding interactions. Biochemistry *9*:1862 (1970).

141. A. J. Feuell, Aflatoxin in groundnuts. IX. Problems of detoxification. Trop. Sci. *8*:61 (1966).

142. T. J. Coomes, P. C. Crowther, A. J. Feuell, and B. J. Francis, Experimental detoxification of groundnut meals containing aflatoxin. Nature *209*:406 (1966).

143. P. N. Newberne, Carcinogenicity of aflatoxin-contaminated peanut meal, p. 187. In Mycotoxins in foodstuffs, G. N. Wogan (ed.). M.I.T. Press, Cambridge, Mass. (1965).

144. F. G. Dollear and H. K. Gardner, Jr., Inactivation and removal of aflatoxin,

p. 72. Proceedings of the 4th National Peanut Research Conference, Tifton, Ga. (1966).

145. G. N. Wogan, G. S. Edwards, and R. C. Shank, Excretion and tissue distribution of radioactivity from aflatoxin B_1-^{14}C in rats. Cancer Res. *27*:1729 (1967).

146. J. Dalezios, G. N. Wogan, and S. M. Weinreb, Aflatoxin P: A new aflatoxin metabolite in monkeys. Science *171*:584 (1971).

147. R. C. Shank and G. N. Wogan, Acute effects of aflatoxin B_1 on liver composition and metabolism in the rat and duckling. Toxicol. Appl. Pharmacol. *3*:468 (1966).

148. J. Gablicks, W. Schaeffer, L. Friedman, and G. Wogan, Effect of aflatoxin B_1 on cell cultures. J. Bacteriol. *90*:720 (1965).

149. M. S. Legator and A. Withrow, Aflatoxin: Effect on mitotic division in cultured embryonic lung cells. J. Assoc. Off. Anal. Chem. *47*:1007 (1964).

150. S. Johasz and E. Greczi, Extracts of mould-infected groundnut samples in tissue culture. Nature *203*:861 (1964).

151. R. Schoental and A. F. White, Aflatoxins and "albinism" in plants. Nature *205*:57 (1965).

152. I. Uritani, T. Asahi, R. Majima, and Z. Mori, The biochemical effects of aflatoxins and other toxic compounds related to parasitic fungi on the metabolism of plant tissues, p. 1. In Conference on Toxic Microorganisms, Honolulu U.J.N.R. (1968).

153. F. Matsumura and S. G. Knight, Toxicity and chemosterilizing activity of aflatoxins against insects. J. Econ. Entomol. *60*:871 (1967).

154. R. T. Godauskas, N. D. Davis, and U. L. Diener, Sensitivity of *Heliothis virescens* larvae to aflatoxin in *ad libitum* feeding. J. Invertebr. Pathol. *9*:132 (1967).

155. A. Ciegler, E. B. Lillehoj, R. E. Peterson, and H. H. Hall, Microbial detoxification of aflatoxin. Appl. Microbiol. *14*:934 (1966).

156. R. S. Portman, K. M. Plowman, and T. C. Campbell, On mechanisms affecting species susceptibility to aflatoxin. Biochim. Biophys. Acta *208*:487 (1970).

157. R. C. Shank, G. N. Wogan, and J. B. Gibson, Dietary aflatoxins and human liver cancer. I. Toxigenic moulds in foods and foodstuffs in tropical South-East Asia. Food Cosmet. Toxicol. *10*:51 (1972).

158. R. C. Shank, G. N. Wogan, J. B. Gibson, and A. Nondasuta, Dietary aflatoxins and human liver cancer. II. Aflatoxins in market foods and foodstuffs of Thailand and Hong Kong. Food Cosmet. Toxicol. *10*:61 (1972).

159. R. C. Shank, J. E. Gordon, G. N. Wogan, A. Nondasuta, and B. Subhamani, Dietary aflatoxins and human liver cancer. III. Field survey of rural Thai families for ingested aflatoxins. Food Cosmet. Toxicol. *10*:71 (1972).

160. R. C. Shank, N. Bhamarapravati, J. E. Gordon, and G. N. Wogan, Dietary aflatoxins and human liver cancer. IV. Incidence of primary liver cancer in two municipal populations of Thailand. Food Cosmet. Toxicol. *10*:171 (1972).

161. R. C. Shank, P. Siddhichai, B. Subhamani, N. Bhamarapravati, J. E. Gordon, and G. N. Wogan, Dietary aflatoxins and human liver cancer. V. Duration of primary liver cancer and prevalence of hepatomegaly in Thailand. Food Cosmet. Toxicol. *10*:181 (1972).

162. C. Wehmer, cited by J. W. Foster, Chemical activities of fungi. Academic Press, New York (1949). P. 327.

163. B. J. Wilson and C. H. Wilson, Oxalate formation in moldy foodstuffs as a possible factor in livestock toxic disease. Am. J. Vet. Res. *22*:961 (1961).

164. M. M. Mershon, Tetany in cattle on winter rations. II. Stresses and mineral metabolism. J. Am. Vet. Med. Assoc. *135*:435 (1959).

165. B. J. Wilson and C. H. Wilson, Toxin from *Aspergillus flavus*: Production on food materials of a substance causing tremors in mice. Science *144*:177 (1964).

166. K. J. van der Merwe, P. S. Steyn, and L. Fourie, Mycotoxins. Part II. The constitution of ochratoxins A, B, and C. Metabolites of *Aspergillus ochraceus* wilh. J. Chem. Soc. (London), 7083 (1965).

167. W. van Walbeek, P. M. Scott, J. Harwig, and J. W. Lawrence, *Penicillium viridicatum* Westling: A new source of ochratoxin A. Can. J. Microbiol. *15*:1281 (1969).

168. H. Tsunoda, Micro-organisms which deteriorate stored cereals and grains, p. 143. In Proceedings of the 1st U.S.–Japan Conference on Toxic Microorganisms. U.J.N.R. Joint Panel on Toxic Microorganisms and U.S. Dep. Interior (1970).

169. L. Stoloff, S. Nesheim, L. Yin, J. Rodricks, M. Stack, and A. D. Campbell, Multimycotoxin detection method for aflatoxins, ochratoxins, zearalenone, sterigmatocystin, and patulin. J. Assoc. Off. Anal. Chem. *54*:91 (1971).

170. I. F. H. Purchase and J. J. van der Watt, Carcinogenicity of sterigmatocystin. Food Cosmet Toxicol. *6*:555 (1968).

171. I. F. Purchase and J. J. van der Watt, Acute toxicity of sterigmatocystin to rats. Food Cosmet. Toxicol. *7*:135 (1969).

172. H. J. Burkhardt and J. Forgacs, O-Methylsterigmatocystin, a new metabolite from *Aspergillus flavus* Link ex Fries. Tetrahedron *24*:717 (1968).

173. J. V. Rodricks, K. R. Henery-Logan, A. D. Campbell, L. Stoloff, and M. J. Verrett, Isolation of a new toxin from cultures of *Aspergillus flavus*. Nature *217*:668 (1968).

174. J. V. Rodricks, E. Lustig, A. D. Campbell, L. Stoloff, and K. R. Henery-Logan, Aspertoxin, a hydroxy derivative of O-methyl sterigmatocystin from aflatoxin-producing cultures of *Aspergillus flavus*. Tetrahedron Lett. *25*:2975 (1968).

175. C. W. Holzapfel, I. F. Purchase, P. S. Steyn, and L. Gouws, The toxicity and chemical assay of sterigmatocystin, a carcinogenic mycotoxin, and its isolation from two new fungal sources. South Afr. Med. J. *40*:1100 (1966).

176. O. D. Shotwell, C. W. Hesseltine, M. Goulden, and E. E. Vandergraft, Survey of corn for aflatoxin, zearalenone and ochratoxin. Cereal Chem. *47*:700 (1970).

177. P. M. Scott, W. van Walbeek, J. Harwig, and D. I. Fennell, Occurrence of a mycotoxin, ochratoxin A, in wheat and isolation of ochratoxin A and citrinin producing strains of *Penicillium viridicatum*. Can. J. Plant Sci. *50*:583 (1970).

178. T. Yokotsuka, Y. Asao, M. Sasaki, and K. Oshita, Pyrazine compounds produced by molds, p. 133. In Proceedings of the 1st U.S.–Japan Conference on Toxic Microorganisms. U.J.N.R. Joint Panel on Toxic Microorganisms and U.S. Dep. Interior (1970).

179. S. C. Werch, Y. T. Oester, and T. E. Friedemann, Kojic acid—A convulsant. Science *126*:450 (1957).

180. A. Beelik, Kojic acid, p. 145. In Advances in carbohydrate chemistry. Vol. 2, W. W. Pigman and M. L. Wolfrom (eds.). Academic Press, New York (1946).

181. B. J. Wilson, C. H. Wilson, and A. W. Hayes, Tremorgenic toxin from *Penicillium cyclopium* grown on food materials. Nature *220*:77 (1968).

182. N. Sakabe, T. Goto, and Y. Hirata, The structure of citreoviridin, a toxic compound produced by *P. citreoviride* on rice. Tetrahedron Lett. *27–28*:1825 (1964).

183. C. W. Holzapfel, The isolation and structure of cyclopiazonic acid, a toxic metabolite of *Penicillium cyclopium* westling. Tetrahedron *24*:2101 (1968).

184. I. H. F. Purchase, The acute toxicity of the mycotoxin cyclopiazonic acid to rats. Toxicol. Appl. Pharmacol. *18*:114 (1971).

185. A. Ciegler and C. T. Hou, Isolation of viridicatin from *Penicillium palitans*. Arch. Mikrobiol. *73*:261 (1970).

186. M. Taniguchi and Y. Satomura, Isolation of viridicatin from *Penicillium crustosum*, and physiological activity of viridicatin and its 3-carboxymethylene derivative on microorganisms and plants. Agric. Biol. Chem. (Japan) *34*:506 (1970).

187. M. O. Moss, F. V. Robinson, and A. B. Wood, Rubratoxin B, a toxic metabolite of *Penicillium rubrum*. Chem. Ind. 587 (1968).

188. M. O. Moss, A. B. Wood, and F. V. Robinson, The structure of rubratoxin A, a toxic metabolite of *Penicillium rubrum*. Tetrahedron Lett. *5*:367 (1969).

189. S. Natori, S. Sakaki, H. Kurata, S. Udagawa, M. Ichinoe, M. Saito, M. Umeda, and K. Ohtsubo, Production of rubratoxin B by *Penicillium purpurogenum* stoll. Appl. Microbiol. *19*:613 (1970).

190. A. W. Hayes and E. P. Wyatt, Survey of the sensitivity of microorganisms to rubratoxin B. Appl. Microbiol. *20*:164 (1970).

191. M. O. Moss and I. W. Hill, Strain variation in the production of rubratoxins by *Penicillium rubrum* stoll. Mycopathol. Mycol. Appl. *40*:81 (1970).

192. C. W. Hesseltine, Mycotoxins. Mycopathol. Mycol. Appl. *39*:371 (1969).

193. B. J.Wilson and C. H. Wilson, Extraction and preliminary characterization of a hepatotoxic substance from cultures of *Penicillium rubrum*. J. Bacteriol. *84*:283 (1962).

194. R. Kinosita and T. Shikata, On toxic moldy rice, p. 117. In Mycotoxins in foodstuffs, G. N. Wogan (ed.). M.I.T. Press, Cambridge, Mass. (1965).

195. J. Singh, p. 621. In Antibiotics 1, D. Gottleib and P. D. Shaw (eds.). Springer-Verlag, Berlin (1967).

196. A. D. Campbell, Chemical methods for mycotoxins, p. 36. In Proceedings of the 1st U.S.–Japan Conference on Toxic Microorganisms. U.J.N.R. Joint Panel on Toxic Microorganisms and U.S. Dep. Interior (1970).

197. B. J. Wilson, T. M. Harris, and A. W. Hayes, Mycotoxin from *Penicillium puberulum*. J. Bacteriol. *93*:1737 (1967).

198. C. L. Alsberg and O. F. Black, Contributions to the study of maize deterioration. U.S. Dep. Agric. Bur. Plant Ind. Bull. 270 (1913).

199. M. W. Miller, p. 772. The Pfizer handbook of microbial metabolites. McGraw-Hill, New York (1961).

200. C. P. Kurtzman and A. Ciegler, Mycotoxin from a blue-eye mold of corn. Appl. Microbiol. *20*:204 (1970).

201. F. Sakai, An experimental study on the toxic effect especially on the kidney of "yellowed rice" polluted by *Penicillium citrinum* thom, as well as of citrinin, a pigment isolated from the mould. Folia Pharmacol. Jap. *51*:431 (1955).

202. Studies on "yellowed rice" of *Penicillium citreo-viride biourge,* 1940–1951. Department of Pharmacology, Faculty of Medicine, University of Tokyo.

203. M. D. Grove, S. G. Yates, W. H. Tallent, J. J. Ellis, I. A. Wolff, N. R. Kosuri,

and R. E. Nichols, Mycotoxins produced by *Fusarium tricinctum* as possible causes of cattle disease. Agric. Food Chem. *18*:734 (1970).

204. N. R. Kosuri, M. D. Grove, S. G. Yates, W. H. Tallent, J. J. Ellis, I. A. Wolff, and R. E. Nichols, Response of cattle to mycotoxins of *Fusarium tricinctum* isolated from corn and fescue. J. Am. Vet. Med. Assoc. *157*:938 (1970).

205. C. J. Mirocha, C. M. Christensen, and G. H. Nelson, Estrogenic metabolite produced by *Fusarium graminearum* in stored corn. Appl. Microbiol. *15*:497 (1967).

206. T. Tatsuno, M. Saito, M. Enomoto, and H. Tsunoda, Nivalenol, a toxic principle of *Fusarium nivale*. Chem. Pharm. Bull. *16*:2519 (1968).

207. Y. Ueno, Y. Ishikawa, K. Amaki, M. Nakajima, M. Saito, M. Entomoto, and K. Ohtsubo, Comparative study on skin-necrotizing effect of scirpene metabolites of fusaria. Jap. J. Exp. Med. *40*:33 (1970).

208. L. Badiali, M. H. Abou-Youssef, A. I. Radwan, F. M. Hamdy, and P. K. Hildebrandt. Moldy corn poisoning as the major cause of an encephalomalacia syndrome in Egyptian equidae. Am. J. Vet. Res. *29*:2029 (1968).

209. B. J. Wilson and R. R. Maronpot, Causative fungus agent of leucoencephalomalacia in equines. Vet. Rec., 484, (May 9, 1971).

210. D. C. Gajdusek, Alimentary toxic aleukia, p. 82. In Acute infectious hemorrhagic fevers and mycotoxicoses in the Union of Soviet Socialist Republics. Med. Sci. Publ. No. 2, Army Med. Ser. Grad. School, Walter Reed Army Med. Cent., Washington, D.C. (1953).

211. J. R. Bamburg, F. M. Strong, and E. B. Smalley, Toxins from moldy cereal. J. Agric. Food Chem. *17*:443 (1969).

212. J. R. Bamburg, N. V. Riggs, and F. M. Strong, The structure of toxins from two strains of *Fusarium tricinctum*. Tetrahedron *24*:3329 (1968).

213. M. Saito, M. Entomoto, and T. Tatsuno, Radiomimetic biological properties of the new scirpene metabolites of *Fusarium nivale*. Gann *60*:599 (1969).

214. J. R. Bamburg and F. M. Strong, 12,13-Epoxytricothecenes, pp. 207–292. In Fungal toxins. Microbial toxins, Vol. VII, S. Kadis, A. Ciegler, and S. Ajl (eds.). Academic Press, New York (1971).

215. M. Saito and K. Okubo, Studies on the target injuries in experimental animals with the mycotoxins, p. 82. In Proceedings of the 1st U.S.–Japan Conference on Toxic Microorganisms. U.J.N.R. Joint Panel on Toxic Microorganisms and U.S. Dep. Interior. (1970).

216. S. G. Yates, H. L. Tookey, J. J. Ellis, and H. J. Burkhardt, Mycotoxins produced by *Fusarium nivale* isolated from tall fescue. Phytochemistry 7:139 (1968).

217. C. M. Christensen, G. H. Nelson, and C. J. Mirocha, Effect on the white rat uterus of a toxic substance isolated from fusarium. Appl. Microbiol. *13*:653 (1965).

218. W. H. Urry, H. L. Wehrmeister, E. B. Hodge, and P. H. Hidy, The structure of zearalone. Tetrahedron Lett. *27*:3109 (1966).

219. V. G. Drobotko, Stachybotryotoxicosis. A new disease of horses and humans. Am. Rev. Sov. Med. *2*:238 (1944–45).

220. M. Palyusik, Biological test for the toxic substance of *Stachybotrys alternans*. Acta Vet. Acad. Sci. Hung. *20*:55 (1970).

221. M. K. Slifkin and J. Spalding, Studies on the toxicity of *Alternaria mali*. Toxicol. Appl. Pharmacol. *17*:375 (1970).

222. B. Doupnik, Jr., and E. K. Sobers, Mycotoxicosis: Toxicity to chicks of *Alternaria longipes* isolated from tobacco. Appl. Microbiol. *16*:1596 (1968).

223. D. G. Crosby (symp. coord.), Natural food toxicants. J. Agric. Food Chem. *17*:413 (1968).

224. R. W. Pero, R. G. Owens, S. Dale, and D. Harvan, Isolation and identification of a new toxin, altenuene from the fungus *Alternaria tenuis*. Biochim. Biophys. Acta *230*:170 (1971).

225. M. Herzberg (ed.), Toxic micro-organisms. U.J.N.R. Joint Panels on Toxic Micro-organisms and the U.S. Dep. Interior, Washington, D.C. (1970).

226. L. A. Goldblatt (ed.), Aflatoxin. Academic Press, New York (1969).

227. B. J. Wilson, D. T. C. Yang, and M. R. Boyd, Toxicity of mould-damaged sweet potatoes (*Ipomoea batatas*). Nature *227*:521 (1970).

228. T. Taira and Y. Fukagawa, Bitter substance separated from alcohol distillation of sweet potato mash. Nippon Nogei Kagaku Kaishi *32*:513 (1958).

229. K. Oshima and I. Uritani, Participation of mevalonate in the biosynthetic pathway of ipomeamarone. Agric. Biol. Chem. (Japan) *32*:1146 (1968).

230. F. Nonaka and K. Yasui, Selective toxicity of ipomeamarone toward phytopathogens. Saga Daigaku Nogaku Iho *22*:39 (1966).

231. M. R. Boyd and B. J. Wilson, Preparative and analytical gas chromatography of ipomeamarone, a toxic metabolite of sweet potatoes (*Ipomoea batatas*). J. Agric. Food Chem. *19*:547 (1971).

232. M. D. Sutherland and R. J. Park, Sesquiterpenes and their biogenesis in *Myoporum deserti*, p. 147. In Terpenoids in plants, J. D. Pridham (ed.). Academic Press, London (1967).

233. B. F. Hegarty, J. R. Kelly, R. J. Park, and M. D. Sutherland, Terpenoid chemistry, XVII. (−)-Ngaione, a toxic constituent of *Myoporum deserti*. The absolute configuration of (−)-ngaione. Aust. J. Chem. *23*:107 (1970).

234. D. T. C. Yang, B. J. Wilson, and T. M. Harris, The structure of ipomeamaronol. A new toxic furanosesquiterpene from moldy sweet potatoes. Phytochemistry *10*:1653 (1971).

235. B. J. Wilson, M. R. Boyd, T. M. Harris, and D. T. C. Yang, A lung oedema factor from mouldy sweet potatoes (*Ipomoea batatas*). Nature *231*:52 (1971).

236. M. R. Boyd, B. J. Wilson, and T. M. Harris. Confirmation by chemical synthesis of the structure of 4-ipomeanol, a lung toxic metabolite of the sweet potato *Ipomoea batatas*. Nature (New Biol.) *236*:158–159 (1972).

237. T. Akazawa, I. Uritani, and H. Kubota, Isolation of ipomeamarone and two coumarin derivatives from sweet potato roots injured by the weevil, *Cyclas formicarius elegantulus*. Arch. Biochem. Biophys. *88*:150 (1960).

238. Food Protection Committee, National Research Council, Reference methods for the microbial examination of foods. National Academy of Sciences, Washington, D.C. (1971).

19 Edward J. Schantz

SEAFOOD TOXICANTS

INTRODUCTION

Marine organisms produce many toxic* substances. Halstead,[1] in a compilation of the poisonous and venomous marine animals of the world, has listed hundreds of species in this category. However, only a relatively small number of these are involved in food poisoning problems of the world. Dack,[2] Russell,[3] and Wills[4] have reviewed various aspects of the poisons and toxins found in seafoods.† In years past, poisoning from eating seafoods such as shellfish was considered a public health problem only in local seacoast areas where people consumed considerable amounts of these products. Modern methods of freezing and shipping seafood throughout the country have broadened this problem and have necessitated controls on shipments to make certain that harmful amounts of poisons are not present. In some areas of the world, Japan, for example, poisoning from seafood has amounted to two thirds of all food poisoning cases. As worldwide distribution of seafood products be-

---

* In this paper, the term *toxicant* refers to any substance causing signs of toxicity in animals or symptoms of toxicity in humans. The term *toxin* is used in reference to a toxic protein capable of producing antibodies and a poison as any other toxic substance as suggested by Bonventre, Lincoln, and Lamanna, Bacteriol. Rev. *31*:95 (1967).

† See also Symposium on Marine Pharmacology[78] and References 79–81.

comes more common, the number of cases of food poisoning in inland areas will naturally increase, unless proper precautions are taken.

Many of the marine toxicants involved in cases of food poisoning are produced by microorganisms, such as various forms of marine algae, and reach the edible marine animals consumed by man through the food chain. These particular poisons are difficult to control from the standpoint of public health safety because of the unpredictable and sporadic occurrence of the organisms producing them. Also, they may cause any one of a number of species of fish consuming the organism to become poisonous. Another important factor regarding safety is that these poisons usually are quite stable to heat processing or cooking and are refractory to the action of the digestive enzymes of man. Some species of fish—for instance, the puffers—are intrinsically poisonous, however. These poisons are more controllable in commercial fisheries, because they can be identified with the species of marine animal. Some other important problems are the bacteria that are particularly adapted to contamination and the production of toxins in seafoods. These toxins are usually proteins; they are readily destroyed by heat but are not sufficiently destroyed by digestive enzymes to prevent poisoning in a person consuming them. In most cases the venomous marine animals are not food-poisoning problems. Venoms are localized in special organs where they do not contaminate the edible portions of marine animals and, because they are proteinaceous, are readily destoryed by heat and by the digestive enzymes.

This chapter will examine the most troublesome worldwide problems of concern to the seafood industry and to public health officials who exercise control over the collection and sale of fishery products. The subjects are covered briefly, but references are given for more detailed information in each case. For the purpose of this text, the various seafood toxins are classed and discussed as: (1) those produced by microscopic marine plankton or algae; (2) those produced inherently in certain species of fish; and (3) those produced by bacteria that usually contaminate fish products.

TOXICANTS PRODUCED BY MICROSCOPIC PLANKTON OR ALGAE

Shellfish Poisons

Occurrence of Poisons and Nature of the Disease   Many species of shellfish become poisonous through the consumption of toxic marine algae,

particularly some of the dinoflagellates. Table 1 lists the various dinoflagellates that are known to be poisonous, with their observed locations
and some of their properties. Paralytic shellfish poisoning is a classical
example of a disease caused by the toxic metabolite produced by
Gonyaulax catenella.[5] This disease also has been caused by the poison
from *Gonyaulax acatenella*,[6] occurring in clams along the Pacific coast;
Gonyaulax tamarensis,[7] occurring in scallops in the Bay of Fundy;
clams in the St. Lawrence estuary; mussels along the northeast coast of
England; and *Pyrodinium phoneus*[8] in mussels along the Belgian coast.
G. catenella appears to be the predominant toxigenic dinoflagellate in

TABLE 1   Characteristics of Toxicants Produced by Various Marine
Dinoflagellates

| Species | Observed Location | Characteristics | |
		Biological	Chemical
Gonyaulax catenella	North Pacific coasts from Central California to Japan	Causes paralytic shellfish poisoning; poison blocks sodium influx in nerve cells	Among most potent poisons; low mol. wt. (372); water-soluble tetrahydropurine (saxitoxin)
Gonyaulax acatenella	Pacific Coast of North America	Similar to *G. catenella* poison	Not characterized
Gonyaulax tamarensis	North American Atlantic Coast and North Sea	Similar to *G. catenella* poison	Not completely charterized (different from *G. catenella* poison)
Pyrimidium phoenus	North Sea	Similar to *G. catenella* poison	Not characterized
Gymnodinium breve	Gulf Coast of United States	Toxic to mice; symptoms similar to ciguatera poisoning	Several poisons; lipid-soluble; mol. wt. 600–1500
Exuviaella mariae lebouriae	Japan	Causes fatty degeneration of liver and kidney	Not characterized
Gonyaulax polyedra[a]	California Coast	Toxic to mice and fish	Not characterized
Gonyaulax monilata[a]	Gulf Coast of United States	Toxic to fish	Not charcaterized
Gymnodium veneficum[a]	English Channel	Toxic to fish and mice	High molecular weight; water-soluble

[a] Not involved in known cases of shellfish or fish poisoning in humans.

the North Pacific areas; *G. tamarensis* appears to be the dominant one from the North Atlantic area. Although the poisons from these two organisms produce the same paralytic effect in man and animals, they are different chemically. The structure for the poison from *G. catenella* (saxitoxin) has been determined, but the structure of the poison from *G. tamarensis* has not been completely elucidated.

Symptoms of paralytic shellfish poisoning begin with a numbness in lips, tongue, and fingertips that may be apparent within a few minutes after eating contaminated shellfish. This feeling is followed by numbness in the legs, arms, and neck, and by general muscular incoordination. The mental symptoms vary, but most patients remain conscious during the illness. As the illness progresses, respiratory distress becomes more severe, and death results from respiratory paralysis within 2–12 h, depending upon the magnitude of the dose. If one survives 24 h, the prognosis is good, and there appear to be no lasting effects from the ordeal. The amount of toxin required to cause sickness or death in humans varies considerably. From accidental cases along the coast of California, Meyer[9] estimated that sickness may result from about 1,000 to 20,000 mouse units (MU) and estimated the minimum amount to cause death at 20,000 MU or more. A mouse unit of poison is defined as the amount that will kill a 20-g white mouse in 15 min. Bond and Medcof,[10] working in the Maritime Provinces, found that sickness occurred with about 600 MU and death at 3,000–5,000 MU. The lower figures are explained on the basis that these persons had not consumed shellfish regularly and had not acquired any tolerance to the poison by consuming small doses; this is most likely the case with many people along the California coast.

Until 1937 the shellfish poison problem was indeed puzzling. Shellfish that might have been edible for generations suddenly, and for no reason apparent at the time, became extremely poisonous. The shellfish would remain so for 1–3 weeks and then again become safe for human consumption. This sporadic occurrence of poisonous shellfish was finally explained in 1937 by Sommer and Meyer,[11] Sommer *et al.*,[5] and co-workers at the University of California. These workers observed the presence of a particular microscopic plankton in the waters around the mussel beds during several outbreaks that occurred between 1920 and 1937 along the central California coast. They identified this organism as the dinoflagellate *Gonyaulax catenella* and found that it contained a poison that produced effects in mice similar to those of extracts of the poisonous mussels. Their work showed that the mussels acquired the poisonous properties through the food chain and that they possessed a mechanism in the dark gland or hepatopancreas that binds the poisons. Mussels gradually destroy or excrete the bound poison, so that within

1–3 weeks after the bloom of the poisonous dinoflagellates subsides, they are free of poison. Whenever environmental conditions are right, the dinoflagellates grow and may persist from 1 to 3 weeks in a particular area. Their growth depends to a great extent upon the temperature of the water, pH, salinity, and the various food products in the water from the growth of other organisms and from upwellings along the coast. These organisms, like many others, will reach concentrations of 30,000 cells/ml or more. At a concentration of about 20,000 cells, the water begins to appear brownish red in color and is called a red tide. The amount of poison in the shellfish depends upon the number of poisonous organisms in the water and the amount of water filtered by the shellfish. Along the coast of California, mussels became too toxic for human consumption when only 200 or more *G. catenella* cells were found per ml of water. In some clams, such as the Alaska butter clam, the poison apparently accumulates in the siphon, where it is bound and may be retained for many months before decreasing to a safe level.[12] Generally, the shellfish do not appear to be harmed by consuming the toxic dinoflagellates. The poison that is bound in the shellfish is readily released when they are consumed by man.

Isolation and Characterization   The poison from California mussels and Alaska butter clams was isolated in pure form in 1954 by Schantz and co-workers.[13] The purification was accomplished by ion-exchange chromatography on carboxylic acid resins, followed by chromatography on acid-washed alumina. By this procedure a white hygroscopic product was obtained that had a potency of 5,500 MU/mg solids. The purified poison, saxitoxin, is a dibasic salt with a pK_a at 8.2 and 11.5 and is very soluble in water. Its molecular formula as a hydrochloride salt is $C_{10}H_{15}N_7O_3 \cdot 2HCl$ (mol. wt. 354).[16] It has no ultraviolet absorption, gives positive Benedict–Behre and Jaffe tests, and is completely detoxified by mild catalytic reduction with the uptake of 1 mol hydrogen/mol of poison at atmospheric pressure.[14]

   The poison was also isolated in pure form from axenic cultures of *G. catenella* obtained through the courtesy of Dr. Luigi Provasoli, Haskins Laboratory. This organism was cultured in sterile seawater for 17 days at 13 °C. When the cell count reached about 30,000/ml, the cells were filtered from the medium and lysed with dilute HCl, pH 2–3, to remove the poison. The poison from the extract of the cells was purified in exactly the same manner that the poison was ioslated from shellfish. A study of its chemical and physical properties showed that it is identical to the poison from clams and mussels.[15] Table 2 lists some of

TABLE 2   Comparison of Properties of Poison from Cultured *Gonyaulax catenella* Cells with Poison from Mussels and Clams[a]

Property	Clam Poison	Mussel Poison	G. catenella Poison
Bioassay (MU/mg)[b]	5,200	5,300	5,100
Specific optical rotation	+128°	+130°	+128°
pK_a	8.3; 11.5	8.3; 11.5	8.2; 11.5
Diffusion coefficient	4.9×10^{-6}	4.9×10^{-6}	4.8×10^{-6}
Absorption in ultra-violet and visible[c]	None	None	None
N content (Kjeldahl)	26.8	26.1	26.3
Sakaguchi	−	−	−
Benedict-Behre	+	+	+
Jaffe	+	+	+
Reduction with H_2	Dihydro derivative, nontoxic	Dihydro derivative, nontoxic	Dihydro derivative, nontoxic

[a] Courtesy American Chemical Society, Biochemistry 5:1191 (1966).
[b] All bioassay values are within experimental error of the value $5,500 \pm 500$ MU/mg solids reported previously for clam and mussel poisons.
[c] Infrared absorption of *G. catenella* poison was identical with that of clam and mussel poisons.

the important properties of these poisons. The basic chemical structure of the purified and clam mussel poisons and the poison from *G. catenella,* studied by Wong et al.,[16] is a substituted tetrahydropurine.

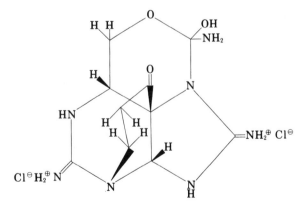

Structure of Saxitoxin (Wong et al.[16])

Physiological Action   Saxitoxin is a neurotoxin and among the most potent of low molecular weight poisons known. In terms of the purified product, 1 MU is equal to 0.18 μg. The intravenous lethal dose for a rabbit weighing 1 kg is 3–4 μg. If it is assumed that 3,000–5,000 MU constitute a lethal dose for man, as suggested from accidental cases, then the weight of poison to cause death in man is 0.54–0.9 mg by oral dose. The paralytic poison has become of special interest to physiologists because it blocks propagation of impulses in nerves and skeletal muscle cells without depolarization. Evans[17] and Kao and Nishiyama[18] found that the block is due to some specific interference with the increase in sodium permeability normally associated with excitation and the passage of a nerve impulse. This action is specific for sodium and appears not to affect any other ion in the cell. The action is similar to that of tetrodotoxin from the pufferfish. There is no known effective antidote for the poisons. However, the Klamath Indians used the gum from the sugar pine tree to overcome the toxic effects. Studies thus far have not proven that the gum is really an effective antidote.[19] Certain substances, such as sodium chloride and ethanol, reduce the effects to some degree when taken with the poison but not sufficiently for use as an antidote. Because muscles of the diaphragm are particularly sensitive to the poison, and death usually results from respiratory failure, artificial respiration has been effective in marginal cases, but not in those where a substantial dose of poison has been ingested.[9]

Other Shellfish Poisons   Recently Konosu *et al.*[20] have found several species of crabs in the Japanese waters to be poisonous. Noguchi *et al.*[21] isolated and purified the poison from some of these crabs and found that it is identical to the poison produced by *G. catenella.* The source of the toxic principle in the crabs is not known, but the identity of the poison with that from *G. catenella* suggest the possibility that crabs are obtaining the poison through the food chain from the dinoflagellates or some similar organism. It is of interest, too, that Jackim and Gentile[22] have found a species of blue-green freshwater algae, *Aphanizomenon flos-aquae,* that produces a poison similar to that produced by *G. catenella.*

Other types of poisons, believed to be cyclic polypeptides, are produced by some blue-green algae, namely, *Anabaena flos-aquae* and *Microcystis aeruginosa,* which have caused poisoning and death in domestic cattle consuming the algae when drinking water from shallow lakes. Such poisonings have occurred throughout the world, notably in northern United States, southern Canada, Brazil, Russia, and Australia. None of these algae is known to have caused food poisoning in humans or to have caused edible fish to become poisonous.[23,24]

Another type of shellfish poisoning resulting from poisonous dino-flagellates, called oyster or asari poisoning, has occurred in the region of Hamana Bay in Japan and has resulted in much sickness and many deaths among people in this area. Nakazima[25] in 1968 found that the dinoflagellate *Exuviaella mariae-lebouriae* was the source of the poison in oysters and that it produced a substance that caused signs in animals similar to those caused by extracts of the oysters. The disease is charac-terized by fatty degeneration of liver and kidney tissue in animals. The first symptoms in man are anorexia, abdominal pain, nausea, vomiting, constipation, and headache within the first few days. These are followed by hemorrhagic spots on the skin, with bleeding from the mucous mem-branes and acute yellow atrophy of the liver. Several hundred cases have been reported in the Hamana Bay area, with more than 100 deaths. The toxic principle is found in the liver or dark gland of the bivalves and has been isolated by the Japanese investigators. It is quite stable to heating and causes intoxication in many animals by both the oral and IP routes. Although the occurrence of this organism seems to have been limited to the one particular area of Japan, the possibility of its occurring in other areas of the world should not be overlooked by public health officials and persons in the shellfish industries.

Other dinoflagellates listed in Table 1 produce poisons, but their rela-tionship to specific types of shellfish poisoning is not clear in most cases. Recently several investigators have reported that *Gymnodinium breve* produces a toxic substance that is extractable with lipid solvents and is poisonous to fish, chicks, and mice. McFarren *et al.*[26] have reported that blooms of this organism along the west coast of Florida caused oysters to become toxic and, when consumed by man, to produce symptoms similar to ciguatera poisoning. The dinoflagellate *Gonyaulax polyedra,* which occurs along the southern coast of California, is reported to be poisonous,[27] but it never has been proven to cause any type of shellfish poisoning. This organism does not appear to produce poison in labora-tory cultures. Because of its rapid growth, it has been proposed as a source of cattle feed.[28] *Gonyaulax monilata,* a dinoflagellate common in the Gulf of Mexico, produces a poison that is toxic to fish. Aldrich *et al.*[29] have found that this poison is not toxic to chicks or, as far as is known, to mice and other warm-blooded animals. Although this orga-nism is toxic to oysters under laboratory conditions, oysters in the Gulf of Mexico do not filter water when exposed to it. Abbott and Ballantine[30] found that *Gymnodinium veneficum,* isolated from the English Channel, produces a poison that is toxic to both fish and mice but has not been known to cause shellfish poisoning.

It should be pointed out that in some cases shellfish may become poisonous by the production of a poison within their bodies. An example of such a case is the poison sometimes found in the red whelk (*Neptunea antiqua*) that is eaten by humans in some areas.[31] Intoxication results from ingesting the whole raw or cooked shellfish. Clinical symptoms include nausea, vomiting, anorexia, weakness, fatigue, dizziness, photophobia, and dryness of the mouth. In some cases either diarrhea or constipation may result. The toxic principle (produced in the salivary gland of the red whelk) is a tetramine (tetramethylammonium hydroxide), which produces typical curare-like effects in mammals and frogs. Some related species, *N. arthritica* and *N. interculpta,* have caused intoxications in Japan.[32] The best method of control is based on knowledge and recognition of the species that are poisonous. Recently, Japanese investigators[33] have reported the identification of a poison in the Japanese ivory shell, *Babylonia japonica,* which has caused intoxications of humans in certain areas of Japan.

Detection and Control of Shellfish Poisons Because the poison does not affect the physiology of the shellfish, there are no distinguishing characteristics between poisonous and nonpoisonous specimens to serve as a guide to a person collecting them. The most practical means for detection of saxitoxin or other paralytic poisons in shellfish products is the bioassay with mice. For the assay, about 10 mussels or clams are collected from a certain area. The meats are removed, weighed, ground, and placed in distilled water; they are then acidified with hydrochloric acid to pH 2 and boiled for a few seconds. Usually 100 g of the meat is added to 100 ml of the acidified water. One ml each of serial dilutions of the clarified supernatant liquid is injected intraperitoneally into white mice weighing between 18 and 22 grams, and the time from challenge to death is measured. The MU, as defined by Sommer and Meyer,[11] is defined as the average minimum amount that will kill a mouse in 15 min. There is a direct relationship between the dose and the time from challenge to death; The curve expressing this is shown in Figure 1. Death times of 3, 4, 5, 6, 7, 8, and 15 min are equivalent to 3.7, 2.5, 1.9, 1.6, 1.4, 1.3, and 1 MU, respectively. Although the MU was originally defined in terms of the amount that will kill a 20-g mouse in 15 min, more consistent results are obtained when the death time is between 4 and 8 min. These times represent the portion of the death-time response curve where the dose is most accurately determined from the time of death. The MU is a variable quantity, depending upon the species and condition of the mice and various other factors. Recent studies have re-

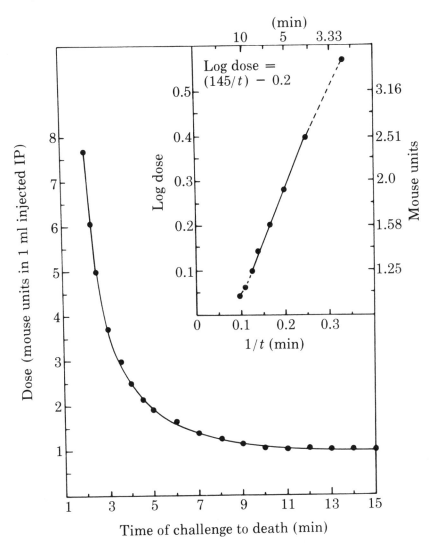

FIGURE 1 Dose and time-to-death relationships for saxitoxin.

sulted in modification of the assay procedure and include using purified shellfish poison as an international reference standard, as described by Schantz and co-workers.[34] By expressing the response of the mice in terms of a definite weight of the reference standard poison, the results of assays from various laboratories of several countries have been found to agree closely. This procedure was made the official method of assay for paralytic shellfish poison (saxitoxin) by the Association of Official Agricultural Chemists[35] and is used by the Food and Drug Administration to determine the poison content of international and intranational shipments of seafood products. To make the assay for shellfish poison more nearly uniform throughout the world and to conform with U.S. Food and Drug Administration assays, small quantities of purified poison solutions are packaged in vials and are available to governmental agencies of the United States and other interested countries as an international standard for the bioassay of the poison in commercial shellfish products. These samples can be obtained free of charge from the U.S. Food and Drug Administration, Division of Microbiology, Washington, D.C.

The hepatotoxic shellfish poison from oysters in Japan can be detected by feeding or injecting water extracts of the oysters into mice and observing them for pathological changes in the liver and other tissues. Observation must be carried out over a period of several days in order to detect small quantities of toxin. The poison in oysters that have been feeding on *G. breve* is detected by making ether extracts of the oysters, evaporating the ether, and taking the residue up in vegetable oil. The oil solution is injected subcutaneously into mice weighing about 20 g. A MU of this poison has been defined on the basis of the amount required to kill 50% of a group of mice in a definite period of time.[36]

Another means of detecting the liklihood of shellfish poisoning caused by dinoflagellates is to examine the water microscopically at intervals near shellfish beds. The occurrence of detectable numbers of the toxic dinoflagellates in the water would indicate that the shellfish should be assayed for the poison with mice. If poison is present in sufficient amounts, the shellfish beds should be excluded from harvesting.

The most practical means of controlling shellfish poisoning is by direct sampling of the beds and assaying these samples for poison content as described above. Many government agencies carry out assays periodically from May to October to check for the poison where shellfish are caught for food. If the shellfish become dangerously poisonous, warnings are posted and publicized. Education of the public by public health agencies regarding the danger of this sporadic occurrence of poison and its cause is very important, especially in the areas where shellfish poisoning is common. This type of education no doubt is responsible for the reduced occurrences of poisoning in recent years. Regulation of the commercial collection and processing of shellfish is described by the U.S. Public Health Service.[37] The U.S. Food and Drug Administration has set the maximum acceptable level of the paralytic poison in fresh, frozen, or canned shellfish at no more than 400 MU, or about 80 μg/100 g of shellfish meat.

As mentioned previously, the poison in the Alaska butter clam and, to some extent, in other species presents a somewhat complicated problem commercially in that the bulk of the poison in the clam is retained in the siphon for long periods of time. The butter clam is one of the most palatable of the species of clams and is an important food item in the economy of Alaska. Another difficulty in handling the problem of poison in clams and in other shellfish is that the poison is quite stable to heating. Canned clams, processed at 240 °F in the normal manner, may still contain 50% or more of the poison. Attempts to destroy the poison in clams by increasing the pH during processing were successful only when the pH was high enough to render the clams unpalatable. Removing the siphons, which contain 60 to 80% of the poison in the clams, will sometimes reduce the poison sufficiently to comply with the maximum limit of 400 M U/100 g of wet meats.

Ciguatera Poisons

Occurrence of the Poison and Nature of the Disease Poisoning from eating certain fish, known now as ciguatera poisoning, was first described in the West Indies by Martyr in 1555. It is common throughout the Caribbean area and much of the Pacific area, particularly in the torrid zones extending 35°N and 35°S latitude. Perhaps as many as 300 species of fish have been implicated in ciguatera poisoning within these areas. These are listed by Fish and Cobb[38] and by Halstead.[1] Several families are usually involved, including snappers, barracudas, surgeon fishes, jacks, groupers, sea basses, sharks, trigger fishes, wrasses, parrot fishes, and eels.

Ciguatera poisoning is without doubt the largest public health problem involving seafood poisons. Although considerable progress has been made recently on the problem, it is still one of the most complicated regarding the source of the poison and its chemical nature. Almost all fish involved in this type of poisoning are reef or shore species, and most are palatable. None appear to be direct plankton-feeders as adults. Most of the poison is found in the liver and other visceral organs, with the least amount in the flesh. All evidence points to the fact that the fish do not produce the poison within their bodies but acquire it through the food chain[39,40] by consumption of smaller fish that feed on algae or plankton or by consumption of plants on which algae are growing. All susceptible species of fish usually become toxic in certain areas, whereas the same species in different environments will not be poisonous. Dawson[41] studied the flora of Palmyra atoll, following its occupation by U.S. forces during World War II, and found that it changed in such a way that the growth of the toxic alga *Lyngbya majuscula* on the reef flats was favored and fish in this area became poisonous to humans.

Studies on extracts of this alga and of poisonous red snappers (*Lutjanus bohar*) showed some differences in the reaction of the poisons in animals,[42] but partial purification indicated that the poisons from two sources were very similar.[43] Cooper[44] has also reported the appearance of an alga that paralleled the reported distribution of toxic fish. The alga was identified as *Schizothrix calcicola*. Both water and lipid extracts of this plant contained poisons that produced signs in mice and mongoose similar to those caused by extracts of the fish.

The first symptoms of the poisoning in humans may be tingling of the lips, tongue, and throat, followed by a numbness in these areas. In other cases, the initial symptoms consist of nausea, vomiting, metallic taste, dryness of the mouth, abdominal cramps, diarrhea, headache, prostration, chills, fever, and general muscular pain. Weakness may become progressively worse until the intoxicated person is unable to walk. Mortality rates are not high in this type of poisoning, but in several cases death has resulted from various complications, mainly cardiovascular collapse.

Detection and Control of Ciguatera Poisons   The detection of ciguatera poison in seafood is difficult and not clear-cut like that for shellfish poison, pufferfish poison, and botulinum toxin. Tests must be carried out on animals—kittens, puppies, mice, and mongooses have been used. The mongoose reacts somewhat like a kitten to the poison, but it is difficult to obtain and handle and does not make a very practical laboratory animal. The mouse IP test and kitten feeding have proved to be most useful. In general, the mouse test is more practical, but it has been subjected to some criticisms in that some of the injected fish proteins complicate the test by giving false positive toxic reactions. Although ciguatera poison (or poisons) are most soluble in lipid solvents, they are sufficiently soluble in water to cause the characteristic reaction of ciguatera intoxication in mice.

Several assay procedures with mice have been used. A practical test involves extracting 100 g of fish with 400 ml of 95% ethanol in a soxhlet extractor for 24 h. Most of the alcohol is evaporated; the remainder is diluted with water, and the residue is extracted with diethyl ether. Evaporation of the ether leaves a thick oil (about 50–70 mg), which is stirred with 25 ml of water to form a stable emulsion. White mice weighing 20–25 g are injected intraperitoneally with 0.5 ml of the emulsion and observed for 36 h. Death in about 1 h indicates a highly poisonous fish; death in 3 h indicates a moderately poisonous fish; and death after 6 h indicates a weakly poisonous fish. A negative test is indicated if the mouse continues to remain unaffected during the test period of 36 h. Challenged mice may develop diarrhea, become inactive, and display excessive salivation and lachrymation. Some investigators dissolve the ether-extracted residue in a vegetable oil (such as peanut oil) and inject this intraperitoneally. The onset of symptoms is somewhat slower with the oil as a solvent, but in general the action is the same. Some of the preparations that cause ciguatera poisoning appear to have anticholine esterase activity, and for this reason the assay for acetylcholine has been proposed as a measure of some of these toxic substances.[45]

Because of the sporadic occurrence of ciguatera poisoning, control for public safety is difficult. Medical and public health officials must be continually alert for cases that might indicate that fish in certain areas are becoming hazardous to health. If symptoms of ciguatera poisoning begin to appear in humans after eating fish, animal assays should be performed at once on the fish to determine the extent of the contamination, and the public should be warned of the situation.

Isolation and Characterization　Several substances that cause ciguatera-like signs in animals have been isolated and partially characterized. These are lipid-soluble substances that are stable to heat used in ordinary cooking, and they can be dried without loss of potency. Scheuer *et al.*[46] in 1967 reported the isolation and partial characterization of the poison, causing ciguatera signs in the mongoose, from the moray eel (*Gymnothorax javanicus*), which they named ciguatoxin. The toxin extracted from the eels with acetone was purified by solvent partition and chromatographic procedures. The potency of the purified material, as determined by the minimum amount to cause death in mice, was 0.5 mg/kg. Analysis of the purified poison indicated an emphirical formula of $C_{35}H_{65}NO_8$ (mol. wt. 627). The toxin is considered to be a lipid containing a quaternary nitrogen, one or more hydroxy groups, and a cyclopentanone moiety.

Physiological Action　The mechanism of action of ciguatera poison is not known. In one particular case the poison was shown to possess anticholinesterase activity as well as several other toxic properties. There is no estimate of the dose required to cause sickness and death in humans.

Other Poisons Obtained through the Food Chain

The phenomenon of ciguatera poison in certain fish consuming toxic algae is paralleled by similar cases with other types of food organisms. Hashimoto *et al.*[47] have found a different toxin in the filefish (*Alutera scripto*) that is believed to originate from the ingestion of a zonatharian,

Palythoa tuberculosa. This organism grows on coral reefs and is consumed by various fish. It produces a poison that, when ingested, causes symptoms in man and animal identical to those caused by the poisonous filefish. Although the filefish is not considered a particularly palatable species, it is consumed for food in certain areas of the western Pacific and, when poisonous, has caused vomiting, diarrhea, and joint ache. Most of the poison appears in the viscera and, when fed to pigs, caused death in less than 2 h. The poison, named aluterin, is water soluble and has been partially purified. Assays for it can be carried out with mice.[47]

There is evidence that several other fish poisons may be acquired through the food chain. Helfrich[48] has reported various syndromes such as dizziness, hallucination, and mental depression in people who ate species of fish that normally are responsible for ciguatera poisoning. Very little is known about the substances that cause such a variety of diseases, and much work is still to be carried out for the clarification of these problems.

TOXICANTS PRODUCED INTRINSICALLY IN FISH

Pufferfish Poison (*Tetrodotoxin*)

Occurrence of the Poison and Nature of the Disease   Reports from China on intoxications from eating pufferfish date back thousands of years, probably to 2000–3000 BC. Although pufferfish have been known to be poisonous, many deaths still occur from eating these fish. Tetrodotoxin is found mainly in the ovaries, liver, intestine, skin, and spawn of various species of pufferfish. The pufferfish are sometimes referred to as blowfish, globefish, or fugu fish because of their ability to distend their abdomen. The most poisonous ones are in the family Tetraodontidae, but not all the fish in this family possess the poison. About 30 species of pufferfish are distributed worldwide, but the most poisonous ones are caught along the coasts of Japan and China, which alone boast 28 species. The choice edible species are those that are most poisonous, and the meat of these species is considered a delicacy by the Japanese and Chinese. According to Ogura,[49] the species used generally for cooking in Japan are *Fugu poecilonotus, F. pardalis, F. vermicularis, F. verm. porphyreus, F. chrusops,* and *F. rubripes,* all of which are among the most poisonous. There is a difference in the species consumed in China and Japan. In China fugu (*F. ocellatus obscurus*) are caught in fresh water when they migrate up various rivers during the spawning season; in Japan all species are marine. The amount of poison in puffers or fugu fish is lowest in the summer months and increases during winter with a peak just before spawning, in the spring. Cases of poisoning in Japan also are higher in the winter months than in the summer.

Symptoms of pufferfish poisoning usually begin with a tingling or prickling sensation of the fingers, toes, lips, and tongue within a few minutes after eating poisonous fish. Nausea, vomiting, diarrhea, and epigastric pain may appear in some cases. As the intoxication deepens, the pupillary and corneal reflexes are lost, progressive paralysis is apparent, and respiratory distress increases. If the dose is sufficient, death results from respiratory paralysis in much the same manner as from shellfish poisoning.

Detection and Control of Pufferfish Poisons   The poisonous species of puffers or fugu fish have been well characterized. Proficiency in the recognition of these species and proper evisceration before eating is the best safeguard against poisoning. It is of interest that the Japanese government licenses trained and experienced persons for species identification and removal of the poisonous visceral organs from the fish without contaminating the white meat. Pufferfish poisoning is a public health problem in Japan and nearby areas. The average number of deaths from eating pufferfish in Japan, over a period of years, is about 100 per year out of 200 reported cases. Over 98% of the deaths occurred because of ignorance and carelessness in the handling and preparation of the poisonous species. It is rare that anyone is poisoned from eating the fish in any of the well-managed restaurants employing licensed handlers.

When it is necessary to determine the amount of tetrodotoxin in the fish, the method used for shellfish poison or saxitoxin can be used. A weighed quantity of the ground meat is extracted with slightly acid (pH 4–5) hot water, cooled, and clarified by filtration or centrifugation. One-milliliter aliquots of the extract are injected intraperitoneally in white mice weighing 18–22 g. The time from challenge to death is measured, and the mouse units are calculated from the data for saxitoxin. The potency of tetrodotoxin and saxitoxin in mice and other experimental animals is very similar. The lethal dose for a mouse is about 0.2 μg and for a rabbit (1 kg) about 3–4 μg. It is assumed that the amount of tetrodotoxin required to cause death in humans is equivalent to the amount of saxitoxin that produces death in humans.

Isolation and Characterization   Tetrodotoxin has been isolated in crystalline form by Japanese investigators, and its chemical structure has been determined by Tsuda *et al.*[50] and Woodward.[51] It is an aminoperhydroquinazoline compound ($C_{11}H_{17}N_3O_8$) with a molecular weight of

319. The cyrstals are colorless prisms that are slightly soluble in water. The toxin is unstable at pH above 7 and pH below 3. Tetrodotoxin from the puffer is identical in chemical structure to a poison found in some species of salamanders such as *Taricha torosa.*[52]

The heat stability of tetrodotoxin has been studied by Halstead and Bunker,[53] who found the usual commercial canning procedure caused a loss in toxicity of cut whole fish, but not enough to allow safe human consumption. Procedures included heating to 100 °C for 10 min and heating under pressures at 116 °C. These steps did not inactivate the poison completely and cannot be relied upon to destroy the poison in canned fish.

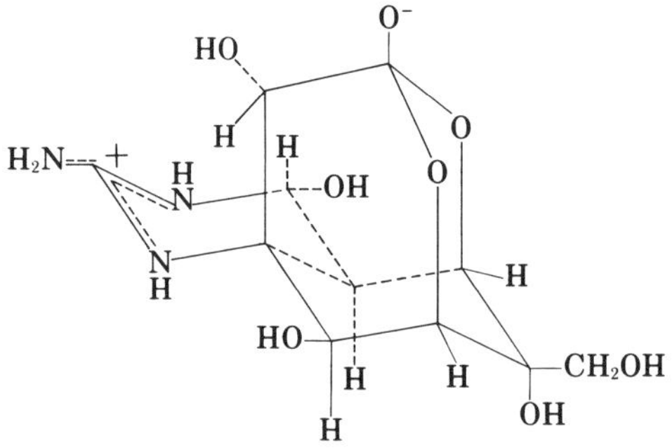

Structure of Tetradotoxin (Tsuda *et al.,*[50] Woodward[51])

Physiological Action   The mechanism of action of tetrodotoxin is very similar in many respects to that of saxitoxin.[54,55] In spite of the marked differences in chemical structures of the two compounds, both appear to act similarly in blocking specifically the influx of sodium into a nerve or muscle cell necessary to propagate an impulse.

Other Fish Poisons   In several instances, poisoning from eating several other types of marine animals has resulted in sickness and in some cases death. The common symptoms are nausea, vomiting, diarrhea, dyspnea, cyanosis, coma, and convulsions. These types have been listed by Wills,[4] Dack,[2] and Halstead[1] and include certain herring-like fishes of the Pacific (clupeoid poisoning), some of the snake mackerels (gempylid poisoning), sharks and dog fishes (elasmo poisoning), lampreys and hagfishes (cyclostome poisoning), squid and octopus (cephalopod poisoning), certain porpoises in the Yangtze (porpoise poisoning), and certain turtles (turtle poisoning). The source of the poison in these marine organisms is not known, but until more information is forthcoming it is assumed that the poison is produced by the animal.

TOXICANTS PRODUCED BY BACTERIA THAT USUALLY CONTAMINATE SEAFOODS

Botulinum Toxin Type E

Occurrence of the Toxin and The Nature of Botulism   This toxin, produced by the gram-positive spore-forming rod *Clostridium botulinum,* Type E, is the main contaminant of seafood products that cause botulism. However, one should not overlook the possibility that other toxins might be produced in seafood products, such as the enterotoxin of *Staphylococcus aureus* and the toxins of the other types of *Cl. botulinum* that have been implicated on rare occasions. There are six immunologically distinct types of *Cl. botulinum,* designated A through F, that are recognized at the present time. Because the type E organism is particularly adapted to the production of toxin in all fishery products, it is described in this chapter. The other types (A, B, C, D, and F) are described in Chapter 18. Type E botulism is now a well-recognized human disease. Koenig and co-workers[56,57] in the United States have made clinical and laboratory observations on Type E botulism in man from several cases of poisoning caused by eating vacuum-packed smoked whitefish. Dolman[58] has carried out similar studies in Canada on various fish products, and Ono *et al.*[59] and Craig *et al.*[60] in Japan have studied Type E botulism in man caused by eating "izushi," a fermented fish food.

Spores of Type E are found generally in soils and marine sediments along the seacoasts of the world, particularly in the northern latitudes, in the lakeshore muds of the inland lakes, and in the muds of some rivers. Boat-docking facilities and fish-processing plants have been found highly contaminated with these spores.[61,62] For this reason, contamination of fish and fishery products with these spores is an ever-present possibility, and great care should be exercised in handling and processing fish that are not consumed fresh. The Type E spores germinate to form vegetative cells and produce toxin at lower temperatures than any of the other types.[56] This process goes on at temperatures as low as 3–5 °C, and with increased growth and toxin production up to 30 °C. This means that food refrigeration is required at all times to preserve fishery products that may be contaminated with the Type E spores.

Characteristics of the Toxin   Type E toxin, as produced in culture at 30 °C, is not highly toxic when injected intraperitoneally into mice, but if treated with trypsin the potency may increase 10- to 100-fold.[63] It is believed that the organism, a nonproteolytic one, produces a progenitor toxin that is activated by the trypsin by breaking a bond and allowing the molecule to assume a toxic form.[64,65] It is quite likely that the situation is the same when the toxin is produced in seafoods. In this case, the foods may not appear highly potent when tested intraperitoneally in mice. However, when eaten by humans, sickness or death may result because of the activation or potentiation of the toxin by the digestive enzymes. There is evidence that the proteolytic types of C. botulinum produce the progenitor toxin also, but the activating enzymes are formed by the organism in culture, thus bringing about the potentiation.

This toxin, like the other types of toxin, is a simple protein with a molecular weight of 200,000 or more in culture.[66] When treated under the proper conditions of pH and ionic strength, the high-molecular-weight toxin dissociates into two main fractions: one fraction (molecular weight 150,000) is the neurotoxic protein, and the other a nontoxic hemagglutinating protein.[65,68] Type E toxin (high molecular weight) has been purified using such techniques as the precipitation of the toxin from the culture with cold ethanol[69,70] and by ammonium sulfate precipitation. The neurotoxic protein has been prepared from the toxin-hemagglutinin complex by dissociation at pH above 7 and at an ionic concentration above 0.13, and also separated by chromatography on DEAE cellulose.[70,71] Gerwing et al.[67] have reported the isolation and purification of the Type E toxin with molecular weight of 18,000, which they claimed was the progenitor toxin. When this toxin was treated with trypsin, a portion of the molecule was split off, leaving the active toxin with a molecular weight of about 10,000. These results have not been confirmed by others. Schantz and Silverman[72] have found that the low-molecular-weight form of Type E toxin is effectively neutralized by Type E toxoid, which is produced by treating the high-molecular-weight forms with formalin. Heimsh et al.[73] have found that the progenitor toxin and the trypsin-activated toxin are both completely neutralized by Type E antitoxin. Antitoxin induced by injection of toxin is more effective in neutralizing the toxicity than is the antitoxin prepared using toxoid. However, antibody production in animals must always be commenced with toxoid injections.

Detection of Toxin and Control of Botulism   The most frequently used assay for all types of botulinum toxin in food products, gastric contents, and blood is the mouse bioassay, although guinea pigs and goldfish also have been employed. Immunological and hemagglutination assays[74,75] have been studied and may yet prove to be of practical value. Tests can be made for Type E toxin in seafoods by the procedures described for the other types (see Chapter 18), except that activation of progenitor toxin with trypsin is necessary prior to the mouse test. Activation is not necessary for immunological tests, because progenitor toxin is neutralized by the antitoxin. Methods for the control of Type E toxin in foods are given in Chapter 18. It should be pointed out here, however, that the best protection against the toxin is heating the food before eating.

Other Toxicants Produced by Bacteria   Another type of poisoning, called scombroid poisoning, is believed to be due to products of bacterial action on the dead flesh of certain scombroid fishes, such as tuna, bonito, mackerel, and skipjack.[2] The toxin is considered to be a histamine-like substance. Poisoning from eating scombroid fishes results in nausea, vomiting, facial flushing, headache, epigastric pain, thirst, labial edema, itching of the skin, and urticaria. The effects usually subside within 12 h, but in some severe cases death has resulted. Geiger *et al.*[76] and Kawabata *et al.*[77] have isolated the active substance and called it "saurine."

REFERENCES

1. B. W. Halstead, Poisonous and venomous marine animals, Vol. 1. U.S. Government Printing Office, Washington, D.C. (1965).
2. G. M. Dack, Food poisoning. University of Chicago Press, Chicago (1956).
3. F. E. Russell, Poisonous marine animals, p. 68. In The safety of foods, H. D. Graham (ed.). Avi, Westport, Conn. (1968).
4. J. H. Wills, Jr., Seafood toxins, pp. 147–163. In Toxicants occurring naturally in foods, National Research Council. National Academy of Sciences, Washington, D.C. (1966).
5. H. Sommer, W. F. Whedon, C. A. Kofoid, and R. Stohler, Relation of paralytic shellfish poison to certain plankton organisms of the genus *Gonyaulax*. Am. Med. Assoc. Arch. Pathol. *24*:537 (1937).
6. A. Prakash and F. J. R. Taylor, A red water bloom of *Gonyaulax acatenella* in the Strait of Georgia and its relation to paralytic shellfish toxicity. J. Fish. Res. Board Can. *23*:1265 (1966).
7. A. Prakash, Source of paralytic shellfish toxin in the Bay of Fundy. J. Fish. Res. Board Can. *20*:983 (1963).
8. H. J. Koch, La cause des empoisonnements paralytiques provoqués par les moules, pp. 654. Assoc. Fr. Av. Sci. Paris 63rd Session (1939).
9. K. F. Meyer, Food poisoning. N. Engl. J. Med. *249*:848 (1953).
10. R. M. Bond and J. C. Medcof, Epidemic shellfish poisoning in New Brunswick. Can. Med. Assoc. J. *79*:19 (1957).
11. H. Sommer and K. F. Meyer, Paralytic shellfish poisoning. Am. Med. Assoc. Arch. Pathol. *24*:560 (1937).
12. E. J. Schantz and H. W. Magnusson, Observations on the origin of the paralytic poison in Alaska butter clams. J. Protozool. *11*:239 (1964).
13. E. J. Schantz, J. D. Mold, D. W. Stanger, J. Shavel, F. J. Riel, J. P. Bowden,

J. M. Lynch, R. S. Wyler, B. Riegel, and H. Sommer, Paralytic shellfish poison. VI. A procedure for the isolation and purification of the poison from toxic clam and mussel tissues. J. Am. Chem. Soc. *79*:5230 (1957).

14. E. J. Schantz, J. D. Mold, W. L. Howard, J. P. Bowden, D. W. Stanger, J. M. Lynch, O. P. Wintersteiner, J. D. Dutcher, D. R. Walters, and B. Riegel, Paralytic shellfish poison. VIII. Some chemical physical properties of purified clam and mussel poisons. Can. J. Chem. *39*:2117 (1961).

15. E. J. Schantz, J. M. Lynch, G. Vayvada, K. Matsumoto, and H. Rapoport, The purification and characterization of the poison produced by *Gonyaulax catenella* in axenic culture. Biochemistry *5*:1191 (1966).

16. J. L. Wong, R. Oesterlin, and H. Rapoport, Structure of saxitoxin. J. Am. Chem. Soc. *93*:7344 (1971).

17. M. H. Evans, Paralytic effects of paralytic shellfish poison on frog nerve and muscle. Br. J. Pharmacol. *22*:478 (1964).

18. C. Y. Kao and A. Nishiyama, Actions of saxitoxin on peripheral neuromuscular systems. J. Physiol. *180*:50 (1965).

19. E. J. Schantz, Studies on shellfish poisons. J. Agric. Food Chem. *17*:413 (1969).

20. S. Konosu, A. Inove, T. Noguchi, and Y. Hashimoto, Comparison of crab toxin with saxitoxin and tetrodotoxin. Toxicon *6*:113 (1968).

21. T. Noguchi, S. Konosu, and Y. Hashimoto, Identity of the crab toxin with saxitoxin. Toxicon *7*:325 (1969).

22. E. Jackim and J. Gentile, Toxins of a blue-green alga: Similarity to saxitoxin. Science *162*:915 (1968).

23. C. T. Bishop, E. F. L. J. Anet, and P. R. Gorham, Isolation and identification of the fast death factor in *Microcystis aeruginosa*. NRC 1. Can. J. Biochem. Physiol. *37*:453 (1959).

24. P. R. Gorham, Laboratory studies on the toxins produced by waterblooms of blue-green algae. Am. J. Public Health *52*:2100 (1962).

25. M. Nakazima, Studies on the source of shellfish poison in Lake Hamana, IV. Identification and collection of the noxious dinoflagellate. Bull. Jap. Soc. Sci. Fish. *34*:130 (1968).

26. E. F. McFarren, H. Tanabe, F. J. Silva, W. B. Wilson, J. E. Campbell, and K. H. Lewis, The occurrence of a ciguatera-like poison in oysters, clams, and *Gymnodinium breve* cultures. Toxicon *3*:111 (1965).

27. J. Schradie and C. A. Bliss, The cultivation and toxicity of *Gonyaulax polyedra*. Lloydia *25*:214 (1962).

28. S. Patton, P. T. Chandler, E. B. Kalan, A. R. Loeblich III, G. Fuller, and A. A. Benson, Food value of a red tide *Gonyaulax polyedra*. Science *158*:789 (1967).

29. D. V. Aldrich, S. M. Ray, and W. B. Wilson, *Gonyaulax monilata*: Population growth and development of toxicity in cultures. J. Protozool. *14*:636 (1967).

30. B. C. Abbott and D. Ballantine, The toxin from *Gymnodinium veneficum*. J. Mar. Biol. Assoc. U.K. *36*:169 (1957).

31. C. Fleming, Case of poisoning from red whelk. Br. Med. J. *3*:520 (1971).

32. M. Asano and M. Ito, Salivary poison of a marine gastropod, *Neptunea arthritica* Bernardi, and the seasonal variation of its toxicity. Ann. N.Y. Acad. Sci. *90*: 674 (1960).

33. T. Kosuge, H. Zenda, and A. Ochiai, Isolation and structure determination of a new marine toxin, surugatoxin from the Japanese ivory shell *Babylonia japonica*. Tetrahed. Lett. No. 25, 2545 (1972).

34. E. J. Schantz, E. F. McFarren, M. L. Schafer, and K. H. Lewis, Purified shell-

fish poison for bioassay standardization. J. Assoc. Off. Anal. Chem. *41*:160 (1958).

35. E. F. McFarren, Report on collaborative studies of the bioassay for paralytic shellfish poison. J. Assoc. Off. Agric. Chem. *42*:263 (1959).

36. J. J. Spikes, S. M. Ray, D. V. Aldrich, and J. B. Nash, Toxicity variations of *Gymnodinium breve* cultures. Toxicon *5*:171 (1968).

37. U.S. Publich Health Service, Manual of recommended practice for sanitary control of the shellfish industry, Part I (1959).

38. C. J. Fish and M. C. Cobb, Noxious marine animals of the central and western North Pacific. U.S. Fish Wildl. Res. Rep. 36. U.S. Government Printing Office, Washington, D.C. (1954).

39. P. Helfrich and A. H. Banner, Experimental induction of ciguatera toxicity in fish through diet. Nature *197*:1025 (1963).

40. J. E. Randall, A review of ciguatera tropical fish poisoning with a tentative explanation of its cause. Bull. Mar. Sci. Gulf Caribb. *8*:236 (1958).

41. Y. E. Dawson, Changes in Palmyra Atoll and its vegetation through the activities of man, 1913–1958. Pac. Natur. *1*:1 (1959).

42. A. H. Banner, P. J. Scheuer, S. Sasaki, P. Helfrich, and C. B. Alender, Observations on ciguatera-type toxin in fish. Ann. N.Y. Acad. Sci. *90*:770 (1960).

43. D. W. Hessel, Marine biotoxins. II. The extraction and partial purification of ciguatera toxin from *Lutjanus bohar* (Forskal). Toxicol. Appl. Pharmacol. *3*: 574 (1961).

44. M. J. Cooper, Ciguatera and other marine poisoning in the Gilbert Islands. Pac. Sci. *18*:411 (1964).

45. K. M. Li, Ciguatera fish poison: A cholinesterase inhibitor. Science *147*:1580 (1965).

46. P. J. Scheuer, W. Tokahashi, J. Tsutsumi, and T. Yoshida, Ciguatoxin: Isolation and chemical nature. Science *155*:1268 (1967).

47. Y. Hashimoto, N. Fusetani, and S. Kimura, Aluterin: A toxin of filefish, *Alutera scripto,* probably originating from a zoantharin, *Palythoa tuberculosa,* Bull. Jap. Soc. Sci. Fisheries *35*:1086 (1969).

48. P. Helfrich, Fish poisoning in the tropical Pacific, University of Hawaii Marine Laboratory, Honolulu (1961).

49. Y. Ogura, Fugu (puffer-fish) poisoning and the pharmacology of crystalline tetrodotoxin in poisoning, p. 139. In Neuropoisons, Vol. 1, L. L. Simpson (ed.). Plenum Press, New York (1971).

50. K. Tsuda, R. Tachikawa, K. Sakai, C. Tamura, O. Amahasu, M. Kawamura, and S. Ikuma, On the structure of tetrodotoxin. Chem. Pharm. Bull. *12*:642 (1964).

51. R. B. Woodward, Structure of tetrodotoxin. Pure Appl. Chem. *9*:49 (1964).

52. H. S. Mosher, F. A. Fuhrman, H. D. Buchwald, and H. G. Fisher, Tarichatoxin–tetrodotoxin: A potent neurotoxin. Science *144*:1100 (1964).

53. B. W. Halstead and N. C. Bunker, The effect of the commercial canning process upon puffer poison. Calif. Fish Game *39*:219 (1953).

54. C. Y. Kao, Tetrodotoxin, saxitoxin, and their significance in the study of excitation phenomena. Pharmacol. Rev. *18*:997 (1966).

55. W.-D. Dettbarn, Mechanism of action of tetrodotoxin (TTX) and saxitoxin (STX), p. 169. In Neuropoisons, Vol. 1, L. L. Simpson (ed.). Plenum Press, New York (1971).

56. M. G. Koenig, The clinical aspects of botulism, p. 283. In Neuropoisons, Vol. I, L. L. Simpson (ed.). Plenum Press, New York (1971).

57. M. G. Koenig, A. Spickard, M. A. Cardella, and D. E. Rogers, 1964. Clinical and laboratory observations on type E botulism in man. Medicine *43*:517 (1964).

58. C. E. Dolman, Type E (fish-borne) botulism: A review. Jap. J. Med. Sci. Biol. *10*:383 (1957).

59. T. Ono, T. Karashimada, and H. Iida, Studies on the serum therapy of type E botulism (Part II). J. Inf. Dis. *120*:534 (1969).

60. J. M. Craig, H. Iida, and K. Inove, A recent case of botulism in Hokkaido, Japan. Jap. J. Med. Sci. Biol. *23*:193 (1970).

61. E. M. Foster, J. S. Deffner, T. L. Bott, and E. McCoy, *Clostridium botulinum* food poisoning. J. Milk Food Technol. *28*:86 (1965).

62. P. J. Pace, E. R. Krumbiegel, R. Angelotti, and H. J. Wisniewski, Demonstration and isolation of *Cl. botulinum* from whitefish chubs collected at fish smoking plants of the Milwaukee area. Appl. Microbiol. *15*:877 (1967).

63. J. T. Duff, G. G. Wright, and A. Yarinsky, Activation of *Clostridium botulinum* type E toxin by trypsin. J. Bacteriol. *72*:455 (1956).

64. G. Sakaguchi and S. Sakaguchi, Some observations on activation of *Cl. botulinum* type E toxin by trypsin, p. 266. In Botulism 1966. Chapman and Hall, London (1967).

65. B. R. DasGupta and H. Sugiyama, A common subunit structure in *Clostridium botulinum* Type A, B, and E toxins. Biochem. Biophys. Res. Comm. *48*:108 (1972).

66. E. J. Schantz, Some chemical and physical properties of *Clostridium botulinum* toxins in culture. Jap. J. Microbiol. *11*:380 (1967).

67. J. Gerwing, C. E. Dolman, and A. Ko, Mechanism of tryptic activation of *Clostridium botulinum* type E toxin. J. Bacteriol. *89*:1176 (1965).

68. K. Masaru, S. Sakaguchi, and G. Sakaguchi, Dissociation of *Clostridium botulinum* type E toxin. Biochem. Biophys. Res. Comm. *28*:892 (1967).

69. M. M. Gordon, M. A. Fiock, A. Yarinsky, and J. T. Duff, Studies on the immunity to toxins of *Clostridium botulinum*. III. Preparation, purification and detoxification of type E toxin. J. Bacteriol. *74*:533 (1957).

70. J. Gerwing, C. E. Dolman, M. E. Reichman, and H. S. Bains, Purification and molecular weight determination of *Clostridium botulinum* type E toxin. J. Bacteriol. *88*:216 (1964).

71. D. A. Boroff and B. R. DasGupta, Study of the toxin of *Clostridium botulinum*. VII. Relation of tryptophan to the biological activity of the toxin. J. Biol. Chem. *239*:3694 (1964).

72. E. J. Schantz and S. Silverman, Unpublished data.

73. R. C. Heimsch, L. A. Chamption, and H. Sugiyama, Botulinal toxin and toxoid as antigens. Proc. Soc. Exp. Biol. Med. *135*:151 (1970).

74. C. A. Miller and A. W. Anderson, Rapid detection and quantitative estimation of type A botulinum toxin by electroimmuno-diffusion. Infect. Immunol. *4*:126 (1971).

75. H. M. Johnson, K. Brenner, R. Angelotti, and H. E. Hall, Serological studies of types A, B, and E botulinal toxins by passive hemagglutination and bentonite flocculation. J. Bacteriol. *91*:967 (1965).

76. E. Geiger, G. Courtney, and G. Schnakenberg, The content and formation of histamine in fish muscle. Arch. Biochem. *3*:311 (1944).

77. T. Kawabata, K. Ishizaka, and T. Miura, Studies on the allergy-like food poisoning associated with putrefaction of marine products. Jap. J. Med. Sci. Biol. *8*: 521 (1955).
78. Pharmacology Society Symposium, Marine pharmacology: Mode of action of toxins on excitable tissues. Fed. Proc. *31*:1115 (1972).
79. T. Noguchi and Y. Hashimoto, Isolation of tetrodotoxin from a goby, *Gobius cringer.* Toxicon *11*:305 (1973).
80. M. Y. Spiegelstein, Z. Paster, and B. C. Abbott, Purification and biological activity of *Gymnodinum breve* toxins. Toxicon *11*:85 (1973).
81. M. Alam, J. J. Sasner, and M. Ikawa, Isolation of *Gymnodinum breve* toxin from Florida red tide water. Toxicon *11*:201 (1973).

20 Richard L. Hall

TOXICANTS OCCURRING NATURALLY IN SPICES AND FLAVORS*

Although historical records are lacking, spices are certainly among the first substances, after salt, that man added to his food. These natural aromatics were seldom valued solely for their flavor, for nearly all enjoyed status as drugs, stimulants, aphrodisiacs, or food preservatives. Without much doubt, in most instances their merit lay chiefly in the mind of the user. As effective pharmacological agents became available, and as our ability to assess their merits developed, the use of naturally occurring drugs, including the spices, declined. The formularies, pharmacopoeias, and dispensatories of today carry only the surviving remnants of a much larger number, and these primarily because of their use as flavors in pharmaceutical preparations. Even the apparent preservative effect actually relied, in most instances, on the spice's ability to mask deterioration that had already occurred.

It is not surprising that almost all of our present spices are devoid of physiological effect even in amounts much greater than are normally used in food. This is partly because those few that might present some hazard have been recognized and dropped from use. Beyond this, however, is the fact that in the majority of instances, a naturally occurring toxicant in food is not only detected by taste, odor, or the common chemical sense, but it becomes distinctly unpalatable at a level several orders of magnitude below that at which toxic effects can be observed.

*Literature reviewed through March 1971.

The exceptions to this generalization form one of the reasons for this book, and flavors contain a few of these exceptions. Even these exceptions, however, can accurately be described as self-limiting. For the purposes of this review, the substances that will be regarded as toxicants naturally occurring in flavors are those in which the customary gap, or safety factor, between levels that are organoleptically acceptable and those that are harmful is markedly narrower than usual, or the constituent in question exhibits unusual features of toxicity, such as vesicant or narcotic action, carcinogenesis, or toxicity at extraordinarily low levels. Since toxicity (the capacity of a substance to cause harm) is an absolute property, there is a hazard only if the state of the organism and the conditions and levels of use permit this capacity to be realized. So far as spices and flavors are concerned, the examples of actual harm resulting from their ingestion are so rare as to be medical curiosities.

Using these general criteria, there are to date 11 substances that occur naturally in flavoring materials in current or recent use that could reasonably be included in a list of substances generally regarded as toxic. These are hydrogen cyanide, found in a number of glycosides; allyl isothiocyanate, in brown mustard; umbellulone, in California bay laurel; capsaicin, in red pepper; glycyrrhizic acid, in licorice; β-asarone, in sweet flag and wild ginger; and coumarin, menthol, myristicin, safrol, and thujone, each of which occurs in a number of different species of plants.

CYANIDE

Hydrogen cyanide (HCN) is released by enzymatic hydrolysis of a number of glycosides found in food. (See Chapter 14.) Oil of bitter almonds, a generic name for pit oils, including also oils of apricot and peach kernels, contains the glycoside amygdalin. The enzyme emulsin is also present, and when the pits are crushed and moistened, the glycoside is cleaved with the liberation of hydrogen cyanide. The leaves of the cherry laurel, *Prunus laurocerasus* L. contain a similar glycoside, prulaurasin, which is also split by emulsin to release benzaldehyde and hydrogen cyanide. While such oils may originally contain glycosides equivalent to as much as 11% of HCN, the usual level is 2–4%.[1] All oils produced commercially for food use are treated chemically to remove the HCN and are designated FFPA (free from prussic acid). Homemade foods containing these materials, and other natural sources of hydrogen cyanide such as cashew nuts, lima beans, and some liqueurs, e.g., Kirsch, result in the continued consumption of usually insignificant quantities of the toxicant.

$$\text{C}_6\text{H}_5-\underset{\underset{\text{CN}}{|}}{\text{CH}}\text{OC}_{12}\text{H}_{21}\text{O}_{10} + 2\text{H}_2\text{O} \xrightarrow{\text{emulsin}}$$

Amygdalin

$$\text{C}_6\text{H}_5-\text{CHO} + \text{HCN} + 2\text{C}_6\text{H}_{12}\text{O}_6$$

Benzaldehyde   Hydrogen   Glucose
                  Cyanide

Toxicologically significant dietary intakes of cyanide result either from improper choice of plant variety, as with some lima beans,[2] inadequate processing, as may occur with cassava,[3] or accidental intake, as in the case of a 3-yr-old girl who incurred cyanide poisoning from eating approximately 15 apricot kernels[4] containing 0.33% available CN^-.

Considerable evidence shows that the body can eliminate small quantities of cyanide (of the order of 10 mg) by its conversion to the much less toxic thiocyanate, in which presumably cystine and methionine act as sulfur donors. Also, cyanide combines with hydroxocobalamin to form cyanocobalamin.[5,6] Failure of this metabolic route may result in a form of tropical (nutritional) ataxia when an excessive intake of cyanide occurs combined with vitamin B_{12} deficiency.[3]

ALLYL ISOTHIOCYANATE

Brown mustard, *Brassica juncea* (L.) Coss., contains the glucoside sinigrin and the enzyme myrosin. When the seeds are moistened and crushed, glucose, potassium bisulfate, and allyl isothiocyanate result. Allyl isothiocyanate is a potent irritant; its usefulness as a local counterirritant accounts for the listing of mustard in the *U.S. Dispensatory.* Allyl isothiocyanate has been isolated from horseradish,[7,8] from several other members of the genus *Brassica* (a large group that includes mustard, broccoli, and cabbage), and also from rocket salad, *Eruca sativa.*[9] Although experience in human use is extensive, there has been only one major toxicological study, that of Hagan *et al.*,[10] which showed that at 50 and 20 mg/kg body weight in dogs, it produced epithelial hyperplasia and ulcers of the stomach and minor inflammatory foci in the liver, whereas in rats at 10,000 ppm (500 mg/kg body weight), there was no effect. Rusch *et al.* report an increase in mitotic activity after a single application to mouse ears,[11] and Cordier and Cordier not surprisingly found 1,500 mg/kg toxic on IP injection in the rabbit.[12] The high levels involved in these adverse effects contrast with those in the human diet.

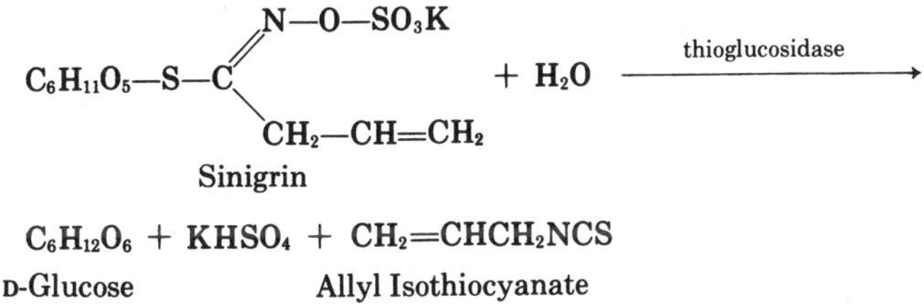

$$C_6H_{11}O_5-S-C \begin{array}{c} N-O-SO_3K \\ \\ CH_2-CH=CH_2 \end{array} + H_2O \quad \xrightarrow{\text{thioglucosidase}}$$

Sinigrin

$$C_6H_{12}O_6 + KHSO_4 + CH_2=CHCH_2NCS$$

D-Glucose $\qquad$ Allyl Isothiocyanate

Sparingly used condiments and highly spiced foods contain 50 to 100 ppm, while those more heavily consumed staple foods that contain it at all have less than 1 ppm. The overall conclusion from both human experience and animal tests is that in high concentration allyl isothiocyanate is a strong irritant, although as normally used in food, there is an entirely adequate margin of safety.

UMBELLULONE

The leaves of the California bay laurel tree (*Umbellularia californica* Nutt.) have had considerable past food use, especially for seasoning game. They contain from 0.5 to 4% of an irritating oil, of which the major constituent, accounting for from 40 to 60%, is umbellulone. According to Guenther,[13] care is advisable to avoid contact injury while collecting the branches. Drake and Stuhr[14] mention that contact with the oil or its vapors has resulted in severe headache, skin irritation, and in some cases unconsciousness. In an experiment on a guinea pig, which received 2 ml of 0.1% umbellulone in olive oil intraperitoneally 3 times a week for 6 weeks, they found it to be markedly hemolytic and compared its effect on the nerves and muscle fibers of frog heart with that of atropine. They concluded that it acted in part by blocking pulmonary

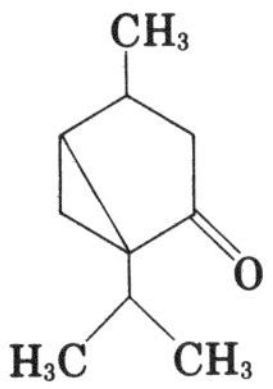

Umbellulone

circulation. Because other spices, including the traditional bay or laurel (*Laurus nobilis* L.), are available without this hazard, the California bay laurel has no currently recognized status as an appropriate food ingredient.

CAPSAICIN

The substance responsible for the heat, or pungency, of all members of the genus *Capsicum*, the red peppers, is the amide capsaicin.[15,16] It is a highly irritating substance, detectable by taste in water at dilutions higher than 1:1,000,000. Applied in concentrated form to the skin, it is a vesicant. Anyone who has had occasion to consume foods high in capsaicin is familiar with its ability to induce sweating and salivation. These reactions and increased gastric flow are apparently reflex actions resulting from the direct effect of capsaicin on the pain fibers in the mucous membranes of the mouth.[17-19]

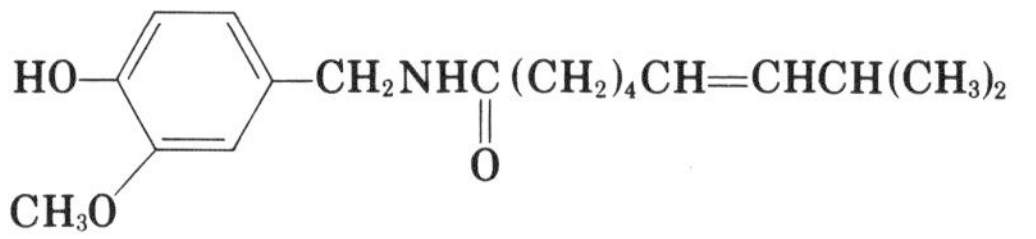

Capsaicin

GLYCYRRHIZIC ACID

The extract of the root of the licorice plant (*Glycyrrhiza glabra* L.) has for many years been used in medicine as a demulcent and expectorant; more recently it has been used in the treatment of gastric ulcer[20] and as a flavor to mask the taste of less palatable ingredients. It is also used widely in confections. The root contains about 5–10% of a glycoside composed of two glucuronic acid units and a polycyclic moiety, glycyrrhetinic acid, which is similar in structure to the plant steroids.[21]

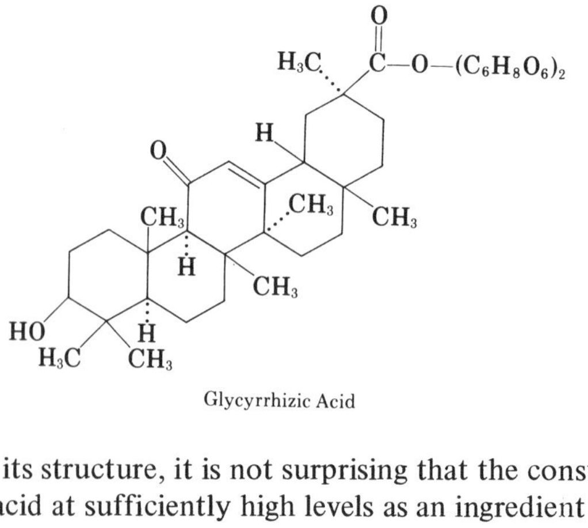

Glycyrrhizic Acid

In view of its structure, it is not surprising that the consumption of glycyrrhizic acid at sufficiently high levels as an ingredient either of medicines or confectionery has produced marked physiological effects. These generally include severe hypertension, sodium retention, and heart enlargement.[22,23] Chamberlain[24] reports a case of fulminant congestive heart failure. In each of the instances cited, consumption of licorice (in the form of candy containing approximately 0.5 g of ammonium glycyrrhizate) approached 100 g/day and continued for extended periods of time. Symptoms disappeared completely after the licorice was withdrawn.

ASARONE

Calamus oil, derived from the roots of the sweet flag (*Acorus calamus* L.) contains from about 5% (European variety) to about 90% (Indian variety) of asarone. This occurs in two isomeric forms, α-(*trans*) and β- (*cis*).[25]

Asarone

Asarone also occurs in several species of the *Asarum* and *Asiasarum* genera, from which its name is derived.[26]

For many years calamus oil had occasional use as a minor ingredient in certain bitter flavors such as vermouth and other flavored wines.

Hagan *et al.* found that dietary levels of 500 to 10,000 ppm of the *Jammu* variety of calamus oil produce growth depression, increased mortality, accumulation of fluid in the abdominal cavity, heart and liver changes, and, in a few cases, malignant intestinal tumors in rats.[10,27] The same type of tumor has been observed as a result of feeding β-asarone.[28] Although human dietary levels could not exceed 1 ppm, calamus oil has been withdrawn from use as a flavor ingredient in the United States and in a number of other countries. At present, its use is not limited in some countries and in Germany continues with the restriction that the content of β-asarone may not exceed 10%.

COUMARIN

Coumarin is found widely distributed in a number of substances that are natural sources of flavors. While neither it nor its principal natural source, tonka beans [*Dipteryx odorata* (Aubl.) Willd.] are now used in food, it is an important flavoring constituent of cassie, *Acacia farnesiana* (L.) Willd.[29] ; lavender, *Lavandula officinalis* Chaix[30,31]; lovage, *Levisticum officinale* Koch[32] ; yellow sweet clover, *Melilotus officinalis*[33] ; *Copaifera lansdorfii*[34] ; deer tongue, *Trilisa odoratissima* (Walt.) Cass.[35] ; and woodruff, *Asperula odorata* L.[36] Traces also occur in citrus oils[37] and in carrot seed oil.[38] Cassie, lavender, and lovage are used

Coumarin

rather widely in candy and liqueur flavors, and woodruff is the principal flavor of May wine.

Coumarin, used as such, disappeared from flavor use in 1954 following reports, initially by Hazleton *et al.*[39] and later by Sporn,[40] of extensive liver damage to rats fed 2,500 ppm in the total diet. Prior to that time, it was widely used as an ingredient of imitation vanilla flavors at use levels in food of about 20 ppm. Total dietary levels were, of course, much lower. It is still used to flavor tobacco. Fortunately, cessation of food use did not, in this case, terminate interest in the study of its toxicity and metabolism, and continued research has developed information of considerable interest.

Hagan *et al.*[10] confirmed in chronic studies that coumarin at high dietary levels (5,000 and 2,500 ppm in rats and 100, 50, and 25 mg/kg in dogs) causes marked growth retardation, testicular atrophy, and extensive liver damage, including enlargement, fatty metamorphosis, and bile duct proliferation with associated fibrosis.

Shilling *et al.*[41] showed that man metabolizes coumarin promptly and nearly completely to 7-hydroxycoumarin (7-OHC), with only traces of *o*-hydroxyphenylacetic acid (oOHPAA). Rats, on the other hand, produce a variety of metabolites, chiefly oOHPAA, but with much less 7-OHC.[42,43] Both oOHPAA, and another rat metabolite, *o*-hydroxyphenyllactic acid, are potent inhibitors of glucose-6-phosphatase in the liver microsomes, while the principal human metabolite, 7-OHC, is inactive in this regard. Thus, it appears that the test animals that provided the evidence on which coumarin was banned are not appropriate models for man.

This conclusion is possible only because the metabolism of coumarin has been the subject of unusually thorough study. It suggests that it might well be profitable to gain a similar degree of understanding of those substances whose metabolic fate is not well established and that have been rejected or cleared solely on the basis of possibly irrelevant animal feeding tests.

The picture has been clouded recently by the report of Bär and Griepentrog that coumarin, at 5,000 ppm in the diet of rats, causes bile-duct carcinoma.[44] Their conclusions conflict with those of Hagan *et al.*,[10] and their interpretation of the bile-duct changes seems at least to call for further investigation.[45]

MENTHOL

Menthol is a major constituent (about 40%) of peppermint oil (*Mentha piperita* L.)[46,47] and is found in small amounts in cocoa[48] and yarrow (*Achillea millefolium* L.).[49] Like many substances, it is capable of sensitizing susceptible individuals. Its widespread use as a flavor and perfume ingredient in candies, liqueurs, chewing gum, cigarettes, toothpaste, mouthwash, and space deodorants, to mention only some of its

Menthol

major uses, virtually ensures sufficient exposure to elicit some sensitization. Several cases of urticaria (hives) and commonly associated symptoms have been reported,[50,51] but these would not normally be regarded as evidence of toxicity.

A few cases of more bizarre reactions have appeared, including two of heart fibrillation from patients addicted to peppermint candy, with intakes over a prolonged period, reaching 225 g of candy per day.[52] In another case, a 58-yr-old woman developed a toxic psychosis from addiction to mentholated cigarettes.[53] In all three cases, symptoms disappeared when the source of menthol was withdrawn.

MYRISTICIN

Nutmeg and mace (both from *Myristica fragrans* Houtt.) contain from 8 to 15% of a volatile oil[54] that was still listed in U.S.P. XVI as Myristica Oil. About 4% of the oil is myristicin, its only physiologically important ingredient. Myristicin is also found in black pepper[55] and in a number of members of the carrot family (Umbelliferae), including carrot,[56] parsley,[57] celery,[58] and dill.[59,60] The medicinal use of nutmeg and mace goes back at least to the early Middle Ages in the Arab world and probably earlier in India. Then, these spices enjoyed high esteem as a treatment for a wide variety of conditions, including toothache, dysentery, cholera, rheumatism, halitosis, and skin diseases. Western medicine fol-

Myristicin

lowed this lead, and improved upon it, until nutmeg came to be considered almost a panacea. Disenchantment did not set in until the nineteenth century, during which the application of these spices was narrowed sharply. At about this time, however, nutmeg acquired in some unknown way the reputation of being an emmenagogue and abortifacient. This wholly unjustified reputation persists even today and is responsible for several cases of nutmeg poisoning.[61] Taken in large quantity, nutmeg and mace exhibit pronounced narcotic and psychomimetic properties, somewhat comparable to alcoholic intoxication.[62] A puzzling aspect of their action is that the effects of the spice are greater than those of an equivalent amount of myristicin and another component, elemicin (5'-allyl-1,2,3-trimethoxybenzene), even though these are the only constituents that separately cause significant physiological response. Very high doses may result in liver damage or death. During the last century, awareness of the narcotic properties of nutmeg led to occasional instances of use for this purpose.[63,64] Nutmeg is the spice usually chosen for the practical reason that it is cheaper and more readily available. The dosage ordinarily involved in attempts at narcotic or abortifacient use is of the order of two whole nutmegs, or half an ounce or more of the grated product—a quantity 50–100 times that encountered in any conceivable flavor use. An 8-oz portion of a food heavily flavored with nutmeg would contain about 175 mg. There is little evidence that those who try the use of nutmeg as a narcotic indulge in much repetition; the side- and after-effects include headache, cramps, and nausea and are reported to be common, severe, and extremely unpleasant (see Chapter 8).

Truitt et al.[62,65,66] advance evidence that myristicin acts as a weak monoamine oxidase inhibitor. If it follows a metabolic pathway similar to that of safrole (see below), it might well be converted *in vivo* into substances similar to or identical with known psychomimetic agents such as 3-methoxy-4,5-methylenedioxyamphetamine.[61,67]

SAFROLE

One of the most widespread of the few essential oil constituents that are now regarded as toxic is safrole. It is the major constituent (85%) of the oil of sassafras, the oil of the root bark of *Sassafras albidum* (Nutt.) Nees.[68] It forms 95% of micranthum oil, from *Cinnamomum micranthum* Hayata, and occurs in several related species and varieties.[69,70] It is a minor or trace constituent in cocoa,[71] mace and nutmeg,[72] Japanese wild ginger,[73] California bay laurel,[74] black pepper (*Piper nigrum* L.),[55] anise (*Pimpinella anisum* L.),[75] and a number of other species.

Safrole

In toxicological studies carried out by the U.S. Food and Drug Administration, Lehman[76] and later Long *et al.*[77] reported that the continuous administration of safrole at 5,000 ppm in the total diet of rats caused liver tumors and that lower levels produced lesser noncancerous damage. Studies in dogs[10] showed extensive liver damage at 80 and 40 mg/kg, lesser damage at lower levels, but no tumors. There was some evidence of adaptation to the stress of safrole ingestion.[78]

Comparative toxicological studies with related compounds seem to indicate that both the three-carbon side chain and the methylene-dioxy group are necessary for heptatotoxicity.[79] It is often assumed that safrole and those oils of which it is the major constituent have been dropped from use because of widespread concern embodied in the provision (the "Delaney Clause") of the Food Additives Amendment of 1958 excluding from use in food substances that, in the diet of man or experimental animals, are found to cause cancer. Aside from its tumorigenic effects, however, the toxicity of safrole appears sufficient to rule out its intentional employment, as such, at the approximately 20 ppm levels at which it was once used in root beer.

Little metabolic work has been done, but piperonylic acid has been found to be a metabolite of safrole and *iso*-safrole after administration to dogs.[80] Safrole stimulates certain of the liver microsomal enzymes but is an effective inhibitor of the metabolism of other drugs.[81]

THUJONE

The flavor constituent that first gained toxilogical notoriety is thujone. It is a major component of oil of wormwood, *Artemisia absinthium* L., the principal flavoring ingredient of the liqueur absinthe.[82] Serious physiological consequences resulting from the excessive use of this beverage, particularly in France, led to a campaign that resulted in its abolition there in 1915. Wormwood continues to be used in trace quantities (less than 10 ppm) in flavored wines such as vermouth. Toxicity studies have shown that, in doses of about 30 mg/kg body weight, thujone produces

Thujone

convulsions associated with lesions of the cerebral cortex.[83-85] Thujone occurs in two stereoisomeric forms, one of which is called α, L, or (−) thujone, and the other β, D, or (+) *iso*-thujone. Both thujones occur in several species of the genus *Artemisia*.[86-89] Both forms are present in oil of wormwood and in oak moss, *Evernia prunastri* (L.) Ach. and *E. furfuracea* (L.) Mann.[90] The α form is the major constituent of cedar leaf oil (oil of thuja), from *Thuja occidentalis* L.,[91,92] and is an important component of sage, *Salvia officinalis* L.[93,94] Tansy, *Tanacetum vulgare* L., contains the β form,[95,96] as does yarrow, *Achillea millefolium* L.[97]

    Little is known of the metabolism of thujone. In the rabbit, at least a portion may be converted by hydroxylative cleavage of the bridge link to the tertiary alcohol, which is excreted as the glucuronide.[98]

    One cannot avoid noting the close relationship in chemical structure between myristicin, asarone, and safrole and between thujone and umbellulone. At this stage of our knowledge, it would be risky to draw conclusions from these relationships, since other substances equally closely related lack the physiological effects of those discussed here.

    It is now evident that while some substances are limited in known occurrence to a single species, others (such as coumarin, safrole, and thujone) are found, at least in traces, in species not merely of several different genera, but of quite unrelated families. Unpublished data indicate, in several cases, far broader distribution than that summarized here. As more sensitive methods of separating and identifying the components of essential oils are developed and applied, one may expect to find that at least some of these relatively toxic materials are nearly ubiquitous and that we must continue to rely upon the remarkable capacity of the human body to deal promptly and effectively with small quantities of toxic materials.

REFERENCES

1. E. Guenther, The essential oils. Van Nostrand, New York (1952). Vol. 5, p. 52.
2. I. E. Liener (ed.), Toxic constituents of plant foodstuffs. Academic Press, New York (1969). P. 144.
3. A. O. Williams and B. O. Osuntokun, Peripheral neuropathy in tropical (nutritional) ataxia in Nigeria. Arch Neurol. *21*:475 (1969).
4. A. E. Gunders, A. Abrahamov, E. Weisenberg, S. Gertner, and S. Shafran, Cyanide poisoning following ingestion of apricot (*Prunus armeniaca*) kernels. J. Isr. Med. Assoc. *76*(12):536 (1969).
5. C. W. Mushett, K. L. Kelley, G. E. Boxer, and J. C. Rickards, Antidotal efficacy of vitamin B_{12a} (hydroxo-cobalamin) in experimental cyanide poisoning. Proc. Soc. Exp. Biol. Med. *81*:234 (1952).
6. C. L. Rose, R. M. Worth, and K. K Chen, Hydroxo-cobalamine and acute cyanide poisoning in dogs. Life Sci. *4*:1785 (1965).
7. A. Guillaume, Horse-radish and its applications. Prod. Pharm. *6*(8):383 (1951).
8. G. Janíček and A. Čapek, Volatile phytonicide of horse-radish. Prumysl. Potravin. *5*:204 (1954).
9. A. Mohammad and S. Ahmad, A note on essential oil of mustard in *Brassica* species and *Eruca sativa*. Indian J. Agric. Sci. *15*:181 (1945).
10. E. C. Hagan, W. H. Hansen, O. G. Fitzhugh, P. M. Jenner, W. I. Jones, J. M. Taylor, E. L. Long, A. A. Nelson, and J. B. Brouwer, Food flavourings and compounds of related structure. II. Subacute and chronic toxicity. Food Cosmet. Toxicol. *5*:141 (1967).
11. H. P. Rusch, D. Bosch, and R. K. Boutwell, The influence of irritants on mitotic activity and tumor formation in mouse epidermis. Acta Unio Int. Contra Cancrum *11*:699 (1955).
12. D. Cordier and G. Cordier, Mode of action of bis (2-chloroethyl) sulfide on the cardiovascular system; effects of chemically similar compounds. C. R. Soc. Biol. *145*:1310 (1951).
13. E. Guenther, The essential oils. Van Nostrand, New York (1950). Vol. 4, p. 207.
14. M. E. Drake and E. T. Stuhr, Some pharmacological and bactericidal properties of umbellulone. J. Am. Pharm. Assoc. Sci. Ed. *24*(3):196 (1935).
15. H. Pella de la Flor, Chemical study of *Capsicum frutescens*. Capsaicine content. An. Fac. Farm. Bio-Quim. Univ. Nac. Mayor San Marcos (Lima) *5*:206 (1954).

16. M. Nuñez-Samper, Capsaicin, its content and colorimetric determination in capsicum. An. Bromatol. (Madrid) *3*:323 (1951).

17. C. C. Toh, T. S. Lee, and A. K. Kiang, The pharmacological actions of capsaicin and analogues. Br. J. Pharmacol. *10*:175 (1955).

18. J. Pórzász, L. Gyorgy, and K. Gibiszer-Pórszász, Cardiovascular and respiratory effects of capsaicin. Acta Physiol. Acad. Sci. Hung. *8*:60 (1955).

19. J. Molnár, Die pharmakologischen Wirkungen des Capsaicins, des scharf schmeckenden Wirkstoffes in Paprika. Arzneimittel-Forsch. *15*:718 (1965).

20. A. Olsol and G. E. Farrar, Jr. (eds.), The dispensatory of the United States of America. 25th ed. Lippincott, Philadelphia (1960). Pp. 618–620.

21. P. G. Stecher (ed.), The Merck index. 8th ed. Merck & Co., Rahway, N.J. (1968). P. 502.

22. M. Koster and G. K. David, Reversible severe hypertension due to licorice ingestion. New Engl. J. Med. *278*(25):1381 (1968).

23. J. W. Conn, D. R. Rovner, and E. L. Cohen, Licorice-induced pseudoaldosteronism. Hypertension, hypokalemia, aldosteronopenia, and suppressed plasma renin activity. J. Am. Med. Assoc. *205*(7):492 (1968).

24. T. J. Chamberlain, Licorice poisoning, pseudoaldosteronism, and heart failure. J. Am. Med. Assoc. *213*(8):1343 (1970).

25. E. Gildemeister and F. Hoffmann, Die Ätherischen Öle. Akademie-Verlag, Berlin (1966). Vol. 3, p. 477.

26. Y. Saiki, Y. Akahori, T. Noro, K. Morinaga, T. Taira, S. Fukushima, and T. Harada, Gas chromatographical studies on natural volatile oils. II. The gas-chromatography on the volatile oils of the plants belonged to *Asiasarum* and *Asarum* genera. Yakugaku Zasshi *87*(12):1529 (1967).

27. J. M. Taylor, W. I. Jones, E. C. Hagan, M. A. Gross, D. A. Davis, and E. L. Cook, Toxicity of oil of calamus (Jammu variety). Toxicol. Appl. Pharmacol. *10*:405 (1967).

28. J. M. Taylor, private communication.

29. D. La Face, The concrete essence of *Acacia farnesiana*. Helv. Chim. Acta *33*: 249 (1950).

30. C. Kleber, Acetates in oil of lavender, Am. Perfum. Essen. Oil 680 (February 1927): and A. St. Pfau, letter of comment. The constituents of lavender oil. Am. Perfum. Essent. Oil Rev. 275 (July 1927).

31. C. F. Seidel, H. Schinz, and P. H. Müller, Lavender oil. III. Monoterpene alcohols and acids occurring as esters in French lavender oil. Helv. Chim. Acta *27*: 663 (1944).

32. Y. R. Naves, Volatile plant materials. XXIV. Composition of the essential oil and resinoid of lovage root. Helv. Chim. Acta *26*:1281 (1943).

33. J. M. Slatensek, Some causes for variation of coumarin content in sweetclover. J. Am. Soc. Agron. *39*:596 (1947).

34. W. B. Mors and H. J. Monteiro, Two coumarins in the seed of *Copaifera Lansdorfii*. An. Assoc. Brasil. Quim. *18*:181 (1959).

35. A. Osol and G. E. Farrar, Jr. (eds.), The dispensatory of the United States of America. 25th ed. Lippincott, Philadelphia (1955). P. 398.

36. P. G. Stecher (ed.), The Merck index. 8th ed. Merck & Co., Rahway, N.J. (1968). P. 1118.

37. A. DiGiacomo, Citrus essential oils. Riechst. Aromen Körperpflegemittel *16*(9): 348 (1966).

38. R. M. Seifert, R. G. Buttery, and L. Ling, Identification of some constituents of carrot seed oil. J. Sci. Food Agric. *19*(7):383 (1968).
39. L. W. Hazleton, T. W. Tusing, B. R. Zeitlin, R. Thiessen, Jr., and H. K. Murer, Toxicity of coumarin. J. Pharmacol. Exp. Ther. *118*:348 (1956).
40. A. Sporn, Toxicity of coumarin as a flavoring agent. Igiena *9*:121 (1960).
41. W. H. Shilling, R. F. Crampton, and R. C. Longland, Metabolism of coumarin in man. Nature Lond. *221*:664 (1969).
42. M. Kaighen and R. T. Williams, The metabolism of [3-^{14}C] coumarin. J. Med. Pharm. Chem. *3*(1):25 (1961).
43. G. Feuer, L. Golberg, and K. I. Gibson, Liver response tests. VII. Coumarin metabolism in relation to the inhibition of rat-liver glucose-6-phosphatase. Food Cosmet. Toxicol. *4*:157 (1966).
44. F. Bär and F. Griepentrog, Die Situation in der gesundheitlichen Beurteilung der Aromatisierungsmittel für Lebensmittel. Med. Ernähr. *8*:244 (1967).
45. Anonymous. Mainly on coumarin. Food Cosmet. Toxicol. *7*:681 (1969).
46. G. H. Beckett and C. R. A. Wright, Isomeric terpenes and their derivatives. Part V. J. Chem. Soc. *29*:1 (1876).
47. D. M. Smith and L. Levi, Treatment of compositional data for the characterization of essential oils. Determination of geographical origins of peppermint oils by gas chromatographic analysis. J. Agric. Food Chem. *9*(3):230 (1961).
48. B. van der Wal, D. K. Kettenes, J. Stoffelsma, G. Sipma, and A. Th. J. Semper, New volatile components of roasted cocoa. J. Agric. Food Chem. *19*(2):276 (1971).
49. E. A. Bejnarowicz and S. J. Smolenski, Gas chromatograhic analysis of the essential oil from *Achillea millefolium* L. J. Pharm. Sci. *57*(12):2160 (1968).
50. C. M. Papa and W. B. Shelley, Menthol hypersensitivity. Diagnostic basophil response in a patient with chronic urticaria, flushing, and headaches. J. Am. Med. Assoc. *189*(7):546 (1964).
51. E. M. McGowan, Menthol urticaria. Arch. Dermatol. *94*:62 (1966).
52. J. G. Thomas, Peppermint fibrillation. Lancet *1*:222 (1962).
53. E. Luke, Addiction to mentholated cigarettes. Lancet *1*:110 (1962).
54. A. T. Shulgin, T. Sargent, and C. Narango, The chemistry and psychopharmacology of nutmeg and of several related phenylisopropylamines, pp. 202–14. In Ethnopharmacologic search for psychoactive drugs, D. H. Efron (ed.). USPHS Publ. No. 1645, U.S. Public Health Service, Washington, D.C. (1967).
55. H. M. Richard and W. G. Jennings, Volatile composition of black pepper. J. Food Sci. *36*:584 (1971).
56. R. G. Buttery, R. M. Seifert, D. J. Guadagni, D. R. Black, and L. C. Ling, Characterization of some volatile constituents of carrots. J. Agric. Food Chem. *16* (6):1009 (1968).
57. J. Small, Parsley seed, Food *18*:268 (1949).
58. M. Karmazin, Critical examination of celery fruit and root on the basis of a colorimetric determination of apiol and myristicin. Pharmazie *10*:57 (1955).
59. Annual Report, Schimmel & Co. (1927). Pp. 36–37.
60. H. Karow, Uber die wertbestimmenden inhaltstoffe einiger Gewürze (II), Reichst. Aromen, Körperpflegemittel *2*:60 (1969).
61. A. T. Weil, Nutmeg as a narcotic. Econ. Bot. *19*:194 (1965).
62. E. B. Truitt, Jr., E. Callaway, III, M. C. Braude, and J. C. Krantz, Jr., The

pharmacology of myristicin, A contribution to the psychopharmacology of nutmeg. J. Neuropsychiatr. 2(4):205 (1961).

63. G. Weiss, Hallucinogenic and narcotic-like effects of powdered Myristica (nutmeg). Psychiatr. Q. 34:346 (1960).

64. H. Jacobziner and H. W. Rayibin, Accidental chemical poisonings. N.Y. State J. Med. 65:2270 (1965).

65. E. B. Truitt and E. M. Ebersberger, Evidence of monoamine oxidase inhibition by myristicin and nutmeg in vivo. Fed. Proc. 21:418 (1962).

66. E. B. Truitt, Jr., The pharmacology of myristicin and nutmeg, pp. 215–222. In Ethnopharmacologic search for psychoactive drugs, D. H. Efron (ed.). USPHS Publ. No. 1645. U.S. Public Health Service, Washington, D.C. (1967).

67. D. A. Kalbhen, Ein Beitrag zur Chemie und Pharmakologie der Muskatnuss (Myristica fragrans). Angew. Chem. 83(11):392 (1971).

68. M. R. Dodsworth, Some considerations on sassafras oil. Biol Divulgaçào Inst. Oleos. 3:21 (1945).

69. E. Guenther, The essential oils. Van Nostrand, New York (1950). Vol. 4, p. 280.

70. T. Naito, The constituents of the volatile oil from the leaf of Cinnamomum camphora var. glaucescens. J. Chem. Soc. Jap. 64:1125 (1943).

71. B. van der Wal, G. Sipma, D. K. Kettenes, and A. Th. J. Semper, Some new constituents of roasted cocoa. Rec. Trav. Chim. Pays-Bas. 87:238 (1968).

72. F. B. Power and A. H. Salway, The constituents of the essential oil of nutmeg. J. Chem. Soc. 91:2037 (1907).

73. T. Harada and Y. Saiki, Pharmaceutical studies of Japanese wild ginger. II. Paper chromatography of essential oils. Pharm. Bull (Tokyo) 4:223 (1956).

74. F. B. Power and F. H. Lees, The constituents of the essential oil of California laurel. J. Chem. Soc. 85:629 (1904).

75. E. Klein, Dragoco Rep. 12:123 (1965).

76. A. J. Lehman, Report on safrole. Assoc. Food Drug Off. U.S. Q. Bull. 25:194 (1961).

77. E. L. Long, A. A. Nelson, O. G. Fitzhugh, and W. H. Hansen, Liver tumors produced in rats by feeding safrole. Arch. Pathol. 75:595 (1963).

78. M. S. Weinberg and S. S. Sternberg, Effect of chronic safrole administration on hepatic enzymes and functional activity in dogs. Toxicol. Appl. Pharmacol. 8(2):363 (1966).

79. J. M. Taylor, P. M. Jenner, and W. I. Jones, A comparison of the toxicity of some allyl, propenyl and propyl compounds in the rat. Toxicol. Appl. Pharmacol. 6:378 (1964).

80. R. T. Williams, Detoxication mechanisms. 2nd ed. Wiley, New York (1959). P. 371.

81. D. V. Parke and H. Rahman, The induction of hepatic microsomal enzymes by safrole. Biochem. J. 119:53P (1970).

82. P. Balavoine, Thujone in absinthe and its imitations. Mitt. Geb. Lebensm. Hyg. 43:195 (1952).

83. F. H. Pike, M. Osnato, and J. Notkin, The combined action of some convulsant agents in small doses and the action of bromides in experimentally induced convulsions. Arch. Neurol. Psychiatr. 25:1306 (1931).

84. H. M. Keith and G. W. Stavraky, Experimental convulsions induced by administration of thujone. A pharmacologic study of the influence of the autonomic nervous system on these convulsions. Arch. Neurol. Psychiatr. 34:1022 (1953).

85. L. Opper, Pathologic picture of thujone and monobromated camphor convulsions. Comparison with pathologic picture of human epilepsy. Arch. Neurol. Psychiatr. *41*:460 (1939).
86. M. I. Goryaev, I. M. Shabanov, and L. A. Ignatova, Essential oil of *Artemisia mogoltavica*. Izv. Akad. Nauk Kaz. SSR, *123*; Ser. Khim. *7*:75 (1953).
87. M. I. Goryaev and Zh. K. Gimaddinov, Essential oil of *Artemisia rutaefolia*. Zh. Prikl. Khim. *32*:1878 (1959).
88. M. I. Goryaev and E. I. Satdarova, Analysis of the essential oil of *Artemisia serotina*. Tr. Inst. Khim. Nauk, Akad. Nauk Kaz. SSR *4*:37 (1959).
89. L. K. Tikhanova and M. I. Goryaev, The chemical composition of the essential oil from *Artemisia ferganensis*. Izv. Akad. Nauk Kaz. SSR, Ser. Khim. *2*:65 (1957).
90. A. St. Pfau, Composition of commercial oakmoss products. Riechst. Kosmet. *12*(9):179; *12*(10):208 (1937).
91. E. Jahns, Über das ätherische Oel von *Thuja occidentalis*. Arch. Pharm. *221*: 748 (footnote) (1883).
92. O. Wallach, Zur Kenntniss der Terpene und der ätherischen Oele. Ann. Chem. *272*:99 (1893).
93. N. Vernazza, Thujone in Dalmation sage oil. Acta Pharm. Jugoslav. *7*:163 (1957).
94. C. H. Brieskorn and E. Wenger, Constituents of *Salvia officinalis* XI. The analysis of ethereal sage oil by means of gas and thin-layer chromatography. Arch. Pharm. *293*:21 (1960).
95. H. Braun, Effect of extracts from *Tanacetum vulgare* on gastric secretion. Med. Monatsschr. *3*:528 (1949).
96. Ya. Maizite, A. Klyava, and L. Kluga, Composition and anthelmintic action of tansy. Latv. PSR Zinat. Akad., Kim. Inst. Zinatn. Raksti. *1*:101 (1950).
97. R. E. Kremers, The chemistry of the volatile oil of milfoil. A study of the application of modern organic chemistry to drug plant investigations. J. Am. Pharm. Assoc. *10*(4):252 (1921); Oil of *Achillea millefolium* L. 1922, J. Am. Pharm. Assoc. *14*(5):399 (1925).
98. R. T. Williams, Detoxication mechanisms. 2nd ed. Wiley, New York (1959). P. 530.

21 A. G. Van Veen

TOXIC PROPERTIES OF CERTAIN UNUSUAL FOODS*

The author has avoided items that are dealt with in other parts of this volume, for example, fungal toxins, alkaloids, lathyrogens, cyanogens, saponins, and favism, and he has dealt with foods that are generally little known in the United States though common enough among certain groups of people.

QUAIL

Quail is a favorite game bird in southern Europe and along the North African coast, but it is little known that this bird is the subject of one of the oldest descriptions of food poisoning.

After their flight from Egypt and during their wanderings through the desert, the Hebrews were twice saved from starvation by manna and by quail descending in huge numbers on their camp (Exodus, Numbers, Psalms).[1] The hungry people collected the birds and started to eat them. Numbers 11 especially mentions quail, and the story is repeated in Psalm 78: "But before they had sated their craving, while the food was still in their mouths, the anger of God rose against them, and He slew the strongest of them and laid low the picked men of Israel." Apparently the Hebrews were punished for their greediness and overeating; the fact

* Literature reviewed through 1970.

464

that it is mentioned that they were punished with the "meat between their teeth" gives the impression of a rather acute poisoning.

In later centuries, numerous authors (Pliny the Elder, Lucretius, Galen, and Avicennus, for example) mention that quail can be poisonous to man; this was attributed to the birds' sometimes eating poisonous plants such as *Helleborus* and *Conium maculatum* (hemlock). However, it has been only in recent times that this interesting and classic problem has been more thoroughly investigated.

Sergent[1] describes signs and symptoms in a number of people of Algeria who were reported to have become ill by the eating of so-called "green" quail (i.e., quail returning in spring from Central Africa to Europe and often quite emaciated). Nausea, vomiting, cold shivers, and partial, slow-spreading paralysis are the main symptoms; usually the patients recover. In fall, the quail migrate from Europe over the Mediterranean to Africa; they are well fed and then do not seem to present any health hazard.

Hemlock was a favored and effective poison in Socrates' time and he himself was poisoned by it. Sergent was able to show that hemlock seed is practically harmless to quail, even in high dosage and in prolonged feeding tests, but very toxic when fed to dogs. He fed the meat of quail that had survived such feeding tests to two dogs, with fatal results. In general, the symptoms of the poisoning were the same as those described in human beings.

More recently Ouzounellis,[2] quoting the observations and conclusions of Sergent, decided that these classical poisonings were probably due to acute myoglobinuria, as was the case with the victims of quail poisoning he observed himself on the island of Lesbos.

Though it is stated nowhere in the literature explicitly, it seems to be generally assumed that the coniine alkaloids are responsible for the toxicity. Coniine is fatal for a human in a quantity of about 100 mg, causing weakness, drowsiness, nausea, labored respiration, paralysis, and asphyxia.[46]

DJENKOL

In certain parts of Indonesia, especially in Java and some parts of Sumatra, the population is fond of eating djenkol beans, the seeds of a leguminose tree, *Pithecolobium lobatum* Benth, that often grows very tall. In size and appearance the seeds resemble horse chestnuts and are brown. Another variety produces much smaller seeds that are black, flat, and compressed together in a relatively small pod.

When maturing, and also after soaking, the beans develop a disagreeable odor, caused mainly by volatile sulfur compounds. By preference, the beans are consumed in this stage with the result that the consumer acquires the same disagreeable odor; however, this does not seem to bother him or his neighbors.

It has been observed that consumers of djenkol beans often suffer from acute kidney trouble, which results in anuria. The urine may contain red blood cells, epithelial cells, and sometimes clusters of white crystals (needles) that disappear upon standing (i.e., when the urine becomes alkaline). Sometimes these needles may clog the ureter, giving rise to such disturbances as necrosis or fistulae. In spite of these disagreeable side effects, which are observed rather often, the djenkol eaters will consume their beloved beans again the following season.

It has been found that the djenkol bean contains a substance, djenkolic acid, that occurs often in a concentration of 1 to 2%.[3] The "black" variety of the bean from Sumatra may even contain 3–4%. This amino acid seems to occur in the bean in the free state and not to be bound to a protein or other high-molecular-weight compound.[4] It is at least partly absorbed from the intestinal tract, and a part is excreted unaltered by the kidneys. If the urine has an alkaline pH, the djenkolic acid

$$S—CH_2—CH(NH_2)—COOH$$
$$CH_2$$
$$S—CH_2—CH(NH_2)—COOH$$

Djenkolic Acid

remains dissolved, but when it has a faintly acid reaction, the djenkolic acid crystallizes with the results mentioned above. It is interesting to note that the djenkol eaters sometimes consume, either for preventive or curative purposes, the alkaline extract of some plant ashes.

It was believed that djenkol intoxication seldom occurred in children, but recently two Indonesian workers[5] described no less than 50 cases in children, varying in age from 1½ to 12 yr.

It has been shown that djenkolic acid can be metabolized by man and also by rabbits. It cannot replace cystine in the diet of white rats.[3] Du Vigneaud and co-workers synthesized djenkolic acid in 1936 and improved the synthesis in 1947.[6]

KAVA-KAVA

Piper methysticum, a plant between 2 and 5 ft high, easily grown in hot swampy areas, is well known in many islands in the Pacific. It is sometimes mentioned that a kind of black or green tea or beer is prepared from it. This drink, to which refreshing and tonic properties are often ascribed, is appreciated by some Westerners who have spent a long time in that part of the world. Sometimes kava-kava is described or used as a drug having healing and even magic properties; as such, it has played an important role in the social and religious life on many Pacific islands. It has sometimes been described as the source of a narcotic drug. In all cases, parts of the root and stem are used; sometimes, especially for "tea," the leaves of the plant are also used.

It is not surprising that more than 75 yr ago a monograph was written on this popular and somewhat mysterious plant.[7] In his publication, Lewin mentions that a water-insoluble resin was extracted that showed strong physiological action when injected into frogs and birds, but no details were given.

From about 1914 to 1933, Borsche isolated a number of constituents from the resin, all of which were derivatives of 6-styryl-2,4-pyronone. But in the thirteenth of a series of 14 papers he stated that none of the substances he had isolated showed any action typical of kava-kava.[8]

Madaus[9] has described some of the uses made of the kava-kava plant. The explanation of the different modes of action has been ascribed to the fact that if a simple aqueous extract is made from roots, stems, and/ or leaves, the resulting liquid contains mainly water-soluble substances with some essential oil and perhaps traces of resin.[10] This liquid usually tastes slightly bitter and is, in essence, the famous kava-kava beer or tea, which seems to be harmless. If, however, the stem and root are chewed carefully, or ground intensively with saliva, lecithin, or some other emulsifying agent, the resulting emulsion, which is very bitter, shows an extremely fast action when given orally to rats, pigeons, monkeys, or humans. Often within 20–30 min the animals are in a deep sleep, which, in the case of monkeys, may last from 24 to 48 h.

This explains the use made of kava-kava by the Marindinese in the southern part of West New Guinea. Young children are given the roots and stems to chew; but they are not allowed to swallow the product. The resulting emulsion is filtered through grass into coconut shells and in the evening consumed by the adults in whom it causes a deep sound sleep during the night. Although the taste is extremely bitter, this potion can be consumed day after day, and, according to medical information, it does not seem to produce any harmful effects.

It has been possible to isolate the causative substance in beautiful crystals called marindinine; however, after purification these appeared to be identical with one of the substances isolated by Borsche, i.e., dihydrokawain, which he stated to be without any pharmacological

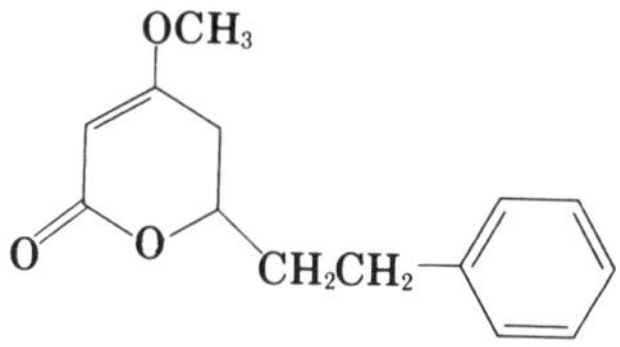

Dihydrokawain

action.[8] And indeed the water-insoluble crystals or powder do not show
any effect when given to test animals. However, when these crystals
were brought into a fine emulsion as described above, they showed the
typical narcotic reaction within a short time.[10]

   More recently the kava-kava problem has drawn attention again.
Singleton and Kratzer[11] state that dihydromethysticin, which differs from
dihydrokawain in that it contains a methylenedioxy group in the benzene ring, produced sleep when given in oil solution to mice in doses of

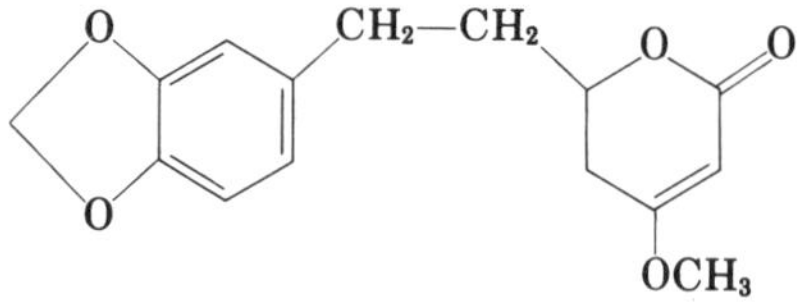

Dihydromethysticin

50–100 mg/kg; in humans, however, a dose of 500 mg/day acted as a
mild tranquilizer.

   It seems, therefore, that more than one of the substances originally
isolated by Borsche[8] is active in emulsion. Which is the most active in
a given case may depend on the concentration of the active principles in
the variety of *Piper methysticum* used.[10]

   An excellent review has been given by Keller *et al.*[12] Aqueous extracts
have been investigated by O'Hara *et al.,*[13] and Sauer and Hänsel[14] investigated the kava lactones in a newly discovered *Piper* variety from
New Guinea.

Leucaena glauca

This is a shrub or low tree belonging to the Leguminosae family and is
found in Central America, South America, and the Far East. It is used as
a shade tree as well as for hedges in tea and coffee plantations. In certain
tropical areas, the pods, seeds, and leaves of *Leucaena glauca* (Benth)

are used as a food for human beings, but more often as an animal feed. There is no exact information about the areas in which *Leucaena glauca* is used in the human diet, but it is eaten more or less regularly in certain parts of Indonesia.

It is an unusual food, as are the others so far described, in the sense that it is eaten by many people in certain areas, although they know that there is risk of certain undesirable side effects. The young leaves and small pods can be eaten raw; the mature small brown seeds can be roasted; leaves, pods, and seeds can be consumed in a soup together with other ingredients.

At the end of the last century it was recorded in South America that sometimes animals (nonruminants) lost some of their hair after eating parts of this shrub.[15] Around 1938 it was discovered in different parts of Indonesia during the course of food-consumption surveys that apparently healthy people in the villages were bald and had only a few new thin, yellowish hairs. Typhoid, protein malnutrition, or other diseases could be excluded as causes of this condition. According to the local population, it was due to the consumption of parts of *Leucaena glauca.* Indeed, a small group of women and children were found about 48 h after they had eaten leaves, pods, and seeds of the plant in a soup, and all had lost their hair within this period of time. They stated that their scalps and eyebrows had been hurting somewhat, and at the time of the investigations the scalp and eyebrows showed slight, very localized edema.[16,17]

Accordingly, experiments with animals (horses, pigs, and rats) were undertaken with rather inconsistent results. Nevertheless, loss of hair was one of the findings, and there were indications that this was due to the amino acid mimosine or leucenine, which occurs in the seed in concentrations of 1–4% and is also found in the leaves and stems.[16,17]

Kostermans proposed two alternatives for the structural formula of this interesting product, which later was synthesized by Adams and Johnson.[18] This synthesis proved the structural formula to be β-[N-(3-hydroxypyridone-4)]-α-aminopropionic acid.

An interesting question arises: If mimosine is the active substance,

CH₂—CH(NH₂)—COOH

Mimosine

why are harmful results, such as loss of hair, so seldom seen among the population eating *Leucaena glauca* more or less regularly?

In Japan and in Formosa some investigators undertook animal experiments, and special mention should be made of the investigations of Jung-Yaw Lin and co-workers,[19] who showed that 1% mimosine in the diet is toxic for mice and rats. Rats show alopecia, retarded growth, and shortened life spans.

Mimosine forms an intensively red iron complex, which is often observed in *Leucaena glauca* extracts and in the feces of *Leucaena glauca* consumers. Jung-Yaw Lin showed that this iron complex has little, if indeed any, toxicity. It is probable, therefore, that if meals containing *Leucaena glauca* are prepared in iron vessels, as is often the case, the product is harmless. The researchers also showed that mimosine [in the same way as DOPA (dihydroxyphenylalanine), with which it has much in common structually] condenses easily under physiological conditions with pyridoxal-5-phosphate and probably inactivates all enzymes containing this compound. This interesting observation may be the basis of the explanation of the pharmacological action of mimosine.

Montagna showed that *Leucaena glauca* extracts cause gross damage to hair follicles of mice in the anagen stage.[20] The matrix of cells of the hair follicles was destroyed, and this continued until the eighth day when the follicles attained a stage similar to catagen. During the ingestion of the extract, the epidermis became very thin and atrophic, but it returned to normal when the animals were placed on a normal diet.

Hegarty *et al.*[21] published a specific and useful method for the determination of mimosine and its degradation product, 3,4-dihydroxypyridine.

BONGKREK

Bongkrek, or tempeh bongkrek, is a product made from coconut press cake or a similar coconut product (e.g., grated coconut) with the help of a fungus, usually *Rhizopus oryzae*. This is the same fungus that is used for the manufacture of better-known products such as tempeh and ontjom, made from soybeans and from peanut press cake, respectively. Bongkrek is eaten mainly in central Java, a part of the country very rich in coconut palms. It consists of flat white cakes covered with a white mold and wrapped in banana or other large leaves. The fungus makes the product more digestible and attractive to eat. Although bongkrek is eaten by millions of people every day without harmful effects, occasionally groups of people do die or become seriously ill after consuming it even in small quantities. It has been found that, especially when the product is not manufactured in the right way, a species of bacteria, apparently present everywhere in that part of the country, gets the upper hand over the fungus after inoculation of the basic material, with usually fatal results for the consumers.[22] In periods of economic depression, when there is no market for the locally produced oil and press cakes, and when unskilled villagers start to manufacture bongkrek, poisonings are much more common than usual. Outbreaks of bongkrek poisoning were reported at the end of the last century. It was found that a newly discovered bacterium, *Pseudomonas cocovenenans,* produces two poisonous substances. One, called bongkrek acid, is especially interesting. In the bongkrek itself, dissolved in residual fat, this poison is very stable and is seldom, if ever, decomposed during heating. It was found that even small quantities cause hypoglycemia in human consumers and in experimental animals (e.g., monkeys, rabbits, and rats). It has been found in animals that the glycogen of liver and muscles is mobilized so that a hyperglycemia precedes the hypoglycemia after which the victim dies, either within a few hours or after 1 or 2 days. Glucose injections only prolong life by a number of hours.

In spite of these outbreaks of poisoning, people go on consuming this palatable and cheap food because they think that the poisonings are due to evil spirits or something comparable.

The same bacteria do not produce bongkrek acid in soybeans and peanut press cake. The pharmacological activity of the preparations depends on the optical rotation. In the purified state the product is extremely unstable.

It is interesting to note that the substance is also an effective antibiotic for the *Rhizopus* fungus,[23] on which it acts in much the same way as on human beings and experimental animals, i.e., it upsets glycogen metabolism. It has been shown by Berends and co-workers that bongkrek acid disturbs oxidative phosphorylation; oxidation of pyruvate and malate was inhibited.[24]

If the coconut press cake is treated with some acid before inoculation with the fungus, for example, with the acid of leaves from a certain variety of *Oxalis* (which is available everywhere in central Java), the pH gets low enough (approximately 5.5) to inhibit the growth of *Pseudomonas cocovenenans,* although the fungus grows extremely fast at this pH. However, it is not easy to convince the population that by the simple method of adding oxalis leaves to bongkrek the health hazard would be reduced.

Bongkrek acid has the properties of an unsaturated fatty acid.[24] More recently the chemical structure of bongkrek acid ($C_{28}H_{38}O_7$) has

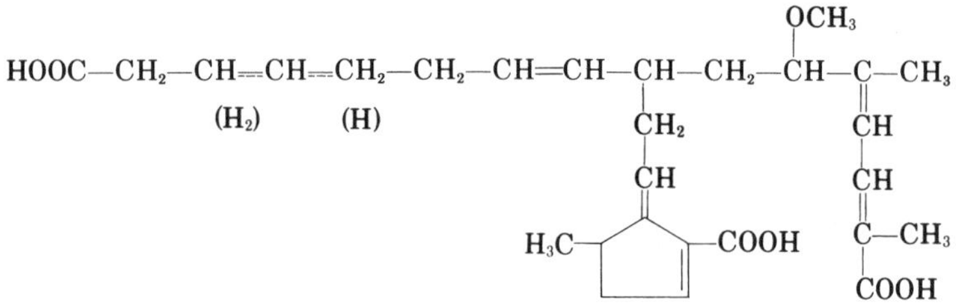

$$HOOC-CH_2-CH=CH=CH_2-CH_2-CH=CH-\underset{\underset{\underset{H_3C-\underset{}{\boxed{}}-COOH}{CH}}{CH_2}}{CH}-CH_2-\underset{\underset{\underset{\underset{COOH}{C-CH_3}}{CH}}{CH}}{\overset{\overset{OCH_3}{|}}{CH}}-\overset{\overset{OCH_3}{|}}{\underset{}{C}}-CH_3$$

(H₂)   (H)

Bongkrek Acid

been elucidated by Lymbach.[25] Henderson, Lardy, et al.[26,27] have described the interaction between the antibiotic with ADP and ATP in
mitochondria. Bongkrek acid is an active inhibitor of adenine nucleotide translocase, but the degree of inhibition depends on a number of
factors. For the interesting details we refer to the literature.

ACKEE

The ackee fruit (*Blighia sapida*) of Jamaica, which is known in Nigeria
as "isin," grows on a tree 15–25 ft high. Even the unripe fruit is attractive, having a bright pinkish red outer pod. The ripe fruit splits open and
then shows two or three light yellow arilli, in the bottom of which are
embedded the hard black seeds. The fruit is an extremely popular food.
A branch of the ackee tree with leaves and fruit is to be found on the
Jamaican "Independence" 5d stamp.

It is said that in general the housewife is aware of the health hazard of
eating the arilli of the unripe fruit, but nevertheless poisonings occur
every now and then when the fruit is not carefully selected. The ackee is
usually boiled, but because the arilli are very delicate, the cooking time
is usually rather short—15–20 min. The cooking water is said to be used
for other dishes. Sometimes ackee is fried in coconut oil. In many public
places it is sold "ready to eat," although such places as supermarkets do
not seem to carry it.

The fruit contains a water-soluble substance, hypoglycin, α-amino-
β-methylenecyclopropanyl propionic acid[28,29] that can cause acute
hypoglycemia, which seems to be responsible for the "vomiting sick-

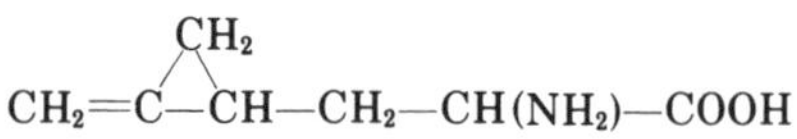

$$CH_2=\overset{\overset{\displaystyle CH_2}{\diagup\diagdown}}{C}-CH-CH_2-CH(NH_2)-COOH$$

Hypoglycin A

ness" that has been reported from Jamaica so often. Jelliffe and Stuart published an excellent review on this disease[30] and at the same time reported on the treatment with intravenous glucose injections on five young patients all having low blood-sugar levels. Although one patient died, the others recovered. This is rather different from the bongkrek poisoning, mentioned elsewhere, in which hypoglycemia is also found but in which glucose injections usually are not effective. The authors report that vomiting sickness usually occurs in winter when food is relatively scarce and when poverty and "subnutrition" are frequent. The mortality is high, death usually occurring after 12 h. It should be kept in mind that the term *vomiting sickness* is used rather loosely in that country and that sometimes other products may be the cause of similar poisonings.[30]

It has been suggested that the ackee toxin (hypoglycin) may act as a riboflavin antimetabolite.[31] (See Chapter 12.)

It has also been suggested that carnitine is the substance inhibited *in vivo*[32] and that a deaminated product--not hypoglycin A--might be the active inhibitor.[33] For the chemistry and synthesis of this interesting substance, its biological activities, etc., one is referred to the original literature.[34,35]

Persaud showed that IP injection of aqueous extracts of hypoglycin A in pregnant rats caused teratogenic effects.[36,37,38]

Ackee poisoning seems to be seldom seen these days, but it is difficult to decide whether this is due to the effect of nutrition education and a better food supply or to improved economic levels.

MIRACLE FRUIT (*Synsepalum dulcificum*)

Miracle fruit is a red berry from a shrub growing in tropical West Africa. The pulp, when chewed, causes sour substances to taste sweet and is therefore locally used to make sour maize-bread, sour beer, and palm wine more palatable. Lemons, limes, etc., taste sweet after the mouth (that is, the tongue) has been exposed to the mucilaginous pulp. Recently the active material, a glycoprotein, has been isolated by two groups of workers.[39,40]

The Florida group mentions[39] that the sweetening of the subsequent taste of acids was observed in a concentration of 5×10^{-8} M, the maximum being reached at 4×10^{-7} M. They also analyzed the amino acid composition of the protein. This remarkable protein itself (molar weight 44,000) has no special taste, but if mixed with acids, the mixture starts to taste sweet if held in the mouth for about 1 min. These researchers believe that the protein binds to the receptors of the taste buds and modifies their function. Indeed, in a recent paper[41] they propose an interesting explanation of the mode of action of this "taste-modifying protein" on the basis of the presence of arabinose and xylose (together present in the protein in a concentration of 6.7%), both sweet-tasting substances that might "fit" as some kind of prosthetic group in the sweet receptor site.

Another natural product, recently mentioned as a possible new sweetening agent, is the glycoside "stevioside," which occurs in concentrations of 6–7% in the leaves of *Stevia rebaudiana.*[42,43] The leaves have long been used as a sweetening agent in Paraguay. Stevioside is said to be about 300 times as sweet as sucrose, but recently Dorfman and Nes[44] showed that the aglucone of this glycoside, steviol (a diterpenoic acid), has anti-androgenic action, which makes this proposal less attractive. For the chemical structure one is referred to *The Merck Index.*[45]

NOTE

Important additional information on the biochemistry mechanism of action and possible public health significance of hypoglycin has been published.[47]

REFERENCES

1. E. Sergent, Les cailles empoisonneuses dans la bible, et en Algerie de nos jours. Arch. Inst. Pasteur Alger. *19*(2):161 (1941).
2. T. Ouzounellis, Some notes on quail poisonings. J. Am. Med. Assoc. *211* (7): 1186 (1970); also Presse Med. *76*:1863 (1968).
3. A. G. van Veen and A. J. Hyman, On the toxic component of the djenkol-bean. Geneeskd. Tydschr. Ned. Indie *73*:991 (1933); *76*:840 (1936).
4. A. G. van Veen and H. E. Latuasan, The state of djenkolic acid in the plant. Chron. Nat. (Indonesia) *105*:288 (1949).
5. Suharjono and Sadatun, Djenkol intoxication in children. Paediatr. Indones. *8* (1):20 (1968).
6. M. D. Armstrong and V. du Vigneaud, A new synthesis of djenkolic acid. J. Biol. Chem. *168*:373 (1947).
7. L. Lewin, Über Piper methysticum (Kawa). August Hirschwald, Berlin (1886).
8. W. Borsche and M. Gerhardt, Untersuchungen über die Bestandteile der Kawa-Wurzel, I. Chem. Ber. *47*:2904 (1914); W. Borsche and B. K. Blount, Untersuchungen über die Bestandteile der Kawa-Wurzel, XIII. Chem. Ber. *66*:803 (1933).
9. G. Madaus, Lehrbuch der biologischen Heilmittel. G. Thieme, Leipzig (1938).
10. A. G. van Veen, Over de bedwelmende stof uit de Kawa-kawa of wati plant (*Piper methysticum*). Geneeskd. Tydschr. Ned. Indie *78*:1941 (1938); Isola-

tion and constitution of the narcotic substance from kawa-kawa (*Piper methysticum*). Rec. Trav. Chim. *58*:521 (1939); On the isolation of the soporific substance from kawa-kawa or wati. Proc. R. Acad. Sci. Amst. *41*:855 (1938).

11. V. L. Singleton and F. H. Kratzer, Toxicity and related physiological activity of phenolic substances of plant origin. J. Agric. Food Chem. *17*:508 (1969).

12. F. Keller and M. W. Klohs, A review of the chemistry and pharmacology of the constituents of *Piper methysticum*. Lloydia *26*:1 (1963).

13. M. J. O'Hara, W. J. Kinnard, and J. P. Buckley, Preliminary characterization of aqueous extracts of *Piper methysticum*. J. Pharm. Sci. *54*:1021 (1965).

14. H. Sauer and R. Hänsel, Kawalaktone und Flavenoide aus einer endemischen Piper-Art Neu Guineas. Plant. Med. *15*:443 (1967).

15. K. Morris, Le Leucaena glauca (tamarin sauvage) faisant tomber les poils des animaux qui s'en nourrissent. Rep. Pharm. *9*:364 (1897); ref. Tropenpflanzer (1897). P. 169.

16. A. G. van Veen, Lamtoro en Kaalhoofdigheid. Natuurwet. Tydschr. Ned. Indie *101*:55 (1941).

17. D. Kostermans, Lamtoro-zaden (Leucaena glauca) en Kaalhoofdigheid, Geneeskd. Tydschr. Ned. Indie *80*:2959 (1941); Notes on mimosine, Rec. Trav. Chim. *65*:319 (1946); The structure of mimosine, Rec. Trav. Chim. *66*:93 (1947).

18. R. Adams and J. L. Johnson, Leucenol (VI), a total synthesis. J. Am. Chem. Soc. *71*:705 (1949).

19. Jung-Yaw Lin and Kuo-Hang Ling, Isolation and identification of mimosine. J. Formosan Med. Assoc. *60*(7):657 (1961); Studies on the mechanism of toxicity of mimosine. J. Formosan Med. Assoc. *61*(10):997 (1962).

20. W. Montagna and J. S. Yun, The effects of the seeds of *Leucaena glauca* on the hair follicles of the mouse. J. Invest. Dermatol. *40*:325 (1963).

21. M. P. Hegarty, R. D. Court, and P. M. Thorne, The determination of mimosine and 3,4-dihydroxy pyridine. Aust. J. Agric. Res. *15*:168 (1964).

22. W. K. Mertens and A. G. van Veen, Die Bongkrek vergiftungen in Panjumas. Meded. Dienst. Volksgezond. Ned. Indie *22*:209 (1933); A. G. van Veen and W. K. Mertens, Über das Toxoflavin, Rec. Trav. Chim. *53*:257 (1934); Uber die Giftstoffe der Bongkrekvergiftungen, *54*:398 (1935); Der Einfluss der Bongkreksäure auf den Kohlenhydrat-stoffwechsel, Arch. Neerl. Physiol. *21*:73 (1936).

23. A. G. van Veen, Bongkrek acid, a new antibiotic. Doc. Neerl. Indon. Morbis Tropicis *2*:185 (1950).

24. W. Welling, J. A. Cohen, and W. Berends, Disturbance of oxidative phosphorylation by an antibioticum produced by *Pseudomonas cocovenenans*. Biochem. Pharmacol. *3*:122 (1960).

25. G. W. M. Lymbach, PhD thesis, University of Delft, Holland (1969).

26. P. J. F. Henderson and H. A. Lardy, Bongkrekic acid, inhibitor of the adenine nucleotide translocase of mitochondria. J. Biol. Chem. *245*:1319 (1970).

27. P. J. F. Henderson, H. A. Lardy, and E. Dorschner, Factors affecting the inhibition of adenine nucleotide translocase by bongkrekic acid. Biochemistry *9*: 3453 (1970).

28. C. H. Hassal, K. Reyle, and P. Feng, Hypoglycin A,B: Biologically active polypeptides from *Blighia sapida*. Nature *173*:356 (1954).

29. E. C. De Renzo, K. W. McKerns, H. H. Bird, W. P. Cekleniak, B. Coulomb, and

E. Kaleita, Some biochemical effects of hypoglycin. Biochem. Pharmacol. *1*: 236 (1959).

30. D. B. Jelliffe and K. L. Stuart, Acute toxic hypoglycemia in the vomiting sickness of Jamaica. Br. Med. J. *1*:75 (1954).

31. H. C. Fox and D. S. Miller, Ackee toxin: A riboflavin antimetabolite. Nature *186*:561 (1960).

32. M. Entman and R. Bressler, The mechanism of hypoglycin in long-chain fatty oxidation. Mol. Biol. *3*:303–310 (1967).

33. H. J. Yardley and G. Godfrey, Some in vitro effects of hypoglycin on skin. Arch. Dermatol. *96*:89–93 (1967).

34. E. V. Ellington *et al.*, Amino acids and peptides: The constitution of hypoglycin A. J. Chem. Soc. *64*:80–85 (1959).

35. R. S. deRopp *et al.*, The structure and biological activities of hypoglycin. J. Am. Chem. Soc. *80*:1004–1005 (1958).

36. T. V. N. Persaud, Hypoglycin A, teratogenic effect in rats. West Indian Med. J. *16*:1903 (1967).

37. T. V. N. Persaud and S. Kaplan, The effects of hypoglycin-A, a leucine analog, on the development of rat and chick embryos. Life Sci. *9*:1305 (1970).

38. T. V. N. Persaud, Mechanism of teratogenic action of hypoglycin-A. Experientia *27*:414 (1971).

39. K. Kurihara and L. M. Beidler, Taste-modifying protein from miracle fruit. Science *161*:1241 (1968).

40. J. N. Brouwer, H. Van Der Weil, A. Francke, and G. J. Henning, Miraculin, the sweetness inducing protein from miracle fruit. Nature *220*:373 (1968).

41. K. Kurihara and L. M. Beidler, Mechanisms of the action of taste-modifying protein. Nature *222*:1179 (1969).

42. Sweetening agents, Nutr. Rev. *28*:97 (1970).

43. Stevioside toxicity, Nutr. Rev. *28*:219 (1970).

44. R. G. Dorfman and W. R. Nes, Anti-androgenic activity of dihydroisosteviol. Endocrinology *67*:282 (1960).

45. The Merck index. 8th ed. P. 981 (1968).

46. The Merck index. 8th ed. P. 282 (1968).

47. K. Tanaka, K. J. Isselbacher, and V. Shih, Isovaleric and α-methylbutyric acidemias induced by hypoglycin A: Mechanism of Jamaican vomiting sickness. Science *175*:69–71 (1972).

22 V. N. Patwardhan* and
Jonathan W. White, Jr.†

PROBLEMS ASSOCIATED WITH PARTICULAR FOODS

Problems associated with foods are many and varied. The four examples discussed in this chapter are typical of the interaction of the host–agent–environment relationship between man and his food. It is clear that constituents of foods normally considered as nutrients (and others not contributing to nutrition of the host but believed to be ordinarily inert, harmless, or capable of being metabolized without causing any harm) can, under certain circumstances arising from inherited or acquired host characteristics, prove deleterious to health or may even cause acute disease. Such a situation emphasizes the need for further studies of the relationship referred to above. These studies can be facilitated in the first instance by a more detailed knowledge of the composition of food, which should extend far beyond its nutrient content and must encompass all constituents, major and minor, including those present in trace amounts.

DISACCHARIDE INTOLERANCE

Lactose intolerance, as a congenital defect, was reported for the first time in 1959 by Holzel et al.,[1] who postulated that it was caused by an

* Deceased, July 8, 1971.
† Authored section on Toxic Honeys only.

enzyme deficiency. Soon thereafter, congenital sucrose intolerance was also demonstrated.[2] Since then, our knowledge concerning disaccharide absorption has progressed rapidly with an improved understanding of the mechanism involved. Disaccharidase deficiencies with specific defects in the absorption of dietary disaccharides have come to light, and the contributory factors have been elucidated.

Carbohydrates are among the natural constituents of human diets. They range from simple mono- and disaccharides to polysaccharides such as starch and, to a very small extent, glycogen. These polysaccharides are hydrolyzed in the gastrointestinal tract by amylases present in the secretions of the salivary gland and pancreas, during which process disaccharides like maltose and isomaltose are formed. Disaccharidases present in the brush border or the microvilli of the epithelial cells of the small intestine hydrolyze these disaccharides—as well as lactose and sucrose ingested with food—into monosaccharides, which are then absorbed.

Procedures such as heat inactivation, selective inhibition, and gel filtration chromatography have been used to identify several disaccharidases in the intestinal mucosa of man.[3,4] Four maltases, two lactases, and trehalase occur normally. Maltase Ia is identical to isomaltase (oligo-1,6-glucosidase), and maltase Ib is identical to sucrase (β-fructosidase). Maltase II and III (α-glucosidases) hydrolyze only maltose. One of the two lactases (β-D-galactosidases) hydrolyzes cellobiose in addition to lactose. Trehalase (a specific α-glucosidase) acts on trehalose, although this nonreducing disaccharide is not a normal constituent of the diet.

Lactose intolerance is due to lactase deficiency, whereas maltose intolerance requires simultaneous deficiency of more than one enzyme.[4] In a deficiency of these enzymes, the digestion of the disaccharides and the absorption of their component monosaccharides are diminished. The unaltered disaccharide remains in the intestinal lumen and causes problems by its continued presence. It may attract water from the tissue to the lumen of the gut, causing osmotic catharsis.[5] In the colon, the undigested lactose is fermented by bacterial enzymes to lactic acid and other short chain acids that raise the osmolarity, lower pH, and interfere with the reabsorption of fluid. The carbon dioxide and hydrogen produced by this fermentation probably contribute to the bloating, frothy diarrhea, and flatulence.

These characteristic stools appear after the ingestion of the disaccharide for which the subject is intolerant.[3,6] Certain observations indicate that acid stools and the presence of low-molecular-weight fatty acids in feces are not necessarily found in disaccharide intolerance in adults.[7] Some individuals who are lactose intolerant do not experience symptoms with one, two, or three glasses of milk. Thus it is possible to have a spectrum of symptomatology from no symptoms to that of a severe reaction.

Disaccharide intolerance may occur as a congenital defect in infants and is due to lack of one or more specific disaccharidases. In these cases the enzymic defect is probably inherited. In addition to lactase deficiency, congenital deficiencies of isomaltase and sucrase have been reported.[8,9] However, lactase deficiency is the commonest of all disaccharidase deficiencies.

Lactose intolerance is also frequently manifested later in childhood, during adolescence, or in adulthood.[10] This is far more common than the manifestations of congenital deficiency seen in early infancy. The significance of the late occurrence of lactose intolerance is discussed later.

Methods for Detection

A history of diarrhea and abdominal pain following the ingestion of certain foods gives an indication of possible intolerance. The offending disaccharide can be identified by noting the effect of its withdrawal from the diet and by feeding tests, during which the onset of symptoms and other signs (e.g., acid stools, presence of reducing sugar in stools, etc.) are noted. However, the tolerance test should not be done when the patient is actually having diarrhea.

The test is accomplished by oral administration of the test sugar in aqueous solution or suspension. The dose for infants and children is 2 g/kg; for adults 50- and 100-g test doses have been used.[4,11] A dose of 50 g sugar per m^2 body surface has also been used for children as well as adults.[6,10] Intolerant subjects experience abdominal pain or diarrhea or both. Abdominal distension may be caused by gas produced through fermentation. The blood sugar curve either is flat or may rise somewhat above the fasting level. The accepted blood sugar rise is usually less than 26 mg/100 ml.[10] Stools collected over several hours will have a low pH (pH 5.5 or less), especially in infants and children, and will contain unaltered disaccharide. The above test should be followed by a tolerance test using the corresponding monosaccharide(s). This helps to differentiate disaccharide intolerance from the general malabsorption syndrome in which the absorption of monosaccharide may also be impaired. In screening large populations, however, additional tests using monosaccharides may be unproductive in revealing lactose intolerance secondary to monosaccharide intolerance.[12]

In recent years peroral biopsy has been utilized to obtain samples of jejunal mucosa for the determination of enzyme activity. The respective disaccharidase activities are estimated in the mucosal homogenate, which is incubated at 37 °C and pH 5.8 with the appropriate substrates. The results are usually expressed as μmoles disaccharide split/min/g wet tissue.

There is considerable variation in the range of activities in the jejunal mucosa from normal individuals, partly because of the variable amounts of epithelial cells and other inactive tissue in the biopsy sample. The results from different laboratories are not always comparable because some authors express them in terms of dry weight of the tissue or per g of protein. However, when expressed as ratios such as sucrase/lactase or maltase/lactase, the results are more comparable. The ratios between the various disaccharidase activities have proved useful in the detection of enzymic defects, first because they vary within comparatively narrow limits in normal individuals, and second because they allow comparison of the findings of different laboratories.[6,13]

Another reason for the lack of comparability of results may lie in the fact that different investigators obtain biopsy samples from different sites in the small intestine. The activities of disaccharidases vary throughout the small intestine. They are low in the proximal parts of the jejunum; they then increase progressively, reaching a peak in adults at about 170 cm (as measured by the length of the tube swallowed) from the teeth and decrease thereafter until minimum values are reached in distal ileum.[13] Although most reported biopsies have been taken in proximal jejunum, there is merit in the suggestion that they should be taken at the ligament of Treitz. Apart from ensuring comparability of results reported from different laboratories, it has also been claimed that values for lactase activity found in specimens taken from this site will correctly diagnose lactase deficiency if it exists. At other sites the values are higher, and the results may be equivocal.[11,13]

Certain caution, however, has to be exercised in interpreting the results of disaccharidase activities, for the biopsy sample may not necessarily be representative of the mucosa of the small intestine. Enzyme assays on biopsy material should preferably be followed by appropriate tolerance tests.

Disaccharidase Deficiency in Infancy

Congenital disaccharide intolerance is manifested as soon as a disaccharide for which intolerance exists or its precursor is found in the food given to infants. Intolerance to breast milk may be seen after breast feeding starts and is often ascribed to allergy, although it could easily be due to lactose, of which human milk contains 6–7 g/100 ml. If the lactase deficiency is not severe, feeding cow's milk and making up calories by adding sugar other than lactose restores the health of the infant. Lactase deficiency of a congenital nature often leads to a rapid downhill course on the part of the newborn, and the deficiency has to be suspected and diagnosed quickly to ensure the survival of the infant. Cow's milk contains only about 4% lactose, and in adapting it for the infant, lactose concentration is still further reduced.

Inherited sucrose intolerance becomes apparent when the food of the infant contains added sucrose. Since the enzymes that split sucrose and isomaltose are often deficient simultaneously, the infant with sucrose intolerance will also be intolerant to dextrin or starch, both of which give rise to isomaltose during digestion.[6,14] In this type of disaccharide intolerance, the child either recovers spontaneously as he gets older, or he learns to live with the condition by avoiding foods containing sucrose. Furthermore, since isomaltase activity is not as depressed as the sucrase— and since the amount of isomaltose formed is relatively small compared to maltose in the digestion of starch and dextrin—isomaltose intolerance does not cause much inconvenience or affect the individual's health even when starchy foods are eaten. In contrast, inherited lactase deficiency persists into adult life.[3,6]

Lactase Deficiency in Children, Adolescents, and Adults

Disaccharidase deficiencies have been known to occur in children, adolescents, and adults. Lactase deficiency is the one most commonly encountered and may occur by itself as an isolated deficiency.[15] Several studies have been published[10,18] on lactose intolerance and lactase deficiency in population groups. Most of them involve adolescents and adults and cover an age span from less than 20 yr to over 60 yr of age.

In the United States a high prevalence of lactose intolerance has been found among blacks; the reported figures vary between 70 and 95%.[10,16,17] On the other hand, the incidence in American whites varies between 6 and 10%.[10,11] The subjects in some studies were healthy volunteers or inpatients of hospitals; in both cases, those investigated were free from diseases of the gastrointestinal tract and associated organs. The microscopic appearance of intestinal mucosa in almost all these subjects has been reported to be normal. In an investigation on healthy children, 14 out of 20 black children and 2 out of 20 white children had a family history of milk intolerance. Of these, 7 black and 2 white children showed intolerance to an oral dose of lactose given at the level of 50 g/m^2 body surface.[10] Although the authors did not determine lactase activity, they postulated that intestinal lactase activity decreases with age in blacks and that this may be responsible for the higher prevalence of lactose intolerance observed in the adult black population.

In Uganda lactase deficiency was found among Baganda children and those of neighboring Bantu tribes, whereas subjects with Hamitic ancestry showed higher levels of lactase activity.[18]

A higher prevalence of lactose intolerance and lactase deficiency than that in American whites has been reported from Britain and in Greek Cypriots, but this may be because the latter studies were done in patients having abdominal pain, diarrhea, or bone disease or megaloblastic anemia.[19,20] Observations on a limited number of healthy Asians suggest a high prevalence of lactose intolerance and lactase deficiency among them.[21,22,23] In an investigation in India on 192 infants and children (up to 5 yr of age) suffering from chronic or recurrent diarrhea, 49 children gave a flat curve after a lactose tolerance test. This suggests that in over 20% of the cases, lactase deficiency may have been the cause for the diarrhea.[24] All these 49 children improved clinically on withdrawal of milk from their food. It is possible, however, that in these cases lactase deficiency may have resulted from chronic and recurrent diarrhea and could have been a contributory factor to lactose intolerance. In Cairo, Egypt, isolated lactase deficiency was found in 5 out of 10 healthy subjects and in 9 out of 13 anemic patients with schistosome and/or hookworm infection with or without pellagra.[25] In biopsy specimens from lactase-deficient patients, sucrase and maltase activities were within the reported normal limits. In most of them (including specimens from healthy controls) the intestinal mucosa showed gross and microscopic abnormalities that ranged from mild to severe.

One can conclude, therefore, that lactose intolerance and presumably lactase deficiency may be far more widespread among apparently healthy subjects than has been realized. However, further studies on healthy population groups are needed to get a correct idea of its worldwide prevalence.

There is some question whether lactose intolerance and lactase deficiency found in adolescents and adults is inherited or acquired. Limited evidence on familial incidence and the different racial distribution are arguments in favor of their being inherited. It has been shown that the incidence of lactase deficiency differs widely in healthy subjects of different racial groups who live under the same conditions, who are comparable in socioeconomic status, and who have no history of malnutrition or a major gastrointestinal (G I) disease. On the other hand, certain observations indicate that intestinal lactase is more drastically affected in disorders of the gastrointestinal tract than in other disorders. Furthermore, there is the suggestion that lactase activity decreases with age. In some cases this decrease may reach a point where lactose intolerance manifests itself. These considerations provide a likely reason to consider lactase deficiency in adolescents and adults as an acquired deficiency.

Secondary Lactase Deficiency

This is associated with diseases of the small intestine, among which can be mentioned infective diarrheas, celiac disease, and tropical malabsorption syndrome, including sprue.[6,26,27,28] In these conditions the gross and microscopic appearance of the intestinal mucosa is abnormal and shows moderate to severe degrees of damage.[29] Second, disaccharidase activities other than lactase are also depressed, and other absorptive defects are found as well. On treatment and recovery from these conditions, absorption defects are rectified, and activities of disaccharidases other than lactase return to normal. The deficiency of lactase, however, may persist.[28]

Diarrhea—infective as well as noninfective—is very often associated with protein–calorie malnutrition (kwashiorkor and marasmus). Some observers have found that it can be exacerbated by treatment of the basic condition with skim milk. Lately it has been demonstrated that lactase deficiency is responsible for milk intolerance in kwashiorkor.[30] Other disaccharidases are also adversely affected but much less so than lactase. Lactose intolerance is believed to be a transient phenomenon in protein–calorie malnutrition. However, recent findings have shown that although lactose absorption improved on recovery, lactase activity of the mucosa did not return to normal, in one case even up to 1 yr on a good protein diet.[31] Thus a lactase deficiency due to malnutrition in infancy and early childhood could become an acquired characteristic.

The finding, admittedly based on limited studies, that lactase deficiency is common among Asians and Africans has led some to question the advisability and wisdom of donating skim milk as food aid to developing countries for supplementary feeding of infants and children.[23] This seems an unfortunate conclusion based on insufficient evidence.[32] Even assuming that lactase deficiency were widespread, proof is still wanting that the reconstituted milk served to infants and children as supplementary food has not been tolerated. It is possible that lactase deficiency may be relative and not absolute. Observations in the United States on healthy subjects have shown that most lactase-deficient subjects are able to tolerate small quantities of milk; several individuals had not had a history of milk intolerance in infancy and childhood. In view of this and the fact that the supplementary milk that any single individual receives is not likely to be more than 10–12 fluid oz per day, the chances that it will cause health problems or will be wasted are extremely remote.

FOODS AND FLATUS

Flatulence is a common complaint even among healthy individuals and is one of the most common causes of abdominal discomfort. Flatulence is also associated with such bowel disorders as dyspepsia, constipation, and diarrhea. This discussion is concerned with the mechanism of flatus and with the factors contributing to its formation in health.

Flatus has been associated in the minds of most people with certain types of food. Consumption of beans (of any kind) and other grain legumes is considered to be conducive to intestinal gas formation. A large variety of other foods has also been incriminated from time to time.[33] Among these may be mentioned such tubers as potatoes, sweet potatoes, and radishes; such other vegetables as cabbage, cauliflower, cucumbers, lettuce, onions, and pumpkins; and such fruits as apples, oranges, strawberries, and tomatoes. Eggs and milk have been included in the list of flatulent foods. Fatty foods and those cooked in fat are also believed to contribute to gas formation.

This association between certain foods and flatulence has been linked with their coarseness and/or their relative indigestibility. This concept was not wrong, although the immediate cause of gas formation was not known. In certain cultures, the capacity to give rise to gas was considered a desirable attribute of some foods, among which grain legumes—including beans and pulses—held the pride of place.

With the discovery of microorganisms, the understanding of microbial action on pure compounds and food components, and the knowledge that some microbes normally inhabit the GI tract, a rational approach to the study of flatulence became possible. Interest in intestinal gas was centered chiefly on its clinical aspects during the first half of this century. Little attention was devoted to the elucidation of the relationship between food and flatus until after the second World War. Flatulence associated with high-altitude flying called for investigation. It was, however, the need arising from man's attempt to conquer space and the possibility of astronauts having to spend days or months in a relatively small enclosed space that provided the powerful impetus setting intensive studies in motion.

Normally, a small amount of gas is found in the lumen of the alimentary tract. This originates from three sources: swallowed air, diffusion of gas into the lumen from across the epithelial border, and gas formed within the lumen by the intestinal flora acting on food residues.[33,34] Gases are also absorbed into the blood from the intestine and are excreted with the expired gases. In addition, the passage of CO_2 across the intestinal barrier is mediated by the enzyme carbonic anhydrase. Nitrogen is absorbed slowly and may cause distress. The quantity of gas found at any time will be the result of the relative contributions from the three sources mentioned above and the gaseous exchange between blood and intestine. However, normally 70% of GI gas is swallowed air. The proportion of gas produced by fermentation and that arising through diffusion from blood vary, with the former predominating.

Methods

Several methods have been used for the study of gas formation. The simplest is that of placing a flatus tube in position up the rectum and collecting the gas passed. This enables one to study the rate and composition of the gas produced in the colon. Other methods have been devised to study the rate of gas formation and its composition at different sites in the GI tract. Among these are: (1) intragastric administration of a known volume of oxygen and collection of flatus as it emerges per rectum through an indwelling catheter; (2) intubation with a specially designed polylumen tube for the withdrawal of gas specimens at predetermined sites and intervals; and (3) an analysis of expired gases, which give information on the contribution of bacterial fermentation to the composition of intestinal gas. The role of intestinal microorganisms has been studied by culturing fresh feces or dejecta from established ileostomies and colostomies followed by fermentation of food constituents or pure compounds and analysis of the gases produced.

Gastrointestinal Flora

The composition and habitat of the microbial population varies in the alimentary tract.[35,36] The stomach itself is believed to be sterile. Any organisms found there are believed to have originated in the mouth and the pharynx. The upper reaches of the small intestine have also been found to be bacteriologically sterile in about 70% of the subjects studied. Microorganisms occur in appreciable numbers in the terminal ileum and include aerobes and anaerobes, with the former predominating. The colon is the normal habitat of a large variety of microorganisms. The non-spore-forming anaerobes predominate, although enterobacteria of the coli-aerogenes group are also found in large numbers.

The composition of the intestinal flora varies from one person to another and depends to a large extent on the habitual diet of the individual. The total identification of G I flora is difficult, for a sample taken from the intestinal tract may not be fully representative. Attempts have been made to identify the organisms by culturing fresh feces on the assumption that these organisms represent G I flora. They probably represent the colonic flora.[37,38] In a recent National Aeronautics and Space Administration-sponsored study, 16 types of anaerobes have been partially characterized and identified as normally occurring in healthy subjects living on a "typical American" diet. The organisms varied in numbers between 1 and 100 billion per g feces. Non-spore-forming anaerobes predominated in fecal bacterial population over the aerobes by a factor 1,000:1.

Aerobic organisms such as the coliforms produce CO_2 and H_2, and the predominating anaerobes produce H_2 and CH_4. Some of the latter also produce NH_3, H_2S, indole, skatole, and butyric and valeric acids, products that are among those responsible for the malodor of flatus. It is thus clear that the composition of G I flora—which in turn depends upon the type of diet and the substrate thus provided—will determine the composition of the flatus. Although microbial action starts in the small intestine, the major contribution to the flatus results from action in the colon, where food residues stay for a long time and the microbial population is comparatively large and varied.

Amount and Composition of Gastrointestinal Gas

Gas normally present in the G I tract does not exceed about 200 ml. However, between 400 and 650 ml of flatus is expelled per day, which is composed of up to 50% of N_2 from swallowed air, about 12–14% of O_2, and a variable proportion of CO_2, H_2, and CH_4 as products of fermentation. Between 1,000 and 1,500 ml of gas per day can normally leave the body without causing discomfort.[37] Products of bacterial fermentation may cause spasm by irritating the intestinal mucosa and thus give rise to abdominal distension and discomfort.[34]

Different observers have given varying values for the concentrations of O_2, CO_2, CH_4, and H_2 in flatus. These variations prbably reflect differences in the techniques of flatus collection, the time of flatus collection in relation to meals, the composition of intestinal flora, the substrate available for bacterial action, and the variability among individuals in the capacity to form gases like H_2 and CH_4.

The amount and composition of G I gas is related to meals and is influenced by microbial action. In observations on nine healthy subjects, using intestinal intubation with a polyluminal tube, it was found that in a fasting state the production of H_2 was negligible.[39] Within 15 min of the introduction of 60 ml of a 10% solution of lactose, H_2 production increased and reached a peak at 1 h. Most H_2 was produced in the cecum and colon and much less in the small intestine. Capacity to produce methane varied in different subjects. In five subjects, no CH_4 could be detected, but in four others 0.55 ml of CH_4/min was produced; this was not influenced by lactose. That some individuals are methane producers and others not has been repeatedly documented. In some people, CH_4 may always be present in breath; in others it may largely appear in flatus.

Incubation of dejecta collected from established ileostomies and colostomies under anaerobic conditions using different substrates showed that whereas CO_2 and H_2 were formed in both, CH_4 was formed only by the colonic dejecta.[40] It seems therefore that CH_4 results from the bacterial action in the colon.

In another series of investigations in which GI gas formation was studied by analysis of expired air, the following observations were made.[41,42] During fasting, the expired air had 4–7 ppm H_2. After a bland meal consisting of egg albumin, sucrose, dextrimaltose, corn starch, corn oil, shortening, and salt mixture, the concentration of H_2 in expired air rose to 25–30 ppm within 1 h. Flatus formed at the rate of 1–4 ml/30 min during fasting; flatus formation then increased to 11–20 ml/30 min after the meal and was associated with the peak in H_2 in the expired air.

Effect of Different Foods on Flatus

A meal of 100 g cooked dried white beans at lunch increased flatus formation, beginning at 5 h after lunch and lasting through 7 hours[41]; 130–170 ml per 30 min of flatus was recorded at the peak. Individual variations in flatus formation were recorded in response to the meals of beans. The authors concluded that large amounts of undigested material can cause flatulence. They found that consumption of 150 g of raw potato starch caused an increase in breath H_2 for over 15 h (amounting to 40 ml/h), whereas raw wheat starch gave a normal breath pattern with an H_2 concentration of 3–7 ppm.

The effect of bean diet on flatus formation and the potency of beans in producing large amounts of gas in the GI tract have been confirmed in other studies.[43,44] Healthy volunteers were fed a bland non-gas-forming basal diet containing the following foods: whole wheat bread, potatoes, lean beef, cottage cheese, butter, skim milk, banana, pear, pineapple, coffee, and cream. The diet provided 2,625 kcal/day and contained

246 g carbohydrate, 88 g fat, 152 g protein, and 7 g crude fiber. Flatus was collected by flatus tube for 2 h after lunch and after dinner on the fourth and seventh day on the diet. The volume of flatus was measured and an aliquot analyzed.

After 7 days on the basal diet, a variable proportion of it was replaced by commercial food preparations, such as pork and beans, green lima beans, and Boston baked beans. Each of these diets was fed for 7 days. The carbohydrate, fat, protein, and calorie contents of the diets were adjusted and were approximately comparable to those of the basal diet. Gas collections were made as in the basal period. The results of these studies are given in Table I.

TABLE 1   Influence of Beans on Flatus Formation[a]

Diet	Average Volume of Flatus (ml/h)	Average Composition of Gas (%)				
		CO_2	O_2	N_2	H_2	CH_4
Basal	15	8.1	3.6	61.2	19.8	7.3
Pork and beans, 57%	176	51.4	1.3	19.1	11.0	17.2
Pork and beans, 27%	66	23.1	1.1	37.7	24.2	13.9
Green lima beans, 28%	127	37.7	0.8	20.2	27.0	14.3
Boston baked beans, 51%	168	49.1	1.1	19.4	8.0	22.4
Basal	14	—	—	—	—	—
Pork and baked beans, 37%	83	—	—	—	—	—
Pork and baked beans, 37% + Mexaform	17	—	—	—	—	—

[a] Adapted from F. R. Steggerda and J. G. Dimmick[43] and F. R. Steggerda.[44]

It was clear that beans were powerful producers of gas in the GI tract. Individual variations in the quantity and composition of the gas produced were again observed. The most notable change in the composition of gas was in CO_2, which was three to six times higher on bean diets than on the basal diet. The form of the bean product fed (i.e., bean flour or homogenates of the above-mentioned commercial preparations) made little difference in gas production. Green lima beans at 27% of the diet produced only 25% less flatus than Boston baked beans fed at the level of 51%. Thus, the beans differed in their capacity to produce flatus. When an antibacterial preparation (Mexaform) was administered to the subjects, flatus production was suppressed, thus showing the influence of bacterial action on flatus production. Antispasmodics and antiprotozoal compounds, however, were found to be without any influence. The authors conclude on the basis of supporting animal experiments that the clostridial group of anaerobes was responsible for flatus formation.[45]

A careful search for a compound or compounds in beans responsible for flatulence led the authors through various stages of fractionation and testing. They concluded that oligosaccharides (such as raffinose and stachyose) are largely responsible for the flatulent properties of beans.

Raffinose is a trisaccharide consisting of galactose, glucose and fructose residues and is O-α-D-galactopyranosyl-$(1 \rightarrow 6)$-O-α-D-glucopyranosyl-$(1 \rightarrow 2)$-β-D-fructofuranoside. Stachyose is a tetrasaccharide also composed of galactose, glucose, and fructose residues and is O-α-D-galactopyranosyl-$(1 \rightarrow 6)$-O-α-D-galactopyranosyl-$(1 \rightarrow 6)$-O-α-D-glucopyranosyl-$(1 \rightarrow 2)$-β-D-fructofuranoside. The intestinal tract does not produce enzymes capable of splitting these oligosaccharides; they are acted upon by some anaerobic microorganisms giving rise to gaseous products. The capacity of stachyose and raffinose to produce gas when fed with a bland, non-gas-producing diet has been confirmed independently.[41]

Another reason for flatulence may be intolerance to food, exemplified best by milk intolerance. Several investigations have shown that milk intolerance of varying degrees exists in certain otherwise healthy people. It is intolerance to lactose that commonly is responsible for milk intolerance, and this is due to a deficiency of lactase in the intestinal mucosa. The basic cause of flatulence in lactose intolerance is identical to that discussed earlier. The undigested lactose forms a good substrate for the intestinal microorganisms for the production of gas and of other symptoms described in the earlier section of this chapter. Hence, lactose in such persons behaves in a manner similar to disaccharides in normal persons and becomes a flatus-producing factor.

It would thus appear that the older belief that less-digestible or indigestible foods cause flatulence has now received scientific support. The compounds in beans responsible for excess flatus formation have been identified. Further investigations are necessary, for there still exists the possibility that there may be other unidentified substances in food that might interfere with the absorption of intestinal gas, causing its accumulation in the digestive tract and passage as flatus. Furthermore, in addition to the type of the diet, other factors such as stress (including emotional stress) may cause flatulence in healthy individuals, Thus, flatulence in health may be associated with certain types of food, but it would be unwise to ascribe it to this single factor alone.

FAVISM

This topic has been the subject of an excellent review by Mager, Razin, and Hershko.[46]

Favism is the term used to describe a hemolytic syndrome in susceptible individuals following the ingestion of seeds or inhalation of the pollen from *Vicia faba*, commonly known as broad bean, horse bean, or fava bean. The hemolysis varies in intensity and is accompanied by hemoglobinuria and jaundice in the more severe cases. In the majority of cases, the onset of the favic crisis is usually 5–24 h after ingestion of the beans. However, symptoms of hemolysis have been reported within a few minutes after pollen inhalation.

The disease is usually self-limiting in adults; the acute stage lasts 24–48 h followed by complete spontaneous recovery. Repeated attacks may occur on renewed exposure. There is a sex difference in favism in which males appear to be more susceptible than females. Male : female ratios between 2.7 and 21.3 have been reported from different countries. Children appear to be more susceptible to favism and often experience severe hemolytic reactions. The most susceptible age group is that between 1 and 5 yr of age, but cases of favism have been reported in nurslings and infants under 1 yr. In early 1900[47] a fatality rate of 6.8% was reported for children under 6 yr of age. With the advent of blood-transfusion therapy, however, the mortality rates have been greatly reduced.

Geographic Distribution

Favism occurs principally in the countries of the Mediterranean littoral.[48-50] In certain of these countries—Egypt, Greece, and Italy—reports of favism go back to antiquity. It would appear that the fava bean was grown and eaten in ancient Egypt, since it was found in the tombs of pharaohs dating from the Fifth and Sixth Dynasties, over 2000 years BC. Fava beans have also been mentioned in the ancient papyri. Priests were prohibited from eating these beans, but in ancient Greece fava beans were considered to be appropriate food for athletes in order to improve their athletic performance.

The highest incidence of favism has been reported in recent times from Sardinia, with five cases of favism per year per 1,000 population. The island of Sicily and Calabria on the mainland in South Italy are other areas where the incidence of favism is fairly high. Statistics from countries bordering on the Eastern Mediterranean are lacking. The disease, however, has been reported from the Greek mainland and islands and from Turkey, Cyprus, Lebanon, and Egypt.

Outside the Mediterranean basin favism has been reported from other Middle Eastern countries, such as Iraq and Iran, and from Bulgaria. Recent reports indicate that in Iran it is far more widespread than had been realized. In 1965 an incidence of favism varying from 2 to 9 per 10,000 population was reported from three provinces of Iran.[49,51] It has also been reported from Szechwan province in western China, and a large number of cases occurred in 1956–1958 in Kwantung province in southern China.[52,53] The disease is observed only sporadically in other European countries and the United States.

Fava bean is cultivated and used as human food in almost all countries of the world. Although it is a well-known and common food, no exact consumption figures are available. According to the 1959/1960 Food and Agriculture Organization Food Balance Sheet, daily consumption of the beans is fairly large in Egypt, with 29 g per capita of various grain legumes available for human consumption. Fava beans formed nearly two thirds of this supply, which would provide about 19 g fava bean per capita per day.[54] Figures for fava beans available in Egypt for human consumption in 1965 were almost identical with the above estimate. It is noteworthy that in spite of such a high daily consumption, cases of favism reported from Egypt are so few as to find little mention in Egyptian medical literature.

Fresh beans are eaten raw or cooked with the skin. Dried beans are usually soaked overnight in water and cooked in several ways, mostly without removing the skin. Beans are commonly consumed by older children and adults. However, fresh beans with or without the skin may be cooked soft, mashed, and fed as supplementary foods to infants during the weaning period.

Favism is most often associated with the consumption of fresh beans with or without skin and cooked or uncooked. Dried beans are also implicated to a lesser extent.

Seasonal Incidence

Seasonal variation in the incidence of favism in endemic areas is well documented. A characteristic peak incidence is associated with the harvesting of the bean. The harvesting season varies from country to country according to local climatic conditions, and the exact time of the highest incidence of the disease varies accordingly. Most cases of favism appear in the spring and early summer when fresh harvested beans are available. A second peak of incidence has been observed in Egypt in the autumn. This peak is associated with the consumption of dried beans that have been stored underground under anaerobic conditions for 6 months after harvest. This practice is peculiar to a certain locality in Egypt.[55] When these beans are taken out from storage, they are white or green and outwardly resemble fresh harvested fava beans, whereas beans stored above ground in sacks become brown, probably due to exposure to light and oxygen.

Mechanism of Toxic Action

Different, usually mixed, strains of *Vicia faba* are cultivated in different countries. It has not been possible so far to associate favism with any particular strain or variety of the bean.

The onset of hemolytic attack on exposure to pollen of the flowering plant has been reported several times in the older literature. Authentic evidence of pollen-causing favism has not appeared in recent publications.

Various early hypotheses to explain the association between fava bean and favism were advanced. The disease was ascribed to infection, food allergy, autoimmune sensitivity, or "toxicity" of the bean. Most of these are now mainly of historical interest. In 1956 Crosby, in reviewing the situation in Sardinia, suggested that hemolysis caused by fava bean resembled that caused by primaquine in certain individuals with an intrinsic abnormality in erythrocytes.[56] The inherent defect leading to drug sensitivity was found to consist of a low concentration and relative instability of reduced glutathione (G-S-H) in erythrocytes, and of a deficiency of the enzyme glucose-6-phosphate dehydrogenase (G-6-PD).[57] In erythrocytes deficient in G-6-PD, the total glutathione content is reduced; however, the glutathione (G-S-S-G) levels are higher and G-S-H levels lower than in normal erythrocytes.[58] It has since been found that all persons with a history of favism have G-6-PD deficiency and that they show the same characteristics of a low level of G-S-H in erythrocytes and an instability of G-S-H toward acetyl phenylhydrazine similar to that found in drug-sensitive G-6-PD–deficient individuals.

G-6-PD deficiency is inherited as a sex-linked trait transmitted by an incompletely dominant gene located on the x chromosome. Two genotypes of individuals can be predicted for males and three for females. Genetic mosaicism may explain the wide variations in enzyme activity in different subjects. Thus, the basic defect that is a prerequisite for susceptibility to favism is inherited.

G-6-PD deficiency occurs with varying degrees of prevalence in different parts of the world, and different variants of G-6-PD have been described, a deficiency of any of which can result in drug sensitivity.[59] Not all G-6-PD–deficient subjects are susceptible to favism, although most of them may be susceptible to drug-induced hemolysis. Among the G-6-PD variants, the Mediterranean one is characterized by the unusually low enzyme activity in erythrocytes of G-6-PD-deficient subjects (less than 5% of the normal) and in addition a low Michaelis constant for glucose-6-phosphate (G-6-P).[60] These characteristics may partly explain the enhanced susceptibility to favism in the Mediterranean type of G-6-PD deficiency. Even then, the reported prevalence of favism shows no relation to that of G-6-PD deficiency in these same countries. For example, in certain agricultural areas of Greece where fava bean is cultivated and consumed, about 20% of the population may be G-6-PD deficient, but cases of favism are comparatively rare in spite of frequent opportunities of exposure to the bean.[61]

The search for toxic factors has thus far yielded information on some active principles in fava bean that may be responsible for hemolysis. Crude or semipurified extracts of fresh young fava beans, on incubation with G-6-PD-deficient erythrocytes and glucose, were found to cause a significant decrease in G-S-H as compared to that in normal erythrocytes.[62,63] Extracts of the pollen or pistils of fava flowers had the same effect. This discriminatory effect of fava bean extracts on erythrocyte G-S-H has been utilized to isolate and identify the compounds in fava bean responsible for favism. Certain similarities between the action of primaquine and fava juice or extract on erythrocytes in G-6-PD deficiency have been demonstrated.[64] They both cause a fall in G-S-H, an increase in osmotic fragility, and a decrease of *in vivo* survival of treated red blood cells from G-6-PD–deficient individuals on transfusion. However, unlike primaquine, fava juice did not cause a loss of potassium from erythrocytes of susceptible subjects.

In the meantime, Lin and Ling claimed that vicine, a nucleoside occurring in fava bean, was responsible for hemolysis and hence for favism.[65,66] They found that vicine had a growth-retarding effect in rats and caused a mild hemoglobinuria when administered to dogs by stomach tube at a dosage level of 0.2 g/kg. Furthermore, vicine inhibited the activity of G-6-PD *in vitro.* Vicine was isolated in 1870 from *Vicia sativa* seeds, and another related compound, convicine, was later isolated from the same source. Vicine and convicine were also found to occur in *Vicia faba.* Vicine is 2,6-diamino-4,5-dihydroxypyrimidine-5-β-D-glucopyranoside,[67] and convicine has been assigned the formula of 2,4,5-trihydroxy-6-aminopyrimidine-5-β-D-glucopyranoside.[68] Both of these glucosides are hydrolyzed by emulsin, a β-glucosidase. Mild acid hydrolysis of the glucosides yields the aglycones divicine and isouramil, respectively. It is possible that the aglycones are released in the GI tract by the action of β-glucosidase prior to their absorption.

Both the aglycones, divicine and isouramil, caused a decrease in G-S-H when incubated with human erythrocytes suspended in phosphate buf-

Divicine   Isouramil

fer saline at pH 7.4.[69] The presence of glucose in the incubating medium abolished this effect on erythrocytes from normal subjects but not on those from G-6-PD–deficient individuals. These effects were about 20–30 times greater than those of acetylphenylhydrazine (APH) and ascorbic acid. There was no stoichiometric relationship between the amounts of aglycone used and the extent to which G-S-H was decreased. This suggested a catalytic mode of action. Furthermore, whereas APH required the presence of hemoglobin to cause a decrease in G-S-H, the aglycones exert this effect on G-S-H in the absence of hemoglobin. The activity of the aglycones is attributed to the presence of a carbonyl conjugated amino–enol system analogous to the endiol in ascorbic acid. The glucosidic linkage at position 5 in the pyrimidine ring disturbs this system and renders the parent glucosides completely inactive.[46]

The presence of another active compound in fava beans has been demonstrated. It is 3,4-dihydroxy-L-phenylalanine or L-DOPA.[70] (See Chapter 7.) It also has the capacity to cause a fall in G-S-H in erythrocytes obtained from G-6-PD–deficient subjects. L-DOPA occurs in fava bean in the free state and also as a glucoside having the formula β-[3-(β-D-glucopyranosyloxy)-4-hydroxyphenyl]-L-alanine. Both compounds are found in the dormant and germinating cotyledons of fava bean.[71] They also occur in garden peas (*Pisum sativum*). However, consumption of peas is rarely associated with the acute hemolytic attacks that occur in favism. Later investigations showed that L-DOPA alone had no effect on G-S-H levels in erythrocytes from G-6-PD–deficient subjects, whereas dopaquinone, formed by the action of tyrosinase on DOPA, did cause a lowering of G-S-H. A synergistic action between divicine and isouramil on the one hand, and L-DOPA on the other, in causing a rapid decrease in G-S-H in G-6-PD–deficient erythrocytes has been described.[72] The suggestion that the active hemolytic principle in fava bean is dopaquinone, produced from the L-DOPA contained in the bean, has to be viewed in this context.[73]

Thus, the presence of more than one active compound responsible for the rapid fall in G-S-H in G-6-PD-deficient erythrocytes has been demonstrated in fava beans. There is a strong probability that they are responsible for the hemolysis that is characteristic of favism, although the actual mechanism of hemolysis has not been elucidated. Additional aspects of favism remain to be clarified. First, that only some of the known G-6-PD –deficient subjects are susceptible to favism needs to be explained. If the active compounds in the bean are responsible for hemolysis, their occurrence in fava pollen remains to be demonstrated, and attacks of favism on inhalation of fava pollen need to be authenticated, for these have been attributed to "cryptoconsumption" of raw fava bean while walking through the fields of ripening fava. Finally, some correlation has to be established between the amounts of fava bean consumed, the form in which it is consumed, and the severity of favism in susceptible individuals. It is possible that, apart from genetic factors in man and the concentration of the active compounds in the bean, other variables (such as the effect of cooking, digestion, absorption and metabolic disposal) may determine the susceptibility to and severity of the toxic effects of fava bean.

TOXIC HONEYS*

Introduction

Honey is a plant product that is gathered, modified, concentrated, and stored by honeybees for their use. Considering the variety of plants that have toxic components, it should not be surprising that materials toxic to humans may occasionally be found in honey. Such occurrences are relatively rare for several reasons: The bees themselves may be poisoned before storing the honey[74] ; and the beekeeping industry sees that honey from known toxic flora in their area does not reach the market.

Toxic honeys have been known since antiquity, the oldest record being the description by Xenophon of the mass poisoning of the expedition of Cyrus in 401 BC (the retreat of the ten thousand) near Trebizonde in Asia Minor. It is presumed that the honey was produced from the nectar of *Rhododendron ponticum*; many more occurrences have been recorded in this area of the world. Nearly 2,300 yr later, Plugge isolated a compound he called andromedotoxin from Trebizonde honey.[75] Honey from Ericaceae (*Rhododendron, Azalea, Andromeda* and *Kalmia* spp.) is implicated in the greatest number of reports.[75,78,79,85,90,96] The beekeeping literature contains detailed descriptions of the experiences of those consuming honey from various members of Ericaceae. A physician described intoxication by mountain laurel honey (*K. latifolia*) as follows[87] :

* Literature reviewed through October 1971.

Symptoms of poisoning—These have varied in severity from a mere tingling in the skin to almost death. No two persons reacted exactly alike, yet they did enough so as to be recognized from a common causative agent. Shortly after eating, within a few minutes to two hours, the person felt a tingling and numbness in the extremities and lost consciousness, sometimes but momentarily and others for several hours. The pulse weakened to imperceptibility and went down to 50 or even 30. The face turned ghastly blue so characteristic of a heart attack but without anginal pain. A cold sweat appeared. These symptoms lasted from a few minutes to four or five hours. Usually there was no nausea or other gastro-intestinal symptoms. Recovery was complete within from a half to 12 hours, usually 6 to 8, except for a numbness or a tingling in the skin of the extremities.

A differing description is found in the review by Howes,[85] who reports a Civil War surgeon's description of the effects on soldiers of presumably the same honey:

It has a highly poisonous effect, being an extremely distressing narcotic, varying in its effects in proportions to the quantity eaten. . . . Some time after eating a queerish sensation of tingling all over, indistinct vision, caused by dilation of the pupils, with an empty, dizzy feeling about the head and a horrible nausea which would not relieve itself by vomiting. The first case or two I saw were entirely overpowered by it, and their appearance was exactly as if they were dead drunk . . . the enervation of all the voluntary muscles was completely destroyed. The usual remedies for narcotics partially restored them in a few hours, but the effects did not completely wear off for two or three days, and I was assured that fatal consequences have been known to follow a too free indulgence.

This resembles more closely the classic description by Xenophon in that vomiting was present.

A review of the relationships among the toxic agents isolated from Ericaceae may be found in the paper of Scott et al.[104] Of the 12 closely related compounds, 4 have been isolated from honey and chemically identified. Acetylandromedol[111] was isolated in a 0.010% yield from an authenticated sample of honey from K. latifolia and identified by paper electrophoresis, mixed melting point, and infrared spectrum. Scott et al.[104] isolated three compounds from a honey of unknown source and identified them by T L C with three solvent systems and four chromogenic reagents. These, and their levels of occurrence, were andromedol (7 ppm), anhydroandromedol (3 ppm), and desacetyl pieristoxin B, which, though quantitative data were not obtained, appeared to be present in amounts greater than andromedol. Carey et al.[75] isolated acetylandromedol from nectar of Rhododendron thomsonii and identified it by melting point, optical rotation, and IR spectrum. Animal toxicity data were obtained by the latter two groups of workers both for the isolated materials and the original nectar or honey. The structures of acetylan-

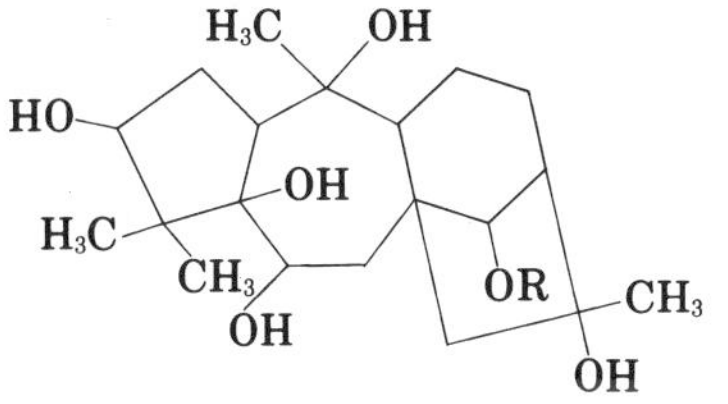

Acetylandromedrol, R = COCH₃
Andromedol, R = H

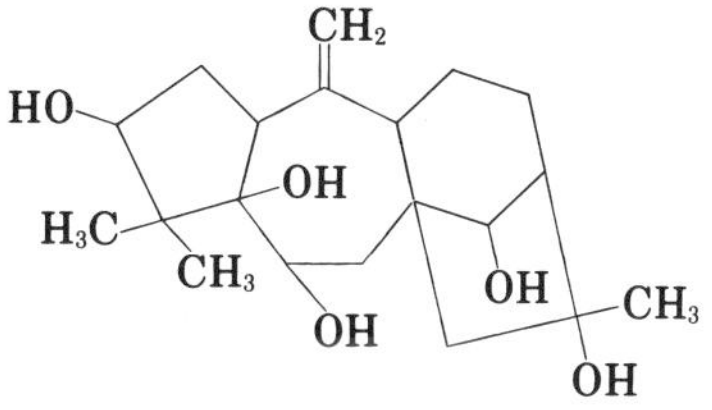

Anhydroandromedol

dromedol, andromedol, and anhydroandromedol[89] are shown above. That of desacetyl pieristoxin B is not known.

Andromedotoxin and Related Substances

Moran *et al.*[93] have reported the most extensive study of the pharmacological actions of andromedotoxin. The material they used (melting point 258–260 °C, $[\alpha]_D^{25}$ –8.4° in ethanol) was isolated from the leaves of *R. maximum* by Wood *et al.*[113]; a later paper from this group[108] named it acetylandromedol. Moran *et al.* concluded:

The rapid intravenous injection of andromedotoxin produces bradycardia, hypotension, and respiratory depression. Atropine prevents the bradycardia, and diminishes the hypotensive component. Vagotomy abolishes the entire response. Three manometer technique studies demonstrate a reflex vasodilation, as well as bradycardia, as contributing to the hypotensive effect. The minimal effective dose in eliciting this reflex is two to three microgm./kgm.

A distinct hypotensive action in vagotomized animals occurs in a dose range of 2 to 20 microgm./kgm., the magnitude of the depressor effect being proportional to the dose. Associated with this response is a blockade of the carotid sinus pressor reflex and the production of postural hypotension. The absence of a peripheral autonomic blocking action, the failure to obtain the response in the spinal cat, and the absence of direct vasodilatation on intra-arterial administration demonstrate a lack of peripheral action. Studies with the three manometer technique indicate a nerve mediated vasodilatation. It is believed that the action is a direct depression of the vasomotor center or a simulation of receptors in the head and neck with a reflex vasodilatation.

Electrocardiographic changes such as ventricular extrasystoles, A-V nodal and ventricular tachycardia, conduction impairment, and ventricular fibrillation occur with doses of 35 microgm./kgm. and greater.

Andromedotoxin in doses of 40 microgm./kgm. and greater causes a rise in blood pressure due largely to the release of epinephrine from the adrenal medulla, as shown by the absence of the greater part of the effect after adrenergic blocking doses of phentolamine and after adrenalectomy. Because of a transient venous pressure lowering effect, the possibility exists of a positive inotropic action on the heart as a contributory factor in this pressor effect.

A veratrine-like action on the isolated frog sartorius muscle appears in concentrations of 1:250,000, along with a progressive decrease in the twitch height. Unlike veratridine there is no significant initial increase in twitch height, only a delayed relaxation. Andromedotoxin also antagonizes the action of veratridine.

Emesis occurs in unanesthetized dogs upon parenteral administration of andromedotoxin in doses of 7 microgm./kgm. and greater.

Respiratory stimulation or depression occur in vagotomized dogs with doses of 20 microgm./kgm. and greater. The mechanisms of these actions are unknown.

Stimulation of the central nervous system followed by depression occurs with high doses.

The actions of andromedotoxin are of short duration, lasting less than one hour even with toxic doses.

The close similarity in actions of andromedotoxin to the veratrum alkaloids has been discussed.

Nothing is known of the metabolic fate of andromedotoxin.[93] Hardikar[80] has reported that at least one third of the poison is eliminated in toxic form in the urine after subcutaneous administration to animals.

Investigating a British Columbia honey that had caused nausea, blurred vision, shortness of breath, and mild paralysis of hands and arms, Scott et al.[104] isolated the three compounds noted above. Aqueous solutions of the isolated materials as well as crystalline standards were injected intraperitoneally into male albino mice (21–44 g). The LD_{50} values for the standard toxins were: acetylandromedol (grayanotoxin I), 1.28 (1.11–1.49) mg/kg (95% confidence levels); andromedol (grayantoxin III), 0.908 (0.805–1.03) ng/kg; anhydroandromedol, not toxic at doses up to 4 mg/kg. Clinical symptoms were dyspnea, periodic clonic convulsions, lordosis, paralysis, exophthalmos, and sedation, with death apparently due to respiratory failure; ventricular fibrillation was noted in animals autopsied shortly after cessation of respiration. The toxic honey extract had an LD_{50} value equivalent to 34 g honey/kg (17.5–65 g/kg) with similar symptoms.

Carey et al.[75] examined the toxicity to honeybees and mice and the pharmacology of nectars from 17 Rhododendron species and 14 hybrids. Andromedotoxin was isolated from R. thomsonii nectar (which itself had an approximate LD_{50} for mice of 10 ml/kg). Toxic nectars when injected into cats (0.1–0.5 ml/kg) caused depression of respiration, associated with contractions of the diaphragm, bradycardia, and either a sharp, short-lived fall in blood pressure (often followed by a smaller rise), or a sustained hypertensive effect; similar effects were obtained by injection of 10–40 µg/kg of andromedotoxin. Bradycardia and hypotension were abolished by 1 mg/kg of atropine sulfate; the pressor response by 2 mg/kg of phentolamine. These results are similar to those reported by Moran et al.[93] and Hardikar.[80]

Ancient and modern literature reports of human poisoning from Ericaceae honey appear to refer most frequently to areas in Asia Minor, U.S.S.R., eastern and Pacific Northwest United States, and Japan. In areas where production of this honey is a recurring problem, biological tests have been proposed for its detection. Pulewka[102] suggested that the andromedotoxin content of honey could be approximated from its action on the respiration of white mice and guinea pigs; a cramp-like contraction of the diaphragm and glottis is observed similar to the action of aconitine, which is used as a standard. Popova *et al.*[101] proposed the use of pollen analysis and biological testing for this purpose.

Sporadic instances of nonfatal human poisoning by honey have occurred in the Bay of Plenty area of New Zealand for about 50 yr. The offending toxic material was traced to honeydew collected by bees from the leaves of *Coriaria arborea* (tree tutu), a plant known to contain a toxic substance, tutin. The honeydew was produced by the passion-vine hopper, *Scolypopa australis*; the flowers do not secrete nectar and the pollen is not toxic.[81,96,97,99,106,107]

Tutin and Related Substances

Sutherland and Palmer-Jones[106] isolated from the honey a crystalline material, different from tutin, which they named mellitoxin, noting that it did not account for all of the toxicity. No mellitoxin could be isolated from the plant,[107] but Palmer-Jones and White[98] demonstrated that tutin was converted to mellitoxin by passage through the passion-vine hopper. Structure of the latter was elucidated[84] and shown to be identical with hyenanchin, a hydroxy tutin.

Tutin, R = H
Hyenanchin, R = OH

Since that time, 1,000 mi^2 of the area have been closed to beekeeping, and samples from that and other areas are periodically assayed for the toxic properties. Assay until 1955 was by oral dosing of guinea pigs with honey extracts. Since then, more sensitive tests, such as intracerebral injection of the mouse[76,92] and a TLC procedure[33] have been used.

These were compared by Turner and Clinch[110] and found to agree under certain interpretative restrictions. Hodges and White[83] isolated both hyenanchin and tutin from the toxic honey and described a TLC procedure for their detection in honey at levels of 40 and 10 μg in 5 g. A honey known to be toxic was estimated to contain 100 μg tutin and 800 μg hyenanchin in 5 g. Clinch and Turner[77] discussed sample testing between 1962 and 1967 by guinea pigs, mice, and TLC methods. In general, tutin, which is nine times more toxic to mice, is present in much smaller amounts than is hyenanchin. Data are generally reported as the tutin equivalent; about 0.10 mg tutin equivalent per 100 g honey is detectable by the mouse test. Approximate quantities in samples are estimated by determining the LD_{50} of toxic honeys, taking the LD_{50} for tutin to be 0.01 mg/kg. Results for 40 samples ranged from <0.1 to 6.7 mg/100 g tutin equivalent. A honey responsible for human poisoning assayed at 4.0 mg/100 g, and on the basis that a 1-mg dose of tutin caused human nausea, vomiting, and incapacity for work for 24 h, this amount would be contained in 25 g of such honey.

Intoxication of the human by the tutin plant causes vomiting, giddiness, delerium, great excitement, stupor, coma, and convulsions, and in several cases loss of memory according to Fitchett (in Palmer-Jones[97]). Physicians' descriptions of symptoms in early cases of honey poisoning in New Zealand stated that the poison was delerient; patients became extremely violent, suffering from giddiness, pains in the abdomen and head, and vomiting, followed by rigidity of the limbs and convulsions, and often coma and loss of memory. No fatalities were seen.[96] Honey that was toxic to man was found on oral ingestion not to affect pigs, sheep, rabbits, mice, rats, or bees. Guinea pigs were quite susceptible, though not as susceptible as are humans, who may be severely affected by a half to one teaspoonful of the toxic honey.[96] The toxicology of tutin, mellitoxin (hyenanchin), and picrotoxin was examined by Palmer-Jones.[97] The honey toxins are closely related to picrotoxin. The toxic dosages were reported as shown in Table 2.

TABLE 2 LD_{50} (mg/kg) for Tutin, Hyenanchin, and Picrotoxin

	Stomach Tube		Subcutaneous		Intraperitoneal	
Toxicant	Guinea Pigs	Rats	Guinea Pigs	Rats	Guinea Pigs	Rats
Tutin	1.2[a]	~20	0.75[a]	~4	0.7	~5
Hyenanchin	12	~40–90	9	~30	9	~30
Picrotoxin	27	15.5	3	4.5	5.5	~3.5

[a] LD_{75}.

Palmer-Jones also examined the antagonism of tutin, hyenanchin, and picrotoxin by barbiturates in guinea pigs. The most satisfactory method of treatment for poisoning by the three toxins was to give the maximum IP dose of pentobarbital sodium (10 mg for guinea pigs) as soon as convulsions commenced, and repeat dosing with 5- or 10-mg amounts when necessary. Two IP injections, each 10 mg of pentobarbital sodium, were sufficient to cause rapid recovery in guinea pigs given lethal doses of the toxic honey by stomach tube.

Other Honey Toxins

Hazslinsky[82] described a toxic effect of a Hungarian honey, which he ascribed to belladonna alkaloids from the nightshade, but Örösi-Pál[94] claimed that the source was Egyptian henbane (*Datura metel*) and that the poisoning was by scopolamine, not atropine. Lehrner[91] and Sviderskaya[105] have described honey poisoning ascribed to atropine; in the latter article the source was said to be *Datura stramonium* and *Hyoscyamus niger.*

Several records of honey poisoning in the United States in the nineteenth century are described by Kebler,[90] including an occurrence at Branchville, S.C., where 3 children died of 20 persons affected. Wiley[112] stated that the honey contained gelsemine, and Howes[85] ascribes the honey origin as the yellow jasmine (false jasmine, jessamine, *Gelsemium sempervirens*), a well-known poisonous climbing vine common to southern United States and Mexico, with yellow fragrant flowers in February and March. A report in Pellett's book[100] describes fatal honeybee poisoning ascribed to this plant. Howes[85] quotes the following course of a case of the Branchville poisoning, presumably from this source: "A boy eleven years old was the first of the family to eat some of the honey. In an hour afterwards the child became giddy and staggered as he walked and could not see. He was affected with general lassitude and slight nausea. In two hours he was seized with convulsions and died." An account of the symptoms of poisoning by *Gelsemium* is given by Osol and Farrar[95] as "dizziness, dimness of vision, dilated pupil, general muscular debility, and unusual prostration, reducing the frequency and force of the pulse and the frequency of respiration." Further details of the course of fatal poisoning are given. Toxicology of the *Gelsemium* alkaloids is also reviewed there but will not be included here, since only one instance of presumed poisoning by honey from *Gelsemium* is recorded.

Juritz[88] discussed so-called Noors honey from several species of South African *Euphorbia*, which produces a strong, burning sensation in the throat and which may have caused poisoning resembling that from belladonna. Sanna[103] reported that a Sardinian honey with a sour, bitter taste was found to contain the glucoside arbutin, derived from *Arbutus unedo* L.

Bitter honeys are not uncommon; Joachim and Kandiah[86] attributed bitterness in a Ceylon honey to alkaloids from pollen of the Ceara rubber plant. Very little chemical work has been done with bitter honeys; likewise, little information is available on the materials responsible for the strong, sometimes nauseating odors and flavors of certain honeys, such as that from *Melaleuca,*[109] *Agave,*[100] and privet.

Even though some 250 million lb of honey are harvested and consumed annually in the United States, the odds are negligibly small of anyone encountering a toxic honey in commercial channels. Beekeepers are well aware of the availability in their areas of sources of toxic honey and take appropriate action to keep any such material out of the markets.

REFERENCES

1. A. Holzel, V. Schwarz, and K. W. Sutcliffe, Defective lactose absorption causing malnutrition in infancy. Lancet *1*:1126 (1959).
2. H. A. Weijers, J. H. Van de Kamer, D. A. A. Mossel, and W. K. Dicke, Diarrhoea caused by deficiency of sugar splitting enzymes. Lancet *2*:296 (1960).
3. A. Dahlquist, Disaccharide intolerance. J. Am. Med. Assoc. *195*:225 (1966).
4. G. Semenza, S. Auricchio, and A. Rubino, Multiplicity of human intestinal disaccharidases; I—chromatographic separation of maltases and of two lactases; II—characterization of the individual maltases. Biochim. Biophys. Acta *96*: 487, 498 (1965).
5. F. Kern, Jr., and J. E. Struthers, Jr., Intestinal lactase deficiency and lactose intolerance in adults. J. Am. Med. Assoc. *195*:927 (1966).
6. A. Prader and S. Auricchio, Defects of intestinal disaccharide absorption. Ann. Rev. Med. *16*:345 (1965).
7. H. B. McMichael, J. Webb, and A. M. Dawson, Jejunal disaccharidases and some observations on the cause of lactase deficiency. Br. Med. J. *2*:1037 (1967).
8. A. Dahlquist, S. Auricchio, G. Semenza, and A. Prader, Human intestinal disaccharidases and hereditary disaccharide intolerance. The hydrolysis of sucrose, isomaltose, palatinose (isomaltulose) and 1,6-α oligosaccharide (isomalto-oligosaccharide) preparation. J. Clin. Invest. *42*:556 (1963).
9. S. Auricchio, A. Rubino, A. Prader, J. Rey, J. Jos, and J. Frezal, Intestinal disaccharidase activity in congenital malabsorption of sucrose and isomaltose. Lancet *2*:914 (1964).
10. S. S. Huang and T. M. Bayless, Lactose intolerance in healthy children. N. Engl. J. Med. *276*:1283 (1967).
11. A. D. Newcomer and D. B. McGill, Disaccharidase activity in the small intes-

tine. Prevalence of lactase deficiency in 100 healthy subjects. Gastroenterology *53*:881 (1967).

12. J. D. Welsh, Isolated lactase deficiency in humans; report on 100 patients. Medicine *49*:257 (1970).

13. A. D. Newcomer and D. B. McGill, Distribution of disaccharidase activity in the small bowel of normal and lactase deficient subjects. Gastroenterology *51*: 481 (1966).

14. S. Auricchio, A. Dahlquist, G. Murset, and A. Parker, Isomaltose intolerance causing decreased ability to utilize dietary starch. J. Pediatr. *62*:165 (1963).

15. S. Auricchio, A. Rubino, M. Landolt, G. Semenza, and A. Prader, Isolated lactase deficiency in the adult. Lancet *2*:324 (1963).

16. P. Cuatrecasas, D. H. Lockwood, and J. R. Caldwell, Lactase deficiency in the adult. A common occurrence. Lancet *1*:14 (1965).

17. T. W. Bayless and N. S. Rosensweig, A racial difference in incidence of lactase deficiency. A survey of milk intolerance and lactase deficiency in healthy adult males. J. Am. Med. Assoc. *197*:968 (1966).

18. G. C. Cook and S. K. Kajubi, Tribal incidence of lactase deficiency in Uganda. Lancet *2*:725 (1966).

19. H. B. McMichael, J. Webb, and A. M. Dawson, Lactase deficiency in adults. A cause of functional diarrhoea. Lancet *1*:717 (1965).

20. H. B. McMichael, J. Webb, and A. M. Dawson, Jejunal disaccharidase and some observations on the cause of lactase deficiency. Br. Med. J. *2*:1037 (1967).

21. S. S. Huang and T. M. Bayless, Milk and lactose intolerance in healthy orientals. Science *160*:83 (1968).

22. M. H. Chung and D. B. McGill, Lactase deficiency in orientals. Gastroenterology *54*:225 (1968).

23. A. E. Davies and T. Bolin, Lactose intolerance in Asians. Nature *216*:1244 (1967).

24. R. K. Chandra, R. R. Pawa, and O. P. Ghai, Disaccharide intolerance in the etiology of chronic and/or recurrent diarrhoea in young children. Indian J. Med. Res. *57*:713 (1969).

25. C. H. Halsted, S. Sheir, N. Sourial, and V. N. Patwardhan, Small intestinal structure and absorption in Egypt. Influence of parasitism and pellagra. Am. J. Clin. Nutr. *22*:744 (1969).

26. K. N. Jeejeebhoy, H. G. Desai, and R. V. Verghese, Milk intolerance in tropical malabsorption syndrome. Role of lactose malabsorption. Lancet *2*:666 (1964).

27. C. E. Rubin, Celiac sprue. Ann. Rev. Med. *12*:39 (1961).

28. T. W. Sheehy, P. R. Anderson, and B. E. Baggs, Carbohydrate studies in tropical sprue. Am. J. Dig. Dis. New Ser. *11*:461 (1966).

29. F. A. Klipstein, Intestinal morphology in tropical sprue, Proc. West. Hemisphere Nutr. Cong. II. American Medical Association, Chicago (1969). P. 78.

30. M. D. Bowie, G. L. Brinkman, and J. D. L. Hansen, Acquired disaccharide intolerance in malnutrition. J. Pediatr. *66*:1083 (1965).

31. M. D. Bowie, G. O. Barbezat, and J. D. L. Hansen, Carbohydrate absorption in malnourished children. Am. J. Clin. Nutr. *20*:89 (1967).

32. N. S. Rosensweig, Adult human milk intolerance and intestinal lactase deficiency. J. Dairy Sci. *52*:585 (1969).

33. W. C. Alvarez, What causes flatulence? J. Am. Med. Assoc. *120*:21 (1942).

34. W. C. Alvarez, What causes gas? Iowa State Med. Soc. J. Des Moines *38*:518 (1948).
35. R. M. Donaldson, Normal bacterial populations of the intestine and their relation to intestinal function. N. Engl. J. Med. *270*:938 (1964).
36. G. H. Bornside, J. S. Welsh, and I. Cohn, Jr., Bacterial flora of the human small intestine. J. Am. Med. Assoc. *196*:1125 (1966).
37. L. S. Gall, The role of intestinal flora in gas formation. Ann. N.Y. Acad. Sci. *150*:27 (1968).
38. L. S. Gall, Normal fecal flora of man. Am. J. Clin. Nutr. *23*:1457 (1970).
39. M. D. Levitt and F. J. Ingelfinger, Hydrogen and methane production. Ann. N.Y. Acad. Sci. *150*:75 (1968).
40. D. H. Calloway, D. J. Colasito, and R. D. Mathews, Gases produced by human intestinal microflora. Nature *212*:1238 (1966).
41. D. H. Calloway and E. L. Murphy, The use of expired air to measure intestinal gas formation. Ann. N.Y. Acad. Sci. *150*:82 (1968).
42. D. H. Calloway, Human ecology in space flight III. Proceedings of the Third International Interdisciplinary Conference. New York Academy of Sciences. (1968). P. 136.
43. F. R. Steggerda and J. G. Dimmick, Effects of bean diets on concentrations of carbon dioxide in flatus. Am. J. Clin. Nutr. *19*:120 (1966).
44. F. R. Steggerda, Gastrointestinal gas following food consumption. Ann. N.Y. Acad. Sci. *150*:57 (1968).
45. E. A. Richards, F. R. Steggerda, and A. Murata, Relationship of bean substrate and certain intestinal bacteria to gas production in the dog. Gastroenterology *55*:502 (1968).
46. J. Mager, A. Razin, and A. Hershko, Favism, p. 293. In Toxic constituents of plant foodstuffs, E. I. Liener (ed.). Academic Press, New York (1969).
47. C. Fermi and P. Martinetti, Studio sul favismo. Ann. Ig. *15*:75 (1905).
48. J. V. Dacie, The hemolytic anaemias: Congenital and acquired, p. 1061. Part 4—Drug induced haemolytic anaemias. 2nd ed. J. & A. Churchill, London (1967).
49. M. A. Belsey, Favism in the Middle East. An epidemiological appraisal of the problem in relationship to infant nutrition and public health. Final Report to the World Health Organization, Geneva, Switzerland, Unpublished (February 1970).
50. A. Luisada. Favism: A singular disease chiefly affecting the red blood cells. Medicine *20*:339 (1941).
51. G. Donoso, H. Hedayat, and H. Khayatian, Favism, with special reference to Iran. Bull. WHO *40*:513 (1969).
52. S. Du, Favism in West China. Chin. Med. J. *70*:17 (1952).
53. S. F. Chung, Studies on favism in Kwantung Province. Pediatr. Indonesia, Suppl. 880, 5. Quoted from Belsey[49] (1965).
54. W. R. Aykroyd and J. Doughty, Legumes in human nutrition, p. 27. FAO Nutritional Studies No. 19. FAO, Rome (1964).
55. M. K. Gabr, Personal communication.
56. W. H. Crosby, Favism in Sardinia. Blood *11*:91 (1956).
57. P. E. Carson, C. L. Flanagan, C. E. Ickes, and A. S. Alving, Enzymatic deficiency in primaquine-sensitive erythrocytes. Science *124*:484 (1956).
58. S. K. Srivastava and E. Beutler, Oxidized glutathione levels in erythrocytes of glucose-6-phosphate dehydrogenase deficient subjects. Lancet *2*:23 (1968).

59. Anonymous, Standardization of procedures for the study of glucose-6-phosphate dehydrogenase. Report of a WHO Scientific Group. WHO Tech. Rep. Ser. 366. WHO, Geneva (1967).

60. H. N. Kirkman, Glucose-6-phosphate dehydrogenase variants and drug induced hemolysis. Ann. N.Y. Acad. Sci. *151*:753 (1968).

61. G. Stamatoyannopoulos, G. R. Fraser, A. G. Motulsky, P. Fessas, A. Akrivakis, and T. Papayannopoulou, On the familial predisposition to favism. Am. J. Hum. Genet. *18*:253 (1966).

62. D. G. Walker and J. E. Rowman, *In vitro* effect of *Vicia faba* extracts upon reduced glutathione of erythrocytes. Proc. Soc. Exp. Biol. Med. *103*:476 (1960).

63. J. E. Bowman and D. G. Walker, Action of *Vicia faba* on erythrocytes: Possible relationship to favism. Nature *198*:555 (1961).

64. F. Panizon and F. Zacchello, The mechanism of hemolysis in favism. Some analogy in the activity of primaquine and fava juice. Acta Haemat. *33*:129 (1965).

65. J. Y. Lin and K. H. Ling, Studies on favism II—Studies on the physiological activities of vicine *in vivo*. J. Formosan Med. Ass. *61*:490 (1962).

66. J. Y. Lin and K. H. Ling, Studies on favism III—Studies on the physiological activities of vicine *in vitro*. J. Formosan Med. Assoc. *61*:579 (1962).

67. A. Bendich and G. Clements, A revision of the structural formulation of vicine and its pyrimidine aglucone, divicine. Biochim. Biophys. Acta *12*:462 (1952).

68. S. Bien, G. Salemnik, and L. Zamir, The structure of convicine. J. Chem. Soc. (C), 496 (1968).

69. J. Mager, G. Glaser, A. Razin, G. Izak, S. Bien, and M. Noam, Metabolic effects of pyrimidines derived from fava beans glycosides on human erythrocytes deficient in glucose-6-phosphate dehydrogenase. Biochem. Biophys. Res. Comm. *20*:235 (1965).

70. N. S. Kosower and E. M. Kosower, Does 3,4-dihydroxyphenylalanine play a part in favism? Nature *215*:285 (1967).

71. R. S. Andrews and J. B. Pridham, Structure of a Dopa glucoside from *Vicia faba*. Nature *205*:1213 (1965).

72. A. Razin, A. Hershko, G. Glaser, and J. Mager, The oxidant effect of isouramil on red cell glutathione and its synergistic enhancement by ascorbic acid or 3,4-dihydroxyphenylalanine. Isr. J. Med. Sci. *4*:852 (1968).

73. E. Beutler, L-Dopa and favism. Blood *36*:523 (1970).

74. C. E. Burnside and G. H. Vansell. Plant poisoning of bees. U.S. Dep. Agric., Bur. Entomol. Plant Q. Bull. *E-398* (1936).

75. F. M. Carey, J. J. Lewis, J. L. MacGregor, and M. Martin-Smith. Chemical and pharmacological observations on some toxic nectars. J. Pharm. Pharmacol. Suppl. *11*:269T–274T (1959).

76. P. G. Clinch, An improved intracerebral injection method for detecting tutin and hyenanchin in toxic honey. N. Z. J. Sci. *9*:433–439 (1966).

77. P. G. Clinch and J. C. Turner, Estimation of tutin and hyenanchin in honey. 2. The toxicity of honey samples from test hives during the period 1962–67. N. Z. J. Sci. *11*:346–351 (1968).

78. H. Fühner, Über den giftigen Honig des pontischen Kleinasien. Naturwissenschaften *14*:1283 (1926).

79. W. Gruch, Zur Frage der Giftwirkung gewisser Honige. Z. Bienenforsch. *4*(2): 47–57 (1957).

80. S. W. Hardikar, Rhododendron poisoning. J. Pharmacol. *20*.17–44 (1922).

81. W. F. Harris and D. W. Filmer, A recent outbreak of honey poisoning. Part VI. Botanical investigation of pollen and nectar flora. N. Z. J. Sci. Technol. 29A: 134–143 (1947).

82. B. Hazslinsky, Toxische Wirkung eines Honigs der Tollkirsche (Atropa belladonna L.). Z. Bienenforsch. 3(5):93–96 (1956).

83. R. Hodges and E. P. White, Detection and isolation of tutin and hyenanchin in toxic honey. N. Z. J. Sci. 9:233–235 (1966).

84. R. Hodges, E. P. White, and J. S. Shannon, The structure of mellitoxin. Tetrahedron Lett. 7:371–381 (1964).

85. F. N. Howes, Poisoning from honey. Food Manuf. 24:459–462 (1949).

86. A. W. R. Joachim and S. Kandiah, The analysis of Ceylon foodstuffs. IX A. The composition of some Ceylon honeys. Trop. Agric. Ceylon 95:339–340 (1940).

87. W. R. Jones, Honey poisoning. Gleanings Bee Cult. 75:76–77 (1947).

88. C. F. Juritz, The problem of Noors honey. J. Dep. Agric. Union S. Afr. 10: 334–337 (1925).

89. H. Kakisawa, T. Kozima, M. Yanai, and K. Nakanishi, Stereochemistry of grayanotoxins. Tetrahedron 21:3091–3104 (1965).

90. L. F. Kebler, Poisonous honey. Am. Pharm. Assoc. Proc. 44:167–174 (1896).

91. L. Lehrner, Többszörös atropinmérgezés méz fogyasztása után. Nepégészségügy 36:315–316 (1955).

92. A. Melville and F. N. Fastier, Detection of certain honey poisons. Proc. Univ. Otago Med. Sch. 42:3–4 (1964).

93. N. C. Moran, P. E. Dresel, M. E. Perkins, and A. P. Richardson, The pharmacological actions of andromedotoxin, an active principle from Rhododendron maximum. J. Pharmacol. Exp. Ther. 110:415–432 (1954).

94. Z. Orösi-Pál, A mérgező méz titka nyomában. Méhészet 4(2):25–27 (1956).

95. A. Osol and G. E. Farrar, Jr., The dispensatory of the United States of America. 24th ed. Lippincott, Philadelphia (1947). P. 498.

96. T. Palmer-Jones, A recent outbreak of honey poisoning. Part I. Historical and descriptive. N. Z. J. Sci. Technol. 29A:107–114 (1947).

97. T. Palmer-Jones, A recent outbreak of honey poisoning. Part III. The toxicology of the poisonous honey and the antagonism of tutin, mellitoxin, and picrotoxin by barbiturates. N. Z. J. Sci. Technol. 29A:121–125 (1947).

98. T. Palmer-Jones and E. P. White, Recent outbreak of honey poisoning. VII. Observations on the toxicity and toxin of the tutu (Coriaria arborea). N. Z. J. Sci. Technol. 31A:46–56 (1949).

99. C. R. Paterson, A recent outbreak of honey poisoning. Part IV. The source of the toxic honey—Field observations. N. Z. J. Sci. Technol. 29A:125–129 (1947).

100. F. C. Pellett, American honey plants. 4th ed. Orange Judd Pub. Co., New York (1947). P. 97.

101. V. M. Popova, M. D. Rozental, M. M. Sadyrin, I. E. Trop, and I. K. Chulovskii, Group poisoning with spring honey and a method of determination of the toxicity by the method of biological testing and pollen analysis. Gig. Sanit. 25: 92–94 (1960).

102. P. Pulewka, Andromedotoxin enthaltenender Honig und eine biologische Methode zur Bestimmung seiner Giftigkeit. Bull. Fac. Med. Istanbul 12:275–286 (1949).

103. A. Sanna, Su una qualità di miele della Gallura di sapone amaro. Ann. Chim. Appl. *21*(8):397–402 (1931).

104. P. M. Scott, B. B. Coldwell, and G. S. Wiberg, Grayanotoxins. Occurrence and analysis in honey and a comparison of toxicities in mice. Food Cosmet. Toxicol. *9*:179–184 (1971).

105. Z. I. Sviderskaya, A case of food poisoning from honey. Gig. Sanit. *24*(5):57 (1959).

106. M. D. Sutherland and T. Palmer-Jones, A recent outbreak of honey poisoning. Part II. The toxic substances of the poisonous honey. N. Z. J. Sci. Technol. *29A*:114–120 (1947).

107. M. D. Sutherland and T. Palmer-Jones, A recent outbreak of honey poisoning. Part V. The source of the toxic honey—Laboratory investigations. N. Z. J. Sci. Technol. *29A*:129–133 (1947).

108. W. H. Tallent, M. L. Riethof, and E. C. Horning, Studies on the occurrence and structure of acetylandromedol (andromedotoxin). J. Am. Chem. Soc. *79*:4548–4554 (1957).

109. P. V. Taylor, Melaleuca trees annoy Florida beekeepers. Am. Bee J. *96*:449 (1956).

110. J. C. Turner and P. G. Clinch, Estimation of tutin and hyenanchin in honey. 1. A comparison of the thin-layer chromatography and intracerebral injection methods. N. Z. J. Sci. *11*:342–345 (1968).

111. J. W. White, Jr., and M. L. Riethof, The composition of honey. III. Detection of acetylandromedol in toxic honeys. Arch. Biochem. Biophys. *79*:165–167 (1959).

112. H. W. Wiley, Foods and adulterants. Part sixth. Sugar, molasses and sirup, confections, honey and beeswax. U.S. Dep. Agric., Div. Chem. Bull. 13 (1892). P. 750.

113. H. B. Wood, Jr., V. L. Stromberg, J. C. Keresztesy, and E. C. Horning, Andromedotoxin. A potent hypotensive agent from *Rhododendron maximum*. J. Am. Chem. Soc. *76*:5689–5692 (1954).

23 James A. Miller

NATURALLY OCCURRING SUBSTANCES THAT CAN INDUCE TUMORS*

INTRODUCTION

This chapter is limited largely to a description of the properties of the naturally occurring nonviral and nonradioactive chemicals that have been tested for carcinogenic activity and found to induce the formation of tumors in experimental animals under specific conditions. Only very limited assessments can be made at this time of the hazards they may pose for man. Although some of these substances occur in certain common human foods, they have been found primarily in unusual food sources and in foods contaminated by certain fungi. It is virtually certain that other naturally occurring compounds with carcinogenic activity exist among the vast number of nonnutritive minor components of common foods. The great majority of these compounds have yet to be isolated, characterized, and tested for biological activity. Some of the compounds described below occur in what may appear to be nonfood sources. They are included since it appears impossible to categorize a naturally occurring compound as one that is not now or will not at some time be contained in a food source of man.

The origin and development of tumors, whether or not they follow exposures to chemicals, are complex subjects, and many critical facts

* Literature reviewed through 1971.

and principles remain to be learned about these processes. The complexities and deficiencies in knowledge of these subjects and of the epidemiology of cancer in man make the evaluation of the carcinogenic hazard of chemicals in the environment for man a truly difficult study. To present these problems and the naturally occurring compounds that can induce tumors in some perspective, it is first necessary to outline pertinent knowledge of chemical carcinogens and carcinogenesis.

TUMORS, CARCINOGENESIS, AND CHEMICAL CARCINOGENS

Extensive discussion and authority for many of the following statements and conclusions could not be provided in the limited space available. Secondary sources[37,63,90,125,126,127] are recommended as guides to the voluminous primary literature.

The Gross Natures and Origins of Tumors

Tumors (originally, swellings of tissue) or, more accurately, neoplasms (new growths) are abnormal masses of host-derived tissue that grow more or less continuously in a manner uncoordinated with normal tissues and organs. Tumors occur in many animal and plant species, but they have been studied primarily in man and certain experimental mammals. Tumors that invade adjacent tissue and spread or metastasize to other parts of the host are known as malignant neoplasms or cancers. Malignant tumors or cancers also frequently exhibit rapid growth, atypical structures, and many mitotic figures. Benign tumors lack these features to a great extent, particularly the ability to metastasize, and are usually encapsulated. However, benign tumors may kill the host through pressure or gross mass. Many tumors occur that possess some characteristics of both the malignant and benign categories, and benign tumors may "progress" and become malignant.

Tumors are further divided into two main types on the basis of their histology and, by inference, their histogenetic derivation. The epithelial tumors derived from ectodermal and endodermal cells include benign tumors (the wart-like papillomas and the gland-like adenomas) and malignant tumors (carcinomas and epitheliomas). The mesenchymal or connective tissue types also include benign tumors (fibromas, myomas, lipomas, osteomas, etc.) and malignant tumors (fibrosarcomas, myosarcomas, liposarcomas, etc.). Some terms are less meaningful. A hepatoma can be a benign or malignant hepatic tumor, and the leukemias are tumors of the blood-cell-forming tissues.

Many tumors occur without known cause, and the majority of these "spontaneous" tumors occur in the last third of the life span in man and in other animals. The incidences of these tumors vary with the species and strain and may be lowered or raised markedly by selective breeding.

Carcinogenic Agents

Agents that cause malignant tumors to develop in greater incidence than would occur spontaneously are known as *carcinogens* or, more accurately, as *oncogens*. The process thereby caused is termed *carcinogenesis* or *oncogenesis*. The terms with the prefix *carcino*, strictly applied, refer only to malignant epithelial neoplasms and their genesis, but carcinogen and carcinogenesis are commonly used also in reference to the genesis of benign epithelial tumors and of malignant connective-tissue tumors. No compound is known that will cause the formation of benign tumors only. The ability of benign tumors to give rise to malignant neoplasms makes it likely that few, if any, such compounds will be found.

Three principal classes of carcinogenic agents exist. A large number of viruses containing either DNA or RNA are known that can induce tumors in experimental animals. It is highly probable that viral oncogens exist that are active in man, but none has been demonstrated unequivocally. The carcinogenic viruses cannot yet be distinguished from other viruses by their physical, chemical, biochemical, or genetic properties, although recent discoveries of RNA-dependent DNA polymerases in RNA tumor viruses suggest that these viruses may be distinguished in this respect from nononcogenic RNA viruses.[10,188,190] A second class is comprised of the "chemical" carcinogens. The chemical carcinogens now constitute a very diverse group of nonviral and nonradioactive organic and inorganic structures with various species and tissue selectivities. Most of these carcinogens are small organic molecules with molecular weights below 500. The inorganic chemical carcinogens consist of a small group of divalent ions (Co^{++}, Ni^{++}, Cd^{++}, Be^{++}, Pb^{++}, $CrO_4^{=}$) and certain complex metal silicates (types of asbestos). A third class of carcinogenic agents consists of radiations and is comprised of ultraviolet light and a variety of ionizing continuous and particulate radiations. The chemical and radiation carcinogens are required only for the times and the dosages needed to induce tumors; their presence is not needed for the continued growth of the induced tumors.

Man has the dubious distinction of being the first species in which carcinogenesis by chemicals and by radiation was demonstrated. The first clear finding, by Pott in 1775, concerned the high incidence of scrotal skin cancer in chimney sweeps who had gross and prolonged contact with coal soot. A number of other chemicals, organic and inorganic, have since been found to be carcinogenic in man, usually in industrial situations. Exposure to large amounts of these chemicals for many years was required to produce incidences of tumors in these small population groups that were significantly above the incidences noted in the general population. Similarly, most skin cancer in man results from overexposure to solar ultraviolet light.

Modern studies on the geographical pathology of cancer in man[82,137] suggest that a large fraction, perhaps as high as 80%, of nonskin cancer in the human is also of environmental origin. Thus, the chemical carcinogens in our total environment, through lifetimes of exposure to small amounts of these compounds, may rank as major causes of human cancer. These agents, and various oncogenic viruses and radiations, may separately and in combination be responsible for the majority of cancers in the human. The recognition and control of chemical, physical, and viral carcinogens in man's total environment have become principal tasks of cancer research.

Biochemical Reactivity of Chemical Carcinogens and Their Metabolites

In carcinogenesis with chemical carcinogens it is axiomatic that these agents must react, directly or indirectly, with critical molecules in cells. The synthetic and naturally occurring chemical carcinogens comprise a very diverse group of structures, and no common structural feature is evident. However, it is now recognized that the reactive forms of these structures are electrophilic (electron-deficient) reactants. Some chemical carcinogens, such as the carcinogenic alkylating agents and the carcinogenic metal ions, are electrophiles per se, and these agents appear to be reactive and carcinogenic as such.

The majority of the chemical carcinogens must be metabolized to form reactive and carcinogenic electrophiles. Many chemical carcinogens have been found to form covalent nucleic acid-bound and protein-bound derivatives in target tissues. It is now clear that these macromolecules contain many nucleophilic (electron-rich) components that combine with the electrophilic metabolites of these carcinogens. It is not difficult to see how the genetic and epigenetic consequences of these interactions might lead to heritable and essentially irreversible changes characteristic of neoplastic transformations and tumors.

Both metabolic activation and deactivation reactions are known for a variety of chemical carcinogens. These metabolic pathways appear to account for much of the species and tissue selectivity exhibited by chemical carcinogens. The electrophilic nature of the reactive and carcinogenic forms of chemical carcinogens provides some order among these varied structures, and it offers some hope for the future recognition of carcinogenic chemicals from their structures and the reactivity of their metabolic products.

Mechanisms of Carcinogenesis

Tumors clearly result from defects in growth control among cells and tissues in the organism. Some of the cellular alterations needed for the eventual formation of tumors may be caused by doses of chemical carcinogens too low to complete the carcinogenic process, and these alterations may remain latent in tissues for a long time. This is evident in the gross stages of "initiation" and "promotion" in skin carcinogenesis by polycylic aromatic hydrocarbons in the mouse. Sufficient dosages of these carcinogens will cause completion of the carcinogenic process with the appearance of skin papillomas and carcinomas in a few months (an appreciable fraction of the mouse life span of about 2 years).

A single sufficiently low dose of some of these hydrocarbons can "initiate" the mouse skin but not cause the appearance of gross tumors in the lifetime of the mouse. The process of skin carcinogenesis can be completed in the usual time if, following initiation, relatively specific and essentially noncarcinogenic "promoters" (e.g., croton oil or its phorbol ester components) are applied. The initiation stage in skin appears to be completed rapidly. It is essentially irreversible, since a year may be permitted to elapse and the promotion of the skin tumors can still be accomplished to the same extent as immediately following initiation. In addition, the interplay of other factors (hormonal, immunological, etc.) may be required to permit the appearance of tumors following dosage with carcinogens.

The cellular and molecular mechanisms by which "spontaneous" processes and carcinogenic viruses, chemicals, and radiations lead to tumor formation are not known. It is not known whether these varied carcinogenic agents induce tumors *de novo,* whether they hasten intrinsic cellular processes leading to the "spontaneous" tumors, whether the "spontaneous" carcinogenic processes are linked with unrecognized environmental carcinogens, or whether each of these mechanisms applies in specific cases.

Most of the hypotheses proposed for the molecular mechanisms of carcinogenesis are based on the interactions of these carcinogenic agents with cellular constituents (DNA's, RNA's, proteins) which, directly or indirectly, lead to heritable and at least quasi-irreversible changes in the content or the expression, or both, of genetic information needed for the control of growth in a cooperative community of cells. Natural selection among the altered cells and their progeny for those with proliferative capacities under little or no host control favors the growth and progression of such cells into gross tumors. The elucidation at the molecular level of the mechanisms of action of carcinogenic agents may well lead to control of the appearance of tumors in humans and to further appreciation of the roles of environmental factors in carcinogenesis in man.

The Detection and Evaluation of the Carcinogenic Activity of Chemicals

The chemicals known to be carcinogenic in man were detected from epidemiological studies on small population groups with high exposures to specific chemicals or chemical mixtures. The chemicals recognized as carcinogenic in man comprise certain soots, tars, and oils, including cigarette smoke tar (which are mixtures of aliphatic and aromatic hydrocarbons and many other compounds) that are active in the skin or lungs, or both; a variety of aromatic amines that are active in the urinary bladder; an aromatic nitrogen mustard active in the urinary bladder; sulfur mustard gas that is active in the lungs; nickel compounds active in the lungs and nasal sinuses; chromium compounds active in the lungs; and forms of asbestos active in the lungs and pleura. All these agents are carcinogenic in experimental animals. Inorganic arsenic compounds are under high suspicion of being carcinogenic in man but have so far proven inactive in experimental animals.

A large variety and number of synthetic chemical carcinogens have been discovered in the past four decades by accident and by design. It is the existence of these chemical carcinogens, the present knowledge of chemical carcinogenesis in man and experimental animals, and the necessary wide and increasing use of chemicals in the modern world that have given rise to concern and to legislation on the carcinogenic hazards to humans of the chemicals in the environment. Now this concern is increased by our knowledge of a small but increasing number of naturally occurring chemical carcinogens.

For both practical and ethical reasons, the carcinogenic activities of chemicals to which humans may be exposed are determined in experimental animals. Rats, mice, and hamsters are used in these tests because of their relatively short (2–3 yr) life span and because most of our knowledge of chemical carcinogenesis has been obtained with these species. Protocols for such tests, their limitations, and their role in the evaluation of carcinogenic hazards of chemicals for man have been considered extensively in the past decade.[7,57,59,62,70,199] The species differences in

activity of various chemical carcinogens are presently not predictable
and constitute a principal limitation to the extrapolation of results from
experimental animals to man. Another major uncertainty in such extrap-
olations derives from the statistical inadequacy of the size of groups of
experimental animals (rarely over 100 animals) that are practical in carcinogenicity tests. Such bioassays are incapable of detecting incidences
below a few percent and thus reveal only the activity of relatively potent
chemical carcinogens. Incidences far below these levels would be unacceptable in human populations. In order to minimize the insensitivity of
tests on small groups of animals and the species differences between man
and experimental animals, it is common to conduct carcinogenicity tests
with dosages at the highest level consistent with survival of the test
species for a large fraction of the normal life span. These dosage levels
may be several orders of magnitude greater than man might experience.
These uncertainties make it necessary to evaluate both positive and negative results in carcinogenicity tests with considerable caution.

Evidence that a substance is carcinogenic in one or more test species
raises the suspicion that it would be carcinogenic in man. Negative
results in these tests pose uncertainties of safety that must be judged from
the stringency of the tests and the level of exposure expected in man.
These uncertainties must be balanced against any benefits to be gained
from any uses of the chemical in question. A great need exists for dis-
criminating studies on the comparative metabolism of chemical carcinogens and their noncarcinogenic congeners in man and in experimental
animals. Some new approaches to these problems have been outlined
recently.[127]

It will be noted that most of the agents described below have been
administered to test animals by the oral route. This is the route of
choice for substances present in foods. Various parenteral routes of administration, especially injection into the subcutaneous tissue, have also
been used in carcinogenicity tests. The results of tests by subcutaneous
injection in rodents must be carefully evaluated, since in the rat and
some other rodents carcinogenesis occurs in connective tissue near intact
and smooth implants of sufficient area of almost every substance studied
(cellophane, nylon, teflon, silver, platinum, etc.). In general, the formation of sarcomas with subcutaneous implants of these substances occurs
late (usually after 1 yr). The incidence of tumor-bearing animals may be
low or as high as 50%. Likewise, sarcomas develop in similar fashion
after repeated subcutaneous injections in rats of certain vehicles (some
oils, cholesterol, etc.) and surface-active solutions. Tumor formation
under such conditions usually follows abnormal connective-tissue responses to the foreign body in the subcutaneous tissue. These phenom-

ena of "smooth surface" or "foreign body" carcinogenesis must be considered in evaluating the results of tests for carcinogenicity that are conducted in the subcutaneous tissue of rodents.[15,33,70,71] As Grasso *et al.*[71] suggest, "such local sarcomas in the rat, produced by long-continued repeated injections into the same subcutaneous site, do not constitute a valid index of chemical carcinogenicity for purposes of safety evaluation."

INDIVIDUAL AGENTS THAT CAN INDUCE TUMORS

From Fungi

Ergot Ergot is a term used to designate the fungus *Claviceps purpurea* that grows on rye and certain other grasses, and it is the name of the dried sclerotia of this fungus. Ergot contains many alkaloids and other physiologically active substances. Nelson *et al.*[132] noted in 1942 that when ergot was fed to rats as 5% of the diet for 2 yr, about one half of the rats developed multiple neurofibromas of the ears. None of these uncommon neoplasms were observed in control rats. When administration of the ergot was stopped, most of these benign tumors regressed and disappeared, but they reappeared when feeding of the ergot was resumed. This observation with ergot does not appear to have been investigated further. Relatively recently, Tannenbaum *et al.*[186] noted a low (7%) incidence of similar tumors in the ears of rats about 1 yr after IP administration of the synthetic chemical carcinogen urethan (ethyl carbamate) during the preweaning period.

Luteoskyrin and Cyclochlorotine Stored rice is quite susceptible to contamination by many fungi, especially *Penicillium* and *Aspergillus* species. Heavy mold growth and accumulation of fungal pigments may color the rice yellow and render it bitter and useless as human food. Such contaminated rice, depending on the fungi present, may produce toxic symptoms upon ingestion by humans or rats and mice. In the past several decades many Japanese workers have intensively investigated the chemical, biochemical, and biological aspects of this problem.

Several fungi that grow on rice produce toxins, and much attention has been devoted to metabolites of *Penicillium* species. Strains of one of these, *P. islandicum* Sopp, have produced hepatotoxic metabolites that can induce liver neoplasms in rats and mice. The initial findings were reported in 1951 by Tsunoda,[191] who noted liver cirrhosis in rats fed diets containing cereals contaminated by the mold. The results of the

many subsequent investigations at the University of Tokyo were summarized in 1965 by the group leaders Miyake and Saito[130] and in 1971
by Saito et al.[157] Continuous feeding of diets containing small to large
percentages of the mold produced a wide range of pathologic changes in
the livers of rats and mice, including acute atrophy at high levels of administration, and nodular hyperplasia, bile duct hyperplasia, fibrosis,
and cirrhosis at lower levels. Rats and mice surviving the lower levels of
intake for more than 1 yr showed low incidences of adenomatous lesions
and hepatomas. Fractionation of the toxic mold revealed a lipophilic
toxin and a hydrophilic toxin. The yellow lipophilic component,

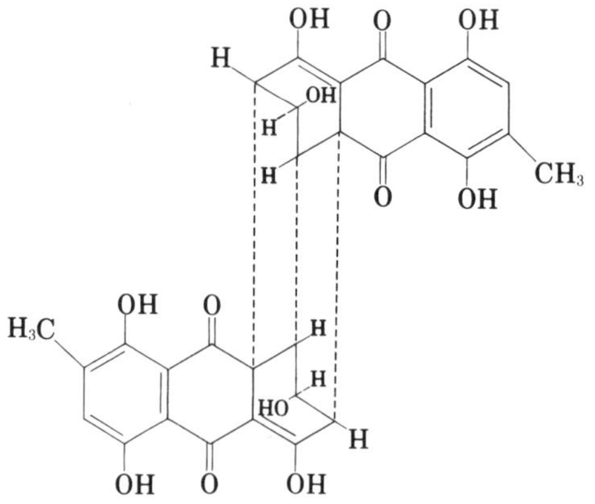

(−)-Luteoskyrin

(−)–luteoskyrin, is a substituted *bis*-polyhydroxydihydroanthraquinone
and the present concept of its structure[162] is shown herein. The hydrophilic component, cyclochlorotine, is a cyclic pentapeptide containing
residues of a dichloroproline, α-aminobutyric acid, serine, β-amino-β-
phenylbutyric acid, and serine—in that order.[95,157] Chronic daily ingestion of a few tenths of a milligram of (−)–luteoskyrin by mice for 2 yr
produced liver adenomas and hepatomas; the hepatoma-inducing property of (−)–luteoskyrin in mice has been confirmed in other experiments. The water-soluble cyclochlorotine is a more potent acute hepatotoxin. Chronic administration of this compound has yielded only a
low incidence of liver tumors in mice. Further data have recently appeared on the hepatocarcinogenicity of (−)–luteoskyrin and cyclochlorotine in mice.[197] Islanditoxin,[157] a toxic cyclic peptide isomeric with
cyclochlorotine, was originally thought to be identical with the latter
compound.

Both (−)–luteoskyrin and cyclochlorotine are cytotoxic to liver and
HeLa cells *in vitro*[196]; (−)–luteoskyrin inhibited DNA synthesis and

produced chromosome aberrations in cultures of Ehrlich ascites tumor cells.[164] $(-)$–Luteoskyrin forms a complex *in vitro* with native DNA in the presence of Mg^{++}, which appears to involve the pyrimidine bases.[192-194] This may be the basis of its inhibition of DNA-dependent RNA polymerase in *E. coli*[195] and of nuclear-RNA synthesis in Ehrlich ascites tumor cells.[195]

Aflatoxins   Aside from its intrinsic value, the story of the aflatoxins is important in that it increased the interest of workers in many disciplines in mycotoxins. Hopefully this interest will be long lasting, because these substances and their biological effects are so poorly known. Furthermore, it is now recognized that monitoring of foods for these substances is a necessary ongoing task. The aflatoxin story began with the outbreak in England in 1960 of "turkey X disease." This acute hepatic disease led to severe losses of turkey poults, and its cause was traced to diets containing peanut meals contaminated with the mold *Aspergillus flavus.* The rapid resolution of this problem and its continuing study is an outstanding example of interdisciplinary cooperation. A massive literature on aflatoxins now exists, and the reader is referred primarily to the collection of reviews entitled *Aflatoxin*[65] and *Mycotoxins in Foodstuffs*[203] and to the recent comprehensive reviews of Lillehoj, Ciegler, and Detroy[113] and Detroy, Lillehoj, and Ciegler[44] on fungal toxins.

Following extraction of contaminated peanut meals and cultures of *A. flavus* strains with solvents, the hepatotoxins (now named the aflatoxins) were recognized by their fluorescence, chromatographic separability, and high biological activity in such sensitive systems as the hepatotoxicity assay in day-old ducklings. Two principal toxins, aflatoxins B_1 and G_1 and their less toxic dihydro derivatives, aflatoxins B_2 and G_2, are formed by the molds. The aflatoxins are relatively stable to heat but can be destroyed by alkali, hypochlorite, and other chemical treatments. The aflatoxins are also formed by some fungi other than strains of *A. flavus.*

The infection of such crops as peanuts with these toxic molds appears to occur during improper harvesting and storage procedures, particularly under conditions of high humidity. Prevention of mold growth by humidity control appears to be the primary need, since no generally satisfactory method of removal of the toxins from feeds and foods is yet available. Peanut oils are free of the aflatoxins because of the alkaline treatment they receive during processing.

The biological properties of the aflatoxins in mammals are manifested primarily in the liver. Acute dosage leads to periportal necrosis and to

death in a few days. The LD$_{50}$ of aflatoxin B$_1$ for such sensitive animals
as the 1-day-old duckling or young rat and rainbow trout is about 0.5
mg/kg of body weight. The values are higher for older animals of these
species and for animals of other species. Except for sheep, which are
relatively resistant, chronic dosage leads to moderate to severe liver
damage in all species that have been studied. In addition to the rat,
duck, and rainbow trout, the sensitive species include the hamster,
mouse, ferret, rabbit, guinea pig, dog, cow, swine, and rhesus monkey.

The hepatic damage includes acute necrosis and hemorrhage, chronic
fibrosis, bile-duct hyperplasia, and regenerative nodules. In addition,
hepatocellular carcinomas have been observed in rats, ducks, rainbow
trout, ferrets, and, to a limited extent, in mice, guinea pigs, and sheep.
The aflatoxins have also been implicated in the formation of limited
numbers of tumors in the glandular stomach, kidney, and some other
tissues of certain animals.[26,205]

Aflatoxin B$_1$ appears to be the most potent hepatocarcinogen known.
Moderate to high incidences of hepatomas and hepatocellular carcinomas have occurred in rats administered continuously only 15 ppb of
aflatoxin in the diet.[205] At this dose level (0.2 μg/day; total dosage of
approximately 100 μg), all of the rats had liver tumors after 476 days.
A single oral dose somewhat above this total dosage did not produce

Aflatoxin B$_1$ (B$_2$)

liver tumors, but single oral doses of 5 mg of aflatoxin/kg of body
weight have induced hepatomas in the rat.[31] Dietary levels of 30 and 2
ppb, respectively, were hepatocarcinogenic in the duckling and rainbow
trout.[30,75] With subcutaneous injections, hepatic lesions are seen only
when large amounts of the aflatoxins are injected, but repeated subcutaneous injections of 10–20 μg of aflatoxins B$_1$ and G$_1$ induced sarcomas in rats and mice.[45] Orally administered aflatoxin G$_1$ appears to be
somewhat less carcinogenic in the rat liver than aflatoxin B$_1$; however,
G$_1$ appeared to be more active than B$_1$ in inducing kidney tumors in
the rat.[27]

Aflatoxin G$_1$ (G$_2$)

Only limited data are available on the metabolism of the aflatoxins *in vivo* and *in vitro*.[113] Ingestion of aflatoxin B$_1$ leads to the appearance of aflatoxins M$_1$ and M$_2$ (4-hydroxy-aflatoxin B$_1$ and 4-hydroxy-aflatoxin B$_2$, respectively) in the milk and urine of several species. Aflatoxin M$_1$ is approximately as toxic as aflatoxin B$_1$. Aflatoxin B$_1$ is metabolized *in vitro* to aflatoxin M$_1$ by an oxidative NADPH-dependent system in rat and mouse liver microsomes.[144] Aflatoxin M$_1$ appears in human urine after the ingestion of peanut butter contaminated with aflatoxin, and its excretion is being studied as a means of evaluating the ingestion of aflatoxin by humans.[29] A new metabolite of aflatoxin B$_1$, aflatoxin P$_1$ (a phenolic desmethyl derivative), has been found in the urine of rhesus monkeys.[43]

Little evidence is available on the possible mechanism of action of aflatoxin B$_1$ as a hepatocarcinogen. Hypophysectomy nearly abolishes the carcinogenicity of the aflatoxins (from contaminated peanut meal) in the rat liver, while the carcinogenicity of dimethylnitrosamine in this tissue is not affected by this endocrine ablation.[66] Aflatoxin B$_1$ binds to proteins and nucleic acids only weakly *in vitro*, but tritiated aflatoxin B$_1$ binds strongly to these molecules in the rat liver *in vivo* although there is no obvious correlation of these gross bindings with carcinogenicity.[111] These and other findings[64,163] suggest that aflatoxin B$_1$, despite its amazing potency as a carcinogen, must be metabolically activated to be carcinogenic and to be reactive *in vivo*. Likewise, treatment with aflatoxin B$_1$ *in vivo* leads to large decreases in hepatic RNA-polymerase activity, but the toxin exhibits little activity against this system *in vitro*.[113] The effects of aflatoxin B$_1$ on the nuclei of cell cultures[47] suggest the action of an alkylating agent; so far, however, metabolic studies of structure versus activity of aflatoxin B$_1$ have provided little idea of what the structures of such alkylating agents might be. The ability of aflatoxin B$_1$ to induce subcutaneous sarcomas upon injection at this site does not constitute evidence that this agent is a carcinogen per se. On the same basis, the polycylic aromatic hydrocarbons were once thought to be carcinogenic per se, but much data from metabolic and carcinogenicity studies have shown that activation of these carcinogens is required.

The marked differences in geographical distribution of liver cancer in humans have long suggested the presence of special contributing factors in areas with high incidences of this neoplasm.[81] The earlier findings on the hepatocarcinogenicity of low doses of the pyrrolizidine alkaloids (see below) in the rat gave rise to the suggestion that these toxins might be involved.[166] Similarly, associations have been suggested for viral hepatitis and for severe protein malnutrition with hepatic neoplasms in the human, but none of these factors has appeared adequate to account for the large differences in incidence of human hepatic tumors in different areas of the world.[82,204] Thus it was natural to causally connect the occurrence of the aflatoxins in parts of Africa with high incidences of hepatic tumors in the native human population.[32,137] Unfortunately there are no direct data that show a parallelism between acute or chronic toxicity or carcinogenic risk in humans and the intake of the aflatoxins. Nevertheless, there are highly suggestive reports[143,152] that associate nonneoplastic liver pathology in humans with aflatoxin intakes. A recent report[29] on the high level of the aflatoxins in some locally manufactured peanut butters in the Philippines is certainly indicative of the possible risk. Surveys are in progress or have been completed in parts of Africa and Thailand to determine the degree of contamination of human foodstuffs with the aflatoxins.[1,176,177,179-181,204] Similar surveys are needed in other areas (such as Central and South America) with similar climatic conditions and with known aflatoxin contamination of peanut crops but with no unusual incidence of human hepatocellular carcinoma. Wogan[204] has provided a useful discussion of these problems.

Sterigmatocystin   This difuranoxanthone is a close relative of the aflatoxins and is formed by several *Aspergillus* species. It is less toxic than aflatoxin B_1 in the rat and is at least an order of magnitude less carcinogenic than aflatoxin B_1, both in the subcutaneous tissue of the rat upon repeated injection[45] and in the liver of this species following oral administration.[147] In the latter study tumors in several other tissues were noted, and papillomatous lesions occurred in the stomachs of most of the treated rats. Sterigmatocystin produced only hepatocellular carcinomas in the rat with no bile-duct proliferation and no cholangiocarcinoma formation. Purchase and van der Watt[147] discuss this and other aspects of the hepatocarcinogenicity of sterigmatocystin in the rat in relation to its possible importance as a hepatocarcinogenic mycotoxin in certain native human populations.

Sterigmatocystin

Griseofulvin Griseofulvin is a polycyclic chlorine-containing antibiotic formed by several *Penicillium* species. Several ring-substituted derivatives of griseofulvin are also produced by these fungi. Griseofulvin is administered in repeated large oral doses for prolonged periods in the therapy of several human cutaneous mycoses for which topical agents are ineffective.[3,5] In the human the ingestion of griseofulvin leads to its occurrence in peripheral keratinized tissues.[3,156] Barich *et al.*[12] found that continuous administration of 1% of griseofulvin in the diet to mice increased the incidence and size of skin tumors that formed following the topical application of the synthetic carcinogen 3-methylcholanthrene. Some cocarcinogenic effect was also noted with 0.01% of the antibiotic in the diet; this level is roughly comparable to the human dosage levels of this agent. Other studies[11,92] with the chronic feeding of 0.05 to 1% of griseofulvin in the diet to male mice demonstrated its ability to induce liver damage and hepatomas in this species. Similar or higher oral doses and duration of administration of griseofulvin are employed in the human. These hepatotoxic effects of griseofulvin were confirmed and extended by a recent report[51] that in male mice several subcutaneous doses of griseofulvin (total dose of 3 mg) before weaning led to liver pathology and a marked increase in hepatoma incidence over that in the control mice.

Griseofulvin

In the rat the injection of griseofulvin leads to arrest of the cells in metaphase in the bone marrow and intestinal crypts.[140] In fungi sensitive to griseofulvin this antibiotic binds to nucleic acids and proteins.[50]

Other Mold Metabolites   A variety of other mold metabolites has been found to induce sarcomas after repeated injections in the subcutaneous tissues of rats and mice. These include various lactones and such related compounds as patulin, penicillin G, and penicillic acid in tests in rats.[36,45] Likewise, some extracts of fungi pathogenic for man have been found to induce sarcomas in mice following repeated injections in the subcutaneous tissue.[16]

From Actinomycetes

The actinomycetes are a group of unicellular branching organisms that reproduce by fission or by forming conidia. They form a mycelium and have been considered as higher filamentous bacteria, possibly occupying a position between bacteria and fungi. The following agents are elaborated by various *Streptomyces* species and were found to induce neoplasia in rats or mice by parenteral administration. Tests of these and similar substances by the oral route are needed.

Actinomycin D   This cyclic polypeptide lactone–phenoxazone forms a specific and tight complex with DNA and is widely employed in biology as an inhibitor of DNA-directed RNA synthesis and as an antitumor agent. Kawamata *et al.*[97] and DiPaolo[46] have obtained sarcomas at the site of subcutaneous injection of repeated μg doses of actinomycin D. Svoboda *et al.*[184] produced invasive mesotheliomas in rats injected repeatedly IP with doses of actinomycin D totaling only a few tenths of a mg. Similar doses of this compound given intravenously did not produce tumors. Similarly, no tumors were produced by heavier IP dosing of rats

Actinomycin D

with actinocylgramicidin S, which has the same chromophore as actinomycin D but a different cyclic peptide component. The latter compound does not complex with DNA. Another *Streptomyces* metabolite, actidione or cycloheximide, was also tested intraperitoneally in rats, and no tumors were noted. This antibiotic is well known to inhibit protein synthesis at the level of translation.

Mitomycin C This antibiotic has also been used in cancer therapy, and it is employed biologically to cross link DNA. It acquires the latter property, and possibly the former too, after its benzoquinone function is reduced and a methoxy group is lost. In the resulting structure the allyic ester and aziridine groups permit the molecule to act as a bifunctional alkylating agent.[185] Thus, it is of interest that Ikegami *et al.*[93] found that repeated injections subcutaneously of μg quantities of mito-

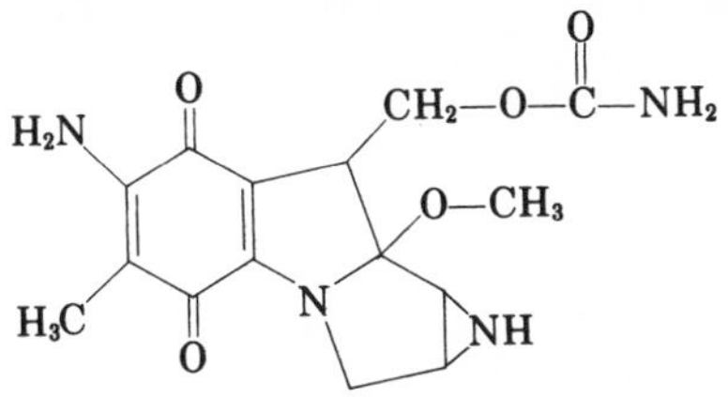

Mitomycin C (Oxidized)

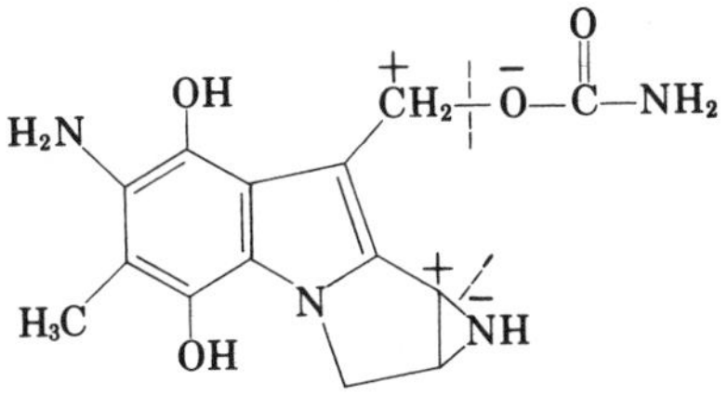

Mitomycin C (Reduced, —CH₃OH)

mycin C produced sarcomas at the site of administration. The active reduced form of mitomycin C is closely related to the reactive metabolic pyrroles derived from the pyrrolizidine alkaloids (see above).

Streptozotocin and Elaiomycin These two *Streptomyces* metabolites are considered together because of similarities in their structures. They should also be compared structurally with the plant metabolite cycasin described elsewhere in this chapter. These nitrosamide and azoxy compounds, respectively, are probably metabolized to form alkylating species *in vivo*. Schoental[168] observed single cases of tumors in a wide variety of tissues in rats 1–2 yr after intragastric or parenteral administration of elaiomycin. Streptozotocin, a broad-spectrum antibiotic and mutagenic agent with antitumor properties, exhibited far stronger carcinogenic properties than elaiomycin. Arison and Feudale[8] found that after a single IV injection of 50 mg/kg, 12 of 23 rats developed kidney cortex tumors during the following 16 months.

Streptozotocin

Elaiomycin

From Bacteria

To the author's knowledge, only the following compounds have been reported as carcinogens formed by bacteria. Few tests for carcinogenic activity have been made with bacterial metabolites, and further examples will surely be found.

Ethionine[58,182] Ethionine, the *S*-ethyl analog of methionine, was designed as a synthetic antagonist of methionine. It is toxic in several rodent species and causes morphological changes in the liver, pancreas, and other tissues that are counteracted by the administration of methionine. It was further noted that chronic feeding of 0.25% of ethionine in the diet of rats results in a high incidence of hepatocellular carcinomas; golden hamsters did not develop tumors under these conditions. In the rat, ethionine is incorporated into protein of several tissues through the pathway normally used for incorporation of methionine. Alkylation of the nucleic acids by the *S*-ethyl group, especially in the tRNA's, occurs essentially only in the liver of the rat. *S*-Adenosyl ethionine is formed in the rat liver from ethionine by the same enzymatic pathway employed for the formation of *S*-adenosyl methionine. However, evidence[139] has been obtained that suggests that *S*-adenosyl ethionine may not be the principal ethyl donor for the transfer nucleic acids in the rat liver.

Many of the above studies with ethionine as a synthetic carcinogen had been completed before it was noted that ethionine is a metabolite of several bacteria, including *E. coli,* grown in a salts–glucose medium containing sulfate ion or methionine.[59] Algal, yeast, or certain tumor cells grown under the same conditions did not form ethionine. The bacterially synthesized ethionine was not incorporated into the bacterial protein. It would be interesting to know the extent to which mammals are exposed to ethionine formed by bacteria in the caecum and large intestine. In the rodent, for example, coprophagy is common and might increase the amount absorbed. A search for ethionine in the rumen contents and milk of ruminants would be worthwhile.

Nitrosamines   The carcinogenic nitrosamines are discussed in some detail below under products of green plants. These compounds are readily formed from various secondary amines and nitrite at acid pH. Nitrosamines are also formed by certain bacteria at neutral pH from these compounds; some bacteria can also reduce nitrate to nitrite. The bacterial synthesis of nitrosamines was first observed by Sander[159] for several nitrate-reducing enterobacteria, and this has been confirmed with the flora of the rat intestine[100] and with human non-nitrate–reducing intestinal bacteria.[78] The nitrosamines synthesized in this way include the potent carcinogen dimethylnitrosamine. Dimethylamine for this synthesis can be derived from the bacterial degradation of choline from lecithin. Bacterially derived nitrosamines should receive consideration in the genesis of colon cancer in the human. The incidence of this disease and the species of gut flora show great geographical variation.[82,83]

Polycyclic Aromatic Hydrocarbons   Recent reports claim that certain bacteria can synthesize polycyclic aromatic hydrocarbons such as the carcinogen benzo(a)pyrene and the noncarcinogen perylene (*peri*-di-naphthalene). Microgram quantities of benzo(a)pyrene appeared to be formed in 100-g samples of sterilized forest soil inoculated with *Cl. putride* or *E. coli* and incubated at room temperature for 6 months.[118] Similarly, peptone broths supplemented with naphthalene acetic acid or vitamin K_1 and incubated with *B. badius* for 7 days at 37 °C formed a few tenths of a μg/liter of benzo(a)pyrene and perylene.[134] The apparent biosynthesis of these hydrocarbons in green plants is described below.

From Green Plants

Pyrrolizidine Alkaloids   Some of these compounds were among the first natural products claimed to be carcinogenic. Although some doubt exists as to their carcinogenicity, there is no doubt that many of these alkaloids are very potent liver and lung toxins. A large literature exists on the chemistry and biological properties of the pyrrolizidine alkaloids, and it has been critically evaluated in a recent monograph by Bull *et al.*[24] and in a more recent review by E. K. McLean,[124] which complement each other. According to Bull *et al.*, the pyrrolizidine alkaloids are the only known hepatotoxic alkaloids.

Acute and chronic poisoning of farm livestock by pyrrolizidine alkaloids from a wide range of plant species (*Senecio, Crotolaria, Heliotropium,* and other genera) has been recognized in many parts of the world and dates back to the latter part of the last century. In man, only acute poisoning has been observed as a result of the occasional contamination of cereals and through the use of native herbal medicines or "bush teas." In laboratory rodents and farm livestock, large doses of the poisons produce acute necrotic and vascular lesions in the liver. Smaller chronic doses produce progressive lesions in the liver and lungs. The liver lesions, especially in young animals, are characterized by the formation of very large parenchymal cells or megalocytes.[23,96] The toxic pyrrolizidine alkaloids appear to have strong antimitotic effects. In man the acute poisoning appears to involve hepatic necrosis and a collagenous occlusion of small branches of the venous tree leading to a "veno-occlusive" disease; progression to a largely nonportal cirrhosis occurs. Megalocytosis of the liver has not yet been observed in young or adult humans.

These alkaloids are derived from the pyrrolizidine nucleus, and the cell toxins are primarily branched-chain esters of the nontoxic unsaturated carbinol retronecine. Toxicity appears to depend on the presence of the nuclear double bond and on the presence of an ester of the carbinol with branched chains in the ester function.[165] These require-

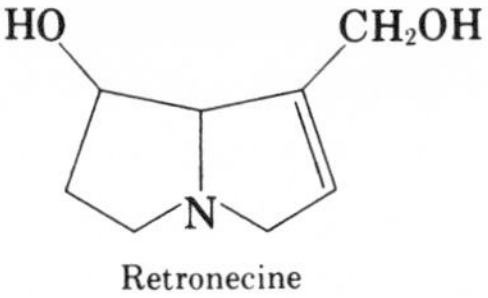

Retronecine

ments for toxicity are exemplified in the structures of heliotrine and the macrocycles senecionine and retrorsine. (See Figure 1.) The toxic pyrrolizidine alkaloids thus are branched-chain allylic esters. In accordance with the susceptibility of allylic esters to attack by strong nucleophiles, heliotrine alkylates benzyl mercaptan in alkaline solution through cleavage of the carbon–oxygen bond under conditions where the competing hydrolytic cleavage of the ester is very slow. This reaction led Culvenor et al.[41] to suggest that this alkylating ability might be the basis of the toxicity of the pyrrolizidine alkaloids in the cell nucleus. The weak reactivity of the pyrrolizidine alkaloids at physiological pH, however, suggested that a metabolic activation step occurred *in vivo*. Recently, Mattocks[121,122] has provided remarkable biochemical and chemical evidence that toxic pyrrolizidine alkaloids are dehydrogenated enzymatically in rat liver to highly reactive pyrroles as shown in Figure 1. (Compare this with the reduced form of mitomycin C discussed above.) These pyrroles act as alkylating agents and become bound to cellular macromolecules. Culvenor and his associates[42] have observed similar

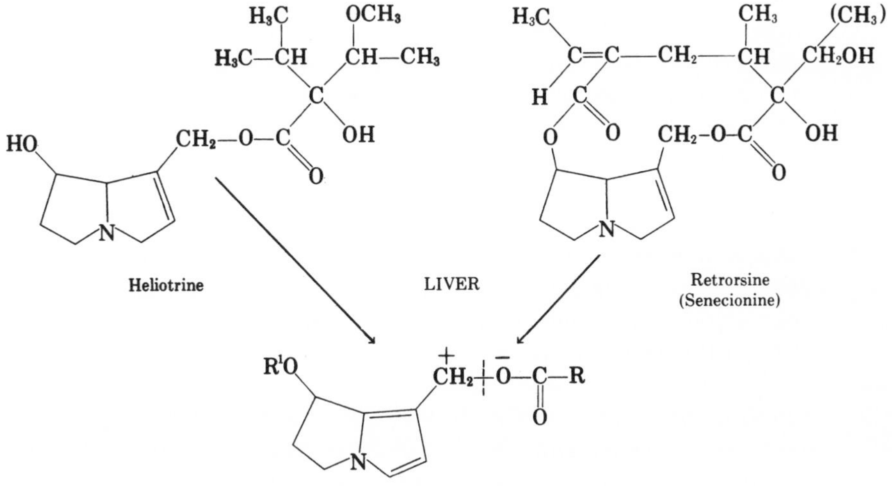

FIGURE 1 Metabolism of toxic pyrrolizidine alkaloids.

reactions. Recent relatively direct evidence obtained by Butler et al.[28] following intravenous injection indicates strongly that these pyrrole metabolites are responsible for the vascular lesions induced in the liver and lungs by the pyrrolizidine alkaloids. Similar data by Mattocks[123] also show that the nature of acid moieties in the pyrrole metabolites is not critical at the sites of toxic action. The recent argument[169] that epoxide metabolites play a role in carcinogenesis by the pyrrolizidine alkaloids is not supported by recent data of Culvenor et al.[40] on the low toxicities of the α- and β-epoxides of monocrotaline.

Most of the evidence for the hepatocarcinogenic activity of pyrrolizidine alkaloids has been obtained by Schoental and her associates[39,170-173]; Schoental,[167] Bull et al.,[24] and McLean[124] have reviewed these data recently. Most of the hepatomas observed have been obtained in the rat with single or interrupted administration of certain of the alkaloids (generally retrorsine and its N-oxide isatidine) in animals surviving for more than 1 yr. Tumor incidences of up to 25% of the animals have been noted, and no such tumors were noted in the control animals. Similar and even higher incidences of liver tumors were more recently described in rats fed intermittently a diet containing 0.5% of dried Senecio longilobus.[77] The negative experiments carried out by Bull et al. did not employ retrorsine or isatidine; frequent small doses of alkaloid derived from Crotolaria and Heliotropium were administered to rats that survived 3–11 months. The lack of reports of liver tumors in livestock poisoned with pyrrolizidine alkaloids is not meaningful, since few of these animals are kept for a major part of the generally long life spans of these species, and few are subjected to careful autopsies. Likewise, although the pyrrolizidine alkaloids have been suspected in the etiology of the high incidences of liver disease and hepatocellular neoplasms in certain human populations in Africa and elsewhere, no sound evidence exists to incriminate them in this regard. Neither megalocytosis nor neoplasms have been reported in the livers of patients exposed to pyrrolizidine alkaloids and with acute and chronic liver disease. In summary, it appears that relatively low interrupted doses of some pyrrolizidine alkaloids are hepatocarcinogenic in the rat and that the reactive electrophilic pyrrole metabolites of these compounds may initiate the chain of events leading to these neoplasms.

Safrole and Related Compounds   Safrole, or 1-allyl-3,4-methylenedioxybenzene (see Figure 2), is a minor constituent of several spices and a frequent and even major component of some essential oils such as oil of sassafras. (See Chapter 20.) It is a natural ingredient of sassafras tea. Until recently, safrole was used as a flavoring agent in root beers, but its

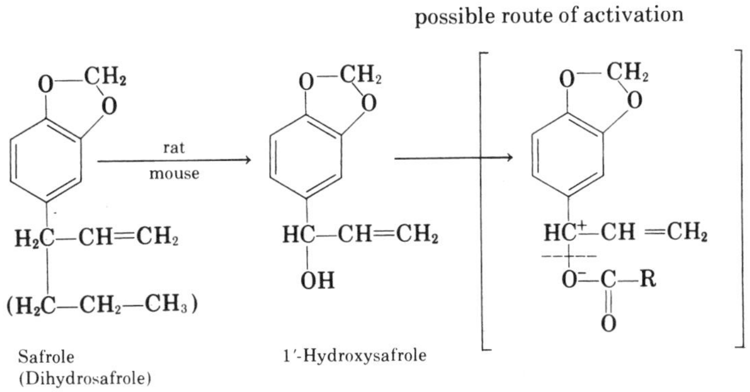

possible route of activation

FIGURE 2 Metabolism of safrole in rats and mice.

use there was withdrawn after it was noted that prolonged ingestion of high levels (0.5% of the diet) of safrole by adult rats led to the formation of liver tumors.[87,88,115] Under these conditions, one group[115] reported the occurrence of liver neoplasms in 19 of 50 rats; 14 of the rats bore malignant hepatomas. No liver pathology was noted in the control rats. Other liver damage was induced in the rat by safrole, which has long been recognized to be hepatotoxic (even in man) at high levels of administration. Subcutaneous injection of safrole in tricaprylin in infant male Swiss mice[52] at total doses of 0.66 and 6.6 mg per mouse led to hepatoma incidences of 50–58% at 1 yr; low incidences of pulmonary tumors were also noted in these mice. The uninjected and solvent-injected control male mice developed a 5–6% incidence of hepatomas and no pulmonary tumors. No hepatomas occurred in untreated or treated female mice under these conditions.

Only a few compounds related to safrole have been tested for carcinogenic activity. Isosafrole (1-propenyl-3,4-methylenedioxybenzene) was only weakly active in inducing liver tumors when fed to male mice.[94] In the same study, dihydrosafrole (*p-n*-propylmethylenedioxybenzene) was moderately active in producing hepatic tumors in male and female mice. In an earlier study[114] administration of 1% of dihydrosafrole (see Figure 2) in the diet to rats gave rise to esophageal tumors but no liver tumors.

Many compounds related to safrole occur naturally, and several such compounds (e.g., sesamol, sesamolin, and sesamin) are minor components of the edible sesame oil. Sesamol (1-hydroxy-3,4-methylenedioxybenzene) appeared to increase the incidence of benign "proliferative lesions" in rats administered 1% of this compound in the diet for several months.[2] Other compounds even more closely related to safrole in structure occur in many essential oils and in spices. These include myristicin (1-allyl-3-methoxy-4,5-methylenedioxybenzene), apiol (1-allyl-3,6-dimethoxy-4,5-methylenedioxybenzene), eugenol (1-allyl-3-methoxy-4-hydroxybenzene), and asarone (1-propenyl-2,4,5-trimethoxybenzene). The latter compound is a major component of oil of calamus (see below).

Relatively little work has been done on the metabolism of safrole and related compounds in relation to carcinogenic activity. These compounds do not appear to contain particularly reactive groups and probably are activated by metabolism. Recently it has been found[19,202] that rats and mice metabolize safrole to the more toxic compound 1′-hydroxysafrole (see Figure 2) and that this metabolite is considerably more carcinogenic than safrole in the livers of rats by the oral route and in the livers of mice upon subcutaneous injection.[202] A synthetic ester of this metabolite, 1′-acetoxysafrole, has electrophilic activity against nucleophiles such as methionine and guanosine-5′-phosphate.

Oil of Calamus   This essential oil is derived from the dried rhizome of *Acorus calamus.* The rhizome and oil are used as flavoring agents in foods at levels below 5 ppm and up to 10–30 ppm in bitters and liqueurs. A recent study[74,187] of the toxicity of oil of calamus in rats fed up to 5,000 ppm for up to 2 yr showed a dose-related formation of malignant mesenchymal tumors of the small intestine. β-Asarone, a structural relative of safrole, is a principal component of oil of calamus.

Cycasin   This toxic glucoside (see Figure 3) occurs in the pulp and husk of the cycad nut as well as in other parts of the palm-like cycad trees (*Cycas circinalis* and other species in the family *Cycadaceae*). Many of these species inhabit tropical and subtropical regions and can survive drought and hurricanes. The cycads have provided emergency and staple food and medicines for natives of these regions for a long time. The native populations have been well aware of the toxic properties (acute jaundice, hemorrhage, and chronic partial paralysis) of food from this source. The toxin is removed from the sliced nuts and pith by repeated soaking in many changes of water. The sun-dried and ground starch, and indeed all parts of the plant, often without extraction by water, have been used as food. The toxicity and the use of cycads as food, medicine, and fodder for livestock have been well reviewed by Whiting.[201]

Many investigations on the toxic principles in the cycads culminated in the isolation of a series of glycosides with a common aglycone by Nishida *et al.*[136] in Japan and by Riggs[150] in Australia. The principal glycoside is cycasin, the β-glucoside of methylazoxymethanol (MAM). (See Figure 3.)

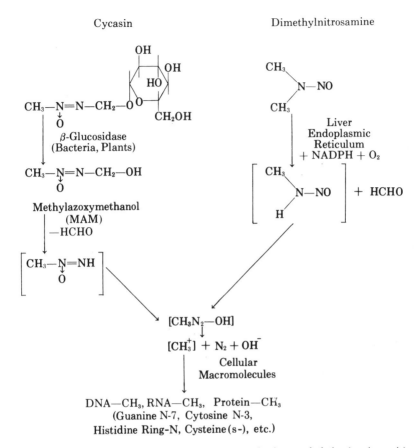

FIGURE 3 Conversion of cycasin and dimethylnitrosamine into methylating (carcinogenic) species.

The recent interest in the cycads and cycasin developed from studies on the paralytic conditions noted in cattle and in natives where cycads are frequently used for food.[201] Attempts to produce neurological damage in experimental animals by cycad nuts or their components have had only limited success, but the unextracted nuts were found to be highly carcinogenic when fed to rats, especially in the liver and kidney.[106] Tumor induction with cycasin has also been noted in mice, guinea pigs, hamsters, and fish. These and many other aspects of the cycads and cycasin have been reviewed recently by Laqueur and Spatz.[107] Cycasin, via conversion to its unstable aglycone, methylazoxymethanol, appears to be responsible for these carcinogenic effects.[84,101,103-105,120] This conversion (see Figure 3) depends on the action of bacterial β-glucosidase in the intestinal tract; this enzyme is absent from rat tissues except for its temporary presence in the subcutaneous tissue of newborn and early postnatal animals. As a result, cycasin has proved to be toxic and carcinogenic when fed to conventional rats but not upon injection into conventional rats or upon feeding or injection into axenic or "germ-free" rats. In the latter cases the cycasin is excreted unchanged in the urine. Methylazoxymethanol, on the other hand, is carcinogenic regardless of the route of administration in both conventional and axenic rats. Methylazoxymethanol induced tumors in the rat at all the sites noted with cycasin and also induced carcinomas of the small intestine if it was administered intraperitoneally. Cycasin and methylazoxymethanol are readily transferred via the placenta to fetuses in pregnant rats, and the offspring later develop tumors. In several of these studies, the relatively more stable ester methylazoxymethanol acetate was employed. This ester is apparently hydrolyzed easily *in vivo; in vitro* it is readily cleaved by serum.[145]

The carcinogenicity of methylazoxymethanol appears to depend on its instability in neutral solution and its decomposition to an electrophilic reactant, which acts as a methylating agent.[119] The carcinogenic and biochemical properties of cycasin are very similar to those of the carcinogen dimethylnitrosamine,[178] as shown in Figure 3. After oxidative demethylation in animal tissues, dimethylnitrosamine—like cycasin— also yields a methylating species, apparently the methyl carbonium ion.[112]

Nitrosamines   Since the discovery of the carcinogenic activity of the synthetic compound dimethylnitrosamine (see Figure 3) in rats in 1956,[117] *N*-nitroso derivatives of a great variety of secondary amines (primarily aliphatic) have been found to be potent and versatile carcinogens. Considerable concern now exists that certain nitrosamines may be environmental carcinogens for man.[110,116,206] This concern derives from:

1. the wide occurrence of secondary amines in plants, plant products, and fish products, together with the wide occurrence of nitrates in water supplies and in plants;

2. the relative ease with which nitrosamines are formed from secondary amines and nitrite,[129] even at low concentrations of these reactants and especially under conditions of relatively low pH as in stomach contents;

3. the formation of nitrosamines from secondary amines and nitrite or nitrate by intestinal bacteria at neutral pH (see above under products derived from bacteria);

4. the occurrence of dimethylnitrosamine in some food plants growing in parts of the Transkei in Africa, where a molybdenum deficiency in the soil results in accumulations of nitrate in plants[25,49];

5. the finding of traces of presumed nitrosamines in grains and other foods[110,116,206];

6. the occurrence of dimethylnitrosamine in fish meals perserved with sodium nitrite and the hepatotoxicity of these meals in mink and sheep[110];

7. the permitted use in some countries (including the United States) of sodium and potassium nitrate and nitrite as preservatives and color fixatives in cured fish and meat products at levels not exceeding 500 and 200 ppm, respectively, in the finished products.

Nitrates and nitrites in animal forages and in human foods have previously been considered from the standpoint of their acute toxic effects such as in methemoglobin formation. Long-term studies with rats fed high levels of sodium nitrite gave no evidence of carcinogenic or teratogenic effects.[48] (See Chapter 1.) On the other hand, rats given high levels of nitrite and certain secondary amines easily nitrosatable at the pH of the rat stomach developed tumors characteristic of the corresponding nitrosamines.[161] A similar finding has been reported for the combined feeding of *N,N'*-dimethylurea and nitrite to rats, with the apparent production in the stomach of a carcinogenic alkyl nitrosamide.[160] The latter compounds are activated by nucleophiles such as thiols and do not require enzymatic activation as do the nitrosamines.

The importance of the nitrosamines as environmental carcinogens for man is not assessable at present, but as Lijinsky and Epstein point out,[110] reduction of human exposure to nitrates and nitrites and to certain secondary amines may be useful prophylactic measures.

Bracken Fern   This fern species (*Pteridium aquilinum*) has been known for some time to damage the bone marrow and intestinal mucosa and to induce polyps in the urinary bladder mucosa of cattle fed the whole plant or extracts thereof. A series of relatively recent reports indicates that diets containing the dried plant at high levels can produce tumors at several sites in a wide range of species: urinary bladder carcinoma in cattle,[146] urinary bladder carcinoma and intestinal adenocarcinoma in rats,[55,141,146] urinary bladder tumors in guinea pigs,[54] pulmonary adenomas in mice,[54] and intestinal adenocarcinomas in Japanese quail.[54] There appeared to be a significantly higher incidence of urinary bladder carcinomas in rats fed bracken fern and supplemented with large amounts of thiamine than in rats fed only the bracken fern diet.[142] This effect did not appear to be attributable to an antithiamine effect of the bracken fern. The thiamine supplementation had no effect on the large incidence of intestinal adenocarcinoma in these rats. A recent report[108] describes the isolation of a substance from bracken fern that is toxic in mice and is stated to be mutagenic and carcinogenic.

Bracken fern is used as human food in greens or salads in New Zealand, in the United States, and especially in Japan,[85,142] and it may contribute to the incidence of tumors in the human gastrointestinal tract in these countries.[56]

Polycyclic Aromatic Hydrocarbons   The occurrence of small amounts of such carcinogenic hydrocarbons as benzo(a)pyrene in tars and oils derived from the incomplete combustion or pyrolysis of organic matter (combustion tars, shale oil, etc.) is now well known and results from the polymerization of small hydrocarbon free radicals.[18] Many attempts have been made to detect the endogenous formation of carcinogenic polycylic aromatic hydrocarbons in animal tissues, but all have been unsuccessful.[18] It therefore comes as an unwelcome surprise to find that evidence is developing that plants can synthesize these hydrocarbons and may contain a level of benzo[a]pyrene amounting to about 10 μg/kg of

Benzo[a]pyrene

dry matter. The occurrence of trace amounts of these hydrocarbons in soil, land plants, and marine flora and fauna has been appreciated for some time[17,18] and often has been assumed to result wholly from contamination by natural and man-made pyrolyses of organic matter. However, recent work by Gräf[67-69] and by Borneff[20,21] and their co-workers suggest strongly that part of the hydrocarbons present are synthesized by the plants themselves and that they exert a strong growth-accelerating effect in plants. In a study by Borneff *et al.*[21] algae were grown in a ^{14}C-acetate medium and found to synthesize benzo(a)pyrene and other hydrocarbons with 10 times higher specific activity than algae from a control system without isotope. The significance of these low levels of carcinogenic hydrocarbons as endogenous components of plant foodstuffs for man is unknown. Man contaminates his environment and person with far greater levels of these hydrocarbons by his use of internal combustion engines, cigarettes, industrial combustions, home heating, etc.

Selenium Derivatives Compounds containing this element, at low levels (0.01–0.1 ppm as Se) in the diet, appear to act as essential nutrients for several mammalian and avian species.[138,175] At high levels in the diet these derivatives can be hepatotoxic and have been reported to induce liver tumors in rats. Inorganic selenium compounds occur naturally in many soils, and the element is incorporated into plant protein, partly as seleno-methionine and seleno-cystine. In some areas the forage contains high amounts of organic selenium compounds and is toxic to live-stock.[131] In other areas the soil is deficient in selenium compounds, and livestock fed on forage grown in these regions develop selenium-deficiency diseases.

In some experiments in the rat, selenium in the form of selenate or selenide, or as seleniferous corn or wheat,[35,133] induced liver cirrhosis and liver tumors when fed in diets at 5–10 ppm for well over a year. A later well-documented attempt[76] to observe hepatocarcinogenesis in another rat strain fed selenate or selenite in a different diet for up to 1–2 yr did not succeed, although hyperplastic liver lesions occurred in rats fed the selenium compounds. A recent report[174] has claimed that 3 ppm of sodium selenite in the drinking water for 2 yr increased the incidence of benign and malignant tumors in rats. For a variety of reasons, none of these findings is conclusive evidence for or against hepatocarcinogenicity of selenium derivatives, and further work, especially with long-term studies of several rat strains in the same laboratory, is desirable.

Antithyroid Compounds Thiourea has been detected in the seeds of certain plants in the genus *Laburnum.*[99] Thiourea is an antithyroid compound that has produced thyroid adenomas and carcinomas, benign liver tumors, and malignant tumors of the eyelid and ear duct gland upon administration in the diet (1–0.1%) to rats.[60,148,155] Another antithyroid compound, (−)-5-vinyl-2-thiooxazolidone, is derived from a precursor (see Chapter 10, p. 212) in turnips, kale, cabbage, and rapeseed.[9] Rats fed a diet containing 45% rapeseed have developed thyroid adenomata.[73]

Tannins (Tannic Acids) During World War II, liver damage was seen in humans treated with tannic acid for burns. Subsequent experiments in rats by Korpassy showed that repeated subcutaneous injection of a hydrolyzable tannin, gallotannic acid, led to hepatotoxicity, cirrhosis, and liver tumors in this species. Korpassy reviewed his extensive work on this subject in 1961.[102] Similarly, three condensed nonhydrolyzable tannins were found to produce liver tumors and sarcomas at the site of injection following repeated subcutaneous injection in mice.[98] High oral doses of gallotannic acid in rats were claimed to result in some pre-cirrhotic lesions in the liver,[102] but no report has been made of the in-duction of tumors by orally administered tannins. Beverages such as coffee, tea, and clarets contain small and varying amounts of tannins. The various tannins are heterogeneous substances and are not well characterized.[91,200]

Carrageenan (Carrageenin) Carrageenan is a hydrophilic colloid that absorbs water easily. It consists of a mixture of high molecular weight sulfated polysaccharides of galactose and anhydrogalactose and is ob-tained from red algae seaweeds (carrageen or Irish moss), notably *Chondrus crispus* and some other species.[71,79] Carrageenan stimulates the formation of fibrous tissue upon subcutaneous injection in the guinea pig,[151] and a single dose of 50 mg of carrageenan dissolved in 5 ml of saline injected into the subcutaneous tissue of rats led to a sig-nificant (11 out of 39) incidence of sarcomas after approximately 2 yr.[34] The appearance of sarcomas induced by multiple subcutaneous injec-tions of carrageenan in rats was accelerated by the simultaneous feeding of the carcinogen 2-acetylaminofluorene.[198] Its carcinogenic activity in the subcutaneous tissue of the rat may be an example of foreign-body carcinogenesis. Oral administration of carrageenan to rats and mice at high levels for 2 yr did not appear to induce tumors,[135] although the survival of the animals for this period was not high. The roles of carra-geenan as a food additive (stabilizer, adding body and bulk to end product), in the treatment of gastric ulcers, and as an agent inducing colonic ulcerations in some studies of herbivorous species have been discussed recently.[4,6]

Sugars A series of early reports from Japan and some later Italian stud-ies indicated that very frequent subcutaneous injections of concentrated solutions of glucose, galactose, fructose, and some di- and polysac-charides in the rat for 2 yr produced low incidences of sarcomas at the site of injection. While these effects could not be repeated by some other workers, the impression has been left in the literature that con-centrated solutions of various sugars indeed have this property. In a recent well-controlled study by Hueper[89] with purified mono- and disac-charides, the positive results obtained earlier could not be verified ex-cept for a borderline result with sorbose. Hueper suggests that the posi-tive results may have been due to carcinogenic impurities, possibly eluted from charcoal frequently employed in the decolorization of sugar preparations. It is also possible that other factors[70,71] were responsible for the earlier results.

Cocarcinogens, Promoting Agents   The actions of these weakly carcinogenic or noncarcinogenic substances have been variously defined. Cocarcinogens generally include compounds that enhance tumor formation when administered with carcinogens; promoting agents induce tumors subsequent to the initiating action of a minimally active dose of a carcinogen.[158] Croton seed oil and latexes from plants of the spurge family or *Euphorbiaceae* contain potent promoting agents for the skin of mice following initiation with single small doses of the carcinogenic hydrocarbons. Hecker and his associates[80] have elucidated the structures of the active components in croton oil and have shown these to be 12,13-diesters of the complex tetracyclic alcohol, phorbol. Phorbol itself is

Phorbol

inactive as a promoter. However, Berenblum, the discoverer of the promoting action of croton oil, and Lonai[13] have recently shown that phorbol has leukemogenic activity in mice. Various citrus oils and one of their components, D-limonene, appear to have weak promoting activity for mouse skin.[86,154] An interesting example of a dietary cocarcinogen for the hepatocarcinogenic activity of aflatoxin B_1 in the rainbow trout has been described recently.[109] The administration of the cyclopropenoid fatty acids (sterculic and malvalic acids) contained in a number of seed oils (including those of cotton and other plants of the order Malvales) enhanced considerably the carcinogenic activity of a low level of aflatoxin B_1 in this species.[109] It is of interest that the cyclopropene group in these fatty acids reacts with the SH groups in cysteine and glutathione.[149]

From Animals

Only a very limited number of components of animal tissues have been reported to induce or enhance the formation of neoplasms in experimental animals. The parenteral administration of estrogens or of growth hormone may lead to the formation of tumors in several tissues. Various metabolites of tryptophan have been implicated in the formation of urinary bladder neoplasms in the human, and they show activity in the mouse urinary bladder implant test.[38] (See Chapter 6, p. 142.) The low incidences of sarcomas induced in rats by repeated subcutaneous injections of cholesterol are probably examples of smooth surface or solid state carcinogenesis as noted above.[15]

Estrogens as Carcinogens

A wide variety of estrogenic substances have been noted as minor components of animal, plant, and fungal cells. (See Chapter 24.[128]) The repeated administration of large amounts of estrogen may lead to hyperplasia and eventually neoplasms in several target tissues such as the mammary gland, uterus, and other hormonally regulated tissues. These effects are strongly conditioned by genetic factors, and such other factors as viruses may be involved. Hormones such as the estrogens may play a permissive, rather than an inductive, role in carcinogenesis.[14,37,63]

Metals

A few nonradioactive metal ions have been tested and found capable of inducing neoplasms in animals, generally after parenteral administration.[37,90,153] Subcutaneous, intramuscular, and intrapleural injections of inorganic compounds of beryllium, cadmium, chromium, cobalt, and nickel have led to the formation of sarcomas at these sites of injection in rats and mice. The ingestion of lead acetate by rats at levels of 0.1 and 1.0% of the diet for 1 yr or longer has led to cystic nephritis and to adenomata and adenocarcinomata of the renal cortex.[22,53] Sunderman[183] has recently reviewed metal carcinogenesis in experimental animals.

PERSPECTIVES

The occurrence of carcinogenic chemicals as products of many forms of life has been clearly established. When one considers variations in foods, food preferences, food processing, etc., it is evident that the degree of exposure of humans, through their food, to these carcinogens is very difficult to estimate. Even were these exposures known, one could only guess at this time about the carcinogenic hazard such exposures would pose for humans of either sex, of various ages, and of various genetic constitutions. The induction time of many years (at least 15–30) for carcinogenesis in the human and the lack of control populations produce very difficult problems in cancer epidemiology. With some of the naturally occurring carcinogens, the low level of their carcinogenicity in experimental animals and the very low human exposures suggest that these substances may not be significant carcinogenic hazards to humans at normal levels of consumption. On the other hand, the carcinogenic hazard may be significant with compounds that are carcinogenic at low dosages and that may induce tumors with only one or a few doses. The aflatoxins and nitrosamines pose such a problem, and human exposures to such carcinogens must be kept as low as practicable. Such food contaminants as the aflatoxins, which occur unevenly and at levels influenced by environmental conditions, can be controlled only by constant monitoring of foods likely to be contaminated.

It is virtually certain that many naturally occurring chemicals with carcinogenic activity remain to be detected. Likely sources of these agents are the fungi and bacteria, and many fungal and bacterial metabolites have not yet been tested for carcinogenic activity. It also seems certain that some carcinogens will be found among the many nonnutritive minor components naturally present in common human foods derived from green plants. These foods should not be exempt from suspicion merely because they have been used for decades or centuries without apparent harm, since—for the first time in history—our modern medical, nutritional, and hygienic age has provided a greatly increased life span for large populations for fuller expression of the possible carcinogenic factors in the environment. Efforts should be made to test the carcinogenicity of concentrates of the minor nonnutritive components of common foods. Furthermore, variations in composition should be expected among different strains of crops. A case in point is the range in cyclic hydroxamic acid content of strains of maize and wheat and its correlation with resistance to insect and fungal attack.[189] Reduction of the amounts of carcinogenic natural products in the diet or intestinal contents of humans may eventually constitute an important weapon in the prevention of cancer.

REFERENCES

1. M. E. Alpert, G. Wogan, and C. S. Davidson, Aflatoxin and hepatoma in Uganda. Am. Assoc. Study Liver Dis. Abstr., Nov., 8 (1967).
2. A. M. Ambrose, A. J. Cox, and F. DeEds, Antioxidant toxicity: Toxicological studies on sesamol. J. Agric. Food Chem. 6:600 (1958).
3. D. W. Anderson, Griseofulvin: Biology and clinical usefulness. Ann. Allergy 23:103 (1965).

4. Anonymous, Carrageenan and the colon. Food Cosmet. Toxicol. *8*:75 (1970).
5. Anonymous, Mycoses in the Americas. WHO Chronicle *24*:512 (1970).
6. Anonymous, Carrageenan. Food Cosmet. Toxicol. *9*:561 (1971).
7. J. Arcos, M. F. Argus, and G. Wolf, Chemical induction of cancer, Vol. I, Part II: The nature of tumors. Concepts and techniques of testing chemical agents for carcinogenic activity. Academic Press, New York (1968).
8. R. N. Arison and E. L. Feudale, Induction of renal tumor by streptozotocin in rats. Nature *214*:1254 (1967).
9. E. B. Astwood, M. A. Greer, and M. G. Ettlinger, L-5-Vinyl-2-thiooxazolidone, an antithyroid compound from yellow turnip and Brassica seeds. J. Biol. Chem. *181*:121 (1949).
10. D. Baltimore, Viral RNA-dependent DNA polymerase. Nature *226*:1209 (1970).
11. L. L. Barich, J. Schwartz, and D. Barich, Toxic liver damage in mice after prolonged intake of elevated doses of griseofulvin, Antibiot. Chemother. *11*:566 (1961).
12. L. L. Barich, J. Schwartz, and D. Barich, Oral griseofulvin: A cocarcinogenic agent to methylcholanthrene-induced cutaneous tumors. Cancer Res. *22*:53 (1962).
13. I. Berenblum and V. Lonai, The leukemogenic action of phorbol. Cancer Res. *30*:2744 (1970).
14. H. A. Bern, Nature of the hormonal influence in mouse mammary cancer. Science *131*:1039 (1960).
15. F. Bischoff and G. Bryson, Carcinogenesis through solid state surfaces. Progr. Exp. Tumor Res. *5*:85 (1964).
16. F. Blank, O. Chin, G. Just, D. R. Meranze, M. B. Shimkin, and R. Wieder, Carcinogens from fungi pathogenic for man. Cancer Res. *28*:2276 (1968).
17. M. Blumer, Benzpyrenes in soil. Science *134*:474 (1961).
18. E. Boger, Formation of carcinogenic polynuclear hydrocarbons. In Biogenesis of natural compounds, P. Bernfeld (ed.). Pergamon Press, New York (1968).
19. P. Borchert, E. C. Miller, and J. A. Miller, 1'-Hydroxy-safrole, a new metabolite, and 1'-acetoxy-safrole, a reactive derivative, of safrole. Proc. Am. Assoc. Cancer Res. *12*:34 (1971). [See Cancer Res. *33*:575 (1973).]
20. J. Borneff and R. Fischer, Kanzerogene Substanzen in Wasser und Boden. IX, X, XI. Arch. Hyg. Bakteriol. *146*:183, 334, 430 (1962).
21. J. Borneff, F. Selenka, H. Kunte, and A. Maximos, Experimental studies on the formation of polycyclic aromatic hydrocarbons in plants. Environ. Res. *2*:22 (1968).
22. E. Boyland, C. E. Dukes, P. L. Grover, and B. C. V. Mitchley, The induction of renal tumors by feeding lead acetate to rats. Br. J. Cancer *16*:283 (1962).
23. L. B. Bull, The histological evidence of liver damage from pyrrolizidine alkaloids. Aust. Vet. J. *31*:33 (1955).
24. L. B. Bull, C. C. J. Culvenor, and A. T. Dick, The pyrrolizidine alkaloids. North-Holland Publishing Co., Amsterdam (1968).
25. R. J. W. Burrell, W. A. Roach, and A. Shadwell, Esophageal cancer in the Bantu of the Transkei associated with mineral deficiency in garden plants. J. Nat. Cancer Inst. *36*:201 (1966).
26. W. H. Butler and J. M. Barnes, Carcinoma of the glandular stomach in rats given diets containing aflatoxin. Nature *209*:90 (1966).

27. W. H. Butler, M. Greenblatt, and W. Lijinksy, Carcinogenesis in rats by aflatoxins B_1, G_1, and B_2. Cancer Res. *29*:2206 (1969).
28. W. H. Butler, A. R. Mattocks, and J. M. Barnes, Lesions in the liver and lungs of rats given pyrrole derivatives of pyrrolizidine alkaloids. J. Pathol. Bacteriol. *100*:169 (1970).
29. T. C. Campbell, J. P. Caedo, Jr., J. Bulato-Jayme, L. Salamat, and R. W. Engel, Aflatoxin M_1 in human urine. Nature *227*:403 (1970).
30. R. B. A. Carnaghan, Hepatic tumours in ducks fed a low level of toxic groundnut meal. Nature *208*:308 (1965).
31. R. B. A. Carnaghan, Hepatic tumours and other chronic liver changes in rats following a single oral administration of aflatoxin. Br. J. Cancer *21*:811 (1967).
32. R. B. A. Carnaghan and M. Crawford, Relationship between ingestion of aflatoxin and primary liver cancer. Br. Vet. J. *120*:201 (1964).
33. R. L. Carter, Induced subcutaneous sarcomata: Their development and critical appraisal, pp. 569–595. In Metabolic aspects of food safety, F. J. C. Roe (ed.). Academic Press, New York (1970).
34. D. B. Cater, The carcinogenic action of carrageenin in rats. Br. J. Cancer *15*: 607 (1961).
35. L. A. Cherkes, S. G. Aptekar, and M. N. Volgarev, Hepatic tumors induced by selenium. Bull. Exp. Biol. Med. *53*:313 (1963).
36. A. Ciegler, R. W. Detroy, and E. B. Lillehoj, Patulin, penicillic acid, and other carcinogenic lactones. In Microbial toxins, Vol. VI, Fungal toxins, A. Ciegler, S. Kadis, and S. J. Ajl (eds.). Academic Press, New York (1971).
37. D. B. Clayson, Chemical carcinogenesis. Little, Brown and Co., Boston (1962).
38. D. B. Clayson and E. H. Cooper, Cancer of the urinary tract. Adv. Cancer Res. *13*:271 (1970).
39. J. W. Cook, E. Duffy, and R. Schoental, Primary liver tumours in the rats following feeding with alkaloids of *Senecio jacoboea*. Br. J. Cancer *4*:405 (1950).
40. C. C. J. Culvenor, J. A. Edgar, L. W. Smith, M. V. Jago, and J. E. Peterson, Active metabolites in the chronic hepatotoxicity of pyrrolizidine alkaloids, including otonecine esters. Nature New Biol. *229*:255 (1971).
41. C. C. J. Culvenor, A. T. Dann, and A. T. Dick, Alkylation as the mechanism by which the hepatotoxic pyrrolizidine alkaloids act on cell nuclei. Nature *195*: 570 (1962).
42. C. C. J. Culvenor, D. T. Downing, J. A. Edgar, and M. V. Jago. Pyrrolizidine alkaloids as alkylating and antimitotic agents. Ann. N.Y. Acad. Sci. *168*:837 (1969).
43. J. Dalezios, G. N. Wogan, and S. M. Weinreb, Aflatoxin P_1: A new aflatoxin metabolite in monkeys. Science *171*:584 (1971).
44. R. W. Detroy, E. B. Lillehoj, and A. Ciegler, Aflatoxin and related compounds. In Microbial toxins, Vol. VI, Fungal toxins, A. Ciegler, S. Kadis, and S. J. Ajl (eds.). Academic Press, New York (1971).
45. F. Dickens, Mold products including antibiotics as carcinogens. In Carcinogenesis: A broad critique. Williams & Wilkins, Baltimore (1967).
46. J. DiPaolo, Experimental evaluation of actinomycin D. Ann. N.Y. Acad. Sci. *89*:408 (1960).
47. D. A. Dolimpio, C. Jacobson, and M. Legator, Effect of aflatoxin on human leukocytes. Proc. Soc. Exp. Biol. Med. *127*:559 (1968).

48. H. Druckrey, D. Steinhoff, H. Beuthner, H. Schneider, and P. Klarner, Prufung von Nitrit auf chronisch toxische Wirkung an Ratten. Arzneimittel-Forsch. *13*:320 (1963).
49. L. S. DuPlessis, J. R. Nunn, and W. A. Roach, Carcinogen in a Transkeian Bantu food additive. Nature *222*:1198 (1969).
50. M. A. El-Nakeeb and J. O. Lampen, Uptake of ^{3}H-griseofulvin by microorganisms and its correlation with sensitivity to griseofulvin. J. Gen. Microbiol. *39*: 285 (1965).
51. S. S. Epstein, J. Andrea, S. Joshi, and N. Mantel, Hepatocarcinogenicity of griseofulvin following parenteral administration. Cancer Res. *27*:1900 (1967).
52. S. S. Epstein, K. Fujii, J. Andrea, and N. Mantel, Carcinogenicity testing of selected food additives by parenteral administration to infant Swiss mice. Toxicol. Appl. Pharmacol. *16*:321 (1970).
53. G. J. van Esch, H. van Genderen, and H. H. Vink, The induction of renal tumours by feeding of basic lead acetate to rats. Br. J. Cancer *16*:289 (1962).
54. I. A. Evans, The radiomimetic nature of bracken toxin. Cancer Res., *28*:2252 (1968).
55. I. A. Evans and J. Mason, Carcinogenic activity of bracken, Nature *208*:913 (1965).
56. I. A. Evans, B. Widdop, R. S. Jones, G. D. Barber, H. Leach, D. L. Jones, and R. Mainwaring-Burton, The possible human hazard of the naturally occurring bracken carcinogen. Biochem. J. *124*:28P (1971).
57. FAO/WHO Expert Committee on Food Additives, Fifth report. Evaluation of the carcinogenic hazards of food additives. Tech. Rep. Ser. No. 220. World Health Organization, Geneva (1961).
58. E. Farber, Ethionine carcinogenesis. Adv. Cancer Res. *7*:383 (1963).
59. J. F. Fisher and M. F. Mallette, The natural occurrence of ethionine in bacteria. J. Gen. Physiol. *45*:1 (1961).
60. O. G. Fitzhugh and A. A. Nelson, Liver tumors in rats fed thiourea or thioacetamide. Science *108*:626 (1948).
61. Food and Drug Administration Advisory Committee on Protocols for Safety Evaluation, Panel on carcinogenesis report on cancer testing in the safety evaluation of food additives and pesticides. Toxicol. Appl. Pharmacol. *20*: 419 (1971).
62. Food Protection Committee, Food and Nutrition Board, National Academy of Sciences–National Research Council, Problems in the evaluation of carcinogenic hazard from use of food additives. Publication No. 749. National Academy of Sciences–National Research Council, Washington, D.C. (1959); Cancer Res. *21*:429 (1961).
63. L. Foulds, Neoplastic development, Vol. 1. Academic Press, New York (1969).
64. R. C. Garner, E. C. Miller, J. A. Miller, J. V. Garner, and R. S. Hanson, Formation of a factor lethal for *S. Typhimurium* TA1530 and TA1531 on incubation of aflatoxin B_1 with rat liver microsomes. Biochem. Biophys. Res. Commun. *45*:774 (1971).
65. L. A. Goldblatt (ed.), Aflatoxin. Academic Press, New York (1969).
66. C. M. Goodall, Endocrine factors as determinants of the susceptibility of the liver to carcinogenic agents. N. Z. Med. J. *67*:32 (1968).
67. W. Gräf, Über natürliches Vorkommen und Bedeutung der kanzerogenen polycyclisher, aromatischen Kohlenwasserstoffe. Med. Klin. Munich *60*(15): 561 (1965).

68. W. Gräf and H. Diehl, Über den naturbedingten Normalpegel kanzerogener, polycyclischer Aromate und seine Ursache, Arch. Hyg. Bakteriol. *150*:49 (1966).

69. W. Gräf and W. Nowak, Wachstumsforderung bei niederen und höheren Pflanzen durch kanzerogene, polycyclischer Aromate, Arch. Hyg. Bakteriol. *150*:513 (1966).

70. P. Grasso and L. Golberg, Subcutaneous sarcoma as an index of carcinogenic potency. Food Cosmet. Toxicol. *4*:297 (1966).

71. P. Grasso, S. D. Gangolli, L. Golberg, and J. Hooson, Physico-chemical and other factors determining local sarcoma production by food additives. Food Cosmet. Toxicol. *9*:463 (1971).

72. P. Gray (ed.), The encyclopedia of the biological sciences. 1st ed. Reinhold Publishing Co., New York (1961). P. 19.

73. W. E. Griesbach, T. H. Kennedy, and H. D. Purves. Studies on experimental goitre. VI. Thyroid adenomata in rats on Brassica seed diet. Br. J. Exp. Pathol. *26*:18 (1945).

74. M. A. Gross, W. I. Jones, E. L. Cook, and C. C. Boone, Carcinogenicity of oil of calamus, Proc. Am. Assoc. Cancer Res. *8*:24 (1967).

75. J. E. Halver, Aflatoxicosis and rainbow trout hepatoma. In Mycotoxins in foodstuffs, G. N. Wogan (ed.). MIT Press, Cambridge (1965).

76. J. R. Harr, J. F. Bone, I. J. Tinsley, P. H. Weswig, and R. S. Yamamoto, Selenium toxicity in rats. II. Histopathology. In Selenium in biomedicine, O. H. Muth (ed.). Avi, Westport, Conn. (1967).

77. P. N. Harris and K. K. Chen, Development of hepatic tumors in rats following ingestion of *Senecio longilobus*. Cancer Res. *30*:2881 (1970).

78. G. Hawksworth and M. J. Hill, The formation of nitrosamines by human intestinal bacteria. Biochem. J. Proc. *122*:28–29 (1971).

79. G. G. Hawley (ed.), The condensed chemical dictionary. 8th ed. Van Nostrand Reinhold, New York (1971).

80. E. Hecker, Cocarcinogenic principles from the seed oil of *Croton tiglium* and from other Euphorbiaceae. Cancer Res. *28*:2338 (1968).

81. J. Higginson, The geographical pathology of primary liver cancer. Cancer Res. *23*:1624 (1963).

82. J. Higginson, Present trends in cancer epidemiology, Can. Cancer Conf. *8*:40 (1969).

83. M. J. Hill, B. S. Drasar, V. Aries, J. S. Crowther, G. Hawksworth, and R. E. O. Williams, Bacteria and aetiology of cancer of large bowel. Lancet, Jan. 16, 7690 (1971).

84. I. Hirono, G. L. Laqueur, and M. Spatz, Tumor induction in Fischer and Osborne-Mendel rats by a single administration of cycasin. J. Nat. Cancer Inst. *40*:1003 (1968).

85. I. Hirono, C. Shibuya, K. Fushimi, and M. Haga, Studies on carcinogenic properties of bracken, *Pteridium aquilinum*. J. Nat. Cancer Inst. *45*:179 (1970).

86. F. Homburger and E. Boger, The carcinogenicity of essential oils, flavors, and spices: A review. Cancer Res. *28*:2372 (1968).

87. F. Homburger, T. Kelley, Jr., T. R. Baker, and A. B. Russfield, Hepatic pathology from a deficient diet and safrole in rats. Arch. Pathol. *73*:118 (1962).

88. F. Homburger, T. Kelley, Jr., G. Friedler, and A. B. Russfield, Toxic and possible carcinogenic effects of 4-allyl-1,2-methylenedioxybenzene (safrole) in rats on deficient diets. Med. Exp. *4*:1 (1961).

89. W. C. Hueper, Are sugars carcinogens? An experimental study, Cancer Res. *25*:440 (1965).

90. W. C. Hueper and W. D. Conway, Chemical carcinogenesis and cancers. C. C Thomas, Springfield, Ill. (1964).

91. S. G. Humphries, The biosynthesis of tannins. In Biogenesis of natural compounds, P. Bernfeld (ed.). 2nd ed. Pergamon Press, Oxford (1967).

92. E. W. Hurst and G. E. Paget, Protoporphyrin, cirrhosis and hepatomas in the livers of mice given griseofulvin. Br. J. Dermatol. *75*:105 (1963).

93. R. Ikegami, Y. Akamatsu, and M. Haruta, Subcutaneous sarcomas induced by mitomycin C in mice: Comparisons of occurrence, transplantability and histology between sarcomas induced by actinomycin S and 3-methylcholanthrene. Acta Pathol. Jap. *17*:495 (1967).

94. J. R. M. Innes, B. M. Ulland, M. G. Valerio, L. Petrucelli, L. Fishbein, E. R. Hart, A. J. Pallotta, R. R. Bates, H. L. Falk, J. J. Gart, M. Klein, I. Mitchell, and J. Peters, Bioassay of pesticides and industrial chemicals for tumorigenicity in mice: A preliminary note. J. Nat. Cancer Inst. *42*:1101 (1969).

95. I. Ishikawa, Y. Ueno, and H. Tsunoda, Chemical determinations of the chlorine-containing peptide, a hepatotoxic mycotoxin of *Penicillium islandicum* Sopp. J. Biochem. (Japan) *67*:753 (1970).

96. M. V. Jago, The development of the hepatic megalocytosis of chronic pyrrolizidine alkaloid poisoning. Am. J. Pathol. *56*:405 (1969).

97. J. Kawamata, N. Nakabayashi, A. Kawai, H. Fujita, M. Imanishi, and R. Ikegami, Studies on the carcinogenic effect of actinomycin. Biken's J. *2*:105 (1959).

98. K. S. Kirby, Induction of tumours by tannin extracts. Br. J. Cancer *14*:147 (1960).

99. G. Klein and E. Farkass, Die mikrochemische Nachweis der Alkaloide in der Pflanze. XIV. Cytisine. Oesterr. Botan. Z. *79*:107 (1930).

100. P. Klubes and W. R. Jondorf, Dimethylnitrosamine formation from sodium nitrite and dimethylamine by bacterial flora of rat intestine. Res. Commun. Chem. Pathol. Pharmacol. *2*:24 (1971).

101. A. Kobayashi and H. Matsumoto, Studies on methylazoxymethanol, the aglycone of cycasin. Arch. Biochem. Biophys. *110*:373 (1965).

102. B. Korpassy, Tannins as hepatic carcinogens. Progr. Exp. Tumor Res. *2*:245 (1961).

103. G. L. Laqueur, Carcinogenic effects of cycad meal and cycasin, methylazoxymethanol glycoside, in rats and effects of cycasin in germfree rats. Fed. Proc. *23*:1386 (1964).

104. G. L. Laqueur and H. Matsumoto, Neoplasms in female Fischer rats following intraperitoneal injection of methylazoxymethanol. J. Nat. Cancer Inst. *37*:217 (1966).

105. G. L. Laqueur, E. G. McDaniel, and H. Matsumoto, Tumor induction in germfree rats with methylazoxymethanol (MAM) and synthetic MAM acetate. J. Nat. Cancer Inst. *39*:355 (1967).

106. G. L. Laqueur, O. Mickelson, M. G. Whiting, and L. T. Kurland, Carcinogenic properties of nuts from *Cycas circinalis* L. indigenous to Guam. J. Nat. Cancer Inst. *31*:919 (1963).

107. G. L. Laqueur and M. Spatz, Toxicology of cycasin. Cancer Res. *28*:2262 (1968).

108. H. Leach, G. D. Barber, I. A. Evans, and W. C. Evans, Isolation of an active

principle from the bracken fern that is mutagenic, carcinogenic and lethal to mice on intraperitoneal injection. Biochem. J. *124*:13P (1971).

109. D. J. Lee, J. H. Wales, J. L. Ayres, and R. O. Sinnhuber, Synergism between cyclopropenoid fatty acids and chemical carcinogens in rainbow trout (*Salmo gairdneri*). Cancer Res. *28*:2312 (1968).

110. W. Lijinsky and S. S. Epstein, Nitrosamines as environmental carcinogens. Nature *225*:21 (1970).

111. W. Lijinsky, K. Y. Lee, and C. H. Gallagher, Interaction of aflatoxins B_1 and G_1 with tissues of the rat. Cancer Res. *30*:2280 (1970).

112. W. Lijinsky, J. Loo, and A. E. Ross, Mechanism of alkylation of nucleic acids by nitrosodimethylamine. Nature *218*:1174 (1968).

113. E. B. Lillehoj, A. Ciegler, and R. W. Detroy, Fungal toxins. In Essays in toxicology, Vol. 2, F. R. Blood (ed.). Academic Press, New York (1970).

114. E. L. Long and P. M. Jenner, Esophageal tumors produced in rats by the feeding of dihydrosafrole. Fed. Proc. *22*:275 (1963).

115. E. L. Long, A. A. Nelson, O. G. Fitzhugh, and W. H. Hansen, Liver tumors produced in rats by feeding safrole. Arch. Pathol. *75*:595 (1963).

116. P. N. Magee, Toxicity of nitrosamines: Their possible human health hazards. Food Cosmet. Toxicol. *9*:207 (1971).

117. P. N. Magee and J. M. Barnes, Carcinogenic nitroso compounds. Adv. Cancer Res. *10*:163 (1967).

118. L. Mallet and M. Tissier, Biosynthèse expérimentale des hydrocarbures polybenzéniques du type benzo 3-4 pyrène aux dépens des terres de forêts. C. R. Soc. Biol. *163*:63 (1969).

119. H. Matsumoto and H. H. Higa, Studies on methylazoxymethanol, the aglycone of cycasin: Methylation of nucleic acids in vitro. Biochem. J. *98*:20C (1966).

120. H. Matsumoto and F. M. Strong, The occurrence of methylazoxymethanol in *Cycas carcinalis* L. Arch. Biochem. Biophys. *101*:299 (1963).

121. A. R. Mattocks, Toxicity of pyrrolizidine alkaloids. Nature *217*:723 (1968).

122. A. R. Mattocks, Dihydropyrrolizidine derivatives from unsaturated pyrrolizidine alkaloids. J. Chem. Soc. Sect. C. Organic *1155* (1969).

123. A. R. Mattocks, Role of the acid moieties in the toxic actions of pyrrolizidine alkaloids on liver and lung. Nature *228*:174 (1970).

124. E. K. McLean, The toxic actions of pyrrolizidine (*Senecio*) alkaloids. Pharmacol. Rev. *22*:429 (1970).

125. E. C. Miller and J. A. Miller, Mechanisms of chemical carcinogenesis: Nature of proximate carcinogens and interactions with macromolecules. Pharmacol. Rev. *18*:805 (1966).

126. J. A. Miller, Carcinogenesis by chemicals: An overview—G. H. A. Clowes Memorial Lecture. Cancer Res. *30*:559 (1970).

127. J. A. Miller and E. C. Miller, Chemical carcinogenesis: Mechanisms and approaches to its control. J. Nat. Cancer Inst. *47*:V–XIV (1971).

128. C. J. Mirocha, C. M. Christensen, and G. H. Nelson, Physiologic activity of some fungal estrogens produced by fusarium. Cancer Res. *28*:2319 (1968).

129. S. S. Mirvish, Kinetics of dimethylamine nitrosation in relation to nitrosamine carcinogenesis. J. Nat. Cancer Inst. *44*:633 (1970).

130. M. Miyake and M. Saito, Liver injury and liver tumors induced by toxins of *Penicillium islandicum* growing on yellowed rice. In Mycotoxins in foodstuffs, G. N. Wogan (ed.). MIT Press, Cambridge (1965).

131. O. H. Muth and W. Binns, Selenium toxicity in domestic animals. Ann. N.Y. Acad. Sci. *111*:583 (1964).

132. A. A. Nelson, O. G. Fitzhugh, and H. O. Calvery, Neurofibromas of rat ears produced by prolonged feeding of crude ergot. Cancer Res. 2:11 (1942).

133. A. A. Nelson, O. G. Fitzhugh, and H. O. Calvery, Liver tumors following cirrhosis caused by selenium in rats. Cancer Res. 3:230 (1943).

134. P. Niaussat, C. Auger, and L. Mallet, Apparition relative de quantités d'hydrocarbures cancérigènes dans des cultures pures de Bacillus badius, en fonction de la présence, dans le milieu, de certains composés chimiques. C. R. Acad. Sci. Paris 270:1042 (1970).

135. H. W. Nilson and J. A. Wagner, Feeding test with carrageenan. Food Res. 24:235 (1959).

136. K. Nishida, A. Kobayashi, and T. Nagahama, Cycasin, a new toxic glycoside of Cycas revoluta Thunb., I. Isolation and structure of cycasin. Bull. Agric. Chem. Soc. Jap. 19:77 (1955).

137. A. G. Oettle, Cancer in Africa, especially in regions south of the Sahara. J. Nat. Cancer Inst. 33:383 (1964).

138. J. E. Oldfield, J. R. Schubert, and O. H. Muth, Implications of selenium in large animal nutrition. J. Agric. Food Chem. 11:388 (1963).

139. B. J. Ortwerth and G. D. Novelli, Studies on the incorporation of L-ethionine-ethyl-1-^{14}C into the transfer RNA of rat liver. Cancer Res. 29:380 (1969).

140. G. E. Paget and A. L. Walpole, The experimental toxicology of griseofulvin. Arch. Dermatol. 81:750 (1960).

141. A. M. Pamukcu and J. M. Price, Induction of intestinal and urinary bladder cancer in rats by feeding bracken fern (Pteris aquilina). J. Nat. Cancer Inst. 43:275 (1969).

142. A. M. Pamukcu, S. Yalciner, J. M. Price, and G. T. Bryan, Effects of coadministration of thiamine on the incidence of urinary bladder carcinomas in rats fed bracken fern. Cancer Res. 30:2671 (1970).

143. M. Payet, J. Cros, C. Quenum, M. Sankalem, and M. Moulanier, Deux observations d'enfants ayants consommés de facon prolongée des farines souillées par Aspergillus flavus. Presse Med. 74:649 (1966).

144. R. S. Portman, K. M. Plowman, and T. C. Campbell, Aflatoxin metabolism by liver microsomal preparations of two different species. Biochem. Biophys. Res. Commun. 33:711 (1968).

145. R. W. Poynter, C. R. Ball, J. Goodban, and T. Thackrah, The influence of physostigmine on the activation of methylazoxymethanol acetate, a potent carcinogen, by a serum factor in vitro. Chem.-Biol. Interactions 4:139 (1971/72).

146. J. M. Price and A. M. Pamukcu, The induction of neoplasms of the urinary bladder of the cow and the small intestine of the rat by feeding bracken fern. Cancer Res. 28:2247 (1968).

147. I. F. H. Purchase and J. J. van der Watt, Carcinogenicity of sterigmatocystin. Food Cosmet. Toxicol. 8:289 (1970).

148. H. D. Purves and W. E. Griesbach, Studies on experimental goitre. VIII. Thyroid tumours in rats treated with thiourea. Br. J. Exp. Pathol. 28:46 (1947).

149. P. K. Raju and R. Reiser, Inhibition of fatty acid desaturase by cyclopropene fatty acids. J. Biol. Chem. 242:379 (1967).

150. N. V. Riggs, Glucosyloxyazoxymethane, a constituent of the seeds of Cycas circinalis L. Chem. Ind. 926 (1956).

151. W. van B. Robertson and B. Schwartz, Ascorbic acid and the formation of collagen. J. Biol. Chem. 201:689 (1953).

152. P. Robinson, Infantile cirrhosis of the liver in India. Clin. Pediatr. *6*:57 (1967).
153. F. J. C. Roe and M. C. Lancaster, Natural, metallic and other substances, as carcinogens. Br. Med. Bull. *20*:127 (1964).
154. F. J. C. Roe and W. E. H. Pierce, Tumor promotion by citrus oils: Tumors of the skin and urethral orifice in mice. J. Nat. Cancer Inst. *24*:1389 (1960).
155. A. Rosin and H. Ungar, Malignant tumors in the eyelids and the auricular region of thiourea-treated rats. Cancer Res. *17*:302 (1957).
156. F. J. Roth and H. Blank, The bioassay of griseofulvin in human stratum corneum. Arch. Dermatol. *81*:662 (1960).
157. M. Saito, M. Enomoto, and T. Tatsuno, Yellowed rice toxins. Luteoskyrin and related compounds, chlorine-containing compounds, and citrinin. In Microbial toxins, Vol. VI, Fungal toxins, A. Ciegler, S. Kadis, and S. J. Ajl (eds.). Academic Press, New York (1971).
158. M. H. Salaman and F. J. C. Roe, Cocarcinogenesis. Br. Med. Bull. *20*:139 (1964).
159. J. Sander, Nitrosaminsynthese durch Bakterien. Hoppe-Seyl. Z. Physiol. Chem. *349*:429 (1968).
160. J. Sander, Induktion maligner Tumoren bei Ratten durch orale Gabe von N,N'-Dimethylharnstoff und Nitrit. Arzneimittel-Forsch. *20*:418 (1970).
161. J. Sander and G. Burkle, Induktion maligner Tumoren bei Ratten durch gleichzeitige Verfutterung von Nitrit und sekundaren Aminen. Z. Krebsforsch. *73*: 54 (1969).
162. U. Sankawa, S. Seo, N. Kobayashi, Y. Ogihara, and S. Shibata, Further studies on the structure of luteoskyrin, rubroskyrin, and rugulosin. Tetrahedron Lett., No. 53, 5557 (1968).
163. J. F. Scaife, Aflatoxin B_1: Cytotoxic mode of action evaluated by mammalian cell cultures. Fed. Eur. Biochem. Soc. *12*:143 (1971).
164. D. O. Schachtschabel, F. Zilliken, M. Saito, and G. E. Foley, Inhibition ascites tumor cells following treatment with luteoskyrin. Exp. Cell Res. *57*:19 (1969).
165. R. Schoental, Hepatotoxic action of pyrrolizidine (*Senecio*) alkaloids in relation to their structure. Nature *179*:361 (1957).
166. R. Schoental, Liver disease and "natural" hepatoxins. Bull. World Health Organ. *29*:823 (1963).
167. R. Schoental, Toxicology and carcinogenic action of pyrrolizidine alkaloids. Cancer Res. *28*:2237 (1968).
168. R. Schoental, Carcinogenic action of elaiomycin in rats. Nature *221*:765 (1969).
169. R. Schoental, Hepatotoxic activity of retrorsine, senkirkine and hydroxysenkirkine in newborn rats, and the role of epoxides in carcinogenesis by pyrrolizidine alkaloids and aflatoxins. Nature *227*:401 (1970).
170. R. Schoental and J. P. M. Bensted, Effects of whole-body irradiation, and of partial hepatectomy, on the liver lesions induced in rats by a single dose of retrorsine, a pyrrolizidine (*Senecio*) alkaloid. Br. J. Cancer *17*:242 (1963).
171. R. Schoental and M. A. Head, Pathological changes in rats as a result of treatment with monocrotaline. Br. J. Cancer *9*:229 (1955).
172. R. Schoental and M. A. Head, Progression of liver lesions produced in rats by temporary treatment with pyrrolizidine (*Senecio*) alkaloids and the effects of betaine and high casein diets. Br. J. Cancer *11*:535 (1957).
173. R. Schoental, M. A. Head, and P. R. Peacock, *Senecio* alkaloids: Primary tumours in rats as a result of treatment with (1) a mixture of alkaloids from S. jacobea a Lin.; (2) retrorsine; (3) isatidine. Br. J. Cancer *8*:458 (1954).

174. H. A. Schroeder and M. Mitchener, Selenium and tellurium in rats: Effect on growth, survival and tumors. J. Nutr. *101*:1531 (1971).
175. K. Schwartz (chairman), Symposium on nutritional significance of selenium (Factor 3). Fed. Proc. *20*:665 (1961).
176. R. C. Shank, N. Bhamarapravati, J. E. Gordon, and G. N. Wogan, Dietary aflatoxins and human liver cancer. IV. Incidence of primary liver cancer in two municipal populations of Thailand. Food Cosmet. Toxicol. *10*:171 (1972).
177. R. C. Shank, J. E. Gordon, G. N. Wogan, A. Nondasuta, and B. Subhamani, Dietary aflatoxins and human liver cancer, III. Field survey of rural Thai families for ingested aflatoxins. Food Cosmet. Toxicol. *10*:71 (1972).
178. R. C. Shank and P. N. Magee, Similarities between the bio-chemical actions of cycasin and dimethylnitrosamine. Biochem. J. *105*:521(1967).
179. R. C. Shank, G. N. Wogan, and J. B. Gibson, Dietary aflatoxins and human liver cancer. I. Toxigenic moulds in foods and foodstuffs of tropical Southeast Asia. Food Cosmet. Toxicol. *10*:51 (1972).
180. R. C. Shank, G. N. Wogan, J. B. Gibson, and A. Nondasuta, Dietary aflatoxins and human liver cancer. II. Aflatoxins in market foods and foodstuffs of Thailand and Hong Kong. Food Cosmet. Toxicol. *10*:61 (1972).
181. R. C. Shank, P. Siddhichai, B. Subhamani, N. Bhamarapravati, J. E. Gordon, and G. N. Wogan, Dietary aflatoxins and human liver cancer. V. Duration of primary liver cancer and prevalence of hepatomegaly in Thailand. Food Cosmet. Toxicol. *10*:181 (1972).
182. J. A. Stekol, Biochemical basis for ethionine effects on tissues. Adv. Enzymol. *25*:369 (1963).
183. F. W. Sunderman, Jr., Metal carcinogenesis in experimental animals. Food Cosmet. Toxicol. *9*:105 (1971).
184. D. Svoboda, J. Reddy, and C. Harris, Invasive tumors induced in rats with actinomycin D. Cancer Res. *30*:2271 (1970).
185. W. Szybalski and V. W. Iyer, The mitomycins and porfiromycins. In Antibiotics I. Mechanism of action, D. Gottlieb and P. D. Shaw (eds.). Springer, New York (1967).
186. A. Tannenbaum, S. D. Vesselinovitch, C. Maltoni, and D. S. Mitchell, Multipotential carcinogenicity of urethan in the Sprague-Dawley rat. Cancer Res. *22*:1362 (1962).
187. J. M. Taylor, W. I. Jones, E. C. Hagan, M. A. Gross, D. A. Davis, and E. L. Cook, Toxicity of oil of calamus (Jammu variety). Toxicol. Appl. Pharmacol. *10*:405 (1967).
188. H. M. Temin and S. Mizutani, RNA-dependent DNA polymerase in virions of Rous sarcoma virus. Nature *226*:1211 (1970).
189. C. L. Tipton, J. A. Klun, R. R. Husted, and M. D. Pierson, Cyclic hydroxamic acids and related compounds from maize. Isolation and characterization. Biochemistry *6*:2866 (1967).
190. J. Tooze, Vintage year for tumour virology. Nature *233*:28 (1971).
191. H. Tsunoda, Studies on a poisonous substance produced on the cereals by a *Pencillium* Sopp under storage. Jap. J. Nutr. (Eigogaku Zasshi) *8*:185 (1951).
192. Y. Ueno, A. Platel, and P. Fromageot, Interaction entre pigments et acides nucleiques. II. Interaction in vitro entre la luteoskyrine et le DNA de thymus de veau. Biochim. Biophys. Acta *134*:27 (1967).
193. Y. Ueno, I. Ueno, K. Ito, and T. Tatsuno, Impairment of RNA synthesis in Erhlich ascites tumour by luteoskyrin, a hepatotoxic pigment of *Pencillium islandicum* Sopp. Experientia *23*:1001 (1967).

194. Y. Ueno, I. Ueno, and K. Mizumoto, The mode of binding of luteoskyrin, a hepatotoxic pigment of *Penicillium islandicum* Sopp, to deoxyribonucleic acid. Jap. J. Exp. Med. *38*:47 (1968).

195. Y. Ueno, I. Ueno, and T. Tatsuno, Inhibition of DNA-dependent RNA polymerase of *E. coli* by luteoskyrin. Seikagaku (Jap. J. Biochem. Soc.) *38*:687 (1966).

196. M. Umeda, Cytotoxic effects of the mycotoxins of *Penicillium islandicum* Sopp, luteoskyrin and chlorine-containing peptide on Chang's liver cells and HeLa cells. Acta Path. Jap. *14*:373 (1964).

197. K. Uraguchi, M. Saito, Y. Noguchi, K. Takahashi, M. Enomoto, and T. Tatsuno, Chronic toxicity and carcinogenicity in mice of the purified mycotoxins, luteoskyrin and cyclochlorotine. Food Cosmet. Toxicol. *10*:193 (1972).

198. A. L. Walpole, Observations upon the induction of subcutaneous sarcomata in rats, pp. 83–88. In The morphological precursors of cancer, L. Severi (ed.). University of Perugia, Perugia, Italy (1962).

199. J. H. Weisburger and E. K. Weisburger, Tests for chemical carcinogens. In Methods in cancer research, Vol. 1, H. Busch (ed.). Academic Press, New York (1968).

200. T. White, K. S. Kirby, and E. Knowles, Tannins. IV. The complexity of tannin extract composition. J. Soc. Leather Trades' Chem. *36*:148 (1952).

201. M. G. Whiting, Toxicity of cycads. Econ. Bot. *17*:271 (1963).

202. P. G. Wislocki, P. Borchert, E. C. Miller, and J. A. Miller, 1'-Hydroxysafrole: A proximate carcinogenic metabolite of safrole. Proc. Am. Assoc. Cancer Res. *13*:12 (1972). [See Cancer Res. *33*:590 (1973).]

203. G. N. Wogan (ed.), Mycotoxins in foodstuffs. MIT Press, Cambridge (1965).

204. G. N. Wogan, Aflatoxin risks and control measures. Fed. Proc. *27*:932 (1968).

205. G. N. Wogan and P. M. Newberne, Dose-response characteristics of aflatoxin B_1 carcinogenesis in the rat. Cancer Res. *27*:2370 (1967).

206. I. A. Wolff and A. E. Wasserman, Nitrates, nitrites, and nitrosamines. Science *177*:15–19 (1972).

24 Martin Stob

ESTROGENS
IN FOODS[*]

The classic review of Bradbury and White[7] first focused attention on the occurrence of estrogens in plants. Subsequent reviews by Moule et al.[36] and Bickoff[2] have emphasized the ubiquitous distribution and diverse chemical types of phytoestrogens. That estrogens in plants may be a contributing factor in cases of infertility of livestock is beyond question,[36] but fortunately for humans, their occurrence in plants, in the majority of cases, is only of academic interest, either because the plants containing the compounds do not constitute a significant portion of the diet or because the quantity of estrogenic compounds is too low to exert physiological effects. Thus, the stilbene compounds from anise and fennel oils,[7] pinosylvin from trees of the genus *Pinus*,[7] chlorophorin from the African tree *Chlorophora excelsa*,[7] or the phenanthrene compound miroestrol from the tuberous roots of a Siamese climbing plant[23] are not likely to be of physiological significance. The steroid estrone has been identified in date seeds,[21] although Jacobson et al.[22] suggest that there is little evidence that any steroidal estrogens occur in plants. Hops, which are used in the brewing of beer, contain four beta bitter acids, three of which have been identified as lupulon, colupulon, and adlupulon; these compounds have been associated with the estrogenic activity of hops, reported[58] to be 12,500 IU/g (Allen–Doisy test). Fortunately, to date there is no evidence that beer is estrogenic.

[*] Literature reviewed to April 1, 1971.

The estrogenic compounds that do warrant scrutiny are the coumestans, isoflavones, and resorcylic acid lactones, not only because of their
reported occurrence in food used for human consumption but also because of their physiological effects.

ISOFLAVONES AND COUMESTANS

The isoflavones and coumestans are biogenetically similar, i.e., they are
formed by similar biosynthetic pathways.[18] The isoflavones commonly
associated with plants are genistein, biochanin A, daidzein, formononetin, and pratensin[53]; the coumestans are coumestrol[3] and 4'-O-methyl-
coumestrol.[4] The chemical characteristics of these compounds are well
documented,[32,33] and methods for their detection by paper or thin-
layer chromatography have been described.[19,29] The isoflavones occur
in plants in a bound form, probably glycosidic.[1] This binding apparently has no effect on the estrogenic activity of genistein versus its
glycoside, genistin.[11] Although all seven of the above-mentioned compounds occur in plants, only genistein and coumestrol will be considered
in detail, because they have the highest estrogenic activity.[5]

Genistein

Genistein was first isolated from soybeans.[56] It is relatively heat stable,
having a melting point of 297 °C. By oral administration, genistein is
100,000 times less effective than diethylstilbestrol, 6,900 times less effective than estrone, and 35 times less effective than coumestrol in stimulating uterine hypertrophy in immature, intact female mice.[5] Genistein
can stimulate protein synthesis in the uterus of ovariectomized rats.[37] It
can displace estradiol from receptor sites in uterine tissue,[43] but it cannot induce ovum implantation in ovariectomized, gestagen-maintained
rats.[40] In sheep, genistein circulates in the blood chiefly as a glucuronide[44]
and is usually rapidly excreted. Isoflavones may accumulate in depot
fat in sheep, but the total isoflavone (genistein, daidzein, biochanin A,

Genistein

formononetin, and coumestrol) concentration in body fat does not exceed 1 ppm.[28] Surprisingly little quantitative data exist regarding genistein in soybeans, which are an important food source for both man and animals. Walter[55] reported that hexane-extracted soybeans contain 0.1% as the glucoside genistein. Wada and Fukushima[51] report the estrogenic activity of soybeans as 6 μg of diethylstilbestrol equivalents per kg. Estrogenically active subterranean clover may contain as much as 0.7 g/ 100 g dry plant material.[13]

Coumestrol

Coumestrol was first isolated from alfalfa.[3] It has also been detected in soybeans and soybean sprouts,[52] both of which may be used in human diets. Coumestrol is a heat-stable compound with a melting point of 385 °C. It is also a weak estrogen, 2,857 times less effective than diethylstilbestrol and 197 times less effective than estrone, but 35 times more effective than genistein in stimulating uterine hypertrophy in immature, intact female mice.[5] Coumestrol can also stimulate protein synthesis in the uterus of ovariectomized rats,[37] and at high levels (500 μg/g diet) it can inhibit hypophysial gonadotropin function.[26] Similar to genistein, coumestrol cannot induce ovum implantation in gestagen-maintained, ovariectomized rats.[40] Coumestrol may accumulate in the body fat of animals consuming forage containing the compound,[28] after circulating in the blood principally in the glucuronide form.[45] The coumestrol content of alfalfa infected with several types of fungal pathogens may be elevated to 115 ppm,[42] and alfalfa leaves affected with physiogenic spotting may contain as much as 2,000 ppm in the spotted areas.[30] Whether this increased coumestrol content would result in the accumulation of increased quantities of the compound in the fat of animals consuming this type of forage is purely speculative. All the chemical and biological properties of coumestrol and related compounds have recently been summarized by Bickoff et al.[6]

Coumestrol

ZEARALENONE

Zearalenone was first isolated by Stob et al.[48] and was chemically identified by Urry et al.[50] as 6-(10-hydroxy-6-oxo-trans-1-undecenyl)-β-resorcylic acid μ-lactone. Its total synthesis has been described,[49] its gas–liquid chromatographic behavior reported,[54] and a method for its detection in a wide variety of foods has been developed.[14] The melting point of zearalenone is 164 °C. The compound is uterotropic in mice[48] and rats[34]; it is anabolic in rats,[34] sheep,[48] and cattle.[41] It is a weak estrogen, only 0.0062 times as effective by subcutaneous injection and 0.016 times as effective by oral administration as estrone in producing uterine hypertrophy in mice, as reported by Dorfman.[35] At doses up to 50 mg/day by oral administration, zearalenone produces effects on the vulva, uterus, ovary, cervix, and mammary glands of swine similar to those caused by the intramuscular injection of up to 2 mg of the steroidal estrogen, estradiol-17-β-cyclopentylpropionate (estradiol cypionate).[25]

Zearalenone

A variety of *Fusarium* species (see Chapter 18) has been shown capable of producing zearalenone. Production per g of autoclaved corn has been reported by Caldwell *et al.*[10] as follows:

F. roseum	0.6–119 μg
F. roseum "Culmorum"	1 –210 μg
F. roseum "Equiseti"	0.6– 2 μg
F. roseum "Gibbosum"	115 –175 μg
F. roseum "Graminearum"	0.2–230 μg
F. tricinctum	0.2– 6 μg

Mirocha *et al.*[34] have reported the detection of as much as 3,500 ppm of zearalenone in stored corn infected with *F. graminearum*. O. L. Shotwell (in Stoloff[46]) reported the presence of a factor in grain extracts that enhances the fluorescence of zearalenone. This factor may explain the difference in the minimum detectable levels (μg/kg) of zearalenone in grains using a multimycotoxin detection method: corn, 200; wheat, 400; barley, 500; oats, 500; and rye, 500.[47] Christensen *et al.*[12] reported possible time and temperature effects on zearalenone production in corn. Caldwell and Tuite[9] reported that ears of corn inoculated with isolates of *Fusarium*, which had produced up to 1,100 ppm of zearalenone on autoclaved corn in the laboratory, did not contain over 5 ppm of the compound, suggesting that it is usually produced in storage and not in developing ears. This suggests that zearalenone production on corn used for human consumption can be prevented by proper storage of the grain.

DISCUSSION

The availability of sensitive methods for the analysis and detection of the major phytoestrogens would seem to guarantee that food containing appreciable quantities of the compounds would not be used for human consumption. Plant breeders must assume responsibility for producing strains of plants low in estrogenic activity.[8,16,20] Food processors are obligated to store grains under proper conditions.[9] Plant pathologists must play a role in identifying organisms and strains of organisms involved in estrogen production.[10] They must also assist in revealing the association of plant diseases with possible estrogen production. For example, Loper et al.[31] and Sherwood et al.[42] reported that the urediospores of the alfalfa rust organism, *Uromyces striatus*, contain from 411 to 746 ppm of coumestrol. Also Noveroske et al.[38,39] reported that phloretin, a weak estrogen,[27] is produced in apple leaves in response to the pathogen *Venturia inaequalis.* The production of phenolic compounds[24] in injured or diseased carrots[15] and potatoes[17] may possibly explain the reported estrogenic activity of these vegetables.

Most of the scientific literature published to date would suggest that estrogens do not occur in plants used for food in quantities that would cause physiological effects. In rare instances, where the quantity of estrogen may be high, the low physiological activity of these compounds provides a safety factor. This, in turn, gives assurance relative to the possible carcinogenic effects of phytoestrogens since, "the carcinogenic effect of a hormone appears to require the presence of increased amounts of the hormone, i.e., more than physiologic levels, and continued exposure to the hormone."[57]

REFERENCES

1. A. B. Beck, The oestrogenic isoflavones of subterranean clover. Aust. J. Agric. Res. *15*:223 (1964).
2. E. M. Bickoff, Estrogenic constituents of forage plants. Commonwealth Agric. Bur. Rev. Ser. No. 1 (1968).
3. E. M. Bickoff, A. N. Booth, R. L. Lyman, A. L. Livingston, C. R. Thompson, and F. DeEds, Coumestrol, a new estrogen isolated from forage crops. Science *126*:969 (1957).
4. E. M. Bickoff, A. L. Livingston, S. C. Witt, R. E. Lundin, and R. R. Spencer, Isolation of 4'-O-methyl-coumestrol from alfalfa. J. Agric. Food Chem. *13*:597 (1965).
5. E. M. Bickoff, A. L. Livingston, A. P. Hendrickson, and A. N. Booth, Relative potencies of several estrogen-like compounds found in forages. J. Agric. Food Chem. *10*:410 (1962).

6. E. M. Bickoff, R. R. Spencer, S. C. Witt, and B. E. Knuckles, Studies on the chemical and biological properties of coumestrol and related compounds. U.S.D.A. Techn. Bull. 1408 (1969).

7. R. B. Bradbury and D. E. White, Estrogens and related substances in plants. Vitam. Horm. *12*:207 (1954).

8. A. H. Burgess, Hops, botany, cultivation and utilization. Interscience, New York (1964).

9. R. W. Caldwell and J. Tuite, Zearalenone production in field corn in Indiana. Phytopathology *60*:1696 (1970).

10. R. W. Caldwell, J. Tuite, M. Stob, and R. Baldwin, Zearalenone production by *Fusarium* species. Appl. Microbiol. *20*:31 (1970).

11. E. W. Cheng, L. Yoder, C. D. Story, and W. Burroughs, Estrogenic activity of some naturally occurring isoflavones. Ann. N.Y. Acad. Sci. *61*:652 (1955).

12. C. M. Christensen, G. H. Nelson, and C. J. Mirocha, Effect on the white rat uterus of a toxic substance isolated from *Fusarium*. Appl. Microbiol. *13*:653 (1965).

13. D. H. Curnow, Oestrogenic activity of subterranean clover. 2. The isolation of genistein from subterranean clover and methods of quantitative estimation. Biochem. J. *58*:283 (1954).

14. R. M. Eppley, Screening method for zearalenone, aflatoxin, and ochratoxin, J. Assoc. Off. Anal. Chem. *51*:74 (1968).

15. R. Ferando, M. M. Guilleus, and A. Guerrilott-Vinet, Oestrogenic content of plants as a function of conditions of culture. Nature *192*:205 (1961).

16. C. M. Francis and A. J. Millington, Varietal variation in the isoflavone content of subterranean clover; its estimation by a microtechnique. Aust. J. Agric. Res. *16*:557 (1965).

17. R. T. Frank, The female sex hormone. Harvey Lect. *26*:1, Williams & Wilkins, Baltimore (1930).

18. H. Grisebach and W. Barz, Zur Biogenese der Isoflavone, VIII. 4,2′,4′-Trihydroxy-chalkon-4′glucosid als Vorstufe fur Cumostrol, Formononetin und Daidzein in der Luzerne (*Medicago sativa L.*). Z. Naturforsch. *19*:569 (1964).

19. J. Guggolz, A. L. Livingston, and E. M. Bickoff, Detection of daidzein, formononetin, genistein, and biochanin A in forages. J. Agric. Food Chem. *9*:330 (1961).

20. C. H. Hanson, G. M. Loper, G. O. Kohler, E. M. Bickoff, K. W. Taylor, W. R. Kehr, E. H. Stanford, J. W. Dudley, M. E. Pedersen, E. L. Sorensen, H. L. Carnahan, and C. P. Wilsie, Variation in coumestrol content of alfalfa as related to location, variety, cutting, year, stage of growth, and disease. U.S.D.A. Techn. Bull. No. 1333 (1965).

21. V. E. Heftman, S. Co, and R. D. Bennett, Identification of estrone in date seeds by thin layer chromatography. Naturwissenschaften *52*:431 (1965).

22. G. M. Jacobson, M. J. Frey, and R. B. Hochberg, The absence of steroid estrogens in plants. Steroids *6*: 93 (1965).

23. H. E. H. Jones and G. S. Pope, A method for the isolation of miroestrol from *Pueraria mirifica*. J. Endocrinol. *22*:303 (1961).

24. J. Kuc, Phenolic compounds and disease resistance in plants. In Phenolics in normal and diseased fruit and vegetables, V. C. Runeckles (ed.). Plant Phenolics Group of North America Symposium, Norwood, Mass. (1964).

25. H. J. Kurtz, M. E. Nairn, G. H. Nelson, C. M. Christensen, and C. J. Mirocha,

Histologic changes in the genital tracts of swine fed estrogenic mycotoxin. Am. J. Vet. Res. *30*:551 (1969).

26. W. W. Leavitt and P. A. Wright, the plant estrogen, coumestrol, as an agent affecting hypophysial gonadotropin function. J. Exp. Zool. *160*:319 (1965).

27. L. J. Lerner, A. R. Turkheimer, and A. Borman, Phloretin, a weak estrogen and estrogen antagonist. Proc. Soc. Exp. Biol. Med. *114*:115 (1963).

28. H. R. Lindner, Study of the fate of phyto-oestrogens in the sheep by determination of isoflavones and coumestrol in the plasma and adipose tissue. Aust. J. Agric. Res. *18*:305 (1967).

29. A. L. Livingston, E. M. Bickoff, J. Guggolz, and C. R. Thompson, Quantitative determination of coumestrol in fresh and dried alfalfa. J. Agric. Food Chem. *9*:135 (1961).

30. G. M. Loper, Accumulation of coumestrol in barrel medic (*Medicago littoralis*). Crop Sci. *8*:317 (1968).

31. G. M. Loper, C. H. Hanson, and J. H. Graham, Coumestrol content of alfalfa as affected by selection for resistance to foliar disease. Crop Sci. *7*:189 (1967).

32. T. J. Mabry, K. R. Markham, and M. B. Thomas, The systematic identification of flavonoids. Springer-Verlag, New York (1970).

33. The Merck Company, Merck index. 8th ed. Rahway, N.J. (1968).

34. C. J. Mirocha, C. M. Christensen, and G. H. Nelson, Estrogenic metabolite produced by *Fusarium graminearum* in stored corn, Appl. Microbiol. *497*:15 (1967).

35. C. J. Mirocha, C. M. Christensen, and G. H. Nelson, Toxic metabolites produced by fungi implicated in mycotoxicoses. Biotech. Bioeng. *10*:469 (1968).

36. G. R. Moule, A. W. H. Braden, and D. R. Lamond, The significance of oestrogens in pasture plants in relation to animal production. Anim. Breeding Abstr. *31*:139 (1963).

37. W. D. Noteboom and J. Gorski, Estrogen effect of genistein and coumestrol diacetate. Endocrinology. *73*:736 (1963).

38. R. L. Noveroske, J. Kuc, and E. B. Williams, Oxidation of phloridzin and phloretin related to resistance of *Malus* to *Venturia inaequalis*. Phytopathology *54*: 92 (1964).

39. R. L. Noveroske, E. B. Williams, and J. Kuc, B-glycosidase and phenoloxidase in apple leaves and their possible relation to resistance to *Venturia inaequalis*. Phytopathology *54*:98 (1964).

40. E. Perel and H. R. Lindner, Dissociation of uterotrophic action from implantation-inducing activity in two non-steroidal oestrogens (coumestrol and genistein). J. Repro. Fert. *21*:171 (1970).

41. T. W. Perry, M. Stob, D. A. Huber, and R. C. Peterson, Effect of subcutaneous implantation of resorcylic acid lactone on performance of growing and finishing beef cattle. J. Anim. Sci. *31*:789 (1970).

42. R. T. Sherwood, A. F. Olah, W. H. Oleson, and E. E. Jones, Effect of disease and injury on accumulation of a flavonoid estrogen, coumestrol, in alfalfa. Phytopathology *60*:684 (1970).

43. D. A. Shutt, Interaction of genistein with oestradiol in the reproductive tract of the ovariectomized mouse. J. Endocrinol. *37*:231 (1967).

44. D. A. Shutt, A. Axelsen, and H. R. Lindner, Free and conjugated isoflavones in the plasma of sheep following ingestion of oestrogenic clover. Aust. J. Agric. Res. *18*:647 (1967).

45. D. A. Shutt, A. W. H. Braden, and H. R. Lindner, Plasma coumestrol levels in sheep following administration of synthetic coumestrol or ingestion of medic hay (*Medicago littoralis*). Aust. J. Agric. Res. *20*:65 (1969).

46. L. Stoloff, Report on mycotoxins. J. Assoc. Off. Anal. Chem. *53*:330 (1970).

47. L. Stoloff, S. Nesheim, L. Yin, J. V. Rodricks, M. Stack, and A. D. Campbell, A multimycotoxin detection method for aflatoxins, ochratoxins, zearalenone, sterigmatocystin, and patulin. J. Assoc. Off. Anal. Chem. *54*:91 (1971).

48. M. Stob, R. S. Baldwin, J. Tuite, F. N. Andrews, and K. G. Gillette, Isolation of an anabolic uterotrophic compound from corn infected with *Gibberella zeae*. Nature *196*:1318 (1962).

49. D. Taub, N. N. Giroda, R. D. Hoffsommer, C. H. Kuo, H. L. Slates, S. Weber, and N. L. Wendler, Total synthesis of the macrolide, zearalenone. Tetrahedron *24*:2443 (1968).

50. W. H. Urry, H. L. Wehrmeister, E. B. Hodge, and P. H. Hidy, The structure of zearalenone. Tetrahedron Lett. *27*:3109 (1966).

51. H. Wada and S. Fukushima, Estrogenic activity in soybeans and its products. Jap. J. Zootech. Sci. *34*:243 (1963).

52. H. Wada and M. Yuhara, Identification of plant estrogens in Chinese milk vetch, soybean and soybean sprout. Jap. J. Zootech. Sci. *35*:87 (1964).

53. E. Wong, Isoflavone contents of red and subterranean clover. J. Sci. Food Agric. *14*:376 (1963).

54. W. J. A. Vandenheuvel, The gas–liquid chromatographic behavior of the zearalenones, A new family of biologically active natural products. Sep. Sci. *3*:151 (1968).

55. E. D. Walter, Genistin (an isoflavone glucoside) and its aglucone, genistein, from soybeans. J. Am. Chem. Soc. *63*:3273 (1941).

56. E. Walz, Isoflavone and saponin glycosides in *Soja hispida*. Liebigs. Ann. *489*:118 (1931).

57. M. X. Zarrow, Carcinogenic action of estrogens. Hormonal relationships and applications in the production of meats, milk and eggs. National Academy of Sciences, National Research Council, Publ. 1415, Washington, D.C. (1966).

58. A. Zenisek and I. J. Bednar, Contribution to the identification of the estrogenic activity of hops. Am. Perfum. *75*:61 (1960).

$$25 \quad \text{Lester D. Scheel}$$

PHOTOSENSITIZING AGENTS*

GENERAL DISCUSSION

In preparing a summary of the scientific work accumulated in the area of food photosensitizers, it is necessary to point out the origin of the observations that, although qualitative and at times speculative, have led to the identification of the combination of light and a toxin as causative agents in the production of the observed pathologic change. The identification of the causative agent and its characterization with regard to its chemical nature and the experimental verification of the photosensitizing ability of the isolated material have made it possible to prove the etiology of many of the pathologic syndromes.

For the purposes of this chapter the materials included will be limited to those that occur in food materials and have been shown to produce a phototoxic effect. Whenever possible, the structure of the toxin, the toxic dose, and the test system used to identify the nature of the phototoxic effect will be reviewed and referenced. In addition, chemical structures will be illustrated whenever sufficient evidence exists for confirmation of their phototoxic effect.

In his book *Photodynamic Action and Diseases Caused by Light*, Blum[1] reviewed a disease in sheep called geeldikkop, which, according to Quin and Rimington,[2] was first observed by Hutcheon in 1886. This

* Literature reviewed to January 1972.

disease, which resulted from eating plants of the genus *Tribulus*, caused the affected animals to avoid sunlight; the disease occurred only during March through December in flocks pasturing on the Karoo veldt in South Africa. Paine[3] noted that the affected sheep avoided sunlight, and he suggested pasturing the flocks at night as a remedy; however, he did not recognize the syndrome as a photosensitization response. Theiler[4] suggested that the lesions that appeared on the face, ears, and hooflines of the sheep were sunburn lesions, but he did not connect food with the production of the sensitivity to sunlight. Quin,[5] while investigating the disease in South Africa, found that the lesions healed if the animals were removed from the sunlight or were placed on other food materials. Thus, he provided the first evidence that both sunlight and the food were necessary to produce the characteristic syndrome in sheep.

This syndrome has been characterized by edema of the skin and head, accompanied by intense jaundice, constipation, and an accumulation of bile pigments that are eliminated in the urine. The animals appear very sick and, when exposed to sunlight, appear stunned. The affected skin turns hard and brown, with the extreme reaction around the eyes causing blindness. The conjunctivae and mucous membranes of the mouth become deep yellow due to the marked jaundice. There has been no evidence reported that the disease is either infectious or associated with secondary infections.

Theiler,[4] in feeding experiments employing *Tribulus terrestris*, produced symptoms of geeldikkop, and Quin[6] confirmed these experiments using *T. ovis*. Quin[7] observed that after feeding two species of *Lippia*, the same signs of disease produced by *Tribulus* occurred; Quin[8] pointed out further that a disease called dikoor also occurred in sheep in the high Transvaal veldt where *Tribulus* is not found. Rimington and Quin[9] extended the previous observations when they reported the disease in sheep feeding on *Pannicum laevifolium* and *P. coloratum*. Thus, the disease is produced by at least three genera of the families *Zygophyllaceae, Verbenaceae*, and *Graminae*.

Quin,[7,10-13] in a series of studies performed to determine the mechanism of the disease, showed that photosensitization in sheep, accompanied by icterus, could be reproduced by ligating the bile duct, thus proving an association between the icterus and the photosensitivity. Included in these studies were feeding trials that involved production of photosensitization by administration of dried *Hypericum ethiopicum*. However, this photosensitization was not accompanied by icterus; therefore, it did not present the same clinical picture as geeldikkop.

In 1934 Rimington and Quin[14] reported the identification of porphyrin in sheep bile and blood following ligation of the bile duct. In studies conducted on sheep during an episode of geeldikkop, the same porphyrin was identified and isolated from the bile of the diseased sheep. Careful studies characterized the porphyrin as phylloerythrin. Parenteral studies using 0.1 g of the crystalline phylloerythrin produced photosensitization of the skin of the injected animal but did not produce the severe icterus seen in the diseased animals.

Fischer[15] discussed the origin and characterization of the porphyrins as derivatives of chlorophyll. In Blum's review of the metabolism of phylloerythrins, he presents evidence showing that the porphyrins are present only in the digestive tract of ruminants when the animals are fed chlorophyll-containing food and that these compounds can be absorbed through the wall of the stomach. He points out further that the normal excretion of these compounds is via the bile; therefore, the appearance of this material in the lower digestive tract is probably from this source.

The careful work of Rimington and Quin[14] established that, if no interference with the bile excretion took place, there was no accumulation of bile in the blood and no icterus. Therefore, in studying the mechanism of the production of phylloerythrin, Quin et al.[16] found that the phylloerythrin is produced normally during the digestive process in the intestinal tract of various animals by the action of the intestinal microorganisms on chlorophyll-containing food. (See Figure 1.)

Since phylloerythrin did not accumulate in the blood and tissues unless a bile duct obstruction took place, these researchers reasoned that geeldikkop results only when liver dysfunction with associated bile duct obstruction takes place. Since the outbreaks of geeldikkop, in general, involved large numbers of sheep in a flock, it was further reasoned that another toxic substance might be the cause of the icterus that is characteristic of this disease.

Rimington et al.[17] isolated a material from *Lippia rehmanni* that, when fed to sheep in doses of 1 g or more, produced bilirubinemia within 24 h. These investigators named their substance "icterogenin" because it produced severe icterus in sheep and caused photosensitization of the skin when the animals were also fed a diet containing chlorophyll. Barton and de Mayo[18] reported that the structure of icterogenin was that of a triterpenoid that was isolated and characterized from *Lippia rehmanni.*

In further experimental studies Heikel and Rimington[19] reported that icterogenin and a closely related compound, rehmannic acid, occur together in *Lippia rehmanni* and in *Lanata camara.* When these two compounds were injected intraperitoneally in doses of 100–150 mg/kg to rabbits with a bile fistula, they caused a marked decrease in bile flow. This decrease in bile flow was accompanied by a severe reduction in

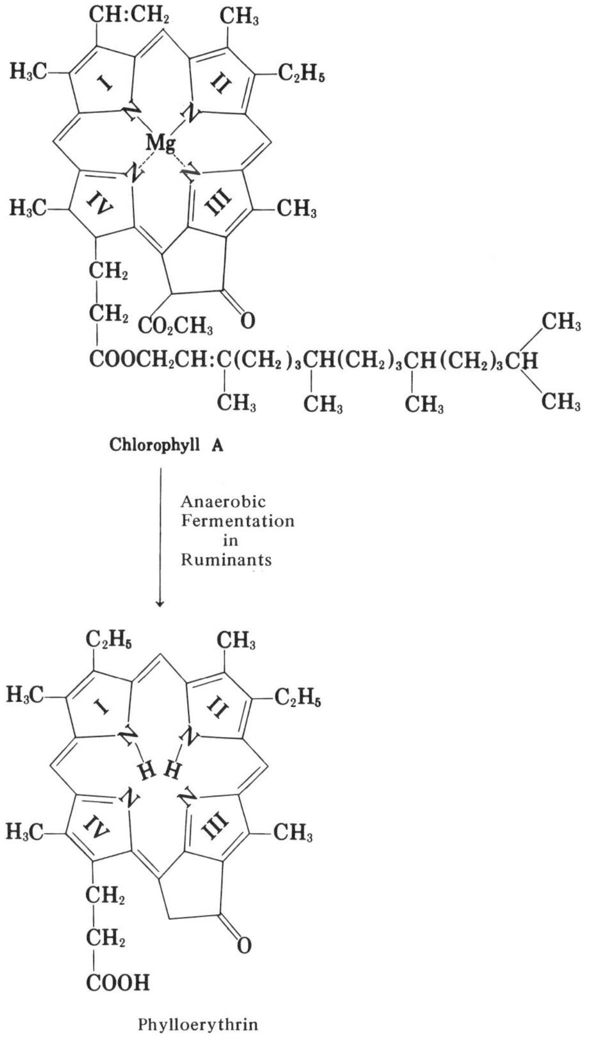

Chlorophyll A

Anaerobic
Fermentation
in
Ruminants

Phylloerythrin

FIGURE 1 The phototoxin phylloerythrin produced from chlorophyll A.

bile pigment and porphyrin excretion. When bilirubin, phylloerythrin, coproporphyrin, or bromsulphalein was injected intravenously at the height of the intoxication, there was little or no elimination of the pigments in the bile, although they were excreted in the urine. Examination of the liver following these studies revealed no severe pathologic changes. Geeldikkop observed in sheep during the summer grazing season has been identified in part as a photosensitive response due to the

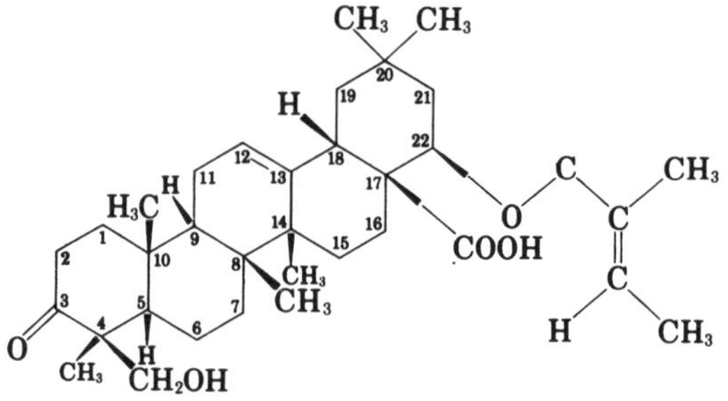

Icterogenin

presence of phylloerythrin in the blood and tissues. This response is caused by the presence of icterogenin, which produces severe constipation and spastic contraction of the bile duct in sheep and thus interferes with the excretion of the chlorophyll degradation products. This response can be prevented by eliminating chlorophyll from the diet, by removing affected animals from direct sunlight, or by pasturing them on plants that are free of icterogenin.

In Australia Dodd[20] observed that shorn sheep displayed symptoms indicating an extreme sensitivity to sunlight. By muzzling the sheep so they could not eat the *Hypericum* (St. John's wort) plants in the pasture, he proved that the external contact with the plant did not cause the disease symptoms. He further showed that the signs of sensitization were only displayed by freshly shorn animals exposed to intense sunlight. These observations were confirmed in Australia by Henry[21] and by Seddon and Belschner,[22] and in South Africa by Quin.[11] In these confirmatory experiments, different samples of plant tissue in the fresh or dried state when fed to sheep did not alter the response observed, thereby proving that age and condition of the plant were of much less importance than the intensity of the sunlight.

Ray[23] reported that an extract of *Hypericum crispum* gave a red fluorescent solution that would produce photosensitization of rabbits

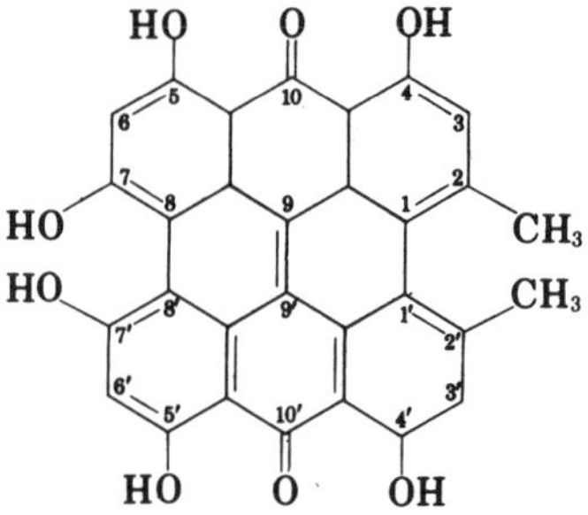

Hypericin

and sheep. These observations were confirmed and extended by Ioannidès[24] and by Horsley.[25] Horsley observed that 4 mg of hypericin administered to a rat produced symptoms of photosensitivity following exposure to sunlight. However, if the dose administered was a 4:1 mixture of a "yellow waxy substance" and hypericin, only 0.8 mg of hypericin was required to produce the same effect. Blum[1] suggests that the yellow substance, also obtained from the plant during extraction, was "undoubtedly quercetin," which did not sensitize the animal when injected without hypericin.

Sampson and Parker[26] described the sick animals as emaciated with a blistering and scabby condition of the muzzle, eyes, and ears and with sloughing of the wool in affected areas. This disease has been reported in widely scattered areas of the world because of the ubiquity of various species of the *Hypericum* plant family. Photosensitive signs have been observed in many different animal species following feeding on pastures containing the *Hypericum* plants.

Brockmann and his co-workers[27-29] extracted the dried flowers of *Hypericum perforatum* with methyl alcohol and obtained a deep red solution that, after acidification and standing for 2 days at a temperature of 0 °C, gave a black powder. When recrystallized from pyridine–methyl alcohol–HCl solution, the black powder yielded red-violet needles that melted with decomposition above 330 °C. Brilliant chemical characterization studies by Brockmann and his students showed the isolated compound to be hexahydroxy-2,2'-dimethylnaphthodianthrone, which was called hypericin.

It was found that the hypericin content of plant tissue increased with the age of the plant and varied with the species of plant studied. The hypericin content of the flowers of *Hypericum perforatum* contained as much as 2,400 mg/kg of dry substance, but the stems contained only 200 mg/kg.

When the isolated material was tested by administering it to rats, followed by exposing the animals to sunlight, it was found that 1–2 mg/rat resulted in death of the animals in 1–2 h. When mice were administered 0.25–0.5 mg of hypericin and exposed to a 2,000-W lamp for 30 min, the animals died within 24 h. Control mice injected with 3–4 mg of hypericin and kept in the dark survived.

The observations of Horsley[25] suggest that secondary factors such as quercetin can enhance the effects of a photosensitizer such as hypericin. Since quercetin is a polyhydroxyflavone that might also be activated by light, it may potentiate the reaction.

The first experiments to demonstrate the photosensitization caused by feeding of *Fagopyrum esculentum* (buckwheat) were carried out in

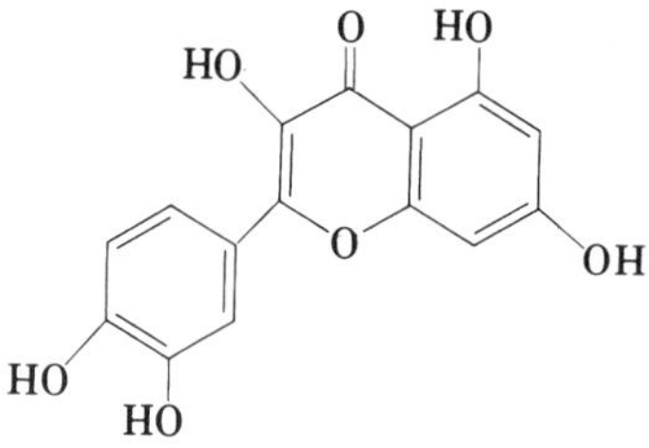

Quercetin

1887 by Wedding.[30] He showed that if sheep and cattle fed on buck-wheat were not exposed to sunlight, no sensory stimulation or skin lesions occurred. Blum[1] reviewed the early literature concerning the confirmation of Wedding's observations.

The work of Brockmann[31] on the helianthrone pigments has resulted in identification of the pigments causing the photosensitization by the *Fagopyrum* plant family. It was shown that the blossoms of the buck-wheat plant contained two pigments, structurally related to hypericin, which could produce photosensitization in the rat. One pigment, fago-pyrin, was a hexahydroxynaphthodianthrone with side chains, $C_7H_{13}NO$, in the 2 and 2' positions replacing the methyl groups of hypericin. The second pigment identified in the buckwheat extract was the helian-throne analog of fagopyrin and was named protofagopyrin.

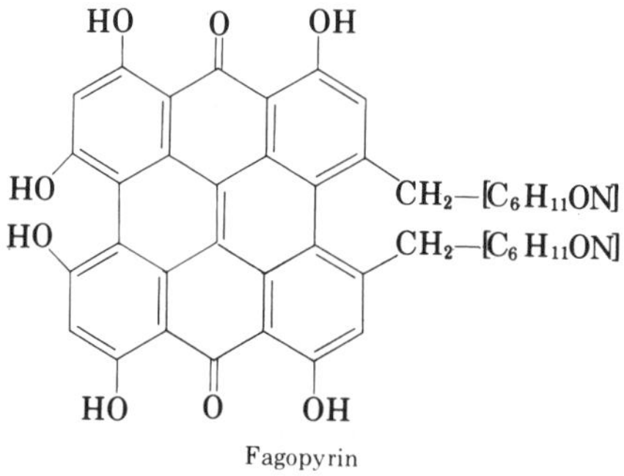

Fagopyrin

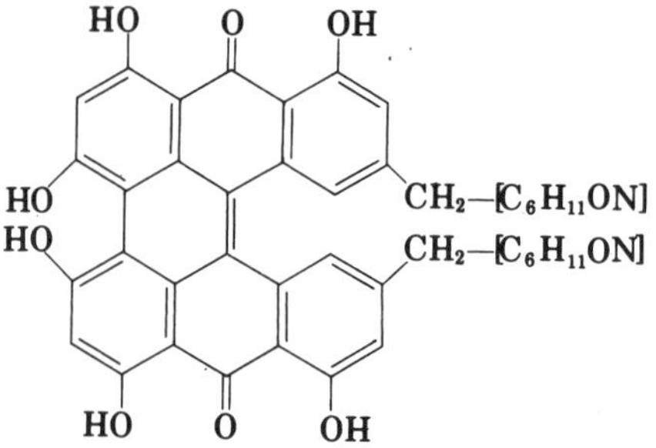

Photofagopyrin

As the result of this work, it was observed that the plant pigments may occur naturally as 7,7'-hydroxy esters.[32] Identification of these groups has not been reported, but their ease of acid hydrolysis during extraction and isolation procedures might indicate that they exist as glycosides.

Brockmann[31] has suggested a scheme for his synthesis of hypericin and for the fagopyrin-type plant pigments. Results of laboratory work indicated that hypericin might be formed by oxidative condensation of two emodin–anthranol molecules. To prove that such condensation could be accomplished, Brockmann and Eggers[33] oxidized a solution of emodin–anthranol in a pyridine–piperidine mixed solvent and chromatographically separated a dark red crystalline compound; upon acetylation, the crystals gave a helianthrene derivative that, on exposure to light, gave hypericin. Thus, starting with known plant products, a spontaneous nonenzymatic condensation leading to the formation of hypericin was demonstrated.

Brockmann and Sanne[34] isolated and identified, from plant sources, the intermediate compounds proposed for the hypericin synthesis. (See Figure 2.)

In addition to the above anthrone pigments, it is known that the buckwheat plant contains significant quantities of flavanol compounds, including quercetin and rutin, that might cause a significant modification of the photosensitizing capacity of the pigments. To date only fragmentary information concerning this type of biological toxicity has been reported.

Rutin

Imai and Furuya,[35] in conducting extraction studies on *Fagopyrum cymosum*, found that the content of the 3-rhamnoglucoside of quercetin (rutin) increased—from about 4% in May to 8.5% in October—with the age of the leaves extracted. More research is needed concerning the interaction of pigments that either increase the effectiveness of photosensitizing materials or are synergistic with photosensitizing compounds.

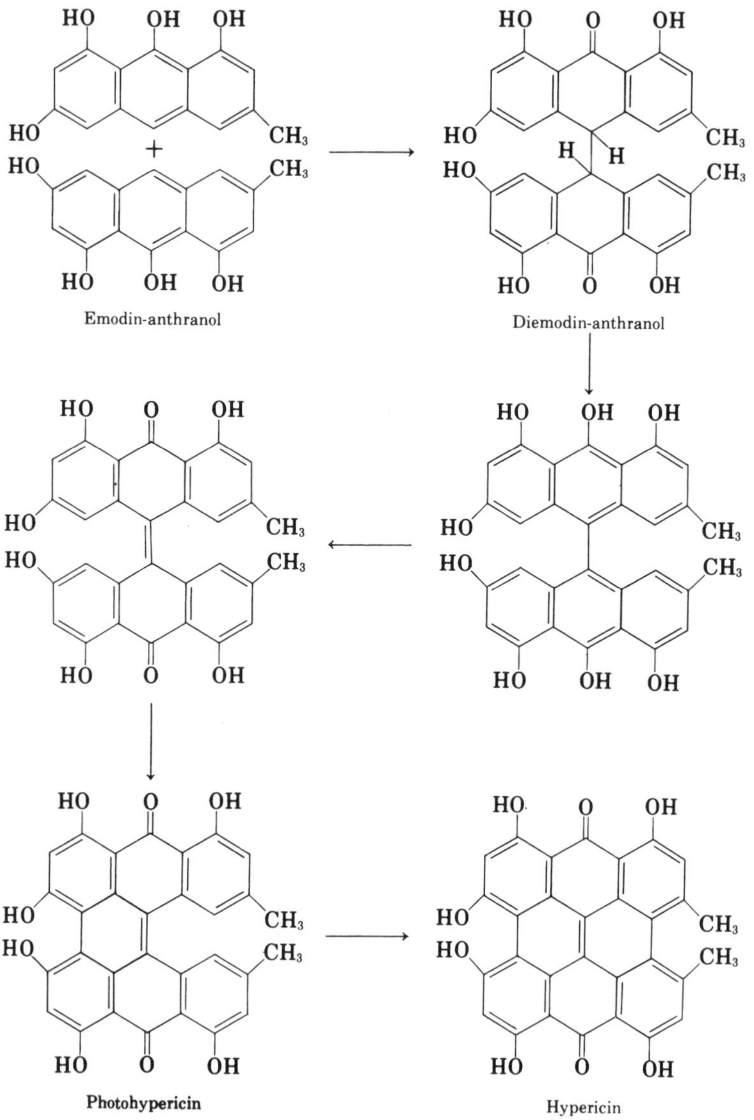

FIGURE 2   Brockmann's proposed hypericin biosynthesis.

PHOTOSENSITIZATION BY PSORALENS

The use of such compounds as *p*-aminobenzoic acid and other sensitizing compounds in suntan oils is based on the principle of induced pigment stimulation following the photosensitization reaction. The identification and characterization of the conditions necessary for primary photosensitization in man have developed around the chemical isolation, characterization, and synthesis of a family of furocoumarin compounds, the psoralens. The naturally occurring parent compounds of this family are psoralen and angelicin.

p-Aminobenzoic Acid   Psoralen   Angelicin

It has been shown by Fitzpatrick *et al.*[36] that, in addition to topical application, man can be sensitized to sunlight by oral administration of the photosensitizer, 8-methoxypsoralen.

These observations raise questions concerning the photosensitizing capacity of food materials, since many of the plants that contain psoralens are used for food. Gryzbowski[37] described a photodermatitic reaction in a starving person following ingestion of goosefoot. Pathak *et al.*[38] reviewed the occurrence of furocoumarins in plants and pointed out that photosensitivity is caused by contact of the skin with such plants as figs, parsley, caraway, and limes. It has not been demonstrated that ingestion of natural furocoumarin-containing food causes photosensitization in man. Such demonstration would be difficult, since man eats a wide variety of cooked foods that may well have been altered in the preparation.

Birmingham *et al.*[39] reported the association of phototoxic sensitization in celery harvesters with the occurrence of a mold (*Sclerotinia sclerotiorum*) on the celery handled by the workers. Later work by Perone *et al.*[40] showed that the phototoxin occurred only in the infected part of the celery plant. They reported that if other molds were grown on celery tissue, the photosensitizers were not produced. The isolation, characterization, and biologic activity studies of 8-methoxypsoralen and 4,5',8-trimethylpsoralen conducted by Scheel *et al.*[41] demonstrated that the photosensitization of the workers was due to this compound.

Because coumarins steam distil, it is suggested that boiling foods greatly reduces the amount of these materials and that man therefore does not ingest a toxic dose except under unusual circumstances.

The extent to which molecular structure influences biologic activity of the photosensitizing furocoumarins has been studied extensively by

Musajo *et al.,*[42] Pathak and Fitzpatrick,[43] and Pathak *et al.*[44] This area has been recently reviewed by Pathak.[45] The linear coumarin structure without substitution is the most active form of this family of compounds. Substitution of positions, 4, 5, 8, 4', or 5' with methyl groups produces less change in photosensitizing activity than substitution with methoxy groups. However, substitution of these positions with hydroxyl groups destroys the photosensitizing activities entirely. Any substituent that causes an interference in the resonance of the furocoumarin molecule alters the activity of the photosensitizer.

The action spectrum of the furocoumarin family of compounds lies between 320 and 380 nm, with a peak of coincident activity at 360 nm. This action spectrum is quite different from that of the hypericin type of sensitizer, which lies between 400 and 600 nm (Brockmann *et al.*[46]). Spikes and Straight[47] have reviewed the sensitized photochemical processes in biological systems and have pointed out that they may be either aerobic or anaerobic.

In the photoautoxidation reactions, the saturated aliphatics and aromatics tend to be resistant to sensitization by active compounds. Heterocyclics and substituted aromatic rings increase the susceptibility to photosensitized oxidation. Thus, such compounds as tyrosine are very sensitive to oxidation, whereas phenylalanine is fairly resistant. These reactions can be activated by such compounds as riboflavin and can produce protein photoautoxidation with accompanying denaturation. A number of materials such as reducing agents, certain metals, and iodide ions protect the cells against this type of photodynamic effect.

The phototoxic reactions have been used to sterilize solutions by the addition of dyes and exposure to appropriate light sources. The dye-sensitized protein denaturations have been found effective against bacteria, protozoa, viruses, plants, and animals and depend only on the dye concentration and the proper radiant energy dose to activate the photosensitized oxidation.

The mechanism of the anaerobic photosensitization, which occurs following contact with the psoralens, has been studied by Musajo[48] and Krauch.[49] These studies have shown that the psoralens react with the flavin mononucleotides and produce an inactivation of their function in cellular respiration. In addition, the psoralens react with DNA and with RNA.[53] This reaction is reported to be located on pyrimidine residues but not on purine residues.[54] Spikes and Straight[47] have reviewed the data available on the mechanism of sensitized photoautoxidation; the reader is referred to their review for further discussion of the subject.

From the above discussion it is obvious that photosensitization of living systems involving the consumption of food materials by animals or man does occur. In addition, as pointed out by the massive research on the psoralens, the phototoxin is active when it comes into contact with the skin; the photosensitized reaction then takes place when the skin is exposed to the sunlight.

Richards,[50] Scheel,[51] and Perone[52] have recently reviewed the chemistry of coumarins associated with mold growth and have shown that many toxic coumarins can be produced during food spoilage by molds. This action includes the furanocoumarins associated with the photosensitization of celery harvesters.

SUMMARY

Although photosensitization associated with food consumption by man is reported, it is not yet a well-established or recognized syndrome that occurs frequently. This may be related to the fact that many of the toxic coumarins would distil out of the food material during the cooking process.

In the case of the animal diseases due to photosensitization, the association between disease and the food is an established fact. Although the isolation and characterization of the chemical compounds that produce the disease have been accomplished, and therefore the mechanism of the disease has been established, the remedy for the situation by elimination of the plants that cause the condition is not a simple procedure.

In addition, as in the case of geeldikkop in sheep, it has been shown that the metabolism of chlorophyll is generally not toxic because the phylloerythrin would be excreted in the bile by the liver. However, in the *Tribulus* plant the triterpene icterogenin occurs, which causes a spastic contraction of the bile duct, thus preventing the normal excretion. Under these conditions the accumulation of the phylloerythrin in the blood and tissues results in the photosensitization. Thus, porphyrins can act as photosensitizers, but the dose level at the site of irradiation may not reach sensitizing concentrations except in the presence of co-factor activity.

Continued effort and keen observation on the part of people connected with the management of situations where exposure to the sun occurs will enlarge our knowledge of suggested photosensitization reactions. This, in turn, should lead to the elucidation of any new phototoxic syndromes that arise.

REFERENCES

1. H. F. Blum, Photodynamic action and diseases caused by light. Hafner Publishing Co., New York (1964).

2. J. I. Quin and C. Rimington, Geeldikkop. A critical review of the problem as it affects sheep farming in the Karoo together with recommendations in the light of newer knowledge. J. S. Afr. Vet. Med. Assoc. 6:16 (1935).

3. R. Paine, Geel Dikkop. J. Comp. Path. Ther. 19:5 (1906).

4. A. Theiler, Geeldikkop in sheep (Tribulosis ovium). Rep. Dir. Vet. Serv. Anim. Ind. Onderstepoort 7–8:1 (1918).

5. J. I. Quin, Recent investigations into geeldikkop affecting sheep and goats in the Cape Province. J. S. Afr. Vet. Med. Assoc. 1:43 (1928).

6. J. I. Quin, Further investigations in geeldikkop (Tribulosis ovium). Rep. Dir. Vet. Serv. Anim. Ind. Onderstepoort 15:765 (1929).

7. J. I. Quin, Studies on the photosensitisation of animals in South Africa. I. The action of various fluorescent dye-stuffs. Onderstepoort J. Vet. Sci. Anim. Ind. 1:459 (1933).

8. J. I. Quin, Further investigations into the problem of geeldikkop (Tribulosis) in small stock. Rep. Dir. Vet. Serv. Anim. Ind. Onderstepoort 16:413 (1930).

9. C. Rimington and J. I. Quin, Dik-oor or geel-dikkop on grass-veld pastures. J. S. Afr. Vet. Med. Assoc. 8:141 (1937).

10. J. I. Quin, Studies on the photosensitisation of animals in South Africa. III. The photodynamic action of Hypericum ethiopicum var. glaucescens Sond. and Hypericum leucoptychodes (Syn. H. lanceolatum Lam.) Onderstepoort J. Vet. Sci. Anim. Ind. 1:491 (1933).

11. J. I. Quin, Studies on the photosensitisation of animals in South Africa. IV. The toxicity of Lopholaena coriifolia (Harv.) Phill. & C. A. Sm. (=L. randii sp. Moore). Onderstepoort J. Vet. Sci. Anim. Ind. 1:497 (1933).

12. J. I. Quin, Studies on the photosensitisation of animals in South Africa. V. The toxicity of Lippia rehmanni (Pears) and Lippia pretoriensis (Pears). Onderstepoort J. Vet. Sci. Anim. Ind. 1:501 (1933).

13. J. I. Quin, Studies on the photosensitisation of animals in South Africa. VI. The effect of surgical obstruction of the normal bile flow. Onderstepoort J. Vet. Sci. Anim. Ind. 1:505 (1933).

14. C. Rimington and J. I. Quin, Studies on the photosensitisation of animals in South Africa. VII. The nature of the photosensitising agent in geeldikkop. Onderstepoort J. Vet. Sci. Anim. Ind. 3:137 (1934).

15. H. Fischer, Chlorophyll. Chem. Rev. 20:41 (1937).

16. J. I. Quin, C. Rimington, and G. C. S. Roets, Studies on the photosensitisation of animals in South Africa. VIII. The biological formaton of phylloerythrin in the digestive tracts of various domesticated animals. Onderstepoort J. Vet. Sci. Anim. Ind. 4:463 (1935).

17. C. Rimington, J. I. Quin, and G. C. S. Roets, Studies on the photosensitisation of animals in South Africa. X. The icterogenic factor in geel-dikkop. Isolation of active principles from Lippia rehmanni Pears. Onderstepoort J. Vet. Sci. Anim. Ind. 9:225 (1937).

18. D. H. R. Barton and P. de Mayo, Triterpenoids. XV. Constitution of icterogenin, a physiologically active triterpenoid. J. Chem. Soc., 887 (1954).

19. T. A. J. Heikel and C. Rimington, Inhibition of biliary secretion by icterogenin and related triterpenes-II. Effect of icterogenin, crude rehmannic acid, oleanolic acetate and "mixed lippia acids" on mitochondria isolated from biliary fistula rabbits receiving the triterpenes. Biochem. Pharmacol. 17:1091 (1968).

20. S. Dodd, St. John's wort and its effects on live stock. Agric. Gaz. N. S. Wales 31:265 (1920).

21. M. Henry, Feeding and contact experiments with St. John's wort, Agric. Gaz. N. S. Wales *33*:205 (1922).
22. H. R. Seddon and H. G. Belschner, The effect of young, immature St. John's wort on sheep. Agric. Gaz. N. S. Wales *40*:914 (1929).
23. G. Ray, Note sur les effets toxiques du Millepertuis à feuilles crispées (*Hypericum crispum*). Bull. Soc. Cent. Méd. Vét. *68*:39 (1914).
24. Z. M. Ioannidès, Le pigment phototoxique de l'*Hypericum crispum*. C. R. Soc. Biol. *105*:349 (1930).
25. C. H. Horsley, Investigation into the action of St. Johns wort. J. Pharmacol. Exp. Ther. *50*:310 (1934).
26. A. W. Sampson and K. W. Parker, St. Johnswort on range lands of California. Univ. Calif. Agric. Exp. Stn. Bull. 503 (1930).
27. H. Brockmann, F. Pohl, K. Maier, and M. N. Haschad, Über das Hypericin, den photodynamischen Farbstoff des Johanniskrautes (Hypericum perforatum). Ann. Chem. *553*:1 (1942).
28. H. Brockmann and F. Kluge, Zur Synthese des Hypericins. Naturwissenschaften *38*:141 (1951).
29. H. Brockmann, F. Kluge, and H. Muxfeldt, Totalsynthese des Hypericins. Chem. Ber. *90*:2302 (1957).
30. M. Wedding, Einfluss des Lichtes auf die Haut der Thiere. Z. Ethnol. *19*, Verh. Berl. Ges. Anthropol. Ethnol. Urgeschichte, 67 (1887).
31. H. Brockmann, Photodynamically active plant pigments. Proc. Chem. Soc., 304 (1957).
32. H. Brockmann, E. Weber, and G. Pampus, Protofagopyrin und Fagopyrin, die photodynamisch wirksamen Farbstoffe des Buchweizens (*Fagopyrum esculenium*). Ann. Chem. *575*:53 (1952).
33. H. Brockmann and H. Eggers, Partialsynthese des Protohypericins und Hypericins aus Emodin-anthron-(9). Angew. Chem. *67*:706 (1955).
34. H. Brockmann and W. Sanne, Zur Biosynthese des Hypericins. Naturwissenschaften *40*:509 (1953).
35. K. Imai and K. Furuya, Study of phytochemical component of *Fagopyrum cymosum* Meisn. J. Pharm. Soc. Jap. *71*:266 (1951).
36. T. B. Fitzpatrick, C. E. Hopkins, D. D. Blickenstaff, and S. Swift, Augmented pigmentation and other responses of normal human skin to solar pigmentation following oral administration of 8-methoxypsoralen. J. Invest. Dermatol. *25*: 187 (1955).
37. M. Gryzbowski, A peculiar, pellagra-like skin sensitization to light in starving persons. Br. J. Dermatol. Syph. *60*:410 (1948).
38. M. A. Pathak, F. Daniels, Jr., and T. B. Fitzpatrick, The presently known distribution of furocoumarins (psoralens) in plants. J. Invest. Dermatol. *39*:225 (1962).
39. D. J. Birmingham, M. M. Key, G. E. Tubich, and V. B. Perone, Phototoxic bullae among celery harvesters. Arch. Dermatol. *83*:73 (1961).
40. V. B. Perone, L. D. Scheel, and R. J. Meitus, A bioassay for the quantitation of cutaneous reactions associated with pink-rot celery. J. Invest. Dermatol. *42*:267 (1964).
41. L. D. Scheel, V. B. Perone, R. L. Larkin, and R. E. Kupel, The isolation and characterization of two phototoxic furanocoumarins (psoralens) from diseased celery. Biochemistry *2*:1127 (1963).
42. L. Musajo, G. Rodighiero, G. Caporale, and C. Antonello, Ulteriori ricerche sui

rapporti fra constituzione e proprietà fotodinamiche nel campo delle furo-
cumarine. Farm. (Pavia) Ed. Sci. *13*:355 (1958).

43. M. A. Pathak and T. B. Fitzpatrick, Relationship of molecular configuration to
the activity of furocoumarins which increase the cutaneous responses following
long wave ultraviolet radiation. J. Invest. Dermatol. *32*:255 (1959).

44. M. A. Pathak, L. R. Worden, and K. D. Kaufman, Effect of structural alterations on the photosensitizing potency of furocoumarins (psoralens) and related
compounds. J. Invest. Dermatol. *48*:103 (1967).

45. M. A. Pathak, Basic aspects of cutaneous photosensitization, pp. 489–511. In
The biologic effects of ultraviolet radiation (with emphasis on the skin). F.
Urbach (ed.). Pergamon Press, Oxford (1969).

46. H. Brockmann, E. H. v. Falkenhausen, R. Neeff, A. Dorlars, and G. Budde, Die
Konstitution des Hypericins. Chem. Ber. *84*:865 (1951).

47. J. D. Spikes and R. Straight, Sensitized photochemical processes in biological
systems, pp. 409–436. In Annual Review of physical chemistry, Vol. 18, H.
Eyring (ed.). Annual Reviews, Inc., Palo Alto (1967).

48. L. Musajo, Photoreactions between flavin coenzymes and skin-photosensitizing
agents. Pure Appl. Chem. *6*:369 (1963).

49. C. H. Krauch, Neuartige strahlen-chemische und-biologische Reaktionen von
Furocumarinen und deren Lenkung. Chimia *20*:59 (1966).

50. D. E. Richards, The isolation and identification of the toxic coumarins, pp. 3–
45. In Microbial toxins, Vol. VIII, S. Kadis, A. Ciegler, and S. J. Ajl (eds.).
Academic Press, New York (1972).

51. L. D. Scheel, The biological action and metabolism of the toxic coumarins, pp.
47–66. In Microbial toxins, Vol. VIII, S. Kadis, A. Ciegler, and S. J. Ajl (eds.)
Academic Press, New York (1972).

52. V. B. Perone, The natural occurrence and uses of the toxic coumarins, pp. 67–
91. In Microbial toxins, Vol. VIII, S. Kadis, A. Ciegler, and S. J. Ajl (eds.)
Academic Press, New York (1972).

53. M. A. Pathak and D. M. Krämer, Photosensitization of skin in vivo by furocoumarins (psoralens). Biochim. Biophys. Acta. *195*:197–206 (1969).

54. L. Musajo and G. Rodighiero, Studies on the photo-C_4-cyclo-addition reactions
between skin-photosensitizing furocoumarins and nucleic acids, pp. 27–35. In
Photochemistry and photobiology, Vol. II. Pergamon Press, Oxford (1970).

26 Julius M. Coon

TOXICOLOGY
OF NATURAL
FOOD CHEMICALS:
A PERSPECTIVE

Any comprehensive consideration of the toxicology of the natural chemical components of foods should take cognizance of the total picture of foods as the most complex part of man's chemical environment. To view in this perspective the toxic substances that occur naturally in foods, the following table is presented to classify the possible origins—man-made as well as natural—of potentially harmful chemical substances in the foods of man. This constitutes a skeleton outline of the subject of food toxicology. Infectious organisms that are important hazards as food contaminants are not included in this outline, because the illnesses they produce are not ordinarily considered to be toxicological processes.

TOXIC CHEMICALS IN FOODS

Natural

    1. Normal components of natural food products
    2. Natural contaminants of natural food products
       a. Microbiological origin—toxins
       b. Nonmicrobiological origin (e.g., Hg, Se), toxicants consumed in feeds by animals used
as food sources

Man-made

    3. Agricultural chemicals (e.g., pesticides, fertilizers)
    4. Food additives
    5. Chemicals derived from food packaging materials
    6. Chemicals produced in processing of foods (e.g., by heat, ionizing radiation)
    7. Inadvertent or accidental contaminants

a. Food preparation accidents or mistakes
b. Contamination from food utensils
c. Environmental pollution
d. Contamination during storage or transport

Categories 1 and 2 in the table will readily be recognized as constituting the subject of this book. The toxins of bacterial origin, such as staphylococcus enterotoxin and botulinum toxin, are considered in Chapter 18, though the presence of these two toxins (as well as some mycotoxins under certain circumstances) in foods as consumed by man is usually the result of man's faulty processing methods or his carelessness or ignorance in their storage or preparation for consumption. On the other hand, the seafood toxins and the other classes of substances designated natural in the outline are present in certain foods *before* they reach the hands of man to be processed for consumption.

Many of the chemical substances present in foods because of natural processes are the same as many that enter foods as a result of man's efforts to produce or process foods or to distribute and prepare them for immediate consumption. For example, a predominant number of the food additives (e.g., vitamins; amino acids; fatty acids and their esters; polysaccharides; inorganic and organic salts of sodium, potassium, calcium, and magnesium; compounds of other essential elements; spices and flavors; and natural coloring materials) are normal constituents of natural food products. Such toxic metals as lead, mercury, cadmium, arsenic, and zinc, which may contaminate foods from utensils or through environmental pollution, are also normally and naturally present in them. In fact, they are unavoidable, since they occur in soil, water, and plants from the natural geochemistry of the earth. Substances generated by chemical changes caused by heat, drying, freezing, pickling, and irradiation are obviously derived from the natural chemical components of the foods subjected to these processing methods.

On a worldwide basis various substances in categories 1 and 2a have produced greater known injury to man than have those in the other categories. Category 7 has also made a substantial, though lesser, contribution to the total incidence of food-borne illness. On the other hand, groups 3 to 6 are not known to have been responsible for adverse effects on human health when such materials have been used in accordance with good agricultural and manufacturing practices. These comparisons of the extent of the known injury to human health caused by the different groups of agents appear to parallel the comparative susceptibility of the groups to regulatory control. Thus, what man has used by design to produce, process, and package foods can be subject to rigid controls, whereas the natural composition of foods and the natural processes of food contamination are relatively immune to legal regulatory measures.

NATURAL CHEMICAL COMPONENTS OF FOODS

The normal components of natural food products constitute more than 99% of the weight of our daily diet. Food additives comprise the bulk of the balance, with pesticide residues and contaminants of both natural and man-made origin contributing only trace amounts of the order of parts per million. When it is considered that most of the food additives are themselves either dietary supplements or materials derived from or present in natural sources, it becomes clear that only a small fraction of 1% of our diet is not derived from natural food products.

Thus, the natural chemical components of foods are placed in the general toxicological context of the modern diet of man as the major part of his chemical environment. The normal and natural constituents of foods contribute by far both the greatest amount and the widest variety of chemical substances consumed by man over his lifetime. No single plant used as a source of food has been as well characterized chemically as has the air we breathe and the water we drink, even when these are quite polluted. The potato, usually thought of as one of man's simpler foods, is a complex chemical aggregate. About 150 distinct chemical substances have been identified in this natural product, among which are the solanine alkaloids, oxalic acid, arsenic, tannins, nitrate, and over a hundred other items of no recognized nutritional significance to man.[1] Forty-two chemical entities have been found in orange oil,[2] including 12 alcohols, 9 aldehydes, 2 esters, 14 hydrocarbons, and 4 ketones. The orange as a whole includes a host of other chemical substances. All vegetables and fruits and other natural food products are similarly complex.

Thus, many chemical components of natural food products have been identified. It is likely, however, that even more have not. The great number of chemical substances discovered in any single food studied itself reflects an almost endless variety of specific chemical compounds that remain to be discovered in all the foods that make up the diet of man. At each step in the continuous increase in the sensitivity of our analytical methods, more and more discrete chemical entities will undoubtedly be found.

TOXICITY VERSUS HAZARD

Relatively few of the specific chemicals known or not known to be naturally present in our foods have been evaluated toxicologically. Furthermore, it is toxicologically axiomatic that if almost any one of this myriad of chemical substances were tested in experimental animals by today's standards of safety evaluation, it would be shown to be toxic.

Thus, it may be said that in the natural foods of our everyday diet there are thousands of toxic substances. This does not imply, however, that a hazard exists in this situation.

The *toxicity* of a substance is its intrinsic capacity to produce injury when tested by itself. The *hazard* of a substance is its capacity to produce injury under the circumstances of exposure. In connection with the safety of natural food products, our concern is not directly with the intrinsic toxicity of their innumerable chemical components but rather with the potential hazards of these materials when we eat the foods in which they are present. For example, arsenic, lead, mercury, and fluorine have high intrinsic toxicities, but no hazard is associated with their natural presence in foods. Oxalate is toxic, but its presence in spinach is not a hazard. The cyanogenetic glycoside in lima beans is a highly toxic substance, but it imposes no hazard under the usual conditions of consumption of this food.

In spite of the multitude of toxic substances consumed daily in a *normal diet* by *normal healthy individuals,* there is yet little evident hazard involved. There are three basic interrelated explanations for this.

First, the concentrations of each of the toxic substances in any commonly accepted food are so low that a grossly exaggerated quantity of consumption of the food, usually over an extended period of time, is required before the toxicity of any single substance can be translated into a hazard. Such a situation has resulted, for example, from the goitrogenic substances in cabbage (Chapter 10) when this food has constituted an excessively large proportion of the diet for a long time, and from lycopene following the daily consumption of a half gallon of tomato juice for several years.[3] If one's diet contains a reasonable diversity of foods and no extraordinary amount of any specific food, then no single chemical is likely to be consumed in a toxic amount.

Second, the toxicities of the thousands of different chemicals present in our diet each day are not additive. For example, on theoretical toxicological grounds, if a hundredth of the lethal dose of each of a hundred different food components of variable biological actions were combined, the mixture would be innocuous. If the subliminal actions of small doses of many of a wide variety of toxic substances were additive, it could be speculated that a single day's normal menu would not be tolerated without adverse effects. The human organism can readily tolerate small amounts of many different chemical substances taken simultaneously, even though any one of them might not be tolerated in a somewhat larger amount.

Third, as pointed out by Underwood (Chapter 3), there are numerous examples among the trace elements in which antagonistic interactions have been demonstrated in animals. Thus the toxicity of one element is offset by the presence of an adequate amount of another. For example, the effects of a toxic level of cadmium in the diet are reduced by an accompanying high level of zinc. The adverse effect of manganese, due to an interference with the absorption of iron, can be offset by additional iron in the diet. Copper antagonizes the toxic effect of high dietary levels of molybdenum. Evidence of antagonisms between selenium and mercury[4] and between cobalt and iron[5] as dietary factors has been reported. Similarly, iodine inhibits the action of some goitrogens. Many other antagonistic interactions among chemicals, including pesticides and drugs, are known.

SAFETY IN NUMBERS

The existence and frequency of these antagonisms among various constituents of foods reinforce the concept of the *safety in numbers* as applied to the chemical components of the diet. The wider the variety of food intake, the greater is the number of different chemical substances consumed and the less is the chance that any one chemical will reach a hazardous level in the diet. This principle has been recognized as applying also to food additives and pesticides.[6] The Joint FAO/WHO Expert Committee on Food Additives stated:

an increase in the number of food additives on a permitted list does not imply an over-all increase in the (total amount of) additives used; the different additives are largely used as alternatives. . . . From the toxicological point of view there is less likelihood of long exposure, or of high or cumulative dose levels being attained if a wide range of substances is available for use. Similar considerations apply to pesticides.

SAFETY THROUGH TECHNOLOGY

Man's technology has obviously been responsible for much of his protection against the potential hazards of the natural chemical composition or contamination of his foods. Heating or other processing methods destroy or remove such toxic components as, for example, the cyanogenetic glycosides and some of the goitrogens. Refrigeration, canning, packaging, and other preservation measures suppress contamination by microbial toxins and chemical changes in foods that might generate toxic materials. Further, as was emphasized in Chapter 3, the widespread geographical distribution of food products results in the consumption by the population in a given geographical area of foods produced in a variety of other areas. Hazards that might arise from geochemical imbalances or other localized environmental factors—if a population consumed only those foods produced in its own area—are thus largely obviated. The food distribution system that has contributed to this protection has been made possible by modern food production and processing technology, including the use of pesticides and food additives.

ABNORMAL OR UNUSUAL CIRCUMSTANCES

It has been explained why a normal healthy individual consuming a reasonably varied diet composed naturally of thousands of toxic chemicals is not poisoned by it. The safety of our foods under these conditions is based on the assumption that, in the context of the total diet, each toxic chemical is present at a "no-adverse-effect" level. In the preceding chapters, however, many examples have been given of three general types of *abnormal* circumstances under which injury has been caused by the chemicals that occur naturally in foods:

1. The seafood (Chapter 19) and microbial toxins (Chapter 18) and the cardioactive glycosides in honey (Chapter 22) are categorized as *abnormal* though natural contaminants that adversely affect the *normal* consumer eating *normal* amounts of the foods in question.

2. The goitrogens, lathyrogens, cyanogenetic glycosides, and avidin (Chapters 10, 7, 14, 12) are *normal* constituents of foods and have caused disease in *normal* people consuming *abnormal* amounts of the foods in which they are present.

3. Numerous *normal* components of foods consumed in *normal* amounts are harmful in *abnormal* individuals who have increased susceptibilities associated with diseased states, malnutrition, allergic sensitivities, inborn errors of metabolism, or nonspecific intolerances.

Even ordinary dietary levels of sodium are considered undesirable in hypertensive patients (Chapter 2). Wilson's disease, a hereditary defect in copper metabolism, can develop from normal intake of dietary copper (Chapter 3). Lactose intolerance (Chapter 22), gluten sensitivity (Chapter 5), favism (Chapter 22), phytanic-acid-storage disease (Chapter 9), and phenylketonuria (Chapter 6) are related to genetic defects in metabolism in which the afflicted individuals cannot tolerate normal dietary levels of specific natural chemical entities in foods eaten by most people with no adverse effects. A keen insight into the human health significance of hereditary metabolic diseases and their control was recently provided by Scriver.[7] Thus, it can be appreciated that either ab-

normal contaminants, abnormal quantities of intake, or abnormal health
or physiological makeup of the individual consumer can reveal the toxic
potential of numerous natural chemical components of foods.

DELAYED EFFECTS

Plants and animals that have served historically as the sources of food
for man were not designed by nature for that purpose. It was necessary
for man to discover for himself, by trial and error, what he could eat
with safety. He discarded things that tasted bad or made him sick. Undoubtedly, most of his decisions to discard were based on what we
would now call acute experiments; the injurious effects occurred so soon
after eating that there was little question about what caused them. However, long-delayed harmful effects of chronically repeated consumption
of certain natural products certainly remained a mystery until relatively
modern times. The relationships of goiter, lathyrism, favism, and ergotism to their specific dietary causes were slow in coming to light. The
problems of establishing the causes of slowly developing or long-delayed
effects have recently increased in number and complexity as new sus-
picions have arisen in the light of new knowledge. It is now suspected,
for example, that dietary sodium and excessive dietary cadmium play
roles in the pathogenesis of hypertension.

Numerous substances that occur naturally in plant food sources are
known or suspected to be carcinogenic in animals (Chapter 23). Among
these are safrole and related compounds, estrogens, antithyroid compounds, lead as normally present in certain foods, and some of the fungal
toxins as natural contaminants. More recently, the discoveries of the
potent carcinogens, the nitrosamines and polycyclic aromatic hydrocarbons, as natural constituents of some plants have intensified the concern that the incidence of cancer in the human population may be
partly attributable to the natural sources of our foods. Added to
such uncertainties is the further suspicion that undiscovered carcinogens
are still lurking among the thousands of known and unknown chemical
compounds that occur naturally in our foods.

In the complex chemical context of our total food supply, attempts
to unravel the cause–effect relationships in respect to carcinogenesis can
hardly be expected to be fruitful. Identification of a carcinogen in a
food may be simple, but ascertaining its carcinogenicity under the conditions of consumption of the food in which it is found will undoubtedly be impossible in most cases. It seems reasonable to assume that efforts to remove from the food supply all carcinogens that are now
present or may be discovered in the future would disrupt that food sup-

ply far out of proportion to any putative benefits that might be derived.

In any case, it is clear that the real challenge that we face is the question of the long-term chronic toxicity, or lifetime effects, of the known and yet unknown natural chemical components of our foods. Such effects that might result from ordinary patterns of consumption are of the greatest potential importance, since they would be expected to affect the largest number of people. Though the problem of carcinogenesis has been emphasized above, similar attention should be focused upon reproductive functions, mutagenesis, cardiovascular–renal diseases, mental disorders, and other chronic ills of mankind of which the causes are unknown.

FOOD ADDITIVES

We have previously presented some comparisons and relationships between the natural chemical components of foods on the one hand and the chemicals entering foods as a result of man's efforts to improve the quantity and quality of his food supply on the other. It was pointed out, for example, that most food additives are derived from natural sources or are identical or closely related to chemical substances that occur in natural foodstuffs. Also, much injury to human health has resulted from natural components of foods, whereas no such injury can yet be attributed to food additives or pesticides when these agents, or the materials to which they have been added, have been used as recommended.

In view of the current public concern about contaminants (additives, pesticides, pollutants) in our food supply and the relative absence of concern about its natural chemical composition that constitutes more than 99.5% of our dietary intake, these two categories of substances should be examined further in relation to each other.

More than 2,000 different substances are used as food additives. Though relatively few of these have been subjected to full-scale toxicological testing, many of them have been scientifically evaluated for their safety under the conditions of their prolonged use. Others have been accepted on the basis of the long history of their use, in spite of the accepted belief that long-continued and widespread dietary intake of a substance with no harmful effects coming to light does not constitute adequate proof of its safety for lifetime consumption. This concept has been applied in the case of saccharin, which has been used extensively in many countries for 80 years with no apparent harm to the consumer. As a synthetic chemical, however, saccharin became subject to a more intensive scientific scrutiny of its safety than is usually considered necessary for food additives that are natural products. Safrole was used as a flavoring agent in root beer until it was found to be a weak carcinogen in rats, but this substance is naturally present in several spices still in wide use. The finding that vinyl thiooxazolidone and related compounds are potent goitrogens readily formed from precursors in cabbage, broccoli, and turnips has not influenced the production or consumption of these vegetables. Thus, safrole and vinyl thiooxazolidone are considered safe when consumed in their natural context in foods, but it is obvious that neither of these agents would be acceptable as a food additive.

If any natural chemical component of a food were found to have a desirable property as a food additive and its biological activity were still unknown, it would now be subject to the same safety evaluation procedures required of a new synthetic chemical compound. Thus, a food or an additive that has had a long history of use with no evidence of harmful effects is usually considered safe until proved harmful, whereas a new food or additive, or even a new use of an old additive, is considered harmful until proved safe.

On superficial grounds it might be asked why, since there are so many known and unknown toxic substances naturally present in our foods, we should be so concerned about the relatively small amounts of additional chemicals that enter our food supply as a result of man's food production, processing, and pollution activities. This question is readily answered by considering that the presence of such an abundance of toxic chemicals is itself an important reason to exercise caution in allowing the entry of any more noxious agents into the food supply. The "safety in numbers" concept described previously does not take care of all contingencies, especially when a toxic chemical entering the food is the same as one already naturally present. For example, the fortification of foods with iron[8,9] or vitamin D has been the subject of much controversy. In the area of pollution, the contamination of fish by mercury in industrial waste might lessen or even obliterate the margin of safety of this toxic element as it is naturally present in the fish.

TOXICOLOGIC INTERACTIONS

It is unlikely, of course, that any of man's synthetic food additives or food-crop pesticides would add in this direct way to natural components of foods. There is the possibility, however, that such agents may participate in additive, synergistic or potentiative toxicologic interactions with natural chemical constituents of foods. The organophosphate insecticides are potent cholinesterase inhibitors and would theoretically be expected to act additively with the cholinesterase inhibitors known to be present in a variety of common foods (Chapter 13). No practical hazard based on this situation, however, is known to exist, nor have there yet been found any other definite dietary hazards based on toxicologic interactions between natural food components and man's food additives or pesticides. Indeed, there is reason to believe that the antagonistic or protective type of interaction between natural and man-added food chemicals may be much more common than the synergistic type. DDT, for example, and most of the other organochlorine insecticides promote the production of enzymes in the body that detoxify many other chemicals, including some of the organophosphate insecticides.[10] The pesticides pyrethrum[11] and piperonyl butoxide[12] have similar enzyme-inducing properties. Nitrites that may arise from nitrates in foods produce a methemoglobinemia that detoxifies the cyanide generated from the cyanogenetic glycosides. Gossypol in cottonseed has recently been found experimentally to promote the detoxification of some carbamate insecticides.[13] Lindane has been reported to antagonize the depressant effect of lead on hemoglobin levels in mice.[14] Numerous examples of antagonistic relationships between trace elements (Chapter 3), amino acids (Chapter 6), and vitamins A and D (Chapter 11) have been described. However, as in the case of the additive or synergistic toxicologic interactions among food chemicals, there is yet no instance in which an experimentally demonstrated antagonistic interaction between a natural food chemical and one added by man has been shown to be of practical significance for man in diminishing any potential hazard in his diet.

Since one chemical may influence the extent to which another chemical affects the toxicologic interaction between two other chemicals, it becomes readily apparent that—in the multitude of molecular entities naturally and artificially comprising the diet of any individual—the problem of potential toxicologic interactions is not a matter of simple pairs of compounds but one of innumerable combinations of many. The unraveling of the intricacies of this situation is further complicated by the incompleteness of our knowledge of the natural chemical composition of most of the foods in our diet.

MARGIN OF SAFETY

When a chemical substance is proposed for use as a food additive or food-crop pesticide, the amount permitted to remain in food products is set at such a level that its estimated percentage in the total diet of the human consumer is a certain fraction of the highest percentage in the diet that can be fed test animals through their lifetime without any deleterious effect. This fraction is an expression of the margin of safety. A much practiced rule of thumb sets the acceptable percentage of the substance in the human diet at one-hundredth of the no-adverse-effect level in the animal test diet, i.e., a 100-fold margin of safety. The margin of safety applied for a given substance, however, may be more or less than 100, depending on the nature of the deleterious effect seen in animals fed high levels of the compound, on the scope of the toxicological knowledge about it, and on a judgment of the reliability of the data available. The possible grounds for increasing or decreasing the margin of safety have been discussed elsewhere.[6]

It is clear that much more attention is given to the margins of safety of food additives and pesticides than to those of chemical substances that occur naturally in foods. The latter have been commonly accepted, not on the basis of scientific tests but because man has learned by experience that he is not hurt when he consumes these materials in the context of the ordinary diet. Very few natural chemical constituents of foods have been tested in animals in such a way that numerical margins of safety for lifetime consumption by man can be stated. It is doubtful, however, that any broad-scale effort to do this would be productive.

It has already been emphasized that it is wholly unrealistic to isolate a chemical substance from a human food, incorporate it into the food of a laboratory test animal, and then expect the toxicity findings in the latter to be a reliable index of the risk of its consumption in the human food in which it occurs naturally. If a substance usually consumed in its natural human food "habitat" is inserted into an animal food for a toxicity study, the opportunities for toxicologic interactions with other substances might be altered and its potential toxicity accordingly altered. The toxicologic balances seen in the cases of cadmium and zinc, copper and molybdenum (Chapter 3), selenium and mercury,[4] vitamins A and D (Chapter 11), and oxalic acid and calcium (Chapter 16) serve to illustrate this principle.

Past experience in man has contributed much more to our knowledge of margins of safety of natural foods than has animal experimentation, though there have been few efforts to express such margins for specific chemical components in quantitative terms. A wide variety of common foods contain known goitrogenic substances or antithyroid activity due to unknown components. Here the margin of safety, assuming a normal well-balanced diet on a chronic basis, is undoubtedly less than 10. A similar estimate for estrogenic activity could probably be made.

It is likely that the daily dietary intake of numerous elements such as iron, zinc, copper, and fluorine could not be increased as much as 5 or 10 times without adverse effects on many people. From data presented by Meneely (Chapter 2) from observations in both the rat and man, the margin of safety of NaCl in the diet, considering the differences between required and hypertensigenic amounts, may be less than 5, though the response in this respect appears to be conditioned to a great extent by hereditary factors and disease. It is well known that the margin of safety of NaCl in the hypertensive segment of the population is less than 1. Sugar has a very narrow margin of safety in the diabetic. The margins for vitamins A and D, in relation to what are considered daily requirements, appear to be about 25–40 in adults and possibly lower than 10 for infants or very young children (Chapter 11).

The real difficulty in making reliable estimates of margins of safety for prolonged consumption of toxic substances from observations on man is based on the lack of true chronicity in scientifically controlled tests. It is not possible to subject human subjects to well-controlled testing procedures for a major part of their lifetime as is done with experimental animals. Epidemiologic approaches are considered more feasible. In any case, it is likely that on a truly long-term basis the above estimates of the margins of safety for various natural food components would be lower than those cited. Thus it is seen that the margins of safety for many natural components of our daily diet are of the same order of magnitude (or in some cases considerably lower) as those legally allowed for food additives and pesticides.

NATURAL VERSUS SYNTHETIC

The process of chemical synthesis does not confer upon the synthesized substance any insidious toxic properties, as is commonly thought. Many of the vitamins, for example, and many important drugs originally derived from plants, are chemically synthesized by man in order to provide an adequate supply for health needs. It is well established that the beneficial or toxic effects of any given substance are identical whether it is derived from natural sources or synthesized in the chemist's laboratory.

A greater suspicion is commonly focused upon chemicals that are synthesized by man and are not known to occur in nature. Most feared by some is the possible deleterious effect of such chemicals on the gene pool of man. It is thought that a single mutation induced by a chemical could ultimately alter the evolutionary process. In 1963 Hermann Muller said,[15] "Today we human beings are exposed to a great number of substances not encountered by our ancestors, to which we therefore have not been specifically adapted by natural selection." Though the theoretical genetic implications of this situation cannot be refuted on the basis of present knowledge, one might submit opposing speculation on equally justifiable grounds.

It is obvious that man has not become fully adapted to the natural chemical components of his foods, certainly not to carcinogenic effects nor to the many other adverse effects described in the preceding chapters of this book. Are we to assume that man has become genetically adapted to the natural products he has eaten through his evolution? More than a hundred hereditary diseases are now known, but there is no reason to believe that there are more such diseases now than there were when man's environment was wholly natural. It seems logical to suppose that if the natural chemical components of our common foods were screened, one by one, for their mutagenic effects, as high a percentage of them would be positive in this respect as would be found among the synthetics that man has added to his food.

Man has added very few totally new synthetic chemicals to his food supply in proportion to the number of different chemical substances that are there naturally. Many, if not most, of even these synthetics may be chemically similar or related to substances in our natural foodstuffs, many of which are still unknown. Considering the great number and variety of chemical substances in natural foods, it is questionable whether man has synthesized anything to add to his diet that is entirely new or baffling, in the amounts used, to the defense mechanisms of the body. There is no reason to believe, for example, that the detoxication mechanisms of the body are less efficient in handling unnatural synthetic chemicals than in handling the natural chemical components of foods. In the final analysis man is only taking advantage of *natural forces* when he synthesizes his molecules in the laboratory, these forces being basically the same, for example, in the synthesis of saccharin as they are in the synthesis of vitamin C. Furthermore, natural chemical synthetic processes are more sophisticated and insidiously productive than are those of man. Many substances have been found in nature that are far more toxic than any synthesized by man.

BENEFIT VERSUS RISK

In balancing the benefits against the risks associated with the consumption of food additives and pesticide residues, the considerations used differ in some respects from those involved in thinking about the benefits and risks associated with the natural chemical constituents of our foods.

The essential justification for the use of an additive in food processing—or of a pesticide that leaves a toxic residue in foods—is some direct or indirect benefit to the food consumer. Furthermore, it is a basic principle that the risks judged to be potentially associated with the use of any such substance should diminish with the importance of the benefit it is designed to achieve. An increased nutritional value, an increased food supply, availability or keeping quality, or a substantially decreased cost to the consumer are benefits that might be considered to justify a small degree of theoretical risk. An improvement in such superficial esthetic qualities of the food, however, as flavor, color, or consistency, that do not benefit the basic health or economic welfare of the consumer, are not acceptable bases for the use of a substance having a known or reasonably suspected risk.

In natural foodstuffs there are innumerable substances, many known and many unknown, that may provide attractive flavors and colors or determine form and consistency. Even a larger number of naturally occurring chemical components have no such functions and provide no known benefits whatever, either to the growth of the natural food source itself or to the human consumer. In the case of many of these substances that are known to have toxic properties, the risks of which are recognized or suspected, it is apparent that such risks are widely accepted, even though known benefits may be totally lacking or at best only of an esthetic nature. The goitrogens, estrogens, and carcinogens naturally present in widely used articles of our diet may be cited as examples.

It is of interest to reflect upon the benefit–risk equation as applied to the essential nutrients in foods. Many of these have toxic properties, but, since they are indispensable to life, their benefits are maximal. Under these circumstances some risk might be thought to be acceptable. We have seen, however, that among the vitamins and essential elements no risk has been recognized as being attributable to the natural presence of these substances in foods. Even though vitamin A has been shown to be teratogenic in several species of animals[16] (and the margin of safety for the hamster, for example, is less than 60), no risk has ever been claimed to be associated with the natural amounts of this vitamin in foods, except in the liver of the polar bear and certain large fishes (see Chapter 11). When certain essential nutrients are used as food additives, however, then the balancing of benefits and risks becomes important. The unquestioned benefits to many people of the judicious addition of vitamin D or iron to foods may be accompanied by an acceptable degree of risk to a few people. Although sodium is an essential element naturally present in foods, the use of sodium chloride as a food additive is not considered to be a benefit to health. On the contrary, the potential risk of the intake of amounts of sodium only a few times greater than those naturally present in our foods has been extensively documented (Chapter 2).

Benefit–risk considerations are also encountered under various circumstances among the caloric nutrients, the proteins and amino acids, fats and fatty acids, and certain disaccharides. Though many of the risks of these materials as they occur naturally in foods are based on inherited errors of metabolism in relatively few people, they are basically beneficial for most of the population. For this type of benefit–risk problem, however, little can be done beyond the medical management and dietary control of the individual at risk.

Much broader implications for major segments of the population arise when one considers the benefits and risks of such things as sucrose and polyunsaturated fats. This has become important for these two materials because of the relatively recent or impending increases in the quantities of their consumption. In neither of these cases, however, is there universal agreement as to either benefits or risks. Though any benefit to human health of a large proportion of the sugar consumed in the United States is held in considerable doubt, the assessment of the risk of this consumption from the results of many experimental and epidemiological studies that specifically relate dietary sugar to coronary heart disease is highly controversial.[17]

In the case of the unsaturated fats, several findings have been reported that confuse the benefit–risk issue. The consumption of unsaturated fats is well known to decrease the concentration of certain lipids in the blood, an effect widely interpreted as beneficial in the prevention or treatment of cardiovascular disease. On the other hand, a diet high in unsaturated fat has been reported to increase the carcinogenic effect of a carcinogen in rats to a greater extent than did a diet high in saturated fat.[18] Another study demonstrated a shortened mean life span of male and female mice and of male rats fed unsaturated fat in comparison with animals fed an isocaloric amount of saturated fat.[19] Thus, if it were to be assumed that these benefits and risks were real and were applied to man, the liberal intake of unsaturated fat would increase his risk of cancer while decreasing his risk of cardiovascular disease so that he might survive long enough to die of a shortened basic aging process. The significance of these findings to man, however, is not known. Even if it were, it is likely that each individual would wish to balance the benefits and risks for himself rather than rely on regulatory control as in the case of pesticides and most food additives. The same would undoubtedly be true of sucrose.

WHAT SHOULD BE DONE?

The value of a varied diet to ensure that the intake of essential nutrients will be *adequate* for good nutrition has long been accepted. We have now further emphasized the value of a varied diet to ensure that the intake of specific chemical substances in foods will be *inadequate* to cause injury. This applies not only to the natural chemical components of foods but also to additives and contaminants and serves as the basis of the concept of the "safety in numbers" as described previously. Thus, public educational programs in nutrition should stress the diverse and balanced diet as the basic approach to the avoidance of toxicologic hazard as well as to the acquisition of the nutritional essentials. It would be hoped that such teaching might provide some nutritional enlightenment for those who have been misguided into the hazards of the so-called Zen macrobiotic diet. This diet is the very antithesis of that considered optimum on the basis of sound nutritional and toxicologic principles. Through a sequence of dietary regimens it progresses to a diet made up of 100% cereals. It is not surprising that such states of malnutrition as scurvy, anemia, hypocalcemia, and others (even death) have been reported in the followers of this dangerous dietary philosophy.[20,21]

Yet the extensively varied diet is not under all conditions the definitive answer to the question of the maximum safety of the foods man eats. First, numerous instances have been cited in which the margins of safety of certain natural components of foods are not wide enough to allow for even normally varied patterns of consumption, as in cases of greatly increased sensitivities associated with inborn errors of metabolism, allergic sensitivities, individual nonspecific intolerances, or a variety of disease states. Under some such conditions it may be necessary to restrict the diversity of the diet, thus offsetting some of the advantages of a widely varied diet as consumed by individuals in good health and of normal constitution.

Second, there are extensive gaps in our knowledge of the identity of many natural chemical components of foods and of their potential toxicologic significance. A further lack of knowledge involves the significance to health of many of the known substances present in natural food products. The principal challenge we face in this regard is the long-term chronic effects on health. For example, are goitrogens, estrogens, safrole, and other known tumorigens of experimental animals responsible for any forms of malignant disease in man by virtue of their presence in many common food items? Do the sodium and cadmium contents of foods play a role in the pathogenesis of hypertension in man? What substances might be responsible for the development of various endocrine or mental disorders? These will be difficult problems to solve, further complicated as they are by many interacting variables. Very likely to be important among these are inadequacies or imbalances themselves. Inscrutable as these problems may be, more intensified efforts should be directed toward a more complete knowledge of the natural chemical composition of our food supply and a better understanding of its long-range significance to human health.

A clear obligation of the food and agricultural industries in their development and production of new or modified food products is to take into account the known chemical composition of the products they work with, especially in regard to those components that have toxic properties, whether or not such substances have yet been known to be harmful to man through his consumption of the foods containing them. The importance of this is illustrated by the recent finding that a new variety of potato, possessing improved chipping and browning properties, unfortunately contained an increased concentration of solanine alkaloids that prevented its further use (Chapter 13).

An awareness of the toxic properties of essential nutrients and of the amounts present in foods being processed should also be maintained by the food industry so that it may avoid the supplementation of its product with hazardous amounts of these agents.

It is wholly reasonable and advisable to resort to methods of selective breeding in order to reduce the levels of toxic substances in plant food sources where potential hazards exist. By such methods the toxic erucic acid has been practically eliminated from a rapeseed oil derived from the rape produced in Canada (Chapter 9), and cottonseed free of gossypol has been developed (Chapter 15). Selective breeding of the lima bean for low cyanogenetic glycoside content has also been encouraged, and the variety of the lima bean grown in the United States or permitted to be imported has a relatively low cyanide-generating capacity (Chapter 14). In procedures of this kind it is obvious that attention should be given to the possible associated changes that might occur in the food product to produce undesirable increases in the contents of other toxic components or a decrease in the nutritional quality.

It is unlikely that it would be either feasible or beneficial, as a general approach in the processing of agricultural food products, to attempt to

extract or remove many of the known toxic components such as goitrogens, cyanogenetic glycosides, oxalates, solanine alkaloids, safrole,
and toxic amino acids and fatty acids. Such procedures would undoubtedly often reduce the consumer acceptability, induce chemical
changes that might introduce other toxic substances, or reduce the nutritional quality, thereby necessitating extensive animal studies to establish the safety of the products for prolonged consumption. To be sure,
some simple processes have long been used to render natural products
safe or acceptable. Cooking destroys the cyanogenetic glycosides and
goitrogens of various plant products, thiaminase in fish, avidin in the
egg, and the hemagglutinins and enzyme inhibitors in beans. Native
populations in the tropics have removed the toxic glucoside, cycasin,
from the cycad nut by a water extraction procedure (Chapter 23). In
areas where cassava is an important food plant a water-soaking and fermenting process has been effective in removing most of the cyanogenetic
glycoside, linamarin (Chapter 14).

Viewing all chemicals that are present in our food supply—the natural
components, agricultural chemicals, food additives, and natural and man-
made contaminants—in perspective, it is clear that the greatest area of
the unknown involves the natural and normal components of our foods.
To achieve a more appropriate balance in the effort applied to the evaluation of the safety of foods in general, it is reasonable that at least as
much attention should be given to the chemical substances that occur
naturally in foods as is given to the additives and pesticide residues that
enter the food supply as a result of man's successful attempts to improve it. This is not to suggest less attention to the latter in comparison
to the former. In fact, due consideration should be given to the potential problems that might arise from the simultaneous presence of these
two groups of chemicals and the resulting chemical and toxicologic
interactions between them, as well as those with miscellaneous contaminants in food. As far as man's food intake is concerned, the ultimate
goal should be to gain an understanding not only of what constitutes
the optimum in nutritional content but also of what involves the minimum of long-range, lifetime toxicologic hazard in the diet.

REFERENCES

1. W. F. Talburt and O. Smith, Potato processing. 2nd ed. Avi, Westport, Conn.
   (1967).
2. R. L. Coleman and P. E. Shaw, Analysis of Valencia orange essence and aroma
   oils. J. Agric. Food Chem. *19*:520 (1971).

3. P. Reich, H. Schwachman, and J. M. Craig, Lycopenemia: A variant of carotenemia. N. Engl. J. Med. *262*:263 (1960).
4. H. E. Ganther, C. Goudie, M. L. Sunde, M. J. Kopecky, P. Wagner, Sang-Hwan Oh, and W. G. Hoekstra, Selenium: Relation to decreased toxicity of methylmercury added to diets containing tuna. Science *175*:1122 (1972).
5. K. N. Chetty and C. H. Hill, In vivo interaction of cobalt and iron in chicks. Fed. Proc. *31*:700 (1972). (Abstr.)
6. Joint FAO/WHO Expert Committee on Food Additives, Procedures for investigating intentional and unintentional food additives. WHO Tech. Rep. Ser. No. 348 (1967).
7. C. R. Scriver, Mutants: Consumers with special needs. Nutr. Rev. *29*:155 (1971).
8. Anonymous, The experts debate the added enrichment of bread and flour with iron. Nutr. Today *7*(2):2 (1972).
9. C. A. Finch and E. R. Monsen, Iron enrichment and the fortification of food with iron. J. Am. Med. Assoc. *219*:1469 (1972).
10. S. W. Bass, A. J. Triolo, and J. M. Coon, Effect of DDT on the toxicity and metabolism of parathion in mice. Toxicol. Appl. Pharmacol. *22*:684 (1972).
11. A. C. Springfield, G. P. Carlson, and J. J. DeFeo, Increased microsomal enzyme activity due to pyrethrum administration. Toxicol. Appl. Pharmacol. *19*:394 (1971).
12. D. J. Wagstaff and C. R. Short, Induction of hepatic microsomal enzymes by technical piperonyl butoxide and some related compounds. Toxicol. Appl. Pharmacol. *19*:395 (1971).
13. M. B. Abou-Donia and J. W. Dieckert, Gossypol: Subcellular localization and stimulation of rat liver microsomal enzymes. Toxicol. Appl. Pharmacol. *18*:507 (1971).
14. C. R. Cress and R. E. Larson, Lead and lindane interaction on heme synthesis in the mouse. Toxicol. Appl. Pharmacol. *17*:293 (1970).
15. Anonymous, Hermann Muller, FDA, and chemical mutagens. FDA Papers *3*(6):15 (1969).
16. J. F. Robens, Teratogenic effects of hypervitaminosis A in the hamster and guinea pig. Toxicol. Appl. Pharmacol. *16*:88 (1970).
17. Anonymous, Sugar: Dangerous to the heart? Med. World News *12*:38 (1971).
18. E. B. Gammal, K. K. Carroll, and E. R. Plunkett, Effects of dietary fat on mammary carcinogenesis by 7,12-dimethylbenz(a)anthracene in rats. Cancer Res. *27*:1737 (1967).
19. H. Denham, Prolongation of life: Role of free radical reactions in aging. J. Am. Geriatr. Soc. *17*:721 (1969).
20. Council on Foods and Nutrition, Zen macrobiotic diets. J. Am. Med. Assoc. *218*:397 (1971).
21. F. J. Stare, This diet can kill. Ladies Home J. (Oct. 1971) (Condensed in Reader's Dig., Feb. 1972).

CONTRIBUTORS

E. A. BELL, Department of Botany, The University of Texas at Austin, Austin, Texas 78712

C. L. COMAR, Department of Physical Biology, New York State Veterinary College, Cornell University, Ithaca, New York 14850

ERIC E. CONN, Department of Biochemistry and Biophysics, University of California, Davis, California 95616

JULIUS M. COON, Department of Pharmacology, Thomas Jefferson University, Philadelphia, Pennsylvania 19107

DAVID W. FASSETT,* 1438 Winton Road South, Rochester, New York 14618

R. E. FEENEY, Department of Food Science and Technology, University of California, Davis, California 95616

RICHARD L. HALL, Vice President, Research and Development, McCormick & Company, Inc., Hunt Valley, Maryland 21031

A. E. HARPER, Department of Nutritional Sciences & Biochemistry, University of Wisconsin, Madison, Wisconsin 53706

A. WALLACE HAYES, University of Alabama, Auburn, Alabama 36830

K. C. HAYES, Department of Nutrition, School of Public Health, Harvard University, Boston, Massachusetts 02115

D. MARK HEGSTED, Department of Nutrition, School of Public Health, Harvard University, Boston, Massachusetts 02115

WERNER G. JAFFÉ, Instituto Nacional de Nutrición, Apartado 2049, Caracas, Venezuela

*Retired

593

F. H. KRATZER, Department of Avian Sciences, University of California, Davis, California 95616

WALTER LOVENBERG, Head, Section on Biochemical Pharmacology, Experimental Therapeutics Branch, National Heart and Lung Institute, Bethesda, Maryland 20014

FRED H. MATTSON, Miami Valley Laboratories, The Proctor & Gamble Company, Cincinnati, Ohio 45239

GEORGE R. MENEELY, Head, Department of Physiology & Biophysics, Louisiana State University Medical Center, Shreveport, Louisiana 71101

JAMES A. MILLER, McArdle Laboratory for Cancer Research, University of Wisconsin Medical Center, Madison, Wisconsin 53706

DONALD OBERLEAS, Department of Medicine, Wayne State University, Detroit, Michigan 48207

V. N. PATWARDHAN,* Division of Nutrition, School of Medicine, Vanderbilt University, Nashville, Tennessee 37203

JOHN H. RUST, A. J. Carlson Animal Research Facility, University of Chicago, Chicago, Illinois 60637

EDWARD J. SCHANTZ, Food Research Institute, University of Wisconsin, Madison, Wisconsin 53706

LESTER D. SCHEEL, National Institute for Occupational Safety and Health, U.S. Department of Health, Education, and Welfare, Cincinnati, Ohio 45202

V. L. SINGLETON, Department of Viticulture & Enology, University of California, Davis, California 95616

J. C. SOMOGYI, Institute for Nutrition Research, Ruschlikon-Zurich, Switzerland

MARTIN STOB, Department of Animal Sciences, Purdue University, Lafayette, Indiana 47906

FRANK M. STRONG, Department of Biochemistry, University of Wisconsin, Madison, Wisconsin 53706

E. J. UNDERWOOD,† W. A. Office of the Executive, CSIRO, Private Bag, P. O., Wembley, Western Australia 6014

C. H. VANETTEN, Northern Regional Research Laboratory, ARS, U.S. Department of Agriculture, Peoria, Illinois 61604

A. G. VAN VEEN, Graduate School of Nutrition, Cornell University, Ithaca, New York 14850

J. R. WHITAKER, Department of Food Science & Technology, University of California, Davis, California 95615

JONATHAN W. WHITE, JR., Eastern Regional Research Center, Northeastern Region, Agricultural Research Service of the U.S. Department of Agriculture, Philadelphia, Pennsylvania 19118

BENJAMIN J. WILSON, Department of Biochemistry, Vanderbilt University School of Medicine, Nashville, Tennessee 37203

I. A. WOLFF, Eastern Regional Research Center, Northeastern Region, Agricultural Research Service of the U.S. Department of Agriculture, Philadelphia, Pennsylvania 19118

*Deceased–July 8, 1971.
†Retired.

INDEX

595